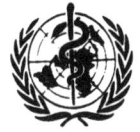

WORLD HEALTH ORGANIZATION

INTERNATIONAL AGENCY FOR RESEARCH ON CANCER

IARC MONOGRAPHS
ON THE
EVALUATION OF CARCINOGENIC RISKS TO HUMANS

Pharmaceutical Drugs

VOLUME 50

This publication represents the views and expert opinions
of an IARC Working Group on the
Evaluation of Carcinogenic Risks to Humans,
which met in Lyon,

17–24 October 1989

1990

IARC MONOGRAPHS

In 1969, the International Agency for Research on Cancer (IARC) initiated a programme on the evaluation of the carcinogenic risk of chemicals to humans involving the production of critically evaluated monographs on individual chemicals. In 1980 and 1986, the programme was expanded to include the evaluation of the carcinogenic risks associated with exposures to complex mixtures and other agents.

The objective of the programme is to elaborate and publish in the form of monographs critical reviews of data on carcinogenicity for agents to which humans are known to be exposed, and on specific exposure situations; to evaluate these data in terms of human risk with the help of international working groups of experts in chemical carcinogenesis and related fields; and to indicate where additional research efforts are needed.

This project is supported by PHS Grant No. 6 UO1 CA33193-06 awarded by the US National Cancer Institute, Department of Health and Human Services. Additional support has been provided since 1986 by the Commission of the European Communities.

©International Agency for Research on Cancer 1990

ISBN 92 832 1250 9

ISSN 0250-9555

All rights reserved. Application for rights of reproduction or translation, in part or *in toto*, should be made to the International Agency for Research on Cancer.

Distributed for the International Agency for Research on Cancer
by the Secretariat of the World Health Organization

PRINTED IN THE UK

CONTENTS

NOTE TO THE READER 5

LIST OF PARTICIPANTS 7

PREAMBLE

    Background 11
    Objective and Scope 11
    Selection of Topics for Monographs 12
    Data for Monographs 13
    The Working Group 13
    Working Procedures 14
    Exposure Data 14
    Biological Data Relevant to the Evaluation of Carcinogenicity to
        Humans 16
    Evidence for Carcinogenicity in Experimental Animals 17
    Other Relevant Data in Experimental Systems and in Humans 19
    Evidence for Carcinogenicity in Humans 21
    Summary of Data Reported 24
    Evaluation 25
    References 29

GENERAL REMARKS 33

THE MONOGRAPHS

    Antineoplastic and immunosuppressive agents

        Azacitidine 47
        Chlorozotocin 65
        Ciclosporin 77
        Prednimustine 115
        Thiotepa 123
        Trichlormethine (Trimustine hydrochloride) 143

CONTENTS

Antimicrobial agents

    Ampicillin 153
    Chloramphenicol 169
    Nitrofural (Nitrofurazone) 195
    Nitrofurantoin 211

Other drugs

    Cimetidine 235
    Dantron (Chrysazin; 1,8-Dihydroxyanthraquinone) 265
    Furosemide (Frusemide) 277
    Hydrochlorothiazide 293
    Paracetamol (Acetaminophen) 307

SUMMARY OF FINAL EVALUATIONS 333

APPENDIX 1. SUMMARY TABLE OF GENETIC AND RELATED EFFECTS 335

APPENDIX 2. ACTIVITY PROFILES FOR GENETIC AND RELATED EFFECTS 337

SUPPLEMENTARY CORRIGENDA TO VOLUMES 1–49 385

CUMULATIVE INDEX TO THE *MONOGRAPHS* SERIES 387

NOTE TO THE READER

The term 'carcinogenic risk' in the *IARC Monographs* series is taken to mean the probability that exposure to an agent will lead to cancer in humans.

Inclusion of an agent in the *Monographs* does not imply that it is a carcinogen, only that the published data have been examined. Equally, the fact that an agent has not yet been evaluated in a monograph does not mean that it is not carcinogenic.

The evaluations of carcinogenic risk are made by international working groups of independent scientists and are qualitative in nature. No recommendation is given for regulation or legislation.

Anyone who is aware of published data that may alter the evaluation of the carcinogenic risk of an agent to humans is encouraged to make this information available to the Unit of Carcinogen Identification and Evaluation, International Agency for Research on Cancer, 150 cours Albert Thomas, 69372 Lyon Cedex 08, France, in order that the agent may be considered for re-evaluation by a future Working Group.

Although every effort is made to prepare the monographs as accurately as possible, mistakes may occur. Readers are requested to communicate any errors to the Unit of Carcinogen Identification and Evaluation, so that corrections can be reported in future volumes.

IARC WORKING GROUP ON THE EVALUATION OF CARCINOGENIC RISKS TO HUMANS: PHARMACEUTICAL DRUGS

Lyon, 17–24 October 1989

LIST OF PARTICIPANTS

Members

I.N. Chernozemsky, National Oncological Centre, Medical Academy, Darvenitza, Sofia 1156, Bulgaria

L. Fiore-Donati, Istituto di Anatomia e Istologia Patologica, Verona University, Policlinico Borgo Roma, 37100 Verona, Italy

G.D. Friedman, Division of Research, Kaiser Permanente Medical Care Program, Northern California Region, 3451 Piedmont Avenue, Oakland, CA 94611, USA

B. Holmberg, Department of Toxicology, National Institute of Occupational Health, 171 84 Solna, Sweden

L.J. Kinlen, Cancer Research Campaign Epidemiology Unit, University of Edinburgh, 15 George Square, Edinburgh EH8 9JZ, UK

M. Marselos, Department of Pharmacology, Medical School, University of Ioannina, Ioannina 45110, Greece

M. Mattila, Department of Clinical Pharmacology, University of Helsinki, Department of Clinical Pharmacology, University of Helsinki, Paasikivenkatu 4, 00250 Helsinki, Finland

G. Obe, Universität GSH Essen, Fachbereich 9, Department of Genetics, PO Box 103 764, 4300 Essen 1, Federal Republic of Germany

J.H. Olsen, Danish Cancer Registry, Rosenvaengets Hovedvej 35, Box 839, 2100 Copenhagen Ø, Denmark

N.V. Popova, Laboratory of Carcinogenic Substances, All-Union Cancer Research Centre, Kashirskoye Shosse 24, 115478 Moscow, USSR

J.P. Seiler[1], Swiss Federal Research Station for Fruit-Growing, Viticulture and Horticulture, 8820 Wädenswil, Switzerland

S. Shapiro, Boston University Medical School, Slone Epidemiology Unit, 1371 Beacon Street, Brookline, MA 02146, USA

S.M. Sieber, Division of Cancer Etiology, National Cancer Institute, Building 31, Room 11A03, Bethesda, MD 20892, USA

M. Sorsa, Institute of Occupational Health, Topeliuksenkatu 41 a A, 00250 Helsinki, Finland (*Vice-Chairperson*)

R. Stahlmann, Institut für Toxikologie und Embryonal Pharmakologie der Freien Universität Berlin, Garystrasse 1-9, 100 Berlin 33, Federal Republic of Germany

B. Stewart, Children's Leukaemia and Cancer Research Unit, The Prince of Wales Children's Hospital, High Street, Randwick, NSW 2031, Australia

F.M. Sullivan, Department of Pharmacology, Guy's Hospital Medical School, London SE1 9RT, UK

J. Weissinger, Office of Drug Evaluation (HFD-502), Center for Drug Evaluation and Research, Food and Drug Administration, 5600 Fishers Lane, Rockville, MD 20857, USA

G.M. Williams, American Health Foundation, Dana Road, Valhalla, NY 10595, USA (*Chairman*)

K. Yokoro, Hiroshima University, Institute of Nuclear Medicine, 1-2-3 Kasumi, Minami-ku, Hiroshima 734, Japan

Representatives and observers[2]

Representative of the International Federation of Pharmaceutical Manufacturers' Associations

E. Longstaff, Safety Medicines Department, ICI Pharmaceuticals, Mereside, Alderley Park, Macclesfield, Cheshire SK10 4TG, UK

Representative of the US Pharmaceutical Manufacturers' Association

M.J. Tidd, Norwich Eaton Pharmaceuticals Inc., PO Box 191, Norwich, NY 13815-0191, USA

---

[1]Present address: Interkantonale Kontrollstelle für Heilmittel (IKS), Erlachstrasse 8, 3000 Bern, Switzerland

[2]Unable to attend, M.-Th. van der Venne, Commission of the European Communities, Health and Safety Directorate, Bâtiment Jean Monnet (C4/83), BP 1907, 2920 Luxembourg, Grand Duchy of Luxembourg

Secretariat

A. Aitio, Laboratory of Biochemistry, Institute of Occupational Health, Arinatie 3, 00370 Helsinki, Finland

H. Bartsch, Unit of Environmental Carcinogenesis and Host Factors

X. Bosch, Unit of Field Intervention Studies

E. Cardis, Unit of Biostatistical Research and Informatics

J. Cheney, Editorial, Translation and Publication Services

M. Coleman, Unit of Descriptive Epidemiology

M. Friesen, Unit of Environmental Carcinogenesis and Host Factors

E. Heseltine, Montignac, France

J. Jongen, Unit of Mechanisms of Carcinogenesis

J. Kaldor, Unit of Biostatistics Research and Informatics

V. Krutovskikh, Unit of Mechanisms of Carcinogenesis

K. L'Abbé, Unit of Analytical Epidemiology

D. McGregor, Unit of Carcinogen Identification and Evaluation

D. Mietton, Unit of Carcinogen Identification and Evaluation

R. Montesano, Unit of Mechanisms of Carcinogenesis

S. Narod, Unit of Mechanisms of Carcinogenesis

G. Nordberg, Unit of Carcinogen Identification and Evaluation

C. Partensky, Unit of Carcinogen Identification and Evaluation

I. Peterschmitt, Unit of Carcinogen Identification and Evaluation, Geneva, Switzerland

D. Shuker, Unit of Environmental Carcinogenesis and Host Factors

L. Shuker, Unit of Carcinogen Identification and Evaluation

L. Tomatis, Director

H. Vainio, Unit of Carcinogen Identification and Evaluation

J. Wilbourn, Unit of Carcinogen Identification and Evaluation

Secretarial assistance

J. Cazeaux

M. Lézère

S. Reynaud

IARC MONOGRAPHS PROGRAMME ON THE EVALUATION OF CARCINOGENIC RISKS TO HUMANS[1]

PREAMBLE

1. BACKGROUND

In 1969, the International Agency for Research on Cancer (IARC) initiated a programme to evaluate the carcinogenic risk of chemicals to humans and to produce monographs on individual chemicals. The *Monographs* programme has since been expanded to include consideration of exposures to complex mixtures of chemicals (which occur, for example, in some occupations and as a result of human habits) and of exposures to other agents, such as radiation and viruses. With Supplement 6(1), the title of the series was modified from *IARC Monographs on the Evaluation of the Carcinogenic Risk of Chemicals to Humans* to *IARC Monographs on the Evaluation of Carcinogenic Risks to Humans*, in order to reflect the widened scope of the programme.

The criteria established in 1971 to evaluate carcinogenic risk to humans were adopted by the working groups whose deliberations resulted in the first 16 volumes of the *IARC Monographs* series. Those criteria were subsequently re-evaluated by working groups which met in 1977(2), 1978(3), 1979(4), 1982(5) and 1983(6). The present preamble was prepared by two working groups which met in September 1986 and January 1987, prior to the preparation of Supplement 7(7) to the *Monographs* and was modified by a working group which met in November 1988(8).

2. OBJECTIVE AND SCOPE

The objective of the programme is to prepare, with the help of international working groups of experts, and to publish in the form of monographs, critical

---

[1] This project is supported by PHS Grant No. 5 UO1 CA33193-07 awarded by the US National Cancer Institute, Department of Health and Human Services, and with a subcontract to Tracor Technology Resources, Inc. Since 1986, this programme has also been supported by the Commission of the European Communities.

reviews and evaluations of evidence on the carcinogenicity of a wide range of human exposures. The *Monographs* may also indicate where additional research efforts are needed.

The *Monographs* represent the first step in carcinogenic risk assessment, which involves examination of all relevant information in order to assess the strength of the available evidence that certain exposures could alter the incidence of cancer in humans. The second step is quantitative risk estimation, which is not usually attempted in the *Monographs*. Detailed, quantitative evaluations of epidemiological data may be made in the *Monographs*, but without extrapolation beyond the range of the data available. Quantitative extrapolation from experimental data to the human situation is not undertaken.

These monographs may assist national and international authorities in making risk assessments and in formulating decisions concerning any necessary preventive measures. The evaluations of IARC working groups are scientific, qualitative judgements about the degree of evidence for carcinogenicity provided by the available data on an agent. These evaluations represent only one part of the body of information on which regulatory measures may be based. Other components of regulatory decisions may vary from one situation to another and from country to country, responding to different socioeconomic and national priorities. *Therefore, no recommendation is given with regard to regulation or legislation, which are the responsibility of individual governments and/or other international organizations.*

The *IARC Monographs* are recognized as an authoritative source of information on the carcinogenicity of chemicals and complex exposures. A users' survey, made in 1988, indicated that the *Monographs* are consulted by various agencies in 57 countries. Each volume is generally printed in 4000 copies for distribution to governments, regulatory bodies and interested scientists. The *Monographs* are also available *via* the Distribution and Sales Service of the World Health Organization.

3. SELECTION OF TOPICS FOR MONOGRAPHS

Topics are selected on the basis of two main criteria: (a) that they concern agents and complex exposures for which there is evidence of human exposure, and (b) that there is some evidence or suspicion of carcinogenicity. The term agent is used to include individual chemical compounds, groups of chemical compounds, physical agents (such as radiation) and biological factors (such as viruses) and mixtures of agents such as occur in occupational exposures and as a result of personal and cultural habits (like smoking and dietary practices). Chemical analogues and compounds with biological or physical characteristics similar to those of suspected carcinogens may also be considered, even in the absence of data on carcinogenicity.

The scientific literature is surveyed for published data relevant to an assessment of carcinogenicity; the IARC surveys of chemicals being tested for carcinogenicity(9) and directories of on-going research in cancer epidemiology(10) often indicate those exposures that may be scheduled for future meetings. An ad-hoc working group convened by IARC in 1984 gave recommendations as to which chemicals and exposures to complex mixtures should be evaluated in the *IARC Monographs* series(11,12).

As significant new data on subjects on which monographs have already been prepared become available, re-evaluations are made at subsequent meetings, and revised monographs are published.

4. DATA FOR MONOGRAPHS

The *Monographs* do not necessarily cite all the literature concerning the subject of an evaluation. Only those data considered by the Working Group to be relevant to making the evaluation are included.

With regard to biological and epidemiological data, only reports that have been published or accepted for publication in the openly available scientific literature are reviewed by the working groups. In certain instances, government agency reports that have undergone peer review and are widely available are considered. Exceptions may be made on an ad-hoc basis to include unpublished reports that are in their final form and publicly available, if their inclusion is considered pertinent to making a final evaluation (see pp. 25 *et seq.*). In the sections on chemical and physical properties and on production, use, occurrence and analysis, unpublished sources of information may be used.

5. THE WORKING GROUP

Reviews and evaluations are formulated by a working group of experts. The tasks of this group are five-fold: (i) to ascertain that all appropriate data have been collected; (ii) to select the data relevant for the evaluation on the basis of scientific merit; (iii) to prepare accurate summaries of the data to enable the reader to follow the reasoning of the Working Group; (iv) to evaluate the results of experimental and epidemiological studies; and (v) to make an overall evaluation of the carcinogenicity of the exposure to humans.

Working Group participants who contributed to the considerations and evaluations within a particular volume are listed, with their addresses, at the beginning of each publication. Each participant who is a member of a working group serves as an individual scientist and not as a representative of any organization, government or industry. In addition, representatives from national and international agencies and industrial associations are invited as observers.

6. WORKING PROCEDURES

Approximately one year in advance of a meeting of a working group, the topics of the monographs are announced and participants are selected by IARC staff in consultation with other experts. Subsequently, relevant biological and epidemiological data are collected by IARC from recognized sources of information on carcinogenesis, including data storage and retrieval systems such as CHEMICAL ABSTRACTS, MEDLINE and TOXLINE—including EMIC and ETIC for data on genetic and related effects and teratogenicity, respectively.

The major collection of data and the preparation of first drafts of the sections on chemical and physical properties, on production and use, on occurrence, and on analysis are carried out under a separate contract funded by the US National Cancer Institute. Efforts are made to supplement this information with data from other national and international sources. Representatives from industrial associations may assist in the preparation of sections on production and use.

Production and trade data are obtained from governmental and trade publications and, in some cases, by direct contact with industries. Separate production data on some agents may not be available because their publication could disclose confidential information. Information on uses is usually obtained from published sources but is often complemented by direct contact with manufacturers.

Six months before the meeting, reference material is sent to experts, or is used by IARC staff, to prepare sections for the first drafts of monographs. The complete first drafts are compiled by IARC staff and sent, prior to the meeting, to all participants of the Working Group for review.

The Working Group meets in Lyon for seven to eight days to discuss and finalize the texts of the monographs and to formulate the evaluations. After the meeting, the master copy of each monograph is verified by consulting the original literature, edited and prepared for publication. The aim is to publish monographs within nine months of the Working Group meeting.

7. EXPOSURE DATA

Sections that indicate the extent of past and present human exposure, the sources of exposure, the persons most likely to be exposed and the factors that contribute to exposure to the agent, mixture or exposure circumstance are included at the beginning of each monograph.

Most monographs on individual chemicals or complex mixtures include sections on chemical and physical data, and production, use, occurrence and analysis. In other monographs, for example on physical agents, biological factors, occupational exposures and cultural habits, other sections may be included, such as: historical perspectives, description of an industry or habit, exposures in the work place or chemistry of the complex mixture.

The Chemical Abstracts Services Registry Number, the latest Chemical Abstracts Primary Name and the IUPAC Systematic Name are recorded. Other synonyms and trade names are given, but the list is not necessarily comprehensive. Some of the trade names may be those of mixtures in which the agent being evaluated is only one of the ingredients.

Information on chemical and physical properties and, in particular, data relevant to identification, occurrence and biological activity are included. A separate description of technical products gives relevant specifications and includes available information on composition and impurities.

The dates of first synthesis and of first commercial production of an agent or mixture are provided; for agents which do not occur naturally, this information may allow a reasonable estimate to be made of the date before which no human exposure to the agent could have occurred. The dates of first reported occurrence of an exposure are also provided. In addition, methods of synthesis used in past and present commercial production and different methods of production which may give rise to different impurities are described.

Data on production, foreign trade and uses are obtained for representative regions, which usually include Europe, Japan and the USA. It should not, however, be inferred that those areas or nations are necessarily the sole or major sources or users of the agent being evaluated.

Some identified uses may not be current or major applications, and the coverage is not necessarily comprehensive. In the case of drugs, mention of their therapeutic uses does not necessarily represent current practice nor does it imply judgement as to their clinical efficacy.

Information on the occurrence of an agent or mixture in the environment is obtained from data derived from the monitoring and surveillance of levels in occupational environments, air, water, soil, foods and animal and human tissues. When available, data on the generation, persistence and bioaccumulation are also included. In the case of mixtures, industries, occupations or processes, information is given about all agents present. For processes, industries and occupations, a historical description is also given, noting variations in chemical composition, physical properties or levels of occupational exposure with time.

Statements concerning regulations and guidelines (e.g., pesticide registrations, maximal levels permitted in foods, occupational exposure limits) are included for some countries as indications of potential exposures, but they may not reflect the most recent situation, since such limits are continuously reviewed and modified.

The absence of information on regulatory status for a country should not be taken to imply that that country does not have regulations with regard to the exposure.

The purpose of the section on analysis is to give the reader an overview of current methods cited in the literature, with emphasis on those widely used for regulatory purposes. No critical evaluation or recommendation of any of the methods is meant or implied. Methods for monitoring human exposure are also given, when available. The IARC publishes a series of volumes, *Environmental Carcinogens: Methods of Analysis and Exposure Measurement(13)*, that describe validated methods for analysing a wide variety of agents and mixtures.

8. BIOLOGICAL DATA RELEVANT TO THE EVALUATION OF CARCINOGENICITY TO HUMANS

The term 'carcinogen' is used in these monographs to denote an agent or mixture that is capable of increasing the incidence of malignant neoplasms; the induction of benign neoplasms may in some circumstances (see p. 18) contribute to the judgement that the exposure is carcinogenic. The terms 'neoplasm' and 'tumour' are used interchangeably.

Some epidemiological and experimental studies indicate that different agents may act at different stages in the carcinogenic process, probably by fundamentally different mechanisms. In the present state of knowledge, the aim of the *Monographs* is to evaluate evidence of carcinogenicity at any stage in the carcinogenic process independently of the underlying mechanism involved. There is as yet insufficient information to implement classification according to mechanisms of action(6).

Definitive evidence of carcinogenicity in humans can be provided only by epidemiological studies. Evidence relevant to human carcinogenicity may also be provided by experimental studies of carcinogenicity in animals and by other biological data, particularly those relating to humans.

The available studies are summarized by the Working Group, with particular regard to the qualitative aspects discussed below. In general, numerical findings are indicated as they appear in the original report; units are converted when necessary for easier comparison. The Working Group may conduct additional analyses of the published data and use them in their assessment of the evidence and may include them in their summary of a study; the results of such supplementary analyses are given in square brackets. Any comments are also made in square brackets; however, these are kept to a minimum, being restricted to those instances in which it is felt that an important aspect of a study, directly impinging on its interpretation, should be brought to the attention of the reader.

For experimental studies with mixtures, consideration is given to the possibility of changes in the physicochemical properties of the test substance during collection, storage, extraction, concentration and delivery. Either chemical or toxicological interactions of the components of mixtures may result in nonlinear dose-response relationships.

An assessment is made as to the relevance to human exposure of samples tested in experimental systems, which may involve consideration of: (i) physical and chemical characteristics, (ii) constituent substances that indicate the presence of a class of substances, (iii) tests for genetic and related effects, including genetic activity profiles, (iv) DNA adduct profiles, (v) oncogene expression and mutation; suppressor gene inactivation.

9. EVIDENCE FOR CARCINOGENICITY IN EXPERIMENTAL ANIMALS

For several agents (e.g., 4-aminobiphenyl, bis(chloromethyl)ether, diethylstilboestrol, melphalan, 8-methoxypsoralen (methoxsalen) plus ultra-violet radiation, mustard gas and vinyl chloride), evidence of carcinogenicity in experimental animals preceded evidence obtained from epidemiological studies or case reports. Information compiled from the first 41 volumes of the *IARC Monographs*(14) shows that, of the 44 agents and mixtures for which there is *sufficient* or *limited evidence* of carcinogenicity to humans (see p. 26), all 37 that have been tested adequately experimentally produce cancer in at least one animal species. Although this association cannot establish that all agents and mixtures that cause cancer in experimental animals also cause cancer in humans, nevertheless, *in the absence of adequate data on humans, it is biologically plausible and prudent to regard agents and mixtures for which there is sufficient evidence (see p. 27) of carcinogenicity in experimental animals as if they presented a carcinogenic risk to humans.*

The monographs are not intended to summarize all published studies. Those that are inadequate (e.g., too short a duration, too few animals, poor survival; see below) or are judged irrelevant to the evaluation are generally omitted. They may be mentioned briefly, particularly when the information is considered to be a useful supplement to that of other reports or when they provide the only data available. Their inclusion does not, however, imply acceptance of the adequacy of the experimental design or of the analysis and interpretation of their results. Guidelines for adequate long-term carcinogenicity experiments have been outlined (e.g., 15).

The nature and extent of impurities or contaminants present in the agent or mixture being evaluated are given when available. Mention is made of all routes of exposure that have been adequately studied and of all species in which relevant experiments have been performed. Animal strain, sex, numbers per group, age at start of treatment and survival are reported.

Experiments in which the agent or mixture was administered in conjunction with known carcinogens or factors that modify carcinogenic effects are also reported. Experiments on the carcinogenicity of known metabolites and derivatives may be included.

(a) Qualitative aspects

An assessment of carcinogenicity involves several considerations of qualitative importance, including (i) the experimental conditions under which the test was performed, including route and schedule of exposure, species, strain, sex, age, duration of follow-up; (ii) the consistency of the results, for example, across species and target organ(s); (iii) the spectrum of neoplastic response, from benign tumours to malignant neoplasms; and (iv) the possible role of modifying factors.

Considerations of importance to the Working Group in the interpretation and evaluation of a particular study include: (i) how clearly the agent was defined and, in the case of mixtures, how adequately the sample characterization was reported; (ii) whether the dose was adequately monitored, particularly in inhalation experiments; (iii) whether the doses used were appropriate and whether the survival of treated animals was similar to that of controls; (iv) whether there were adequate numbers of animals per group; (v) whether animals of both sexes were used; (vi) whether animals were allocated randomly to groups; (vii) whether the duration of observation was adequate; and (viii) whether the data were adequately reported. If available, recent data on the incidence of specific tumours in historical controls, as well as in concurrent controls, should be taken into account in the evaluation of tumour response.

When benign tumours occur together with and originate from the same cell type in an organ or tissue as malignant tumours in a particular study and appear to represent a stage in the progression to malignancy, it may be valid to combine them in assessing tumour incidence. The occurrence of lesions presumed to be preneoplastic may in certain instances aid in assessing the biological plausibility of any neoplastic response observed.

Of the many agents and mixtures that have been studied extensively, few induced only benign neoplasms. Benign tumours in experimental animals frequently represent a stage in the evolution of a malignant neoplasm, but they may be 'endpoints' that do not readily undergo transition to malignancy. However, if an agent or mixture is found to induce only benign neoplasms, it should be suspected of being a carcinogen and it requires further investigation.

(b) Quantitative aspects

The probability that tumours will occur may depend on the species and strain, the dose of the carcinogen and the route and period of exposure. Evidence of an increased incidence of neoplasms with increased level of exposure strengthens the inference of a causal association between the exposure and the development of neoplasms.

The form of the dose-response relationship can vary widely, depending on the particular agent under study and the target organ. Since many chemicals require metabolic activation before being converted into their reactive intermediates, both metabolic and pharmacokinetic aspects are important in determining the dose-response pattern. Saturation of steps such as absorption, activation, inactivation and elimination of the carcinogen may produce nonlinearity in the dose-response relationship, as could saturation of processes such as DNA repair(16,17).

(c) *Statistical analysis of long-term experiments in animals*

Factors considered by the Working Group include the adequacy of the information given for each treatment group: (i) the number of animals studied and the number examined histologically, (ii) the number of animals with a given tumour type and (iii) length of survival. The statistical methods used should be clearly stated and should be the generally accepted techniques refined for this purpose(17,18). When there is no difference in survival between control and treatment groups, the Working Group usually compares the proportions of animals developing each tumour type in each of the groups. Otherwise, consideration is given as to whether or not appropriate adjustments have been made for differences in survival. These adjustments can include: comparisons of the proportions of tumour-bearing animals among the 'effective number' of animals alive at the time the first tumour is discovered, in the case where most differences in survival occur before tumours appear; life-table methods, when tumours are visible or when they may be considered 'fatal' because mortality rapidly follows tumour development; and the Mantel-Haenszel test or logistic regression, when occult tumours do not affect the animals' risk of dying but are 'incidental' findings at autopsy.

In practice, classifying tumours as fatal or incidental may be difficult. Several survival-adjusted methods have been developed that do not require this distinction(17), although they have not been fully evaluated.

10. OTHER RELEVANT DATA IN EXPERIMENTAL SYSTEMS AND HUMANS

(a) *Structure-activity considerations*

This section describes structure-activity correlations that are relevant to an evaluation of the carcinogenicity of an agent.

(b) *Absorption, distribution, excretion and metabolism*

Concise information is given on absorption, distribution (including placental transfer) and excretion. Kinetic factors that may affect the dose-reponse relationship, such as saturation of uptake, protein binding, metabolic activation, detoxification and DNA repair processes, are mentioned. Studies that indicate the metabolic fate of the agent in experimental animals and humans are summarized briefly, and comparisons of data from animals and humans are made when possible. Comparative information on the relationship between exposure and the dose that reaches the target site may be of particular importance for extrapolation between species.

(c) *Toxicity*

Data are given on acute and chronic toxic effects (other than cancer), such as organ toxicity, immunotoxicity, endocrine effects and preneoplastic lesions. Effects on reproduction, teratogenicity, feto- and embryotoxicity are also summarized briefly.

(d) *Genetic and related effects*

Tests of genetic and related effects may indicate possible carcinogenic activity. They can also be used in detecting active metabolites of known carcinogens in human or animal body fluids, in detecting active components in complex mixtures and in the elucidation of possible mechanisms of carcinogenesis.

The adequacy of the reporting of sample characterization is considered and, where necessary, commented upon. The available data are interpreted critically by phylogenetic group according to the endpoints detected, which may include DNA damage, gene mutation, sister chromatid exchange, micronuclei, chromosomal aberrations, aneuploidy and cell transformation. The concentrations (doses) employed are given and mention is made of whether an exogenous metabolic system was required. When appropriate, these data may be represented by bar graphs (activity profiles), with corresponding summary tables and listings of test systems, data and references. Detailed information on the preparation of these profiles is given in an appendix to those volumes in which they are used.

Positive results in tests using prokaryotes, lower eukaryotes, plants, insects and cultured mammalian cells suggest that genetic and related effects (and therefore possibly carcinogenic effects) could occur in mammals. Results from such tests may also give information about the types of genetic effect produced and about the involvement of metabolic activation. Some endpoints described are clearly genetic in nature (e.g., gene mutations and chromosomal aberrations), others are to a greater or lesser degree associated with genetic effects (e.g., unscheduled DNA synthesis). In-vitro tests for tumour-promoting activity and for cell transformation may detect changes that are not necessarily the result of genetic alterations but that may have specific relevance to the process of carcinogenesis. A critical appraisal of these tests has been published(15).

Genetic or other activity detected in the systems mentioned above is not always manifest in whole mammals. Positive indications of genetic effects in experimental mammals and in humans are regarded as being of greater relevance than those in other organisms. The demonstration that an agent or mixture can induce gene and chromosomal mutations in whole mammals indicates that it may have the potential for carcinogenic activity, although this activity may not be detectably expressed in any or all species tested. Relative potency in tests for mutagenicity and related effects is not a reliable indicator of carcinogenic potency. Negative results in tests for mutagenicity in selected tissues from animals treated *in vivo* provide less weight, partly because they do not exclude the possibility of an effect in tissues other than those examined. Moreover, negative results in short-term tests with genetic endpoints cannot be considered to provide evidence to rule out carcinogenicity of agents or mixtures that act through other mechanisms. Factors may arise in many tests that could give misleading results; these have been discussed in detail elsewhere(15).

The adequacy of epidemiological studies of reproductive outcomes and genetic and related effects in humans is evaluated by the same criteria as are applied to epidemiological studies of cancer.

11. EVIDENCE FOR CARCINOGENICITY IN HUMANS

(a) *Types of studies considered*

Three types of epidemiological studies of cancer contribute data to the assessment of carcinogenicity in humans—cohort studies, case-control studies and correlation studies. Rarely, results from randomized trials may be available. Case reports of cancer in humans are also reviewed.

Cohort and case-control studies relate individual exposures under study to the occurrence of cancer in individuals and provide an estimate of relative risk (ratio of incidence in those exposed to incidence in those not exposed) as the main measure of association.

In correlation studies, the units of investigation are usually whole populations (e.g., in particular geographical areas or at particular times), and cancer frequency is related to a summary measure of the exposure of the population to the agent, mixture or exposure circumstance under study. Because individual exposure is not documented, however, a causal relationship is less easy to infer from correlation studies than from cohort and case-control studies.

Case reports generally arise from a suspicion, based on clinical experience, that the concurrence of two events—that is, a particular exposure and occurrence of a cancer—has happened rather more frequently than would be expected by chance. Case reports usually lack complete ascertainment of cases in any population, definition or enumeration of the population at risk and estimation of the expected number of cases in the absence of exposure.

The uncertainties surrounding interpretation of case reports and correlation studies make them inadequate, except in rare instances, to form the sole basis for inferring a causal relationship. When taken together with case-control and cohort studies, however, relevant case reports or correlation studies may add materially to the judgement that a causal relationship is present.

Epidemiological studies of benign neoplasms and presumed preneoplastic lesions are also reviewed by working groups. They may, in some instances, strengthen inferences drawn from studies of cancer itself.

(b) Quality of studies considered

It is necessary to take into account the possible roles of bias, confounding and chance in the interpretation of epidemiological studies. By 'bias' is meant the operation of factors in study design or execution that lead erroneously to a stronger or weaker association than in fact exists between disease and an agent, mixture or exposure circumstance. By 'confounding' is meant a situation in which the relationship with disease is made to appear stronger or to appear weaker than it truly is as a result of an association between the apparent causal factor and another factor that is associated with either an increase or decrease in the incidence of the disease. In evaluating the extent to which these factors have been minimized in an individual study, working groups consider a number of aspects of design and analysis as described in the report of the study. Most of these considerations apply equally to case-control, cohort and correlation studies. Lack of clarity of any of these aspects in the reporting of a study can decrease its credibility and its consequent weighting in the final evaluation of the exposure.

Firstly, the study population, disease (or diseases) and exposure should have been well defined by the authors. Cases in the study population should have been identified in a way that was independent of the exposure of interest, and exposure should have been assessed in a way that was not related to disease status.

Secondly, the authors should have taken account in the study design and analysis of other variables that can influence the risk of disease and may have been related to the exposure of interest. Potential confounding by such variables should have been dealt with either in the design of the study, such as by matching, or in the analysis, by statistical adjustment. In cohort studies, comparisons with local rates of disease may be more appropriate than those with national rates. Internal comparisons of disease frequency among individuals at different levels of exposure should also have been made in the study.

Thirdly, the authors should have reported the basic data on which the conclusions are founded, even if sophisticated statistical analyses were employed. At the very least, they should have given the numbers of exposed and unexposed cases and controls in a case-control study and the numbers of cases observed and expected in a cohort study. Further tabulations by time since exposure began and other temporal factors are also important. In a cohort study, data on all cancer sites and all causes of death should have been given, to avoid the possibility of reporting bias. In a case-control study, the effects of investigated factors other than the exposure of interest should have been reported.

Finally, the statistical methods used to obtain estimates of relative risk, absolute cancer rates, confidence intervals and significance tests, and to adjust for confounding should have been clearly stated by the authors. The methods used should preferably have been the generally accepted techniques that have been refined since the mid-1970s. These methods have been reviewed for case-control studies(19) and for cohort studies(20).

(c) *Quantitative considerations*

Detailed analyses of both relative and absolute risks in relation to age at first exposure and to temporal variables, such as time since first exposure, duration of exposure and time since exposure ceased, are reviewed and summarized when available. The analysis of temporal relationships can provide a useful guide in formulating models of carcinogenesis. In particular, such analyses may suggest whether a carcinogen acts early or late in the process of carcinogenesis(6), although such speculative inferences cannot be used to draw firm conclusions concerning the mechanism of action and hence the shape (linear or otherwise) of the dose-response relationship below the range of observation.

(d) *Criteria for causality*

After the quality of individual epidemiological studies has been summarized and assessed, a judgement is made concerning the strength of evidence that the agent, mixture or exposure circumstance in question is carcinogenic for humans. In making their judgement, the Working Group considers several criteria for causality. A strong association (i.e., a large relative risk) is more likely to indicate causality than a weak association, although it is recognized that relative risks of small magnitude do not imply lack of causality and may be important if the disease is common. Associations that are replicated in several studies of the same design or using different epidemiological approaches or under different circumstances of exposure are more likely to represent a causal relationship than isolated observations from single studies. If there are inconsistent results among investigations, possible reasons are sought (such as differences in amount of exposure), and results of studies judged to be of high quality are given more weight than those from studies judged to be methodologically less sound. When suspicion of carcinogenicity arises largely from a single study, these data are not combined with those from later studies in any subsequent reassessment of the strength of the evidence.

If the risk of the disease in question increases with the amount of exposure, this is considered to be a strong indication of causality, although absence of a graded response is not necessarily evidence against a causal relationship. Demonstration of a decline in risk after cessation of or reduction in exposure in individuals or in whole populations also supports a causal interpretation of the findings.

Although a carcinogen may act upon more than one target, the specificity of an association (i.e., an increased occurrence of cancer at one anatomical site or of one morphological type) adds plausibility to a causal relationship, particularly when excess cancer occurrence is limited to one morphological type within the same organ.

Although rarely available, results from randomized trials showing different rates among exposed and unexposed individuals provide particularly strong evidence for causality.

When several epidemiological studies show little or no indication of an association between an exposure and cancer, the judgement may be made that, in the aggregate, they show evidence of lack of carcinogenicity. Such a judgement requires first of all that the studies giving rise to it meet, to a sufficient degree, the standards of design and analysis described above. Specifically, the possibility that bias, confounding or misclassification of exposure or outcome could explain the observed results should be considered and excluded with reasonable certainty. In addition, all studies that are judged to be methodologically sound should be consistent with a relative risk of unity for any observed level of exposure and, when considered together, should provide a pooled estimate of relative risk which is at or near unity and has a narrow confidence interval, due to sufficient population size. Moreover, no individual study nor the pooled results of all the studies should show any consistent tendency for relative risk of cancer to increase with increasing level of exposure. It is important to note that evidence of lack of carcinogenicity obtained in this way from several epidemiological studies can apply only to the type(s) of cancer studied and to dose levels and intervals between first exposure and observation of disease that are the same as or less than those observed in all the studies. Experience with human cancer indicates that, in some cases, the period from first exposure to the development of clinical cancer is seldom less than 20 years; latent periods substantially shorter than 30 years cannot provide evidence for lack of carcinogenicity.

12. SUMMARY OF DATA REPORTED

In this section, the relevant experimental and epidemiological data are summarized. Only reports, other than in abstract form, that meet the criteria outlined on p. 13 are considered for evaluating carcinogenicity. Inadequate studies are generally not summarized: such studies are usually identified by a square-bracketed comment in the text.

(a) Exposures

Human exposure is summarized on the basis of elements such as production, use, occurrence in the environment and determinations in human tissues and body fluids. Quantitative data are given when available.

(b) Experimental carcinogenicity data

Data relevant to the evaluation of carcinogenicity in animals are summarized. For each animal species and route of administration, it is stated whether an increased incidence of neoplasms was observed, and the tumour sites are indicated. If the agent or mixture produced tumours after prenatal exposure or in single-dose experiments, this is also indicated. Dose-response and other quantitative data may be given when available. Negative findings are also summarized.

(c) Human carcinogenicity data

Results of epidemiological studies that are considered to be pertinent to an assessment of human carcinogenicity are summarized. When relevant, case reports and correlation studies are also considered.

(d) Other relevant data

Structure-activity correlations are mentioned when relevant.

Toxicological information and data on kinetics and metabolism in experimental animals are given when considered relevant. The results of tests for genetic and related effects are summarized for whole mammals, cultured mammalian cells and nonmammalian systems.

Data on other biological effects in humans of particular relevance are summarized. These may include kinetic and metabolic considerations and evidence of DNA binding, persistence of DNA lesions or genetic damage in exposed humans.

When available, comparisons of such data for humans and for animals, and particularly animals that have developed cancer, are described.

13. EVALUATION

Evaluations of the strength of the evidence for carcinogenicity arising from human and experimental animal data are made, using standard terms.

It is recognized that the criteria for these evaluations, described below, cannot encompass all of the factors that may be relevant to an evaluation of carcinogenicity. In considering all of the relevant data, the Working Group may assign the agent, mixture or exposure circumstance to a higher or lower category than a strict interpretation of these criteria would indicate.

(a) *Degrees of evidence for carcinogenicity in humans and in experimental animals and supporting evidence*

It should be noted that these categories refer only to the strength of the evidence that an exposure is carcinogenic and not to the extent of its carcinogenic activity (potency) nor to the mechanism involved. A classification may change as new information becomes available.

An evaluation of degree of evidence, whether for a single substance or a mixture, is limited to the materials tested, and these are chemically and physically defined. When the materials evaluated are considered by the Working Group to be sufficiently closely related, they may be grouped for the purpose of a single evaluation of degree of evidence.

(i) *Human carcinogenicity data*

The applicability of an evaluation of the carcinogenicity of a mixture, process, occupation or industry on the basis of evidence from epidemiological studies depends on the variability over time and place of the mixtures, processes, occupations and industries. The Working Group seeks to identify the specific exposure, process or activity which is considered most likely to be responsible for any excess risk. The evaluation is focused as narrowly as the available data on exposure and other aspects permit.

The evidence relevant to carcinogenicity from studies in humans is classified into one of the following categories:

Sufficient evidence of carcinogenicity: The Working Group considers that a causal relationship has been established between exposure to the agent, mixture or exposure circumstance and human cancer. That is, a positive relationship has been observed between the exposure and cancer in studies in which chance, bias and confounding could be ruled out with reasonable confidence.

Limited evidence of carcinogenicity: A positive association has been observed between exposure to the agent, mixture or exposure circumstance and cancer for which a causal interpretation is considered by the Working Group to be credible, but chance, bias or confounding could not be ruled out with reasonable confidence.

Inadequate evidence of carcinogenicity: The available studies are of insufficient quality, consistency or statistical power to permit a conclusion regarding the presence or absence of a causal association.

Evidence suggesting lack of carcinogenicity: There are several adequate studies covering the full range of levels of exposure that human beings are known to encounter, which are mutually consistent in not showing a positive association between exposure to the agent, mixture or exposure circumstance and any studied cancer at any observed level of exposure. A conclusion of 'evidence suggesting lack of carcinogenicity' is inevitably limited to the cancer sites, conditions and levels of exposure and length of observation covered by the available studies. In addition, the possibility of a very small risk at the levels of exposure studied can never be excluded.

In some instances, the above categories may be used to classify the degree of evidence for carcinogenicity for specific organs or tissues.

(ii) *Experimental carcinogenicity data*

The evidence relevant to carcinogenicity in experimental animals is classified into one of the following categories:

Sufficient evidence of carcinogenicity: The Working Group considers that a causal relationship has been established between the agent or mixture and an increased incidence of malignant neoplasms or of an appropriate combination of benign and malignant neoplasms (as described on p. 18) in (a) two or more species of animals or (b) in two or more independent studies in one species carried out at different times or in different laboratories or under different protocols.

Exceptionally, a single study in one species might be considered to provide sufficient evidence of carcinogenicity when malignant neoplasms occur to an unusual degree with regard to incidence, site, type of tumour or age at onset.

In the absence of adequate data on humans, it is biologically plausible and prudent to regard agents and mixtures for which there is *sufficient evidence* of carcinogenicity in experimental animals as if they presented a carcinogenic risk to humans.

Limited evidence of carcinogenicity: The data suggest a carcinogenic effect but are limited for making a definitive evaluation because, e.g., (a) the evidence of carcinogenicity is restricted to a single experiment; or (b) there are unresolved questions regarding the adequacy of the design, conduct or interpretation of the study; or (c) the agent or mixture increases the incidence only of benign neoplasms or lesions of uncertain neoplastic potential, or of certain neoplasms which may occur spontaneously in high incidences in certain strains.

Inadequate evidence of carcinogenicity: The studies cannot be interpreted as showing either the presence or absence of a carcinogenic effect because of major qualitative or quantitative limitations.

Evidence suggesting lack of carcinogenicity: Adequate studies involving at least two species are available which show that, within the limits of the tests used, the agent or mixture is not carcinogenic. A conclusion of evidence suggesting lack of carcinogenicity is inevitably limited to the species, tumour sites and levels of exposure studied.

(iii) *Supporting evidence of carcinogenicity*

Other evidence judged to be relevant to an evaluation of carcinogenicity and of sufficient importance to affect the overall evaluation is then described. This may include data on tumour pathology, genetic and related effects, structure-activity relationships, metabolism and pharmacokinetics, physicochemical parameters, chemical composition and possible mechanisms of action. For complex exposures, including occupational and industrial exposures, the potential contribution of carcinogens known to be present as well as the relevance of materials tested are considered by the Working Group in its overall evaluation of human carcinogenicity. The Working Group also determines to what extent the materials tested in experimental systems are relevant to those to which humans are exposed. The available experimental evidence may help to specify more precisely the causal factor(s).

(b) *Overall evaluation*

Finally, the body of evidence is considered as a whole, in order to reach an overall evaluation of the carcinogenicity to humans of an agent, mixture or circumstance of exposure.

An evaluation may be made for a group of chemical compounds that have been evaluated by the Working Group. In addition, when supporting data indicate that other, related compounds for which there is no direct evidence of capacity to induce cancer in animals or in humans may also be carcinogenic, a statement describing the rationale for this conclusion is added to the evaluation narrative; an additional evaluation may be made for this broader group of compounds if the strength of the evidence warrants it.

The agent, mixture or exposure circumstance is described according to the wording of one of the following categories, and the designated group is given. The categorization of an agent, mixture or exposure circumstance is a matter of scientific judgement, reflecting the strength of the evidence derived from studies in humans and in experimental animals and from other relevant data.

Group 1—The agent (mixture) is carcinogenic to humans.
The exposure circumstance entails exposures that are carcinogenic to humans.

This category is used only when there is *sufficient evidence* of carcinogenicity in humans.

Group 2

This category includes agents, mixtures and exposure circumstances for which, at one extreme, the degree of evidence of carcinogenicity in humans is almost sufficient, as well as those for which, at the other extreme, there are no human data but for which there is experimental evidence of carcinogenicity. Agents, mixtures and exposure circumstances are assigned to either 2A (probably carcinogenic) or 2B (possibly carcinogenic) on the basis of epidemiological, experimental and other relevant data.

Group 2A—The agent (mixture) is probably carcinogenic to humans.
The exposure circumstance entails exposures that are probably carcinogenic to humans.

This category is used when there is *limited evidence* of carcinogenicity in humans and *sufficient evidence* of carcinogenicity in experimental animals. Exceptionally, an agent, mixture or exposure circumstance may be classified into this category solely on the basis of *limited evidence* of carcinogenicity in humans or of *sufficient evidence* of carcinogenicity in experimental animals strengthened by supporting evidence from other relevant data.

Group 2B—The agent (mixture) is possibly carcinogenic to humans.
The exposure circumstance entails exposures that are possibly carcinogenic to humans.

This category is generally used for agents, mixtures and exposure circumstances for which there is *limited evidence* of carcinogenicity in humans in the absence of *sufficient evidence* of carcinogenicity in experimental animals. It may also be used when there is *inadequate evidence* of carcinogenicity in humans or when human data are nonexistent but there is *sufficient evidence* of carcinogenicity in experimental animals. In some instances, an agent, mixture or exposure circumstance for which there is *inadequate evidence* of or no data on carcinogenicity in humans but *limited evidence* of carcinogenicity in experimental animals together with supporting evidence from other relevant data may be placed in this group.

Group 3—The agent (mixture, exposure circumstance) is not classifiable as to its carcinogenicity to humans.

Agents, mixtures and exposure circumstances are placed in this category when they do not fall into any other group.

Group 4—The agent (mixture, exposure circumstance) is probably not carcinogenic to humans.

This category is used for agents, mixtures and exposure circumstances for which there is *evidence suggesting lack of carcinogenicity* in humans together with *evidence suggesting lack of carcinogenicity* in experimental animals. In some instances, agents, mixtures or exposure circumstances for which there is *inadequate evidence* of or no data on carcinogenicity in humans but *evidence suggesting lack of carcinogenicity* in experimental animals, consistently and strongly supported by a broad range of other relevant data, may be classified in this group.

References

1. IARC (1987) *IARC Monographs on the Evaluation of Carcinogenic Risks to Humans,* Supplement 6, *Genetic and Related Effects: An Updating of Selected* IARC Monographs *from Volumes 1 to 42*, Lyon
2. IARC (1977) *IARC Monographs Programme on the Evaluation of the Carcinogenic Risk of Chemicals to Humans. Preamble* (IARC intern. tech. Rep. No. 77/002), Lyon

3. IARC (1978) *Chemicals with Sufficient Evidence of Carcinogenicity in Experimental Animals* — IARC Monographs *Volumes 1-17* (IARC intern. tech. Rep. No. 78/003), Lyon

4. IARC (1979) *Criteria to Select Chemicals for* IARC Monographs (IARC intern. tech. Rep. No. 79/003), Lyon

5. IARC (1982) *IARC Monographs on the Evaluation of the Carcinogenic Risk of Chemicals to Humans*, Supplement 4, *Chemicals, Industrial Processes and Industries Associated with Cancer in Humans (IARC Monographs, Volumes 1 to 29)*, Lyon

6. IARC (1983) *Approaches to Classifying Chemical Carcinogens According to Mechanism of Action* (IARC intern. tech. Rep. No. 83/001), Lyon

7. IARC (1987) *IARC Monographs on the Evaluation of Carcinogenic Risks to Humans*, Supplement 7, *Overall Evaluations of Carcinogenicity: An Updating of* IARC Monographs *Volumes 1 to 42*, Lyon

8. IARC (1988) *Report of an IARC Working Group to Review the Approaches and Processes Used to Evaluate the Carcinogenicity of Mixtures and* Groups of Chemical *(IARC intern. tech. Rep. No. 88/002), Lyon*

9. IARC (1973-1988) *Information Bulletin on the Survey of Chemicals Being Tested for Carcinogenicity*, Numbers 1-13, Lyon

    Number 1 (1973)   52 pages
    Number 2 (1973)   77 pages
    Number 3 (1974)   67 pages
    Number 4 (1974)   97 pages
    Number 5 (1975)   88 pages
    Number 6 (1976)   360 pages
    Number 7 (1978)   460 pages
    Number 8 (1979)   604 pages
    Number 9 (1981)   294 pages
    Number 10 (1983) 326 pages
    Number 11 (1984) 370 pages
    Number 12 (1986) 385 pages
    Number 13 (1988) 404 pages

10. Coleman, M. & Wahrendorf, J., eds (1988) *Directory of On-going Studies in Cancer Epidemiology 1988* (IARC Scientific Publications No. 93), Lyon, IARC [and previous annual volumes]

11. IARC (1984) *Chemicals and Exposures to Complex Mixtures Recommended for Evaluation in* IARC Monographs *and Chemicals and Complex Mixtures Recommended for Long-term Carcinogenicity Testing* (IARC intern. tech. Rep. No. 84/002), Lyon

12. IARC (1989) *Chemicals, Groups of Chemicals, Mixtures and Exposure Circumstances to be Evaluated in Future IARC Monographs, Report of an ad hoc Working Group* (IARC intern. tech. Rep. No. 89/004), Lyon

13. *Environmental Carcinogens. Methods of Analysis and Exposure Measurement*:
    Vol. 1. *Analysis of Volatile Nitrosamines in Food* (IARC Scientific Publications No. 18). Edited by R. Preussmann, M. Castegnaro, E.A. Walker & A.E. Wasserman (1978)

Vol. 2. *Methods for the Measurement of Vinyl Chloride in Poly(vinyl chloride), Air, Water and Foodstuffs* (IARC Scientific Publications No. 22). Edited by D.C.M. Squirrell & W. Thain (1978)

Vol. 3. *Analysis of Polycyclic Aromatic Hydrocarbons in Environmental Samples* (IARC Scientific Publications No. 29). Edited by M. Castegnaro, P. Bogovski, H. Kunte & E.A. Walker (1979)

Vol. 4. *Some Aromatic Amines and Azo Dyes in the General and Industrial Environment* (IARC Scientific Publications No. 40). Edited by L. Fishbein, M. Castegnaro, I.K. O'Neill & H. Bartsch (1981)

Vol. 5. *Some Mycotoxins* (IARC Scientific Publications No. 44). Edited by L. Stoloff, M. Castegnaro, P. Scott, I.K. O'Neill & H. Bartsch (1983)

Vol. 6. *N-Nitroso Compounds* (IARC Scientific Publications No. 45). Edited by R. Preussmann, I.K. O'Neill, G. Eisenbrand, B. Spiegelhalder & H. Bartsch (1983)

Vol. 7. *Some Volatile Halogenated Hydrocarbons* (IARC Scientific Publications No. 68). Edited by L. Fishbein & I.K. O'Neill (1985)

Vol. 8. *Some Metals: As, Be, Cd, Cr, Ni, Pb, Se, Zn* (IARC Scientific Publications No. 71). Edited by I.K. O'Neill, P. Schuller & L. Fishbein (1986)

Vol. 9. *Passive Smoking* (IARC Scientific Publications No. 81). Edited by I.K. O'Neill, K.D. Brunnemann, B. Dodet & D. Hoffmann (1987)

Vol. 10. *Benzene and Alkylated Benzenes* (IARC Scientific Publications No. 85). Edited by L. Fishbein & I.K. O'Neill (1988)

14. Wilbourn, J., Haroun, L., Heseltine, E., Kaldor, J., Partensky, C. & Vainio, H. (1986) Response of experimental animals to human carcinogens: an analysis based upon the IARC Monographs Programme. *Carcinogenesis*, 7, 1853-1863

15. Montesano, R., Bartsch, H., Vainio, H., Wilbourn, J. & Yamasaki, H., eds (1986) *Long-term and Short-term Assays for Carcinogenesis — A Critical Appraisal* (IARC Scientific Publications No. 83), Lyon, IARC

16. Hoel, D.G., Kaplan, N.L. & Anderson, M.W. (1983) Implication of nonlinear kinetics on risk estimation in carcinogenesis. *Science*, 219, 1032-1037

17. Gart, J.J., Krewski, D., Lee, P.N., Tarone, R.E. & Wahrendorf, J. (1986) *Statistical Methods in Cancer Research*, Vol.3, *The Design and Analysis of Long-term Animal Experiments* (IARC Scientific Publications No. 79), Lyon, IARC

18. Peto, R., Pike, M.C., Day, N.E., Gray, R.G., Lee, P.N., Parish, S., Peto, J., Richards, S. & Wahrendorf, J. (1980) Guidelines for simple, sensitive significance tests for carcinogenic effects in long-term animal experiments. In: *IARC Monographs on the Evaluation of the Carcinogenic Risk of Chemicals to Humans*, Supplement 2, *Long-term and Short-term Screening Assays for Carcinogens: A Critical Appraisal*, Lyon, pp. 311-426

19. Breslow, N.E. & Day, N.E. (1980) *Statistical Methods in Cancer Research*, Vol. 1, *The Analysis of Case-control Studies* (IARC Scientific Publications No. 32), Lyon, IARC

20. Breslow, N.E. & Day, N.E. (1987) *Statistical Methods in Cancer Research*, Vol. 2, *The Design and Analysis of Cohort Studies* (IARC Scientific Publications No. 82), Lyon, IARC

GENERAL REMARKS ON THE SUBSTANCES CONSIDERED

This fiftieth volume of the *IARC Monographs* comprises monographs on five antineoplastic agents, four antimicrobial agents, two diuretics, ciclosporin (an immunosuppressant), cimetidine (used in the treatment of gastric and duodenal ulcers), paracetamol (a popular analgesic and antipyretic drug) and dantron (a laxative). Many pharmaceutical drugs were evaluated in previous *IARC Monographs* (see Table 1), including some of those covered in this volume. Azacitidine and trichlormethine—both antineoplastic agents—and nitrofural—an antibacterial drug—were re-evaluated because new data on carcinogenicity in experimental animals had been published since the earlier evaluations; thiotepa and chloramphenicol were re-evaluated largely because of new data on carcinogenicity in humans.

Table 1. Pharmaceutical agents evaluated in the *IARC Monographs*

Agent	Vol. no.	Year	Evaluation[a]		
			Human	Animal	Overall
Anaesthetics					
Anaesthetics (unspecified mixtures)	Suppl. 7	1987	I	–	3
Chloroform	Suppl. 7	1987	I	S	2B
Cyclopropane	Suppl. 7	1987	I	ND	3
Diethyl ether	Suppl. 7	1987	I	ND	3
Divinyl ether	Suppl. 7	1987	I	ND	3
Enflurane	Suppl. 7	1987	I	I	3
Fluroxene	Suppl. 7	1987	I	ND	3
Halothane	Suppl. 7	1987	I	I	3
Isoflurane	Suppl. 7	1987	I	I	3
Methoxyflurane	Suppl. 7	1987	I	I	3
Nitrous oxide	Suppl. 7	1987	I	I	3
Trichloroethylene	Suppl. 7	1987	I	L	3
Analgesics and anti-inflammatory agents					
Aurothioglucose	13	1977	ND	L	3
Oxyphenbutazone	13	1977	ND	ND	3

Table 1 (contd)

Agent	Vol. no.	Year	Evaluation[a]		
			Human	Animal	Overall
Analgesics and anti-inflammatory agents (contd)					
Paracetamol (Acetaminophen)	50	1990	I	L	3
Phenacetin	Suppl. 7	1987	L	S	2A
Analgesic mixtures containing phenacetin	Suppl. 7	1987	S	L	1
Phenazopyridine hydrochloride	Suppl. 7	1987	I	S	2B
Phenylbutazone	Suppl. 7	1987	I	ND	3
Antibacterial drugs					
Ampicillin	50	1990	I	L	3
Chloramphenicol	50	1990	L	I	2A
Chrysoidine	Suppl. 7	1987	I	L	3
Dapsone	Suppl. 7	1987	I	L	3
Dihydroxymethylfuratrizine	24	1980	ND	I	3
Ethionamide	13	1977	ND	L	3
Isoniazid (Isonicotinic acid hydrazide)	Suppl. 7	1987	I	L	3
Nitrofural (Nitrofurazone)	50	1990	I	L	3
Nitrofurantoin	50	1990	I	L	3
1-[(5-Nitrofurfurylidene)amino]-2-imidazolidinone (Nifuradene)	7	1974	ND	S	2B
N-[4-(5-Nitro-2-furyl)-2-thiazolyl]acetamide (Furothiazole)	7	1974	ND	S	2B
Panfuran S (a formulation with dihydroxymethylfuratrizine and several other compounds)	24	1980	ND	S	2B
Penicillic acid	10	1976	ND	L	3
Rifampicin	24	1980	ND	L	3
Sulfafurazole (Sulphisoxazole)	Suppl. 7	1987	I	I	3
Sulfamethoxazole	Suppl. 7	1987	I	L	3
Antineoplastic drugs					
Actinomycin D (Dactinomycin)	Suppl. 7	1987	I	L	3
Adriamycin (Doxorubicin)	Suppl. 7	1987	I	S	2A
Azacitidine (5-Azacytidine)	50	1990	ND	S	2A
Azaserine	10	1976	ND	S	2B
N,N-Bis(2-chloroethyl)-2-naphthylamine (Chlornaphazine)	Suppl. 7	1987	S	L	1
Bischloroethyl nitrosourea (BCNU)	Suppl. 7	1987	L	S	2A
Bleomycins	Suppl. 7	1987	I	L	2B
1,4-Butanediol dimethanesulfonate (Myleran)	Suppl. 7	1987	S	L	1
Chlorambucil	Suppl. 7	1987	S	S	1

Table 1 (contd)

Agent	Vol. no.	Year	Evaluation[a]		
			Human	Animal	Overall
Antineoplastic drugs (contd)					
1-(2-Chloroethyl)-3-cyclohexyl-1-nitrosourea (CCNU) (Lomustine)	Suppl. 7	1987	I	S	2A
1-(2-Chloroethyl)-3-(4-methylcyclohexyl)-1-nitrosourea (Methyl-CCNU)	Suppl. 7	1987	S	L	1
Chlorotrianisene (*see* Hormones)					
Chlorozotocin	50	1990	ND	S	2A
Cisplatin	Suppl. 7	1987	I	S	2A
Cyclophosphamide	Suppl. 7	1987	S	S	1
Dacarbazine	Suppl. 7	1987	I	S	2B
Daunomycin (Daunorubicin)	10	1976	ND	S	2B
Diethylstilboestrol (*see* Hormones)					
Ethynodiol diacetate (*see* Hormones)					
5-Fluorouracil	Suppl. 7	1987	I	I	3
17α-Hydroxyprogesterone caproate (*see* Hormones)					
Isophosphamide	26	1981	ND	L	3
Mannomustine	9	1975	ND	L	3
Medphalan	9	1975	ND	I	3
Megestrol acetate (*see* Hormones)					
Melphalan	Suppl. 7	1987	S	S	1
6-Mercaptopurine	Suppl. 7	1987	I	I	3
Merphalan	9	1975	ND	S	2B
Methotrexate	Suppl. 7	1987	I	I	3
Mitomycin C	10	1976	ND	S	2B
MOPP[b] and other combined chemotherapy including alkylating agents	Suppl. 7	1987	S	I	1
Nitrogen mustard	Suppl. 7	1987	L	S	2A
Nitrogen mustard *N*-oxide	9	1975	ND	S	2B
Norethisterone (*see* Hormones)					
Prednimustine	50	1990	ND	I	3
Prednisone (*see* Hormones)					
Procarbazine hydrochloride	Suppl. 7	1987	I	S	2A
Streptozotocin (Streptozocin)	17	1978	ND	S	2B
Treosulphan	Suppl. 7	1987	S	ND	1
Trichlormethine (Trimustine hydrochloride)	50	1990	ND	S	2B
Triethylene glycol diglycidyl ether (Ethoglucid)	11	1976	ND	L	3
Tris(aziridinyl)-*para*-benzoquinone (Triaziquone)	Suppl. 7	1987	I	L	3

Table 1 (contd)

Agent	Vol. no.	Year	Evaluation[a]		
			Human	Animal	Overall
Antineoplastic drugs (contd)					
Tris(1-aziridinyl)phosphine sulphide (Thiotepa)	50	1990	S	S	1
2,4,6-Tris(1-aziridinyl)-*s*-triazine	9	1975	ND	L	3
Uracil mustard (Uramustine)	Suppl. 7	1987	I	S	2B
Vinblastine sulphate	Suppl. 7	1987	I	I	3
Vincristine sulphate	Suppl. 7	1987	I	I	3
Antifungal, antiprotozoan and antiparasitic agents					
Chloroquine	13	1977	ND	I	3
DDT (Clofenotane)	Suppl. 7	1987	I	S	2B
Furazolidone (*also antibacterial*)	31	1983	ND	I	3
Griseofulvin	Suppl. 7	1987	ND	S	2B
γ-Hexachlorocyclohexane (Lindane)	Suppl. 7	1987	I	L	2B
Hycanthone mesylate	13	1977	ND	I	3
Metronidazole (*also antibacterial*)	Suppl. 7	1987	I	S	2B
Niridazole	13	1977	ND	S	2B
Pyrimethamine	13	1977	ND	L	3
Trichlorfon (Metrifonate)	30	1983	ND	I	3
Antiseptic agents					
Acridine orange	16	1978	ND	I	3
Acriflavinium chloride	13	1977	ND	I	3
Benzoyl peroxide (*see* Dermatological agents)					
Chrysoidine	Suppl. 7	1987	I	L	3
Eugenol (*used in dentistry*)	36	1985	ND	L	3
Hexachlorophene	20	1979	ND	I	3
Hydrogen peroxide	36	1985	ND	L	3
Phenol	47	1989	I	I	3
Proflavine salts	24	1980	ND	I	3
β-Propiolactone	4	1974	ND	S	2B
Scarlet Red	8	1975	ND	I	3
Tannic acid and tannins	10	1976	ND	L	3
Dermatological agents					
para-Aminobenzoic acid	16	1978	ND	I	3
Arsenic salts (Fowler's solution) (*also antineoplastic*)	Suppl. 7	1987	S	L	1[c]
Benzoyl peroxide (*also antiseptic*)	36	1985	I	I	3
Cantharidin	10	1976	ND	L	3
Coal-tars	Suppl. 7	1987	S	S	1

Table 1 (contd)

Agent	Vol. no.	Year	Evaluation[a]		
			Human	Animal	Overall
Dermatological agents (contd)					
Diacetylaminoazotoluene	8	1975	ND	I	3
Dithranol (Anthralin)	13	1977	ND	I	3
Hydroquinone	15	1977	ND	I	3
8-Hydroxyquinoline (*also antiseptic*)	13	1977	ND	I	3
5-Methoxypsoralen	Suppl. 7	1987	I	S	2A
8-Methoxypsoralen (Methoxsalen) + UV	Suppl. 7	1987	S	S	1
Resorcinol	15	1977	ND	I	3
Safrole (Oil of Sassafras)	10	1976	ND	S	2B
Selenium and selenium compounds	9	1975	I	I	3
Tannic acid and tannins (*see* Antiseptic agents)					
4,5',8-Trimethylpsoralen	Suppl. 7	1987	I	I	3
Drugs for treating anaemia					
Iron-dextran complex	Suppl. 7	1987	I	S	2B
Iron-dextrin complex	2	1973	ND	L	3
Iron-sorbitol-citric acid complex	2	1973	ND	I	3
Saccharated iron oxide	2	1973	ND	L	3
Drugs for treating cardiovascular disorders					
Clofibrate (hypercholesterolaemia)	Suppl. 7	1987	I	L	3
Furosemide (Frusemide) (hypertension)	50	1990	I	I	3
Hydralazine (hypertension)	Suppl. 7	1987	I	L	3
Hydrochlorothiazide (hypertension)	50	1990	I	I	3
Phenoxybenzamine hydrochloride (hypertension)	24	1980	ND	S	2B
Reserpine (hypertension)	Suppl. 7	1987	I	L	3
Spironolactone (hypertension)	Suppl. 7	1987	I	L	3
Drugs for treating central nervous disorders					
Diazepam (anxiety)	Suppl. 7	1987	I	I	3
Oxazepam (anxiety)	13	1977	ND	L	3
Phenelzine sulphate (depression)	Suppl. 7	1987	I	L	3
Phenobarbital (epilepsy)	Suppl. 7	1987	I	S	2B
Phenytoin (epilepsy)	Suppl. 7	1987	L	L	2B
Drugs for treating thyroid disorders					
Methylthiouracil	7	1974	ND	S	2B
Propylthiouracil	Suppl. 7	1987	I	S	2B
Thiouracil	7	1974	ND	L	3
Thiourea	7	1974	ND	S	2B

Table 1 (contd)

Agent	Vol. no.	Year	Evaluation[a]		
			Human	Animal	Overall
Hormones					
Androgenic (anabolic) steroids					
Oxymetholone	Suppl. 7	1987	L	ND	2A
Testosterone	Suppl. 7	1987	L	S	2A
Oestrogens, progestins and combinations	Suppl. 7	1987			
Oestrogens					
Nonsteroidal oestrogens			S		1[c]
Diethylstilboestrol			S	S	1
Dienoestrol				L	
Hexoestrol				S	
Chlorotrianisene				I	
Steroidal oestrogens			S		1[c]
Oestrogen replacement therapy			S		1[c]
Conjugated oestrogens				L	
Oestradiol-17β and esters				S	
Oestriol				L	
Oestrone				S	
Ethinyloestradiol				S	
Mestranol				S	
Progestins			I		2B[c]
Medroxyprogesterone acetate			I	S	2B
Chlormadinone acetate				L	
Dimethisterone				I	
Ethynodiol diacetate				L	
17α-Hydroxyprogesterone caproate				I	
Lynoestrenol				I	
Megestrol acetate				L	
Norethisterone				S	
Norethynodrel				L	
Norgestrel				I	
Progesterone				S	
Oestrogen-progestin combinations					
Sequential oral contraceptives			S		1[c]
Dimethisterone and oestrogens				I	
Combined oral contraceptives			S		1[d]
Chlormadinone acetate and oestrogens				L	
Ethynodiol diacetate and oestrogens				L	
Lynoestrenol and oestrogens				I	

Table 1 (contd)

Agent	Vol. no.	Year	Evaluation[a]		
			Human	Animal	Overall
Hormones (contd)					
Megestrol acetate and oestrogens				L	
Norethisterone and oestrogens				L	
Norethynodrel and oestrogens				S	
Norgestrel and oestrogens				I	
Progesterone and oestrogens				L	
Oestrogen-progestin replacement therapy			I		3
Anti–oestrogens					
Clomiphene citrate	Suppl. 7	1987	I	I	3
Other hormones					
Prednisone	Suppl. 7	1987	I	I	3
Immunosuppressants					
Azathioprine	Suppl. 7	1987	S	L	1
Ciclosporin (Cyclosporin A)	50	1990	S	L	1
Traditional remedies of herbal origin					
Dantron (Chrysazin, 1,8-Dihydroxyanthraquinone) (*Aloe* sp., *Cassia senna*, *Rhamnus purshianus* or *Cascara sagrada*, and *Rheum officinale*)	50	1990	ND	S	2B
Hydroxysenkirkine (*Crotalaria* sp.)	10	1976	ND	I	3
Isatidine (*Senecio* sp.)	10	1976	ND	L	3
Jacobine (*Senecio* sp.)	10	1976	ND	I	3
Monocrotoline (*Crotalaria* sp.)	10	1976	ND	S	2B
Petasitenine (*Petasites japonicus*)	31	1983	ND	L	3
Retrorsine (*Senecio* sp.)	10	1976	ND	L	3
Riddelliine (*Crotalaria* sp.)	10	1976	ND	I	3
Seneciphylline (*Senecio* sp. and *Crotalaria* sp.)	10	1976	ND	ND	3
Senkirkine (*Senecio kirkii*)	31	1983	ND	L	3
Symphytine (*Symphytum officinale*)	31	1983	ND	I	3
Miscellaneous drugs and experimental agents					
2-Amino-5-(5-nitro-2-furyl)-1,3,4-thiadiazole (gastritis)	7	1974	ND	S	2B
Angelicin + UVA (skin disorders)	40	1986	ND	L	3
Cimetidine (peptic ulcer)	50	1990	I	I	3
4,4'-Dimethylangelicin + UVA (skin disorders)	40	1986	ND	ND	3
4,5'-Dimethylangelicin + UVA (skin disorders)	40	1986	ND	L	3

Table 1 (contd)

Agent	Vol. no.	Year	Evaluation[a]		
			Human	Animal	Overall
Miscellaneous drugs and experimental agents (contd)					
Disulfiram (alcoholism)	12	1976	ND	I	3
Investigational oral contraceptives	Suppl. 7	1987	S	L	1[d]
Lasiocarpine (emetic)	10	1976	ND	S	2B
5-Methylangelicin + UVA (skin disorders)	40	1986	ND	L	3
N-Methyl-N-nitrosourea (antineoplastic)	17	1978	ND	S	2A
7-Methylpyrido[3,4-c]psoralen (skin disorders)	40	1986	ND	I	3
Nafenopin (hypercholesterolaemia)	24	1980	ND	S	2B
Pyrido[3,4-c]psoralen (skin disorders)	40	1986	ND	I	3
Sodium diethyldithiocarbamate (nickel poisoning)	12	1976	ND	I	3
4,4',6-Trimethylangelicin + UVA (skin disorders)	40	1986	ND	ND	3
Veterinary drugs					
Acriflavinium chloride (*see* Antiseptic agents)					
para-Aminobenzoic acid (*see* Dermatological agents)					
5-Amino-2-nitrothiazole	31	1983	ND	L	3
Arsanilic acid	Suppl. 7	1987	S	L	1[c]
Diacetylaminoazotoluene (*see* Dermatological agents)					
Furazolidone (*see* Antifungal, antiprotozoan and antiparasitic agents)					
Hexachloroethane	20	1979	ND	L	3
Hexachlorophene (*see* Antiseptic agents)					
Iron–dextran complex (*see* Drugs for treating anaemia)					
Lead arsenate	Suppl. 7	1987	S	L	1[e]
5-(Morpholinomethyl)-3-[(5-nitrofurfurylidene)amino]-2-oxazolidinone (Furaltadone)	7	1974	ND	S	2B
Nithiazide	31	1983	ND	L	3
5-Nitro-2-furaldehyde semicarbazone	7	1974	ND	I	3
N-[4-(5-Nitro-2-furyl)-2-thiazolyl] acetamide (*see* Antibacterial drugs)					

Table 1 (contd)

Agent	Vol. no.	Year	Evaluation[a]		
			Human	Animal	Overall
Veterinary drugs (contd)					
Nitrovin	31	1983	ND	I	3
Selenium (*see* Dermatological agents)					
Urethane	7	1974	ND	S	2B

[a]I, inadequate; S, sufficient; L, limited. For definitions of the symbols used, see Preamble, pp. 26-29.
[b]Combined therapy with nitrogen mustard, vincristine, procarbazine and prednisone
[c]This evaluation applies to the group of chemicals as a whole and not necessarily to all individual chemicals within the group.
[d]There is also conclusive evidence that these agents have a protective effect against cancers of the ovary and endometrium.
[e]According to the overall evaluation of arsenic compounds

Derivatives of chloramphenicol without the NO_2 moiety have been developed; of these, thiamphenicol has been used extensively, but florfenicol is not used in man. Thiamphenicol and florfenicol were not considered in this volume, however, because there appear to be no published data with regard to their carcinogenicity. Similarly, ranitidine and famotidine are used therapeutically like cimetidine; but monographs on ranitidine and famotidine and their nitrosated derivatives were also not prepared due to a lack of relevant published studies.

In clinical use and in formulations, salts, esters and complexes of drugs are often designated by the name of the parent compound; this is the case with ampicillin and chloramphenicol. In the case of nitrofurantoin, products of different crystal size have been synthesized. While the Working Group attempted to distinguish these alternative forms, in some instances insufficient information was available to do so.

The primary source of human exposure to drugs is from their use in therapy. Other types of exposure may also occur, however: persons employed in the manufacture of drugs may be exposed, as well as nursing and other staff responsible for the preparation and administration of compounds and staff responsible for the care of treated patients. Veterinary use of drugs may result in their entry into the human food chain.

For the drugs considered here, as for many others, studies of human carcinogenicity present difficult problems. The symptoms of an undiagnosed cancer may prompt the use of drug, which is subsequently suspected as its cause. Alternatively, the condition for which the drug therapy is prescribed may itself be a risk factor for cancer. An additional problem is that patients commonly receive more than one drug, and determination of the carcinogenicity of any single drug may not be feasible. Repeated reference is made in this volume to hypothesis-generating studies. These refer to sets of data containing information on many drugs and many outcomes, in which multiple comparisons are made. Statistically significant associations ($p < 0.05$) are noted, but in terms of probability theory many such associations may be due to chance. For this reason, the p values given in the text must be interpreted with caution, and independent examination of associations identified in hypothesis-generating studies is particularly desirable. This situation is substantially different from that in which a prior hypothesis exists before the data are analysed.

An increasing number of agents, including pharmaceutical drugs, have been shown to inhibit cancer development in animal models. Such properties may lead to new possibilities for cancer treatment and prevention. The Working Group noted that in long-term experiments with paracetamol, nitrofurantoin and nitrofural, reductions in tumour incidence were seen at some sites in some animal species, although such reductions may have other interpretations than an inhibition of tumour induction.

Exposure can generally be much more accurately measured for drugs than for other agents suspected or identified as human carcinogens, and therapeutic doses used in humans are often close to those tested in experimental animals. However, as is the policy in the *IARC Monographs*, no attempt was made to quantify cancer risk at specific dose levels. As stated in the Preamble, the *Monographs* represent the first stage in carcinogenic risk assessment. Subsequent stages, not attempted in the *Monographs*, may involve quantitative determinations. By extrapolation of available epidemiological data, and possibly experimental data, estimations of risk may be attempted for specific populations in respect of particular carcinogens. Such information may be a factor in regulatory or legislative processes, but no recommendation concerning these processes is given in the *Monographs*. However, the Working Group responsible for the present monographs observed that inference of carcinogenic hazard was likely to be a major factor in decision-making regarding the usage of many of the drugs considered.

Many (if not most) regulatory decisions concerning putative carcinogens necessitate consideration not only of perceived hazard but also of the benefit derived from particular chemicals. It is crucial, therefore, that decisions on the availability of drugs include assessment not only of potential carcinogenicity but also the health benefit derived from their usage.

THE MONOGRAPHS

ANTINEOPLASTIC AND IMMUNOSUPPRESSIVE AGENTS

AZACITIDINE

This substance was considered by a previous Working Group, in October 1980, under the title 5-azacytidine (IARC, 1981). Since that time, new data have become available, and these have been incorporated into the monograph and taken into consideration in the present evaluation.

1. Chemical and Physical Data

1.1 Synonyms

Chem. Abstr. Services Reg. No.: 320-67-2

Chem. Abstr. Name: 1,3,5-Triazin-2(1*H*)-one, 4-amino-1-β-ribofuranosyl

Synonyms: Antibiotic U 18496; 5-azacytidine; ladakamycin; NSC 102816; U-18496; WR-183027

1.2 Structural and molecular formulae and molecular weight

$C_8H_{12}N_4O_5$ Mol. wt: 244.2

1.3 Chemical and physical properties of the pure substance

From Winkley and Robins (1970), unless otherwise specified

(*a*) *Description*: White crystalline powder

(b) *Melting-point*: 235-237°C (decomposes)

(c) *Optical rotation*: $[\alpha]_D^{26}$ = +26.6°C (c = 1.00; in water)

(d) *Solubility*: Soluble in warm water (40 mg/ml), cold water (14 mg/ml), 0.1 N hydrochloric acid (28 mg/ml) and 0.1 N sodium hydroxide (43 mg/ml); soluble in 35% ethanol (14.2-15.0 mg/l), acetone (1 mg/ml), chloroform (1 mg/ml), hexane (1 mg/ml) and dimethyl sulfoxide (52.7 mg/ml) (von Hoff *et al.*, 1975)

(e) *Spectrosocopy data*: Ultraviolet, infrared and nuclear magnetic resonance spectra have been reported (Beisler, 1978).

(f) *Stability*: Very unstable in aqueous media, rapid degradation to complex products occurring within hours of dissolution in intravenous solutions at room temperature (Reynolds, 1989)

1.4 Technical products and impurities

Trade name: Mylosar

Azacitidine is available as a lyophilized powder in vials containing 100 mg of the compound with 100 mg mannitol for reconstitution as injections of 5 mg/ml (von Hoff *et al.*, 1975).

2. Production, Occurrence, Use and Analysis

2.1 Production and occurrence

(a) *Production*

Azacitidine, a pyrimidine analogue of cytidine with a nitrogen substituted for a 5-carbon, can be isolated from a culture of the bacterium *Streptoverticillium ladakanus*, but has also been prepared by synthetic methods. One reported method involved treatment of the trimethylsilyl derivative of 4-amino-1,3,5-triazin-2-one with 2,3,5-tri-*O*-acetyl-D-ribofuranosyl bromide, followed by deacetylation to give azacitidine (Winkley & Robins, 1970).

Azacitidine is synthesized in the Federal Republic of Germany (Chemical Information Services, 1989-90).

(b) *Occurrence*

Azacitidine is produced by the bacterium *Streptoverticillium ladakanus* (Winkley & Robins, 1970).

2.2 Use

Azacitidine is a cytostatic agent. It has been used mainly in the treatment of acute leukaemia, either as intravenous or intramuscular injections or as intravenous infusions at a daily level of 40-750 mg/m² (Weiss *et al.*, 1972; Skoda, 1975; von Hoff *et al.*, 1975, 1976; von Hoff & Slavik, 1977; Wade, 1977; Glover *et al.*, 1987; Reynolds, 1989). It is used alone, or in combination with vincristine, vinblastine, prednisone, cytarabine or amsacrine, at a daily dose of 50-150 mg/m² azacitidine. It has also been tested for use in the treatment of a variety of solid tumours (Glover *et al.*, 1987).

2.3 Analysis

Azacitidine can be quantified in blood by microbiological assay (Pittillo & Woolley, 1969) and in plasma by high-performance liquid chromatography with ultraviolet detection (Rustum & Hoffman, 1987).

3. Biological Data Relevant to the Evaluation of Carcinogenic Risk to Humans

3.1 Carcinogenicity studies in animals

(a) Intraperitoneal injection

Mouse: In a screening assay based on the accelerated induction of leukaemia in a strain highly susceptible to development of this neoplasm, 40 AKR female mice, two months of age, were given six intraperitoneal injections of azacitidine at 1.5 mg/kg bw [purity unspecified] over 20 days, and, because of toxicity, six injections of azacitidine at 0.8 mg/kg bw over the following 30 days. All treated mice had died of leukaemia by 60 days. A control group of 40 females survived free of disease for the observation time of 120 days (Vesely & Cihák, 1973).

In a screening assay based on the accelerated induction of lung tumours in a strain highly susceptible to development of this neoplasm, three groups of ten male and ten female A/He mice, six to eight weeks of age, received intraperitoneal injections of azacitidine [purity unspecified], in a vehicle composed of saline, polysorbate-80, carboxymethyl cellulose and benzyl alcohol, three times a week for eight weeks (total doses, 33, 62 and 90 mg/kg bw (which was the maximum tolerated dose)). Control groups received 24 intraperitoneal injections of 0.1 ml vehicle or were untreated. All animals were killed 24 weeks after the first injection. The numbers of mice with lung tumours, calculated on the basis of survivors of each sex, were 6/11 (54%), 5/15 (33%) and 8/19 (42%) in the groups receiving the high, mid and low doses, respectively. The results for untreated and vehicle-treated groups were expressed only as per cent tumour incidence; thus, 22% (males) and 17% (females) of untreated controls and 26% (males) and 23% (females) of vehicle-treated controls developed lung tumours. The number of lung tumours per mouse (counted grossly) in animals of each sex treated with the highest dose was 0.73 ± 0.22 (SE), which was significantly higher ($p < 0.05$) than that in untreated (males, 0.22 ± 0.03; females, 0.17 ± 0.02) or vehicle-treated (males, 0.25 ± 0.05; females, 0.23 ± 0.04) control mice. With lower doses, the increase in the number of lung tumours per mouse was not statistically significant (Stoner et al., 1973).

Groups of 35 male and 35 female B6C3F1 mice, 38 days of age, received intraperitoneal injections of azacitidine at 2.2 or 4.4 mg/kg bw (>99% pure) in buffered saline three times a week for 52 weeks. Groups of 15 male and 15 female mice were untreated or received the vehicle only. Surviving mice were killed at 81 or 82 weeks. All high-dose females died before week 62, with no significant increase in the incidence of any tumour; of the low-dose females, 17/35 survived until termination of the experiment. Among males, 7/35 of the high-dose group and 13/35 of the low-dose group survived to the end of the study. The overall numbers of survivors in untreated and vehicle-treated groups were 25/30 and 20/30, respectively. In female mice of the low-dose group, lymphocytic and granulocytic neoplasms of the haematopoietic system were observed in 17/29 animals examined histologically, at a highly significant incidence ($p < 0.001$) compared with the vehicle-control group (0/14); 10 of the treated animals had granulocytic tumours (nine sarcomas, one leukaemia). A malignant lymphocytic lymphoma was observed in 1/15 untreated controls. No increase in the incidence of tumours was observed in male mice (National Cancer Institute, 1978).

Groups of 50 male and 50 female BALB/c/Cb/Se mice, eight weeks of age, were given intraperitoneal injections of azacitidine at 2.0 mg/kg bw in saline (99% pure) once a week for 50 weeks. Control groups received injections of saline. After 25 weeks, survival was reduced in exposed animals of each sex. The incidence of lymphoreticular neoplasms was increased, occurring in 12/50 ($p < 0.01$) males and 36/50 ($p < 0.001$) females, compared to 3/50 and 6/50 in control males and females, respectively. The incidence of lung adenomas was increased in treated males (27/50 versus 12/50 [$p < 0.01$]) but not in females. Mammary gland adenocarcinomas and adenoacanthomas were found in 7/50 treated females and in none of the controls. The incidence of skin tumours was increased in treated animals of each sex, occurring in 3/50 treated males compared to 0/50 controls [$p < 0.05$] and in 7/50 treated females compared to 1/50 controls [$p < 0.01$, log rank test] (Cavaliere et al., 1987). [The Working Group noted that adenocanthomas are not described as mammary tumours in reference sources; see Turusov (1973, 1976).]

Rat: Two groups of 12 or 8 male Fischer rats, weighing 160-180 g, were given intraperitoneal injections of azacitidine at 2.5 or 10 mg/kg bw [purity unspecified] in saline twice a week for nine months. A control group of 12 male rats was maintained without treatment. All rats were killed at 18 months. Interstitial-cell testicular tumours were found in 1/8 high-dose animals and 9/12 low-dose animals compared to 0/12 controls. In the high-dose group, two squamous-cell carcinomas of the skin and one skin appendage tumour at the site of injection were found, compared to none in controls (Carr et al., 1984). [The Working Group noted the small number of animals tested, and the absence in controls of testicular tumours, which occurred commonly in a second, shorter study by the same investigators (see below).]

Groups of 10, 10 or 100 young adult male Fischer rats, weighing 100-160 g, received intraperitoneal injections of azacitidine at 0.025, 0.25 or 2.5 mg/kg bw in saline [purity unspecified] three times a week for one year. A control group of 50 rats was injected with saline. At one year, when the study was terminated, 87/100 of animals at the high dose and 10/10 in each of the lower-dose groups were still alive. The highest dose increased the incidence of testicular interstitial-cell tumours to 56/87, compared to 10/49 in controls ($p < 0.001$). No other tumour was observed in controls. In the highest dose group, other tumours noted were four lymphomas, four renal tumours, one lung tumour, three skin tumours, two mesotheliomas and two sarcomas (Carr et al., 1988). [The Working Group noted the short duration of the experiment and the small numbers of animals in some groups.]

(b) *Transplacental administration*

Mouse: Groups of 32-37 pregnant NMRI mice received intraperitoneal injections of azacitidine at 1 or 2 mg/kg bw in saline [purity unspecified] on day 12, 14 or 16 of gestation. A group of 53 control dams was injected with saline. The number of stillbirths was increased at the high dose; survival of offspring was decreased in all exposed groups. In exposed progeny, increased percentages of tumour-bearing animals and increased incidences of leukaemias and lymphomas, lung tumours and liver tumours were seen in some groups (see Table 1). Some increases in the incidence of soft-tissue sarcomas were also seen (Schmahl et al., 1985).

(c) *Administration in combination with other compounds*

Rat: In the experiment by Carr et al. (1984), described above, groups of 6-10 male Fischer rats were given *N*-nitrosodiethylamine at 50 mg/kg bw 18 h after partial hepatectomy, alone or with azacitidine at 2.5 or 10 mg/kg bw by intraperitoneal injection. Liver tumours were found in 2/10 and 8/10 animals given the low and the high dose of azacitidine, respectively, but not in the group given the nitroso compound alone.

Table 1. Incidences of tumours in the progeny of NMRI mice given azacitidine by intraperitoneal injection[a]

Treatment		Sex	No. of animals	Leukaemias and lymphomas		Lung tumours		Liver tumours	
mg/kg bw	day of gestation			No.	%	No.	%	No.	%
1	12	Males	165	81	49.1	30	18.2	15	9.1
		Females	158	80	50.6	33	20.9	6	3.8
2	12	Males	113	28	24.8	22	19.5	11	9.7
		Females	110	26	23.6	22	20.0	9	8.2
1	14	Males	178	42	23.6	29	16.3	12	6.7
		Females	171	26	15.2	31	18.1	20	11.7
2	14	Males	97	9	9.3	46	47.4	11	11.3
		Females	101	14	13.9	43	42.6	7	6.9
1	16	Males	153	97	63.4	81	52.9	14	9.2
		Females	160	98	61.3	99	61.9	8	5.0
2	16	Males	158	67	42.4	78	49.3	18	11.4
		Females	151	57	37.7	82	54.3	5	3.3
Controls		Males	293	84	28.7	57	19.5	14	4.8
		Females	279	82	29.4	53	19.0	11	3.9

[a]From Schmähl et al. (1985)

3.2 Other relevant data

(a) *Experimental systems*

(i) *Absorption, distribution, excretion and metabolism*

Blood levels of azacitidine, determined by biological activity, in mice peaked within 0.5 h after intraperitoneal or oral administration. Maximal concentrations of azacitidine in blood after administration at 50 mg/kg bw were about 2 μg/ml after oral administration and 43 μg/ml after intraperitoneal injection (Neil et al., 1975).

In a study using a microbiological assay, maximal concentrations were found in blood 15 min after intraperitoneal injection of 9.5 and 4.75 mg/kg bw (LD_{10} and $0.5 LD_{10}$) to mice. Elimination was rapid, and no azacitidine was detected in blood 1 h after injection of the high dose or 30 min after injection of the low dose. No drug was detected in liver, lung, brain, spleen or kidneys (Pittillo & Woolley, 1969).

In a further study, ^{14}C activity in blood diminished rapidly in mice after intraperitoneal administration of labelled azacitidine (Raska et al., 1965). The half-time for azacitidine and its radioactive metabolites was calculated by von Hoff and Slavic (1977) to be 3.8 h; radioactivity was retained in lymphatic organs.

As reported in an abstract, 50% of a dose [amount and route unspecified] administered to mice was excreted in the urine within 8 h; of the excreted radioactive material, 4% was associated with unchanged azacitidine. Six additional radioactive metabolites were found (Coles et al., 1975). In beagle dogs, azacitidine, 5-azacytosine, urea and guanidine were observed after intravenous administration of azacitidine at 0.5 mg/kg bw; 33% of the administered dose was excreted in urine by 4 h (Coles et al., 1974). In rabbits, most of the radioactivity (25-40%) was excreted in the urine after intravenous administration of labelled azacitidine at 15 mg/kg bw; only small amounts were excreted via the bile (Chan et al., 1977).

Azacitidine is phosphorylated and inhibits uridine kinase and orotidylic acid hydroxylase (von Hoff et al., 1975, 1976). It is readily deaminated in biological systems to 5-azauridine, which is degraded further (Cihák, 1974; Neil et al., 1975; Glover & Leyland-Jones, 1987).

(ii) *Toxic effects*

As reported in an abstract, the intraperitoneal LD_{50} for azacitidine in mice was 116 mg/kg bw and the oral LD_{50}, 572 mg; five daily doses increased the toxicity considerably (Palm & Kensler, 1971).

After phosphorylation, azacitidine is incorporated into DNA and RNA in L1210 leukaemia cells *in vitro* (Li et al., 1970); it inhibits DNA synthesis in the liver of partially hepatectomized rats. Intraperitoneal injection of azacitidine at 10 μmol/100 g bw inhibited thymidine kinase and thymidylate kinase in rat liver (Cihák & Vesely, 1972).

Azacitidine is cytotoxic to Friend erythroleukaemia cells (Hickey et al., 1986), L1210 leukaemia cells (Li et al., 1970) and normal rat hepatocytes (Carr et al., 1988) *in vitro*; after a dose of 1×10^{-4} M, 32% survival of rat hepatocytes was observed within 24 h.

(iii) *Hypomethylation and effects on gene expression*

After incorporation into DNA, azacitidine inhibits DNA methyl transferase noncompetitively, blocking cytosine methylation in newly replicated DNA. Since hypomethylation patterns in DNA are related to gene expression, this may be the mechanism by which azacytidine induces a range of biological effects (Glover et al., 1987). A number of in-vitro and in-vivo studies have shown that azacitidine treatment affects both differentiation (Constantinides et al., 1978; Taylor & Jones, 1979; Tsao et al., 1984; Csordas & Schauenstein, 1986; Liu et al., 1986; Sémat et al., 1986; Rothrock et al., 1988) and gene expression (Tennant et al., 1982; Harrison et al., 1983; Rothrock et al., 1983; Sugiyama et al., 1983; del Senno et al., 1984; Waalkes & Poirier, 1985; Castelazzi et al., 1986; Hickey et al., 1986; Hoshino et al., 1987; Ishikawa et al., 1987; Price-Haughey et al., 1987; Carr et al., 1988; Stephanopoulos et al., 1988; Wagner et al., 1988).

(iv) Effects on reproduction and prenatal toxicity

Intraperitoneal administration of azacitidine at 1.5-2.5 mg/kg bw to mice for various periods during pregnancy induced very high or total resorption of conceptuses when treatment was given in the preimplantation period up to day 6; after this time, the incidence of resorptions was only slightly greater than the control level (Svata *et al.*, 1966; Seifertová *et al.*, 1968). Other workers have shown that single intraperitoneal doses of 1-2 mg/kg to mice during the period of embryogenesis can cause a high resorption rate and malformations in the majority of surviving fetuses, including major central nervous system defects, facial clefts and limb defects (Schmahl *et al.*, 1984; Takeuchi & Takeuchi, 1985).

Intraperitoneal injection of azacitidine at 1-4 mg/kg to mice at later stages of pregnancy, especially on day 15, can result in morphological changes in the brain (Langman & Shimada, 1971), and behavioural changes can be detected in offspring when tested as adults (Rodier *et al.*, 1973; Langman *et al.*, 1975; Rodier, 1979).

The primary mechanism by which azacitidine causes malformations in rats is thought to be induction of cell death, but inhibition of some but not all of the effects of azacitidine by administration of caffeine indicates that more than one mechanism may be involved (Kurishita & Ihara, 1987a,b).

(v) Genetic and related effects

In *Escherichia coli*, azacitidine caused DNA damage (Bhagwat & Roberts, 1987) and prophage induction (Barbe *et al.*, 1986). It was mutagenic to *E. coli* (Fucik *et al.*, 1965; Lal *et al.*, 1988) and induced base-pair but not frameshift mutations in *Salmonella typhimurium* (Marquardt & Marquardt, 1977; Podger, 1983; Call *et al.*, 1986; Levin & Ames, 1986; Schmuck *et al.*, 1986).

Azacitidine induced mitotic recombinations, mitotic gene conversions and reverse mutations but not mitotic chromosome loss in *Saccharomyces cerevisiae* (Zimmermann & Scheel, 1984). It induced mitotic recombinations, deletions and gene mutations in the wing spot assay in *Drosophila melanogaster* (Katz, 1985) and chromosomal aberrations in root meristem cells of *Vicia faba* (Fucik *et al.*, 1970).

Azacitidine inhibited DNA synthesis in Chinese hamster CHO cells (Tobey, 1972) and induced DNA strand breaks in HeLa cells (Snyder & Lachmann, 1989). It induced mutations at the *hprt* locus in Chinese hamster V79 cells in one study (at 5 µM; Marquardt & Marquardt, 1977) but not in another (at 40 µM; Landolph & Jones, 1982). It did not induce mutation at the *hprt* locus in Syrian hamster BHK cells (Bouck *et al.*, 1984), primary rat tracheal epithelial cells (Walker & Nettesheim, 1986) or mouse lymphoma L5178Y cells (at 4 µM; McGregor *et al.*, 1989). Azacitidine induced mutations at the *hprt* and *tk* loci in human fibroblasts (Call *et al.*, 1986) and at the *tk* locus of mouse lymphoma L5178Y cells (Amacher & Turner, 1987; McGregor *et al.*, 1989). It did not induce ouabain-resistant mutations in mouse C3H 10T½, Chinese hamster V79 (Landolph & Jones, 1982), Syrian hamster BHK (Bouck et al., 1984) or primary rat tracheal epithelial cells (Walker & Nettesheim, 1986).

Azacitidine induced sister chromatid exchange in a cloned hamster cell line (Banerjee & Benedict, 1979), in CHO cells (Hori, 1983) and in human peripheral lymphocytes in vitro [only one concentration, 8 μM, was tested] (Lavia et al., 1985). In another study, azacitidine did not induce sister chromatid exchange in human lymphocytes (up to 9 μM; Ioannidou et al., 1989). It induced chromosomal aberrations in Chinese hamster Don cells (Karon & Benedict, 1972) and in human peripheral lymphocytes in vitro [only one concentration, 8 μM, was tested] (Lavia et al., 1985) but not in human lymphoblasts (10 μM; Call et al., 1986).

Azacitidine induced transformation in mouse C3H/10T½ (Benedict et al., 1977), Syrian hamster BHK (Bouck et al., 1984), mouse BALB/3T3 (Yasutake et al., 1987) and primary rat tracheal epithelial cells (Walker & Nettesheim, 1986).

Azacitidine did not induce dominant lethal mutation in male mice after administration at 5 and 10 mg/kg bw intraperitoneally (Epstein et al., 1972).

(b) *Humans*

The toxicity, cytostatic activity and mechanism of action of azacitidine have been reviewed (Cihák, 1974; von Hoff & Slavik, 1977; Glover & Leyland-Jones, 1987).

(i) *Pharmacokinetics*

After an intravenous injection of radiolabelled azacitidine, the α-phase half-time of radioactivity was 16-33 min (Israeli et al., 1976), and the β-phase half-time was 3.4-6.2 h (Troetel et al., 1972; Israeli et al., 1976). After 30 min, less than 2% of the plasma radioactivity cochromatographed with azacitidine; at least two different metabolites or decomposition products were detected by thin-layer chromatography (Israeli et al., 1976), and 73-98% of the injected radioactivity was detected in the urine within three days (Israeli et al., 1976). Similar results were obtained by Troetel et al. (1972).

Less than 1% of radiolabelled azacitidine was bound to human serum albumin in vitro (Israeli et al., 1976).

(ii) *Adverse effects*

The major toxic effects of the clinical use of azacitidine have been gastrointestinal, haematological and hepatic (von Hoff et al., 1976; von Hoff & Slavik, 1977; Reynolds, 1989). Leukopenia is generally the dose-limiting toxicity; in a compilation of several studies with a total of 821 patients, the incidence of leukopenia (total leukocyte count, less than $1500/mm^3$) was 34% and was dose-related. Thrombocytopenia has been reported less frequently (von Hoff et al.,

1976; von Hoff & Slavik, 1977). Fatal hepatic damage was reported in four patients with previous hepatic dysfunction, who had been treated with azacitidine (Bellet *et al.*, 1973).

(iii) *Effects on reproduction and prenatal toxicity*

No data were available to the Working Group.

(iv) *Genetic and related effects*

No adequate study was available to the Working Group.

3.3 Case reports and epidemiological studies of carcinogenicity to humans

No data were available to the Working Group.

4. Summary of Data Reported and Evaluation

4.1 Exposure data

Azacitidine is a cytostatic agent that has been used since the 1970s for the treatment of acute leukaemia.

4.2 Experimental carcinogenicity data

Azacitidine was tested for carcinogenicity by intraperitoneal injection in four studies in mice and in two studies in rats and by transplacental exposure in one study in mice. In one study in mice, it accelerated the development of leukaemias; in the two long-term studies and in the transplacental study, it increased the incidence of lymphoid neoplasms. In one of the long-term studies, the incidence of lung adenomas was increased in male mice and that of skin tumours in mice of each sex. In the transplacental study in mice, it also increased the incidences of lung and liver tumours. It accelerated the induction of lung tumours in mice. In rats, it increased the incidence of testicular tumours.

Intraperitoneal administration of azacitidine to rats enhanced the development of liver tumours induced by *N*-nitrosodiethylamine.

4.3 Human carcinogenicity data

No data were available to the Working Group.

4.4 Other relevant data

During the early stages of gestation, azacitidine induces embryomortality in mice; during the organogenesis period, multiple, gross structural malformations can be induced; and during later stages of gestation, mainly central nervous system defects have been induced in mice.

Azacitidine is readily deaminated to azauridine and further degraded. It is incorporated into DNA and alters gene expression. In humans, it causes leukopenia.

Azacitidine causes hypomethylation of DNA both *in vivo* and *in vitro*.

In one study, azacitidine did not induce dominant lethal mutations in mice. Contradictory results have been reported with respect to the induction of chromosomal aberrations and sister chromatid exchange in human cells. In single studies, azacitidine induced gene mutations and DNA strand breaks in human cells. It induced chromosomal aberrations in Chinese hamster cells, sister chromatid exchange in cloned Chinese hamster cells, gene mutations in Chinese hamster and mouse lymphoma cells and transformation in various cell lines. It induced mitotic recombination and mutations in *Drosophila*. Azacitidine induced chromosomal aberrations in *Vicia faba*. In *Saccharomyces cerevisiae*, it induced gene mutations and mitotic recombination but not chromosomal loss. It induced mutations and DNA damage in *Salmonella typhimurium* and *Escherichia coli*. (See Appendix 1.)

4.5 Evaluation[1]

There is *sufficient evidence* for the carcinogenicity of azacitidine in experimental animals.

No data were available from studies in humans on the carcinogenicity of azacitidine.

In making the overall evaluation, the Working Group also took note of the following information. Azacitidine is active in a broad spectrum of assays for genetic and related effects, including those involving mammalian cells. Furthermore, azacitidine, a pyrimidine analogue, is incorporated into DNA, causing hypomethylation.

Overall evaluation

Azacitidine *is probably carcinogenic to humans (Group 2A)*.

---

[1] For description of the italicized terms, see Preamble, pp. 26–29.

5. References

Amacher, D.E. & Turner, G.N. (1987) The mutagenicity of 5-azacytidine and other inhibitors of replicative DNA synthesis in the L5178Y mouse lymphoma cell. *Mutat. Res.*, *176*, 123-131

Banerjee, A. & Benedict, W.F. (1979) Production of sister chromatid exchanges by various cancer chemotherapeutic agents. *Cancer Res.*, *39*, 797-799

Barbe, J., Gilbert, I. & Guerrero, R. (1986) 5-Azacytidine: survival and induction of the SOS response in *Escherichia coli* K12. *Mutat. Res.*, *166*, 9-16

Beisler, J. (1978) Isolation, characterization, and properties of a labile hydrolysis product of the antitumor nucleoside 5-azacytidine. *J. med. Chem.*, *21*, 204-208

Bellet, R.E., Mastrangelo, M.J., Engstrom, P.F. & Custer, R.P. (1973) Hepatotoxicity of 5-azacytidine (NSC-102816) (A clinical and pathologic study). *Neoplasma*, *20*, 303-309

Benedict, W.F., Banerjee, A., Gardner, A. & Jones, P.A. (1977) Induction of morphological transformation in mouse C3H/10T½ clone 8 cells and chromosomal damage in hamster A(T_1)C1-3 cells by cancer chemotherapeutic agents. *Cancer Res.*, *37*, 2202-2208

Bhagwat, A.S. & Roberts, R.J. (1987) Genetic analysis of the 5-azacytidine sensitivity of *Escherichia coli* K-12. *J. Bacteriol.*, *169*, 1537-1546

Bouck, N., Kokinakis, D. & Ostrowsky, J. (1984) Induction of a step in carcinogenesis that is normally associated with mutagenesis by nonmutagenic concentrations of 5-azacytidine. *Mol. Cell Biol.*, *4*, 1231-1237

Call, K.M., Jensen, J.C., Liber, H.L. & Thilly, W.G. (1986) Studies of mutagenicity and clastogenicity of 5-azacytidine in human lymphoblasts and *Salmonella typhimurium*. *Mutat. Res.*, *160*, 249-257

Carr, B.I., Reilly, J.G., Smith, S.S., Winberg, C. & Riggs, A. (1984) The tumorigenicity of 5-azacytidine in the male Fischer rat. *Carcinogenesis*, *5*, 1583-1590

Carr, B.I., Rahbar, S., Asmeron, Y., Riggs, A. & Winberg, C.D. (1988) Carcinogenicity and haemoglobin synthesis induction by cytidine analogues. *Br. J. Cancer*, *57*, 395

Castellazzi, M., Vielh, P. & Longacre, S. (1986) Azacytidine-induced reactivation of adenosine deaminase in a murine cytotoxic T cell line. *Eur. J. Immunol.*, *16*, 1081-1086

Cavaliere, A., Bufalari, A. & Vitali, R. (1987) 5-Azacytidine carcinogenesis in Balb/c mice. *Cancer Lett.*, *37*, 51-58

Chan, K.K., Staroscik, J.A. & Sadée, W. (1977) Synthesis of 5-azacytidine-6-C and 6-^{14}C. *J. med. Chem.*, *20*, 598-600

Chemical Information Services (1989-90) *Directory of World Chemical Producers*, Oceanside, NY

Cihák, A. (1974) Biological effects of 5-azacytidine in eukaryotes. A review. *Oncology*, *30*, 405-422

Cihák, A. & Vesely, J. (1972) Prolongation of the lag period preceding the enhancement of thymidine and thymidylate kinase activity in regenerating rat liver by 5-azacytidine. *Biochem. Pharmacol.*, *21*, 3257-3265

Coles, E., Thayer, P.S., Reinhold, V. & Gaudio, L. (1974) Pharmacokinetics of excretion of 5-azacytidine (NSC 102816) and its metabolites (Abstract No. 286). *Proc. Am. Assoc. Cancer Res.*, *15*, 72

Coles, E., Wodinsky, I. & Gaudio, L. (1975) The effects of drug combinations on the metabolism and excretion of 5-azacytidine (5-Aza Sr, NSC 102816) in BDF_1 mice (Abstract No. 362). *Proc. Am. Assoc. Cancer Res.*, *16*, 91

Constantinides, P.G., Taylor, S.M. & Jones, P.A. (1978) Phenotypic conversion of cultured mouse embryo cells by aza pyrimidine nucleosides. *Dev. Biol.*, *66*, 57-71

Csordas, A. & Schauenstein, K. (1986) Thymus involution induced by 5-azacytidine. *Biosci. Rep.*, *6*, 603-612

Epstein, S.S., Arnold, E., Andrea, J., Bass, W. & Bishop, Y. (1972) Detection of chemical mutagens by the dominant lethal assay in the mouse. *Toxicol. appl. Pharmacol.*, *23*, 288-325

Fucik, V., Zadrazil, S., Sormova, Z. & Sorm, F. (1965) Mutagenic effects of 5-azacytidine in bacteria. *Coll. Czech. chem. Commun.*, *30*, 2883-2886

Fucik, V., Michaelis, A. & Rieger, R. (1970) On the induction of segment extension and chromatid structural changes in *Vicia faba* chromosomes after treatment with 5-azacytidine and 5-azadeoxycytidine. *Mutat. Res.*, *9*, 599-606

Glover, A.B. & Leyland-Jones, B. (1987) Biochemistry of 5-azacytidine: a review. *Cancer Treat. Rep.*, *71*, 959-964

Glover, A.B., Leyland-Jones, B.R., Chun, H.G., Davies, B. & Hoth, D.F. (1987) 5-Azacytidine 10 years later. *Cancer Treat. Rep.*, *71*, 737-746

Halle, S. (1968) 5-Azacytidine as a mutagen for arboviruses. *J. Virol.*, *2*, 1228-1229

Harrison, J.J., Anisowicz, A., Gadi, I.K., Raffeld, M. & Sager, R. (1983) Azacytidine-induced tumorigenesis of CHEF/18 cells: correlated DNA methylation and chromosome changes. *Proc. natl Acad. Sci. USA*, *80*, 6606-6610

Hickey, I., Jones, S. & O'Neill, K. (1986) Azacytidine induces reversion of thymidine kinase deficiency in Friend erythroleukemia cells. *Exp. Cell Res.*, *164*, 251-255

von Hoff, D.D. & Slavik, M. (1977) 5-Azacytidine — a new anticancer drug with significant activity in acute myeloblastic leukemia. *Adv. Pharmacol. Chemother.*, *14*, 285-326

von Hoff, D.D., Handelsman, H. & Slavik, M. (1975) *5-Azacytidine (NSC 102816), Clinical Brochure*, Bethesda, MD, National Cancer Institute, Division of Cancer Treatment

von Hoff, D.D. Slavik, M. & Muggia, F.M. (1976) 5-Azacytidine. A new anticancer drug with effectiveness in acute myelogenous leukemia. *Ann. intern. Med.*, *85*, 237-245

Hori, T.-A. (1983) Induction of chromosome decondensation, sister-chromatid exchanges and endoreduplications by 5-azacytidine, an inhibitor of DNA methylation. *Mutat. Res.*, *121*, 47-52

Hoshino, J., Frahm, J. & Kröger, H. (1987) Suppression of nuclear ADP-ribosyltransferase activity in Ehrlich ascites tumor cells by 5-azacytidine and its analogs. *Biochem. biophys. Res. Commun.*, *142*, 468-474

IARC (1981) *IARC Monographs on the Evaluation of the Carcinogenic Risk of Chemicals to Humans*, Vol. 26, *Some Antineoplastic and Immunosuppressive Agents*, Lyon, pp. 37-46

Ioannidou, E., Lialiaris, T., Mourelatos, D. & Dozi-Vassiliades, J. (1989) Synergistic induction of cytogenetic damage by alkylating antineoplastics and 5-azacytidine in human lymphocytes. *Environ. mol. Mutagenesis, 14*, 6-12

Ishikawa, M., Okada, F., Hamada, J., Hosokawa, M. & Kobayashi, H. (1987) Changes in the tumorigenic and metastatic properties of tumor cells treated with quercetin or 5-azacytidine. *Int. J. Cancer, 39*, 338-342

Israeli, Z.H., Vogler, W.R., Mingioli, E.S., Pirkie, J.L., Smithwick, R.W. & Goldstein, J.H. (1976) The disposition and pharmacokinetics in humans of 5-azacytidine administered intravenously as a bolus or by continuous infusion. *Cancer Res., 36*, 1453-1461

Karon, M. & Benedict, W.F. (1972) Chromatid breakage: differential effect of inhibitors of DNA synthesis during G_2 phase. *Science, 178*, 62

Katz, A.J. (1985) Genotoxicity of 5-azacytidine in somatic cells of Drosophila. *Mutat. Res., 143*, 195-199

Kurishita, A. & Ihara, T. (1987a) Inhibitory effect of caffeine on azacitidine-induced digital malformations in the rat. *Teratology, 35*, 247-252

Kurishita, A. & Ihara, T. (1987b) Histological study of inhibitory effect of caffeine on azacitidine induced digital malformations. *Teratology, 35*, 452-453

Lal, D., Som, S. & Friedman, S. (1988) Survival and mutagenic effects of 5-azacytidine in *Escherichia coli*. *Mutat. Res., 193*, 229-236

Landolph, J.R. & Jones, P.A. (1982) Mutagenicity of 5-azacytidine and related nucleosides in C3H 10T½ clone 8 and V79 cells. *Cancer Res., 42*, 817-823

Langman, J. & Shimada, M. (1971) Cerebral cortex of the mouse after prenatal chemical insult. *Am. J. Anat., 132*, 355-374

Langman, J., Rodier, P.M., Webster, W., Crowley, K., Cardell, E.L. & Pool, R. (1975) The influence of teratogens on cellular and tissue behavior during the second half of pregnancy and their effect on postnatal behavior. In: Neubert, D. & Merker, H.-J., eds, *New Approaches to the Evaluation of Abnormal Embryonic Development*, Stuttgart, Georg Thieme, pp. 439-468

Lavia, P., Ferraro, M., Micheli, A. & Olivieri, G. (1985) Effect of 5-azacytidine (5-azaC) on the induction of chromatid aberrations (CA) and sister-chromatid exchanges (SCE). *Mutat. Res., 149*, 462-467

Levin, D.E. & Ames, B.N. (1986) Classifying mutagens as to their specificity in causing the six possible transitions and transversions: a simple analysis using the Salmonella mutagenicity assay. *Environ. Mutagenesis, 8*, 9-28

Li, L.H., Olin, E.J., Buskirk, H.H. & Reineke, L.M. (1970) Cytotoxicity and mode of action of azacitidine on L1210 leukemia. *Cancer Res., 30*, 2760-2769

Liu, L., Harrington, M. & Jones, P.A. (1986) Characterization of myogenic cell lines derived by azacitidine treatment. *Dev. Biol., 117*, 331-336

Marquardt, H. & Marquardt, H. (1977) Induction of malignant transformation and mutagenesis in cell cultures by cancer chemotherapeutic agents. *Cancer, 40*, 1930-1934

McGregor, D.B., Brown, A.G., Cattanach, P., Shepherd, W., Riach, C., Daston, D. & Caspary, W.J. (1989) TFT and 6TG resistance of mouse lymphoma cells to analogs of azacytidine. *Carcinogenesis, 10*, 2003-2008

National Cancer Institute (1978) *Bioassay of 5-Azacytidine for Possible Carcinogenicity* (NCI Publ. No. 279-526), Bethesda, MD

Neil, G.L., Moxley, T.E., Kuentzel, S.L., Manak, R.C. & Hanka, L.J. (1975) Enhancement by tetrahydrouridine (NSC-112907) of the oral activity of azacitidine (NSC-102816) in L1210 leukemic mice. *Cancer Chemother. Rep.*, 59, 459-465

Palm, P.E. & Kensler, C.J. (1971) Toxicology of a new pyrimidine antimetabolite, azacitidine in mice, hamsters, and dogs (Abstract No. 55). *Toxicol. appl. Pharmacol.*, 19, 382-383

Pittillo, R.F. & Woolley, C. (1969) 5-Azacytidine: microbiological assay in mouse blood. *Appl. Microbiol.*, 18, 284-286

Podger, D.M. (1983) Mutagenicity of 5-azacytidine in *Salmonella typhimurium*. *Mutat. Res.*, 121, 1-6

Price-Haughey, J., Bonham, K. & Gedamu, L. (1987) Metallothionein gene expression in fish cell lines: its activation in embryonic cells by 5-azacytidine. *Biochim. biophys. Acta*, 908, 158-168

Raska, K., Jurovcik, M., Sormova, Z. & Sorm, F. (1965) On the metabolism of 5-azacytidine and 5-aza-2'-deoxycytidine in mice. *Coll. Czech. chem. Commun.*, 30, 3001-3006

Reynolds, E.F., ed. (1989) *Martindale. The Extra Pharmacopoeia*, 29th ed., London, The Pharmaceutical Press, p. 599

Rodier, P.M. (1979) A comparison of gross malformations and quantitative measures as indicants of teratogenicity. *Anat. Rec.*, 193, 665

Rodier, P.M., Webster, W. & Langman, J. (1973) Morphological and behavioral anomalies after 5-azacytidine treatment of fetal and neonatal mice. *Teratology*, 7, A-25

Rothrock, R., Perry, S.T., Isham, K.R., Lee, K.-L. & Kenney, F.T. (1983) Activation of tyrosine aminotransferase expression in fetal liver by 5-azacytidine. *Biochem. Biophys. Res. Commun.*, 113, 645-649

Rothrock, R., Lee, K.-L., Isham, K.R. & Kenney, F.T. (1988) Changes in hepatic differentiation following treatment of rat fetuses with 5-azacytidine. *Arch. Biochem. Biophys.*, 263, 237-244

Rustum, A.M. & Hoffman, N.E. (1987) High-performance liquid chromatographic determination of 5-azacytidine in plasma. *J. Chromatogr.*, 421, 387-391

Schmahl, W., Török, P. & Kriegel, H. (1984) Embryotoxicity of 5-azacytidine in mice. Phase- and dose-specificity studies. *Arch. Toxicol.*, 55, 143-147

Schmahl, W., Geber, E. & Lehmacher, W. (1985) Diaplacental carcinogenic effects of 5-azacytidine in NMRI-mice. *Cancer Lett.*, 27, 81-90

Schmuck, G., Pechan, R., Wild, D., Schiffmann, D. & Henschler, D. (1986) SOS-dependent mutagenic activity of 5-azacytidine in Salmonella. *Mutat. Res.*, 175, 205-208

Seifertová, M., Veselý, J. & Sorm, F. (1968) Effect of 5-azacytidine on developing mouse embryo. *Experientia*, 24, 487-488

Sémat, A., Duprey, P., Vasseur, M. & Darmon, M. (1986) Mesenchymal-epithelial conversions induced by 5-azacytidine: appearance of cytokeratin endo-A messenger RNA. *Differentiation*, 31, 61-66 del Senno, L., Conconi, F., Barbieri, R., Amelotti, F., Bernardi, F., Piva, R., Viola, L. & Gambari, R. (1984) Human leukemic K562 cells: differential effects of 5-azacytidine on DNA methylation of ϵ-, γ-globin and 7SL RNA genes. *Boll. Soc. ital. Biol. sper.*, 60, 1613-1619

Skoda, J. (1975) Azapyrimidine nucleosides. In: Sartorelli, A.C. & Johns, D.G., eds, *Antineoplastic Immunosuppressive Agents*, Part II, New York, Springer, pp. 361-372

Snyder, R.D. & Lachmann, P.J. (1989) Differential effects of 5-azacytidine and 5-azadeoxycitidine on cytotoxicity, DNA-strand breaking and repair of X-ray-induced DNA damage in HeLa cells. *Mutat. Res.*, 226, 185-190

Stephanopoulos, D.E., Kappes, J.C. & Bernstein, D.I. (1988) Enhanced *in vitro* reactivation of herpes simplex virus type 2 from latently infected guinea-pig neural tissues by 5-azacytidine. *J. gen. Virol.*, 69, 1079-1083

Stoner, G.D., Shimkin, M.B., Kniazeff, A.J., Weisburger, J.H., Weisburger, E.K. & Gori, G.B. (1973) Test for carcinogenicity of food additives and chemotherapeutic agents by the pulmonary tumor response in strain A mice. *Cancer Res.*, 33, 3069-3085

Sugiyama, R.H., Arfin, S.M. & Harris, M. (1983) Properties of asparagine synthetase in asparagine-independent variants of Jensen rat sarcoma cells induced by azacitidine. *Mol. cell. Biol.*, 3, 1937-1942

Svata, M., Raska, K., Jr & Sorm, F. (1966) Interruption of pregnancy by azacitidine. *Experientia*, 22, 53

Takeuchi, I.K. & Takeuchi, Y.K. (1985) Azacitidine-induced exencephaly in mice. *J. Anat.*, 140, 403-412

Taylor, S.M. & Jones, P.A. (1979) Multiple new phenotypes induced in 10T½ and 3T3 cells treated with azacitidine. *Cell*, 17, 771-779

Tennant, R.W., Otten, J.A., Myer, F.E. & Rascati, R.J. (1982) Induction of retrovirus gene expression in mouse cells by some chemical mutagens. *Cancer Res.*, 42, 3050-3055

Tobey, R.A. (1972) Effects of cytosine arabinoside, daunomycin, mithramycin, azacytidine, adriamycin and camptothecin on mammalian cell cycle traverse. *Cancer Res.*, 32, 2720-2725

Troetel, W.M., Weiss, A.J., Stambaugh, J.E., Lucius, J.F. & Manthei, R.W. (1972) Absorption, distribution and excretion of 5-azacytidine (NSC-102816) in man. *Cancer Chemother. Rep.*, 56, 405-411

Tsao, M.-S., Nelson, K.G. & Grisham, J.W. (1984) Biochemical effects of 12-O-tetradecanoylphorbol-13-acetate, retinoic acid, phenobarbital, and azacitidine on a normal rat liver epithelial cell line. *J. cell. Physiol.*, 121, 1-6

Turusov, V.S., ed. (1973) *Pathology of Tumours in Laboratory Animals*, Vol. 1, *Tumours of the Rat, Part 1* (IARC Scientific Publications No. 5), Lyon, IARC

Turusov, V.S., ed. (1976) *Pathology of Tumours in Laboratory Animals*, Vol. 1, *Tumours of the Rat, Part 2* (IARC Scientific Publications No. 6), Lyon, IARC

Veselý, D. & Cihák, A. (1973) High-frequency induction in vivo of mouse leukemia in AKR strain by 5-azacytidine and 5-iodo-2'-deoxyuridine. *Experientia*, 15, 1132-1133

Waalkes, M.P. & Poirier, L.A. (1985) Induction of hepatic metallothionein following azacitidine administration. *Toxicol. appl. Pharmacol.*, 79, 47-53

Wade, A., ed. (1977) *Martindale, The Extra Pharmacopoeia*, 27th ed., London, The Pharmaceutical Press, p. 1724

Wagner, G., Pott, U., Bruckschen, M. & Sies, H. (1988) Effects of azacitidine and methyl-group deficiency on NAD(P)H:quinone oxidoreductase and glutathione S-transferase in liver. *Biochem. J.*, *251*, 825-829

Walker, C. & Nettesheim, P. (1986) *In vitro* transformation of primary rat tracheal epithelial cells by 5-azacytidine. *Cancer Res.*, *46*, 6433-6437

Weiss, A.J., Stambaugh, J.E., Mastrelango, M.J., Laucius, J.F. & Bellet, R.E. (1972) Phase I study of 5-azacytidine (NSC-102816). *Cancer Chemother. Rep.*, *56*, 413-419

Winkley, M.W. & Robins, R.K. (1970) Direct glycosylation of 1,3,5-triazinones. A new approach to the synthesis of the nucleoside antibiotic azacitidine (4-amino-1-β-D-ribofuranosyl-1,3,5-triazin-2-one) and related derivatives. *J. org. Chem.*, *35*, 491-495

Yasutake, C., Kuratomi, Y., Ono, M., Masumi, S. & Kuwano, M. (1987) Effect of 5-azacytidine on malignant transformation of a mutant derived from the mouse BALB/c 3T3 cell line resistant to transformation by chemical carcinogens. *Cancer Res.*, *47*, 4894-4899

Zimmermann, F.K. & Scheel, I. (1984) Genetic effects of 5-azacytidine in *Saccharomyces cerevisiae*. *Mutat. Res.*, *139*, 21-24

CHLOROZOTOCIN

1. Chemical and Physical Data

1.1 Synonyms

Chem. Abstr. Services Reg. No.: 54749-90-5

Chem. Abstr. Name: D-Glucose, 2-({[(2-chloroethyl)nitrosoamino]carbonyl}-amino)-2-deoxy-

Synonyms: D-Glucopyranose, 2-({[(2-chloroethyl)nitrosoamino]carbonyl}-amino)-2-deoxy-1-(2-chloroethyl)-1-nitroso-3-(D-glucos-2-yl)urea; 2-[3-(chloroethyl)-3-nitrosoureido]-2-deoxy-D-glucopyranose; DCNU; NSC-178248

1.2 Structural and molecular formulae and molecular weight

$C_9H_{16}ClN_3O_7$ Mol. wt: 313.69

1.3 Chemical and physical properties of the pure substance

From Windholz (1983), unless otherwise specified

(a) *Description*: Ivory crystals

(b) *Melting-point*: 147-148°C (decomposes); 140-141°C (decomposes)

(c) *Solubility*: Soluble in water; decomposition in aqueous solution has been studied (Montgomery *et al.*, 1975).

(d) *Spectroscopy data*: Infra-red and nuclear magnetic resonance spectra have been reported (Johnston *et al.*, 1975).

(e) *Stability:* Stable (<5% decomposition by ultraviolet spectroscopy) in solution at room temperature (22-25°C) for 3 h and at 2-8°C for 24 h; powder is stable for 24 months under refrigeration

(f) *Partition coefficient:* Pc = 3 (octanol:water) (Johnston et al., 1975)

1.4 Technical products and impurities

Trade name: Dome

Chlorozotocin is available as a lyophilized powder in vials containing 50 mg of the compound with 48 mg citric acid and sodium hydroxide to adjust the pH (National Cancer Institute, 1988).

2. Production, Occurrence, Use and Analysis

2.1 Production and occurrence

Chlorozotocin is synthesized by nitrosation of the urea derivative prepared from D-glucosamine and 2-chloroethylisocyanate (Johnston et al., 1975). It is reported to be produced in the USA.

Chlorozotocin is not known to occur naturally.

2.2 Use

Chlorozotocin is a cytostatic agent. It can be used in the treatment of cancers of the stomach, large bowel, pancreas and lung, melanoma and multiple myeloma. It has been given intravenously, at doses of 100-225 mg/m^2 (Samson et al., 1982; Smith et al., 1982; Bukowski et al., 1983; Haas et al., 1983; Forman et al., 1984; Gastrointestinal Tumor Study Group, 1985). No indication for its use was given by Reynolds (1989).

2.3 Analysis

A colorimetric method for the analysis of chlorozotocin in plasma has been reported (Hoth et al., 1978; Kovach et al., 1979).

3. Biological Data Relevant to the Evaluation of Carcinogenic Risk to Humans

3.1 Carcinogenicity studies in animals

(a) *Intraperitoneal administration*

Rat: Groups of 20 male and 20 female Sprague-Dawley rats, 100 days old, were given intraperitoneal injections of chlorozotocin (synthesized according to standard methods) at 0.4 or 2.0 mg/kg bw once a week for up to 800 days. Control groups of 20 rats of each sex received injections of Cremophor EL: ethanol:saline in a ratio of 1:1:2 volume parts. The median survival times in days were as follows: control males, 724; low-dose males, 463; high-dose males, 307; control females, 750; low-dose females, 694; high-dose females, 346. Sarcomas and mesotheliomas of the peritoneal cavity occurred in 13/20 [$p < 0.001$] and 14/20 [$p < 0.001$, Fisher's exact test] high- and low-dose males, respectively, compared to 0/20 controls, and in 16/20 [$p < 0.001$] and 10/20 [$p = 0.002$, Fisher's exact test] high- and low-dose females, respectively, compared to 1/20 controls (Habs *et al.*, 1979).

(b) *Intravenous administration*

Rat: Groups of 30 male Wistar rats [age unspecified] were given intravenous injections of chlorozotocin at 9.5, 19 or 38 mg/m^2 every six weeks for 10 applications. A group of 120 controls received Cremophor EL:ethanol:water in a ratio of 1.5:1.5:20 volume parts. The median survival times in days were as follows: high dose, 474; median dose, 590; low dose, 583; controls, 621. Animals were observed for life. Malignant tumours of the nervous system, lung and forestomach were found in 4, 5 and 4% of treated animals compared to 1, 0 and 1% of controls, respectively (Eisenbrand & Habs, 1980; Eisenbrand *et al.*, 1981; Zeller *et al.*, 1982). [The Working Group noted the poor survival and limited reporting.]

3.2 Other relevant data

(a) *Experimental systems*

The toxicity of chlorozotocin has been reviewed (Schein *et al.*, 1976; Macdonald *et al.*, 1980; Wang *et al.*, 1981; Eisenbrand, 1984; Eisenbrand *et al.*, 1986; Johnston & Montgomery, 1986).

(i) *Absorption, distribution, excretion and metabolism*

No data were available to the Working Group.

(ii) *Toxic effects*

The LD$_{50}$ of chlorozotocin within 60 days in Sprague-Dawley rats was 27.2 mg/kg bw after intraperitoneal injection and 22.5 mg/kg bw after intravenous injection (Fiebig *et al.*, 1980).

In one study of acute toxicity, the LD$_{50}$ after intravenous injection in BDF$_1$ mice was 24.9 mg/kg bw for males and 30.3 mg/kg bw for females. In animals of each sex, tubular necrosis of the kidney and cast formation were observed, as well as splenic lymphoid atrophy. In the same study, a dose of 6 mg/kg bw was lethal to beagle dogs after five days, and 3 mg/kg bw after 19 days. Renal dysfunction with tubular necrosis also occurred in these animals. Elevated serum levels of alanine aminotransferase and alkaline phosphatase were observed in dogs injected repeatedly with chlorozotocin. Nephrotoxicity was also seen in rhesus monkeys given 40 mg/kg intravenously (Gralla et al., 1979).

In Fischer rats, a lethal subcutaneous injection of chlorozotocin at 40 mg/kg bw caused renal necrosis in the cortex and, subsequently, necrosis of papillary collecting ducts. At sublethal doses, hypertrophy and karyomegaly were observed in collecting duct cells (Kramer et al., 1986). In Fischer rats given a subcutaneous injection of chlorozotocin at 25 or 40 mg/kg bw, no necrosis was observed in papillary collecting ducts, although karyomegaly was observed (Dees & Kramer, 1986).

Central nervous system vascular necrosis was observed in beagle dogs treated with chlorozotocin at 1.5-2.0 mg/kg bw once a week for two weeks or with a single intraventricular dose of 10 mg/kg bw (Levin et al., 1985).

Chlorozotocin affects cell cycle progression in Chinese hamster CHO cells. Non-cycling G1-arrested cells were the most sensitive; traverse from G1 to S was not affected, and chlorozotocin doubled the time for completion of DNA synthesis. Small quantities of polyploid cells were produced (Tobey et al., 1975). Chlorozotocin at a concentration of 200 µM induced differentiation and inhibited cell growth of mouse neuroblastoma N-18 cells (Yoda et al., 1982). DNA synthesis in L1210 leukaemia cells was almost completely inhibited (96%) within 24 h of an intraperitoneal administration to $BD2F_1$ mice (Anderson et al., 1975). In vitro, DNA synthesis in L1210 leukaemia cells was inhibited by 68% (Fox et al., 1977).

Single intraperitoneal injections of chlorozotocin at 15 mg/kg bw (maximal nonlethal dose) to BDF_1 mice slightly decreased peripheral white blood cell counts (Schein et al., 1976). Similar observations were made in $CD2F_1$ mice (Fox et al., 1977; Macdonald et al., 1980). Intraperitoneal injections of chlorozotocin at 20 mg/kg bw to mice reduced peripheral lymphocyte counts by 50% in three days. Spleen weights were decreased by about 40%, and the response to mitogens was markedly reduced (Fisher et al., 1980).

In another study in mice, chlorozotocin was shown to have immunomodulating activity. The IgM plaque-forming cell response was suppressed when the drug was injected four days before immunization; furthermore, hypersensitivity to oxazolone treatment was increased by about 30% when animals were injected intraperitoneally with chlorozotocin four days before sensitization. Treatment with chlorozotocin in vivo inhibited the proliferative response of spleen cells to mitogens and stimulated the chemiluminescence of peritoneal macrophages (Florentin et al., 1983).

Chlorozotocin exerts its toxic and other adverse effects through the formation of mono- and bifunctional alkylating agents. It also carbamoylates proteins via an isocyanate intermediate formed upon decomposition (Eisenbrand, 1984).

Alkylation of nuclear chromatin in HeLa cells has been observed, and there was preferential alkylation of DNA associated with the nucleosome core particle (Tew et al., 1978).

(iii) *Effects on reproduction and prenatal toxicity*

No data were available to the Working Group.

(iv) *Genetic and related effects*

Chlorozotocin induced base-pair substitutions but not frameshift mutations in *Salmonella typhimurium* in the presence and absence of an exogenous metabolic system (Zimmer & Bhuyan, 1976; Franza et al., 1980; Suling et al., 1983). It induced mitotic gene conversion in *Saccharomyces cerevisiae* (Siebert & Eisenbrand, 1977) and sex-linked recessive mutations in *Drosophila melanogaster* (Kortselius, 1978).

Chlorozotocin alkylated DNA in mouse leukaemia L1210 cells (Panasci et al., 1979; Ahlgren et al., 1982). It induced DNA strand breaks in L1210 cells (Ewig & Kohn, 1977; Alexander et al., 1986) and in V79 Chinese hamster cells (Erickson et al., 1978), and interstrand cross-links in DNA of mouse leukaemia L1210 cells (Ewig & Kohn, 1977) and of human embryo cells (Erickson et al., 1980). It induced mutation at the *hprt* locus in V79 Chinese hamster cells (Bradley et al., 1980) and sister chromatid exchange in mouse leukaemia L1210 cells (Siddiqui et al., 1988) and in 9L rat brain tumour cells (Tofilon et al., 1983).

Chlorozotocin at a single intraperitoneal dose of 100 μmol/kg induced DNA strand breaks and interstrand cross-links in bone-marrow cells of Wistar rats treated *in vivo* (Bedford & Eisenbrand, 1984).

(b) *Humans*

(i) *Pharmacokinetics*

After an intravenous dose of chlorozotocin at 120 mg/m^2, the disappearance curve of the *N*-nitroso group from the circulation exhibited three successive exponential phases, with half-times of 3-4.5 min, 6-12 min and 18-30 min. Twenty-four hours after administration of either ethyl- or glucose-labelled chlorozotocin, 82-84% of the blood-borne radioactivity was bound to protein; after seven days, 2% of the peak radioactivity value was detected in the blood. By 48 h, 50% of the radioactivity from [ethyl-^{14}C]chlorozotocin and 58% of that from [glucose-^{14}C]chlorozotocin was excreted in the urine; only 5-8% was excreted as the intact drug (Hoth et al., 1978).

(ii) *Adverse effects*

Thrombocytopenia, leukopenia, elevated aminotransferase activity, nausea and vomiting were seen in patients after intravenous administration of chlorozotocin, generally at doses of 120 mg/m^2 or higher (Hoth et al., 1978;

Bukowski *et al.*, 1983; Haas *et al.*, 1983; Forman *et al.*, 1984; Schutt *et al.*, 1984; Gastrointestinal Tumor Study Group, 1985).

(iii) *Effects on reproduction and prenatal toxicity*

No data were available to the Working Group.

(iv) *Genetic and related effects*

No data were available to the Working Group.

3.3 Case reports and epidemiological studies of carcinogenicity to humans

No data were available to the Working Group.

4. Summary of Data Reported and Evaluation

4.1 Exposure data

Chlorozotocin has been used as a cytostatic drug for the treatment of cancers at a variety of sites.

4.2 Experimental carcinogenicity data

Chlorozotocin was tested for carcinogenicity in single experiments in rats by intraperitoneal and intravenous injection. Intraperitoneal administration induced a high incidence of sarcomas and mesotheliomas in the peritoneal cavity in rats of each sex. The study by intravenous administration was inadequate for evaluation.

4.3 Human carcinogenicity data

No data were available to the Working Group.

4.4 Other relevant data

Chlorozotocin alkylates DNA and protein and causes DNA interstrand cross-links. In humans, it induces leukopenia and thrombocytopenia; in animals, it suppresses the bone marrow and affects immune response.

It is hepatotoxic in both humans and experimental animals.

Chlorozotocin induced DNA damage in bone-marrow cells of rats *in vivo*. It induced DNA damage in human, mouse and Chinese hamster cells *in vitro*, sister chromatid exchange in mouse and rat cells and gene mutation in Chinese hamster cells. It induced sex-linked recessive lethal mutations in *Drosophila* and gene conversion in *Saccharomyces cerevisiae*. Chlorozotocin induced mutations in *Salmonella typhimurium*. (See Appendix 1.)

4.5 Evaluation[1]

There is *sufficient evidence* for the carcinogenicity of chlorozotocin in experimental animals.

No data were available from studies in humans on the carcinogenicity of chlorozotocin.

In making the overall evaluation, the Working Group also took note of the following information. Chlorozotocin is an alkylating agent and is structurally related to other chloroethyl nitrosoureas, one of which, 1-(2-chloroethyl)-3-(4-methylcyclohexyl)-1-nitrosourea (methyl-CCNU), is carcinogenic to humans (Group 1) and two of which, bischloroethyl nitrosourea (BCNU) and 1-(2-chloroethyl)-3-cyclohexyl-1-nitrosourea (CCNU), are probably carcinogenic to humans (Group 2A) (IARC, 1987). Chlorozotocin has given consistently positive results in a broad spectrum of assays for genetic and related effects, including those involving mammalian cells.

Overall evaluation

Chlorozotocin *is probably carcinogenic to humans (Group 2A)*.

5. References

Ahlgren, J.D., Green, D.C., Tew, K.D. & Schein, P.S. (1982) Repair of DNA alkylation induced in L1210 leukemia and murine bone marrow by three chloroethylnitrosoureas. *Cancer Res.*, *42*, 2605-2608

Alexander, J.A., Bowdon, B.J. & Wheeler, G.P. (1986) DNA damage in cultured L1210 cells by 2-haloethyl esters of (methylsulfonyl)methanesulfonic acid. *Cancer Res.*, *46*, 6024-6028

Anderson, T., McMenamin, M.G. & Schein, P.S. (1975) Chlorozotocin, 2-[3-(2-chloroethyl)-3-nitrosoureido]-D-glucopyranose, an antitumor agent with modified bone marrow toxicity. *Cancer Res.*, *35*, 761-765

Bedford, P. & Eisenbrand, G. (1984) DNA damage and repair in the bone marrow of rats treated with four chloroethylnitrosoureas. *Cancer Res.*, *44*, 514-418

Bradley, M.O., Sharkey, N.A., Kohn, K.W. & Layard, M.W. (1980) Mutagenicity and cytotoxicity of various nitrosoureas in V-79 Chinese hamster cells. *Cancer Res.*, *40*, 2719-2725

---

[1]For description of the italicized terms, see Preamble, pp. 26–29.

Bukowski, R.M., McCracken, J.D., Balcerzak, S.P. & Fabian, C.J. (1983) Phase II study of chlorozotocin in islet cell carcinoma. A Southwest Oncology Group study. *Cancer Chemother. Pharmacol., 11*, 48-50

Dees, J.H. & Kramer, R.A. (1986) Sequential morphologic analysis of the nephrotoxicity produced in rats by single doses of chlorozotocin. *Toxicol. Pathol., 14*, 213-231

Eisenbrand, G. (1984) Anticancer nitrosoureas: investigations on antineoplastic, toxic and neoplastic activities. In: O'Neill, I.K., von Borstel, R.C., Miller, C.T., Long, J. & Batsch, H., eds, *N-Nitroso Compounds: Occurrence, Biological Effects and Relevance to Human Cancer* (IARC Scientific Publications No. 57) Lyon, IARC, pp. 695-708

Eisenbrand, G. & Habs, M. (1980) Chronic toxicity and carcinogenicity of cytostatic N-nitroso(2-chloroethyl)ureas after repeated intravenous application to rats. In: Holmstedt, B., Lauwerys, R., Mercier, M. & Roberfroid, M., eds, *Mechanisms of Toxicity and Hazard Evaluation*, Amsterdam, Elsevier, pp. 273-278

Eisenbrand, G., Habs, M., Zeller, W.J., Fiebig, H., Berger, M., Zelensy, O. & Schmahl, D. (1981) New nitrosoureas—therapeutic and long-term toxic effect of selected compounds in comparison to established drugs. In: Serrous, B., Schein, P.S. & Imbach, J.L., eds, *Nitrosoureas in Cancer Treatment* (INSERM Symposium No. 19), Amsterdam, Elsevier, pp. 175-190

Eisenbrand, G., Müller, N., Schreiber, J., Stahl, W., Sterzel, W., Berger, M.R., Zeller, W.J. & Fiebig, H. (1986) Drug design: nitrosoureas. In: Schmähl, D. & Kaldor, J.M., eds, *Carcinogenicity of Alkylating Cytostatic Drugs* (IARC Scientific Publications No. 78), Lyon, IARC, pp. 281-292

Erickson, L.C., Bradley, M.O. & Kohn, K.W. (1978) Measurements of DNA damage in Chinese hamster cells treated with equitoxic and equimutagenic doses of nitrosoureas. *Cancer Res., 38*, 3379-3384

Erickson, L.C., Bradley, M.O., Ducore, J.M., Ewig, R.A.G. & Kohn, K.W. (1980) DNA crosslinking and cytotoxicity in normal and transformed human cells treated with antitumor nitrosoureas. *Proc. natl Acad. Sci. USA, 77*, 467-471

Ewig, R.A.G. & Kohn, K.W. (1977) DNA damage and repair in mouse leukemia L1210 cells treated with nitrogen mustard, 1,3-bis(2-chloroethyl)-1-nitrosourea, and other nitrosoureas. *Cancer Res., 37*, 2114-2122

Fiebig, H.H., Eisenbrand, G., Zeller, W.J. & Zentgraf, R. (1980) Anticancer activity of new nitrosoureas against Walker carcinosarcoma 256 and DMBA-induced mammary cancer of the rat. *Oncology, 37*, 177-183

Fisher, R.I., Mandell, G.L., Bostick, F., McMenamin, M.G. & Anderson, T. (1980) Chlorozotocin, an anti-tumour agent lacking bone marrow toxicity at therapeutic doses: effects on lymphocyte subpopulations in mice. *Clin. exp. Immunol., 39*, 416-425

Florentin, I., Hayat, M., Kiger, N. & Mathé, G. (1983) Comparative analysis of the immunopharmacological properties of three new nitrosourea analogues: RPCNU, RFCNU and chlorozotocin. *Int. J. Immunopharmacol., 5*, 201-210

Forman, W.B., Cohen, H.J., Bartolucci, A.A. & Manning, G. (1984) Phase II evaluation of chlorozotocin in refractory multiple myeloma. *Cancer Treat. Rep., 68*, 1409-1410

Fox, P.A., Panasci, L.C. & Schein, P.S. (1977) Biological and biochemical properties of 1-(2-chloroethyl)-3-(β-D-glucopyranosyl)-1-nitrosourea (NSC D 254157), a nitrosourea with reduced bone marrow toxicity. *Cancer Res.*, 37, 783-787

Franza, B.R., Jr, Oeschger, N.S., Oeschger, M.P. & Schein, P.S. (1980) Mutagenic activity of nitrosourea antitumor agents. *J. natl Cancer Inst.*, 65, 149-154

Gastrointestinal Tumor Study Group (1985) Phase II trials of maytansine, low-dose chlorozotocin, and high-dose chlorozotocin as single agents against advanced measurable adenocarcinoma of the pancreas. *Cancer Treat. Rep.*, 69, 417-420

Gralla, E.J., Fleischman, R.W. & Luthra, Y.K. (1979) Toxicology studies in mice, beagle dogs and rhesus monkeys given chlorozotocin (NSC 178,248). *Toxicology*, 12, 31-40

Haas, C.D., Stephens, R.L., Bukowski, R.M., Studkey, W.J., McCracken, J.D., Gagliano, R.G., Lehane, D.E. & Pugh, R.P. (1983) High-dose chlorozotocin in lung cancer: a Southwest Oncology Group phase II study. *Cancer Treat. Rep.*, 67, 705-707

Habs, M., Eisenbrand, G. & Schmahl, D. (1979) Carcinogenic activity in Sprague-Dawley rats of 2-[3-(2-chloroethyl)-3-nitrosoureido]-D-glucopyranose (chlorozotocin). *Cancer Lett.*, 8, 133-137

Hoth, D., Woolley, P., Green, D., MacDonald, J. & Schein, P. (1978) Phase I studies on chlorozotocin. *Am. J. clin. Oncol.*, 23, 712-722

Johnston, T.P. & Montgomery, J.A. (1986) Relationship of structure to anticancer activity and toxicity of the nitrosoureas in animal systems. *Cancer Treat. Rep.*, 70, 13-30

Johnston, T.P., McCaleb, G.S. & Montgomery, J.A. (1975) Synthesis of chlorozotocin, the 2-chloroethyl analog of the anticancer antibiotic streptozotocin. *J. med. Chem.*, 18, 104-106

Kortselius, M.J.H. (1978) Mutagenicity of BCNU and related chloroethylnitrosoureas in Drosophila. *Mutat. Res.*, 57, 297-305

Kovach, J.S., Moertel, C.G., Schutt, A.J., Frytak, S., O'Connell, M.J., Rubin, J. & Ingle, J.N. (1979) A phase I study of chlorozotocin (NSC 178248). *Cancer*, 43, 2189-2196

Kramer, R.A., Boyd, M.R. & Dees, J.H. (1986) Comparative nephrotoxicity of 1-(2-chloroethyl)-3-(*trans*-4-methylcyclohexyl)-1-nitrosourea (MeCCNU) and chlorozotocin: functional-structural correlations in the Fischer 344 rat. *Toxicol. appl. Pharmacol.*, 82, 540-550

Levin, V.A., Byrd, D., Campbell, J., Giannini, D.D., Borcich, J.K. & Davis, R.L. (1985) Central nervous system toxicity and cerebrospinal fluid pharmacokinetics of intraventricular 3-[(4-amino-2-methyl-5-pyrimidinyl)ethyl]-1-(2-chloroethyl)-1-nitrosourea and other nitrosoureas in beagles. *Cancer Res.*, 45, 3803-3809

Lown, J.W. & McLaughlin, L.W. (1979) Nitrosourea-induced DNA single-strand breaks. *Biochem. Pharmacol.*, 28, 1631-1638

Macdonald, J.S., Hoth, D. & Schein, P.S. (1980) Preclinical and clinical studies on chlorozotocin, a new nitrosourea with decreased bone marrow toxicity. *Recent Results Cancer Res.*, 70, 83-89

Montgomery, J.A., Janes, R., McCaleb, G.S., Kirk, M.C. & Johnston, T.P. (1975) Decomposition of *N*-(2-chloroethyl)-*N*-nitrosoureas in aqueous media. *J. med. Chem.*, 18, 568-571

National Cancer Institute (1988) *National Cancer Institute Investigational Drugs, Pharmaceutical Data 1988*, Bethesda, MD

Panasci, L.C., Green, D.C. & Schein, P.S. (1979) Chlorozotocin. Mechanism of reduced bone marrow toxicity in mice. *J. clin. Invest.*, *64*, 1103-1111

Reynolds, J.E.F., ed. (1989) *Martindale. The Extra Pharmacopoeia*, 29th ed., London, The Pharmaceutical Press, p. 607

Samson, M.K., Baker, L.H., Cummings, G., Talley, R.W., McDonald, B. & Bhathena, D.B. (1982) Clinical trial of chlorozotocin, DTIC, and Dactinomycin in metastatic malignant melanoma. *Cancer Treat. Rep.*, *66*, 371-373

Schein, P.S., Panasci, L., Woolley, P.V. & Anderson, T. (1976) Pharmacology of chlorozotocin (NSC-178248), a new nitrosourea antitumor agent. *Cancer Treat. Rep.*, *60*, 801-805

Schutt, A.J., Hoth, D., Moertel, C.G., Schein, P.S., Rubin, J. & O'Connel, M.J. (1984) A phase II study of chlorozotocin in advanced large bowel carcinoma. A cooperative study between two institutions. *Am. J. clin. Oncol.*, *7*, 507-511

Siddiqui, K.M., Alexander, J.A. & Struck, R.F. (1988) Induction of sister-chromatid exchanges in L1210 leukemia cells by new antitumor 2-haloethyl(methylsulfonyl)-methanesulfonate compounds. *Mutat. Res.*, *207*, 179-183

Siebert, D. & Eisenbrand, G. (1977) Genetic effects of some new bifunctional and water-soluble analogs of the anti-cancer agent 1,3-bis(2-chloroethyl)-1-nitrosourea (BCNU) in *Saccharomyces cerevisiae*. *Mutat. Res.*, *42*, 45-50

Smith, F.P., Rustgi, V.K., Schertz, G., Woolley, P.V. & Schein, P.S. (1982) Phase II study of 5-FU, doxorubicin, and mitomycin (FAM) and chlorozotocin in advanced measurable pancreatic cancer. *Cancer Treat. Rep.*, *66*, 2095-2096

Suling, W.L., Rice, L.S. & Shannon, W.M. (1983) Increased mutagenicity of chloro-ethylnitrosoureas in the presence of a rat liver S9 microsome mixture. *J. natl Cancer Inst.*, *70*, 767-769

Tew, K.D., Sudhakar, S., Schein, P.S. & Smulson, M.E. (1978) Binding of chlorozotocin and 1-(2-chloroethyl)-3-cyclohexyl-1-nitrosourea to chromatin and nucleosomal fractions of HeLa cells. *Cancer Res.*, *38*, 3371-3378

Tobey, R.A., Oka, M.S. & Crissman, H.A. (1975) Differential effects of two chemotherapeutic agents, streptozotocin and chlorozotocin on the mammalian cell cycle. *Eur. J. Cancer*, *11*, 433-441

Tofilon, P.J., Williams, M.E. & Deen, D.F. (1983) Nitrosourea-induced sister chromatid exchanges and correlation to cell survival in 9L rat brain tumor cells. *Cancer Res.*, *43*, 473-475

Vadi, H.V. & Reed, D.J. (1983) Effect of 2-chloroethylnitrosoureas on plasmid DNA including formation of strand breaks and interstrand cross-links. *Chem.-biol. Interact.*, *46*, 67-84

Wang, A.L., Tew, K.D., Byrne, P.J. & Schein, P.S. (1981) Biochemical and pharmacologic properties of nitrosoureas. *Cancer Treat. Rep.*, *65* (Suppl. 3), 119-124

Windholz, M., ed. (1983) *The Merck Index*, 10th ed., Rahway, NJ, Merck & Co., p. 307

Yoda, K., Shimizu, M. & Fujimura, S. (1982) Induction of morphological differentiation in cultured mouse neuroblastoma cells by alkylating agents. *Carcinogenesis*, *3*, 1369-1371

Zeller, W.J., Ivankovic, S., Habs, M. & Schmahl, D. (1982) Experimental chemical production of brain tumors. *Ann. N.Y. Acad. Sci., 381*, 250-263

Zimmer, D.M. & Bhuyan, B.K. (1976) Mutagenicity of streptozotocin and several other nitrosourea comounds in *Salmonella typhimurium. Mutat. Res., 40*, 281-288

CICLOSPORIN

1. Chemical and Physical Data

1.1 Synonyms

Chem. Abstr. Services Reg. No.: 59865-13-3 (cyclosporin A); 79217-60-0 (cyclosporine)

Chem. Abstr. Name: {R-[R*,R*-(E)]}-L-Cyclic(L-alanyl-D-alanyl-*N*-methyl-L-leucyl-*N*-methyl-leucyl-*N*-methyl-L-valyl-3-hydroxy-*N*,4-dimethyl-L-2-amino-6-octenoyl-L-α-aminobutyryl-*N*-methylglycyl-*N*-methyl-L-leucyl-L-valyl-*N*-methyl-L-leucyl)

Synonyms: Cyclosporin A; cyclosporine; dyclosporin; OL-27-400; cyclo{[(E)-(2S,3R,4R)-3-hydroxy-4-methyl-2-(methylamino)-6-octenoyl]-L-2-aminobutyryl-*N*-methylglycyl-*N*-methyl-L-leucyl-L-valyl-*N*-methyl-L-leucyl-L-alanyl-D-alanyl-*N*-methyl-L-leucyl-*N*-methyl-L-leucyl-*N*-methyl-L-valyl}; cyclo{[4-(E)-but-2-enyl-*N*,4-dimethyl-L-threonyl]-L-homoalanyl(*N*-methyl-glycyl) (*N*-methyl-L-leucyl)-L-valyl(*N*-methyl-L-leucyl)-L-alanyl-D-alanyl-(*N*-methyl-L-leucyl)(*N*-methyl-L-leucyl)(*N*-methyl-L-valyl)}

1.2 Structural and molecular formulae and molecular weight

$C_{62}H_{111}N_{11}O_{12}$ Mol. wt: 1202.64

1.3 Chemical and physical properties of the pure substance

From Ruegger *et al.* (1976), Windholz (1983) and Hassan and Al Yahya (1987)

(a) *Description*: White prismatic crystals from acetone; neutral, hydrophobic, cyclic non-polar oligopeptide composed of 11 amino acid residues. The X-ray crystallographic structure is known.

(b) *Melting-point*: 148-151°C (natural); 149-150°C (synthetic)

(c) *Optical rotation*: $[\alpha]_D^{20} = -244°$ (c = 0.6 in chloroform); $[\alpha]_D^{20} = -189°$ (c = 0.5 in methanol)

(d) *Solubility*: Neutral; rich in hydrophobic amino acids; insoluble in water and *n*-hexane; very soluble in all other organic solvents

(e) *Spectroscopy data*: Ultraviolet, infrared, nuclear magnetic resonance and mass spectra have been reported.

(f) *Stability*: Stable in solution at temperatures below 30°C; sensitive to light, cold and oxidization (Reynolds, 1989)

1.4 Technical products and impurities

Trade names: Sandimmun; Sandimmune

Ciclosporin is available in bottles containing 100 mg/ml in an olive oil-based solution and 12.5% ethanol for oral administration, and in ampoules containing 50 mg/ml with 33% ethanol and 650 mg polyoxethylated castor oil for intravenous injection (Barnhart, 1989).

2. Production, Occurrence, Use and Analysis

2.1 Production and occurrence

The isolation of cyclosporins A and C from the fungus *Tolypocladium inflatum* Gams has been described (Rüegger *et al.*, 1976), and the biosynthesis of ciclosporin has been reported (Kobel & Traber, 1982; Kobel *et al.*, 1983; Billich & Zocher, 1987). It is also produced synthetically from *N*-methyl-*C*-9-amino acid with subsequent additions of appropriate peptides, followed by cyclization (Hassan & Al-Yahya, 1987).

Ciclosporin is manufactured commercially in Switzerland (Reynolds, 1989).

Cyclosporins (mostly A and C) are produced by the fungi *Tolypocladium inflatum* Gams and *T. cylindrosporum* and by other fungi isolated from soil.

2.2 Use

Ciclosporin is an immunosuppressive agent. It is used extensively in the prevention and treatment of graft-*versus*-host reactions in bone-marrow transplantation, and for the prevention of rejection of kidney, heart and liver transplants. It has also been tested for the therapy of a large variety of other diseases in which immunological factors may have a pathogenetic role, including Graves' disease, uveitis, Crohn's disease, ulcerative colitis, chronic active hepatitis, primary biliary cirrhosis, diabetes mellitus, myasthenia gravis, sarcoidosis, dermatomyositis, systemic lupus erythematosus and psoriasis (Calne et al., 1978, 1979; Powles et al., 1980; Merion et al., 1984; Kahan et al., 1985; Reynolds, 1989).

The usual oral dose of ciclosporin is 18 mg/kg daily, beginning 12 h before transplantation and continuing for one to two weeks. Dosage may subsequently be reduced to 5-10 mg/kg or less. Ciclosporin may also be given intravenously, usually at one-third of the oral dose. This drug is often given for several months to transplant recipients (Reynolds, 1989).

2.3 Analysis

Ciclosporin has been measured in pharmaceutical preparations by high-performance liquid chromatography (HPLC; US Pharmacopeial Convention, Inc., 1989).

Ciclosporin and its metabolites have also been measured in biological fluids using HPLC (Awni & Maloney, 1988; Christians et al., 1988a,b; Birckel et al., 1988), and ciclosporin has been monitored in whole blood by radioimmunoassay (Donatsch et al., 1981; Vine & Bowers, 1987). Vine and Bowers (1987) provided a critical summary of HPLC methods used to measure ciclosporin in biological fluids, and Hassan and Al-Yahya (1987) reviewed the methods for analysing ciclosporin. Radioimmunoassay kits for the analysis of ciclosporin in plasma are available, and their performance has been compared to that of HPLC analyses (Vernillet et al., 1989; Wolf et al., 1989).

3. Biological Data Relevant to the Evaluation of Carcinogenic Risk to Humans

3.1 Carcinogenicity studies in animals

(a) Oral administration

Mouse: Groups of 50 male and 50 female OF1 mice, weighing 26-39 and 19-28 g, respectively, were fed ciclosporin at 1, 4 or 16 mg/kg of diet for 78 weeks, at which time all survivors were killed. An untreated group of 50 males and 50 females served as controls. All mice were necropsied, and all macroscopic lesions were examined histologically. Mortality was higher in high-dose females (60%) than in controls (40-50%) and in other treated groups (42-52%). No increase in the incidence of tumours was observed in treated mice (Ryffel et al., 1983).

In a screening assay based on the accelerated induction of leukaemia in a strain highly susceptible to development of this neoplasm, 30 male AKR mice, six weeks of age, were fed ciclosporin at 150 mg/kg of diet. The first thymic lymphoma in treated mice was noted at week 17; these tumours occurred in 13/18 animals killed between 20 and 29 weeks [$p = 0.004$] and in 9/9 killed between 30 and 34 weeks [$p = 0.005$, Fisher's exact test]. In 22 mice that received the basal diet only, the first thymic lymphoma was noted at week 23, and the incidences of these tumours in animals killed between 20 and 29 weeks and 30 and 34 weeks were 2/12 and 3/9, respectively (Hattori et al., 1986).

Rat: Groups of 50 male and 50 female OFA rats, weighing 242-326 and 169-244 g, respectively, were fed ciclosporin at 0.5, 2 or 8 mg/kg bw of diet for 95 weeks (males) and 105 weeks (females), at which time the experiment was terminated. An untreated group of 50 males and 50 females served as controls. All animals were necropsied, and all macroscopic lesions were examined histologically. Mortality rates were 68% in controls, 74% in low- and mid-dose groups, and 86% in the high-dose group. No increase in tumour incidence was observed in treated rats (Ryffel et al., 1983). [The Working Group noted the high incidence of tumours in the controls, which may have reduced the sensitivity of the assay.]

(b) *Administration with other treatments*

Mouse: A group of 39 male Swiss Webster mice and 13 male C57Bl/6J mice, six to seven weeks of age, were given a single whole-body γ-irradiation of 350 rad and ten days later were fed ciclosporin [purity unspecified] at 150 mg/kg of diet for 35 weeks, at which time all survivors were killed and autopsied. A group of 26 male Swiss Webster and 14 male C57Bl/6J mice received the same irradiation and were maintained on basal diet. Two groups of 18 male Swiss Webster and 12 male C57Bl/6J mice received no irradiation and were maintained on control diet or were given ciclosporin at 150 mg/kg of diet. No tumour was observed in either of the strains of mice irradiated and maintained on basal diet alone or in either strain that received no radiation and were fed diets containing ciclosporin. Of the Swiss Webster mice that were irradiated and fed diets containing ciclosporin, 18/39 (46%) [$p < 0.001$, Fisher's exact test] developed lymphoid tumours, primarily in the spleen and mesenteric lymph nodes, within an average latent period of 24 weeks. The tumours were interpreted as B-immunoblastic lymphomas with plasmacytoid features. Four of the 39 (10%) mice developed classical thymic lymphomas within an average latent period of 23.7 weeks. Of the C57Bl/6 mice irradiated and fed diets containing ciclosporin, 7/13 (54%) [$p < 0.002$, Fisher's exact test] developed thymic lymphomas within an average latent period of 27.4 weeks. No spleen or lymph node lymphoma developed in this strain (Hattori *et al.*, 1988).

Two groups of 13 male Swiss Webster mice, six to seven weeks old, received a single intraperitoneal injection of 1 g/kg bw urethane. One week later, ciclosporin [purity unspecified] was administered at 150 mg/kg of diet. Two groups of 15 or 14 mice not receiving injections of urethane were fed the basal diet or ciclosporin at 150 mg/kg of diet. All animals were killed 22 weeks after the beginning of treatment. No significant difference in the number of lung adenomas was found between the groups receiving urethane and ciclosporin and those receiving urethane alone (Shinozuka *et al.*, 1988). [The Working Group noted the small number of animals used and the short duration of the study.]

Groups of 28-41 male Swiss Webster mice, six to seven weeks of age, received a single intraperitoneal injection of *N*-methyl-*N*-nitrosourea (MNU) at 0, 12.5 or 25 mg/kg bw [vehicle unspecified] and one week later were fed either basal diet or ciclosporin [purity unspecified] at 150 mg/kg of diet for 35 weeks. Mice treated with MNU and ciclosporin had four- and eight-fold higher incidences of thymic lymphomas, respectively, than mice treated with either dose of MNU alone (<2%) [figures not given]. Thymic lymphomas did not develop in mice treated with ciclosporin alone or maintained on basal diet (Shinozuka *et al.*, 1988). [The Working Group noted the incomplete reporting of the study.]

Rat: Groups of 10-12 male Sprague-Dawley rats, weighing 100-120 g, received a single intraperitoneal injection of 0 or 25 mg/kg bw MNU in 10% ethanol and citrate buffer; one week later, they were fed basal diet or ciclosporin [purity unspecified] at 110 mg/kg of diet for 34 weeks, at which time the experiment was terminated. Autopsies were carried out on all rats killed during the course or at the end of the experiment, and tissues from the thymus, mesenteric lymph nodes, intestinal lymphoid plaques, spleen, lung, kidney and liver were examined histologically. Of the rats receiving MNU and ciclosporin, 6/10 developed intestinal adenocarcinomas in the region of intestinal lymphoid plaques: two in the lower portion of the ileum and four in the ascending and transverse colon; two of the latter had two tumours each in the colon. The first tumour appeared in week 23 of the study. Of the rats receiving MNU alone, 1/12 developed an intestinal adenocarcinoma in week 33 of the study ($p < 0.05$). No intestinal tumour was observed in rats receiving ciclosporin or basal diet alone, but in rats treated with ciclosporin alone, atypical epithelial proliferations of the intestinal mucosa associated with hyperplasia of gut-associated lymphoid structures was observed (Perera *et al.*, 1986). [The Working Group noted the small number of animals used.]

Rat: Young male Wistar rats, weighing 62-80 g, were divided into six groups: group 1 (five animals) received daily subcutaneous injections of ciclosporin [purity unspecified] at 10 mg/kg bw in olive oil during week 1; group 2 (15 animals) received daily subcutaneous injections of ciclosporin at 10 mg/kg bw in olive oil during week 1, followed by administration of N-methyl-N'-nitro-N-nitrosoguanidine (MNNG) at 83 μg/ml in the drinking-water *ad libitum* from week 3 to 28; group 3 (15 animals) received MNNG in the drinking-water from week 3 to 28; groups 4 and 5 (15 animals per group) received MNNG in the drinking-water in weeks 3-28 and daily subcutaneous injections of ciclosporin at 10 mg/kg bw during week 15 or during week 30; group 6 (ten animals) served as untreated controls. All surviving animals were sacrificed in week 39. No rat in group 1 or 6 died during the experiment, and no tumour was found in any animal in these groups. In group 2, 7/9 surviving rats had a total of 14 tumours (one intestinal carcinosarcoma, 13 adenocarcinomas of the stomach and small intestine; mean number of tumours per rat, 1.56). In group 3, 8/12 survivors had a total of 12 tumours (mostly adenocarcinomas of the stomach, small intestine or both; mean number of tumours per rat, 1.00). In group 4, 10/13 survivors had a total of 19 tumours (18 adenocarcinomas of the stomach, small intestine or both, and one large-cell lymphoma involving coeliac lymph nodes, liver and spleen; mean number of tumours per rat, 1.46). In group 5, 10/12 survivors had a total of 20 tumours (one carcinosarcoma, 19 adenocarcinomas of the stomach, small intestine or both; mean number of tumours per rat, 1.67). No statistical difference in the incidence of tumours was observed among groups 2-5 (Johnson *et al.*, 1984).

Monkey: A group of 55 macaques [age and sex unspecified] that had received cardiac or heart-lung allografts and had survived the first two post-operative weeks received daily intramuscular injections of ciclosporin [purity unspecified] at 25 mg/kg bw in miglyol 812 (an oil base) for 14 days, after which they were treated either every other day or daily with intramuscular injections of 17 mg/kg bw ciclosporin continuously. Eight subgroups were formed: group 1 (16 animals) received no treatment other than ciclosporin; group 2 (nine animals) was treated concurrently with 2 mg/kg bw azathioprine; group 3 (six animals) had previously received daily injections of 10 mg/kg bw rabbit antithymocyte globulin on post-operative days 0-7; group 4 (13 animals) received concurrent weekly treatment with 14 mg/kg bw antithymocyte globulin, azathioprine and methylprednisolone; group 5 (11 animals) had received total lymphoid radiation at a dose of 100 rads per day (total dose, 600-1800 rads) prior to operation; group 6 (ten animals) received injections of azathioprine plus methylprednisolone; group 7 (23 animals) received azathioprine, methylprednisolone and antithymocyte globulin; and group 8 (nine animals) received azathioprine, antithymocyte globulin and total lymphoid irradiation. No lymphoma was observed among animals receiving treatment other than with ciclosporin (groups 6-8). Of the animals treated with ciclosporin alone or in combination with other immunosuppressive agents, B-cell lymphomas developed in 12/55 monkeys [$p < 0.001$, Fisher's exact test]: 2/16 treated with ciclosporin alone (group 1), 4/9 with ciclosporin plus azathioprine (group 2), 1/6 with ciclosporin plus antithymocyte globulin (group 3), 2/13 with ciclosporin, antithymocyte globulin, azathioprine and methylprednisolone (group 4), and 3/11 with ciclosporin and total lymphoid radiation (group 5). Viral particles were noted within the endoplasmic reticulum of plasmacytoid cells in 6/8 tumours from animals treated with ciclosporin alone or in combination with other immunosuppressive agents. The authors noted that the incidence of spontaneous haematopoietic neoplasms in nonhuman primates is generally considered to be low, although outbreaks of lymphomas have been reported among macaques (Bieber et al., 1982).

3.2 Other relevant data

(a) Experimental systems

The experimental toxicology of ciclosporin has been widely reviewed (e.g., Feutren & Bach, 1987; Aszalos, 1988; Grace, 1988; de Groen, 1988; Humes & Jackson, 1988; Kahan et al., 1988a,b; Mihatsch et al., 1988a,b).

(i) *Absorption, distribution, excretion and metabolism*

The toxicokinetics and toxicodynamics of ciclosporin have been reviewed (Wood et al., 1983; Maurer, 1985; Wood & Lemaire, 1985; Grevel, 1986a,b; Lemaire et al., 1986).

Orally administered ciclosporin (in olive oil) was rapidly absorbed in dogs and rats. About 50% of a single dose reached the circulation (plasma levels determined by radioimmunoassay) in both species; there was no tendency for accumulation in beagle dogs after repeated daily administration for a year (Ryffel et al., 1983).

A single oral administration of 82 mg/kg bw to WAG/Rij rats resulted in levels of 80 µg/g in liver, kidney and brain 3 and 7 h after administration. Slow elimination occurred thereafter: even after five days, significant amounts (10 µg/g) were detected. A short time after oral administration, 3.5 µg/ml of ciclosporin were detected in blood, and the levels remained almost the same for about two days; 2% of the administered dose was eliminated unchanged in bile and 2% in urine (Nooter et al., 1984a). About 2% of an oral dose of ciclosporin was absorbed into the intestinal lymphatic system in rats (Ueda et al., 1983).

Pharmacokinetic studies were also performed after intravenous administration of 20, 40 or 80 mg/kg bw to WAG/Rij rats (Nooter et al., 1984b). Elimination of ciclosporin at the lowest dose was best described by a two-compartment model (t½: 6 min and 16.5 h); at the higher dose levels, a three-compartment model best described the observed data. Urine and bile excretion was 10 and 20% of the total administered dose. The bioavailability of ciclosporin in Wistar rats increased with increasing oral dose. Daily oral administration of 4 mg/kg bw was necessary to maintain plasma levels at about 130 ng/ml in very young rats, while 7.5 mg/kg bw per day were needed in one-month-old animals (Levy-Marchal *et al.*, 1988).

Absorption of orally administered tritium-labelled ciclosporin by Sprague-Dawley and Wistar rats was slow and was not affected by the vehicle. The degree of absorption was about 30%. Labelled ciclosporin was widely distributed throughout the body. The terminal elimination half-time of the radiolabel was 46 h after dosing with 10 mg/kg bw daily in olive oil for 21 days; elimination from kidney and liver had a half-time of 70-100 h. Accumulation of the parent compound was evident after repeated treatments, with high levels in kidney, liver, blood and lymph nodes and particularly in skin and adipose tissue (Wagner *et al.*, 1987).

In male CD-COBS rats treated intravenously, blood concentrations during elimination were best described by a three-compartment model, with half-times of 0.11 h, 1.8 h and 23.8 h. The apparent distribution volume ranged from 4.88 to 6.84 l/kg. Elimination was almost entirely by hepatic metabolism (Sangalli *et al.*, 1988). Total body clearance was lower in obese rats than in lean Zucker rats (Brunner *et al.*, 1988).

A non-linear pharmacokinetic behaviour was seen in New Zealand white rabbits injected intravenously. The volume of distribution at steady state increased with increasing dose (Awni & Sawchuk, 1985). The mean half-time after intravenous administration of 15 mg/kg bw to male New Zealand rabbits was 229.7 min (D'Souza *et al.*, 1988).

In rabbits, the concentrations of ciclosporin in blood were about 100 ng/ml from day 43 to 120 after repeated subcutaneous injections; the calculated absorption half-time was 33 days following injection with 20 mg/kg twice a week during days 7-29 of the experiment (Shah *et al.*, 1988). In BALB/c mice injected subcutaneously with 12.5, 50 or 200 mg/kg bw, ciclosporin was detected (by radioimmunoassay) in every organ investigated (Boland *et al.*, 1984). The organs in mice that are susceptible to toxicity (e.g., brain, kidney, liver) retained ciclosporin after intraperitoneal injection (Belitsky *et al.*, 1986).

Following oral, intraperitoneal, subcutaneous or intravenous administration of radiolabelled ciclosporin to C57Bl mice, a high initial concentration of radiolabel was observed in liver, pancreas, salivary glands, spleen and fat tissue by whole-body autoradiography. Relatively high levels were retained in liver, bone marrow, thymus and lymph nodes. In kidney, the radiolabel was confined to the outer zone and outer medulla. No radioactivity was seen in the central nervous system or in fetuses (Bäckman *et al.*, 1987, 1988).

When ciclosporin was mixed with human or rat blood *in vitro*, 50% was found in erythrocytes, 15% in leukocytes and 30-40% in plasma. At concentrations of

25-100 ng/ml in human plasma, 65-80% of tritiated ciclosporin was associated with lipoproteins (Lemaire & Tillement, 1982; Niederberger et al., 1983).

Ciclosporin is extensively metabolized by cytochrome P450-mediated oxidation, hydroxylation and N-demethylation (Maurer et al., 1984; Maurer, 1985; Burke & Whiting, 1986; Maurer & Lemaire, 1986; Bertault-Peres et al., 1987; Wagner et al., 1987). Figure 1 shows some characteristics of the metabolites that have been isolated. The numbers in the following text refer to the amino acids and metabolites identified in the figure.

Fig. 1. Structures and molecular weights of metabolites of ciclosporin that have been isolated[a]

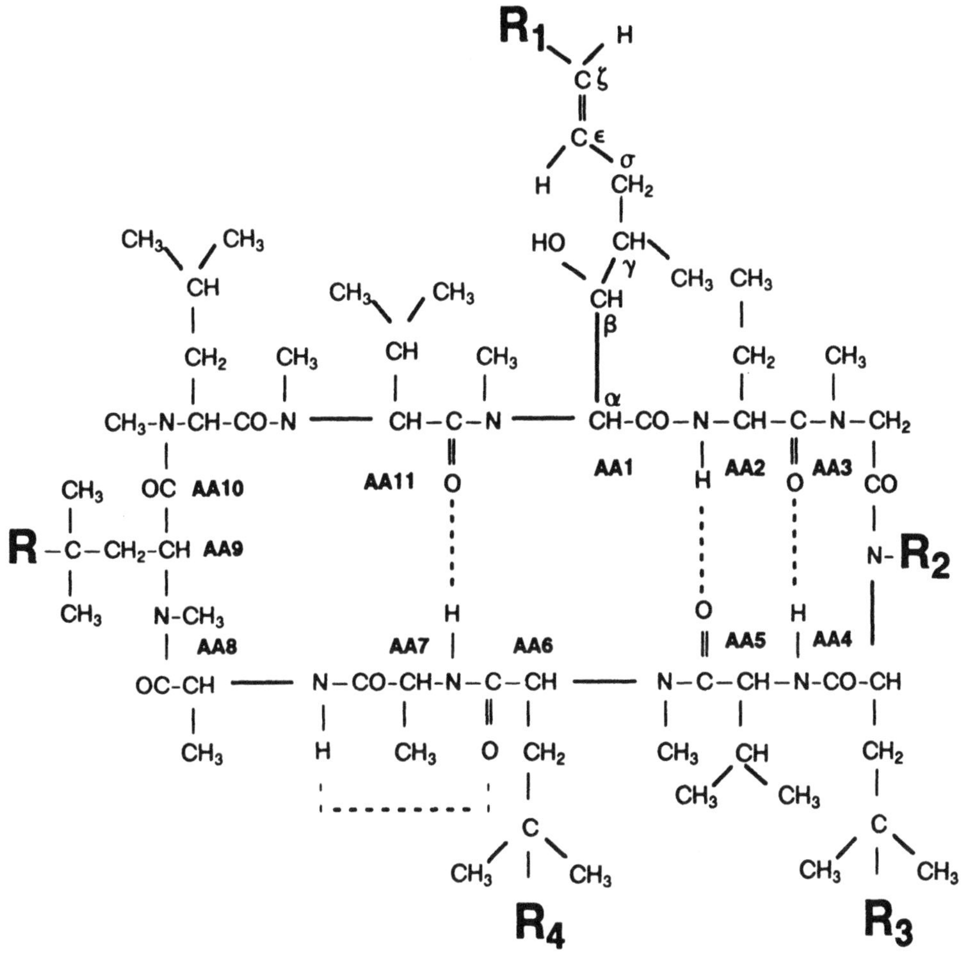

Fig. 1 (contd)

Metabolite no.	R	R₁	R₂	R₃	R₄	Other modification	Molecular weight
Ciclosporin	H	CH₃	CH₃	H	H		1202.64
1	OH	CH₃	CH₃	H	H		1218.64
8	OH	CH₂OH	CH₃	H	H		1234.64
9	OH	CH₃	H	H	OH		1220.62
10	OH	CH₃	CH₃	OH	H		1234.64
13	Hydroxylated and N-demethylated derivative of ciclosporin						1204.62
16	OH	CH₃	CH₃	H	OH		1234.64
17	H	CH₂OH	CH₃	H	H		1218.64
18	H	CH₂OH	CH₃	H	H	$\overset{O}{\overset{/\ \backslash}{\underset{\beta\ \ \epsilon\ \ \ \zeta}{CH\ \ CH\text{-}CH_2}}}$ of AA1	1218.64
22	H	CH₃	H	H	H		1188.62
25	H	CH₂OH	H	H	H		1202.64
26	OH	CH₂OH	CH₃	H	H	$\overset{O}{\overset{/\ \backslash}{\underset{\beta\ \ \epsilon\ \ \ \zeta}{CH\ \ CH\text{-}CH_2}}}$ of AA1	1204.62
203-218	H	COOH	CH₃	H	H		1234.64

ᵃFrom Maurer & Lemaire (1986)

All ciclosporin metabolites from dog urine and from rat bile and faeces retained the intact cyclic oligopeptide structure of ciclosporin. Conjugations with sulfuric or glucuronic acid were not detected (Maurer *et al.*, 1984). Using perfused rabbit liver, 27 metabolites were characterized, including three dihydrodiol metabolites probably derived from epoxide intermediates (Wallemacq *et al.*, 1989a).

An α,β-unsaturated carboxylic acid metabolite of amino acid **9** (AA9) was isolated in rabbit urine after intravenous administration of ciclosporin (Hartman *et al.*, 1985). In a study on ciclosporin metabolism in rats, parent ciclosporin predominated over metabolites in blood. Metabolite **1** was found to be the major one in this species. Intraperitoneal injections of phenobarbital and methyl prednisolone to Wistar rats receiving daily subcutaneous treatments with ciclosporin decreased ciclosporin levels in blood (Pell *et al.*, 1988). In rats injected intravenously, covalently bound ciclosporin was detected in protein fractions of liver and kidney homogenates, and phenobarbital treatment enhanced adduct formation.

Covalent binding to protein was found *in vitro* after incubation of labelled ciclosporin with a rat liver microsomal fraction in the presence of NADPH. Binding also occurred in isolated hepatocytes. SKF-525A inhibited the covalent binding, and glutathione depletion increased ciclosporin binding to protein (Nagelkerke *et al.*, 1987).

No association of radioactivity was observed with cellular proteins or with DNA in liver homogenates from mice administered the drug parenterally (Bäckman *et al.*, 1987, 1988).

(ii) *Toxic effects*

The LD_{50}s for ciclosporin after a single oral administration to mice, rats and rabbits were 2.3, 1.5 and > 1.0 g/kg bw, respectively. The corresponding figures after a single intravenous administration were 107, 25 and > 10 mg/kg bw. Toxic signs were hyperventilation, drowsiness and muscular spasms. After oral administration, weight loss and diarrhoea were noted (Ryffel *et al.*, 1983, 1986).

Daily subcutaneous injections of ciclosporin into BALB/c mice at a dose of 200 mg/kg bw per day resulted in a median survival time of about 13 days. Nephrotoxicity, hypocellularity of the thymus, lymph nodes and spleen and fatty changes in the liver were observed; no abnormality of femoral bone marrow was found (Boland *et al.*, 1984).

Histological findings in OFA rats fed a diet containing ciclosporin for 13 weeks included leukocytosis, lymphopenia, hypochromic anaemia, monocytosis and eosinopenia without myelotoxic effects. Lymphoid tissues were atrophied. Doses of 45 mg/kg bw per day and more produced nephrotoxicity and hepatotoxicity. A chronic nonspecific gingivitis with atrophy of periodontal tissue was observed in treated rats. Nephrotoxicity and hepatotoxicity were also observed among rats administered ciclosporin orally for 104 weeks (Ryffel *et al.*, 1983).

OF1 mice were given ciclosporin in the diet at 1.4 and 16 mg/kg per day for 78 weeks. Females given the high dose had higher mortality rates than other mice and had haematological changes without myelotoxic signs (Ryffel *et al.*, 1983).

NZW and RB rabbits treated subcutaneously with ciclosporin at 15 mg/kg bw daily had weight loss and reduced food and water intake. High mortality was observed within 60 days of treatment, and animals had distended stomachs and intestines (Gratwohl *et al.*, 1986).

After intravenous treatment at 45 mg/kg bw day for four weeks, cynomolgus monkeys showed blood chemistry changes, marked neurological side-effects, and degenerative changes in kidney and liver. Rhesus monkeys tolerated high oral doses of ciclosporin (200-300 mg/kg bw) for 13 weeks, with small functional and histopathological changes (Ryffel *et al.*, 1983).

The renal effects of ciclosporin in experimental systems have been studied extensively and reviewed (Sullivan et al., 1985; Ryffel & Mihatsch, 1986; Humes & Jackson, 1988).

The severity of histological changes in the kidneys of rats receiving subcutaneous injections daily for up to 30 days were directly correlated with tissue levels of ciclosporin (Kumar et al., 1988).

Ciclosporin induced marked renal vasoconstriction in rats (Kaskel et al., 1988; Monaco et al., 1988; Stanley Nahman et al., 1988) and sheep (Friedman et al., 1988). Various defects in renal function accompanied the vasoconstriction, including decreased glomerular filtration rate (Whiting et al., 1982; Sabbatini et al., 1988; Tejani et al., 1988), decreased sodium reabsorption (Whiting & Simpson, 1988), impairment of the diluting capacity of the thick ascending limb of the loop of Henle (Gnutzmann et al., 1986) and release of cellular enzymes into the urine (Whiting et al., 1986).

Sprague-Dawley rats given ciclosporin at 50 or 100 mg/kg bw per 48 h over 21 days by gastric intubation had elevated serum urea and creatinine levels, and urinary N-acetyl-β-D-glucosaminidase activity was increased (Thomson et al., 1981; Whiting et al., 1982). The renal and hepatic functional disturbances were reversible (Thomson et al., 1981). There was cytoplasmic vacuolization of the proximal tubule, swollen cells and cell necrosis—the latter at the higher dose. Vacuolization was due to dilatation of smooth and rough endoplasmic reticulum. The number of lysosomes was increased, and myeloid bodies were present (Whiting et al., 1982).

Rats given ciclosporin at 20 or 40 mg/kg bw in the diet showed augmentation of autoplagic vacuoles, lipid drops and loss of microvilli in the proximal nephron as well as prenecrotic damage of proximal tubular S2 and S3 cells (Pfaller et al., 1986). Similar observations were made by Verani (1986), Jackson et al. (1987), Dieperink et al. (1988), Gillum et al. (1988), Jackson et al. (1988) and Starklint et al. (1988a,b), although strain differences have been reported (Duncan et al., 1986).

When ciclosporin was given by gavage at 30 mg/kg bw per day to Sprague-Dawley rats for four weeks, serum testosterone levels were decreased by 50%; this change was reversible (Sikka et al., 1988).

Rats injected intraperitoneally with ciclosporin at 5, 10 or 15 mg/kg bw for one or three weeks had significantly raised levels of serum bile acids. Both bile salt-dependent and independent-flow were decreased (Stone et al., 1988).

Ciclosporin markedly decreased pancreatic insulin content and insulin release in rats administered the drug by intramuscular injection for two weeks (Hahn et al., 1986). Electron microscopy demonstrated cytoplasmic degranulation, nuclear inclusions and cisternal dilatation of endoplasmic reticulum and of the Golgi apparatus in pancreatic β cells (Hamaguchi *et al.*, 1988).

When Sprague-Dawley rats were fed ciclosporin at 150 mg/kg of diet, their thymuses and lymph nodes were smaller after eight weeks. Proliferative changes were observed in gut-associated lymphoid tissue, with mitotically active lymphocytes that displayed local tissue invasion and destruction (Demetris *et al.*, 1984).

Oral administration of immunosuppressive doses of ciclosporin reduced the trabecular bone volume of Sprague-Dawley rats. Osteoclast number and bone resorption were significantly increased at low (7.5 mg/kg bw per day) and high (15 mg/kg bw per day) doses of ciclosporin (Movsowitz *et al.*, 1988).

Thromboxane synthesis in rats and its excretion in urine were increased by ciclosporin treatment (Perico *et al.*, 1986a,b; Coffman *et al.*, 1987; Benigni *et al.*, 1988; Rogers *et al.*, 1988). Prostaglandin production was stimulated by ciclosporin (Coffman *et al.*, 1987), and administration of prostaglandin E_2 (Ryffel *et al.*, 1986) or its analogues (Paller, 1988a,b) reduced the nephrotoxicity of ciclosporin. A thromboxane synthetase inhibitor (CGS 12970) also prevented nephrotoxicity in rats (Smeesters *et al.*, 1988a,b).

Ciclosporin affected protein synthesis *in vivo* and *in vitro* (Bäckman *et al.*, 1988; Buss *et al.*, 1988), altered hepatic glycogen metabolism (Betschart *et al.*, 1988) and inhibited P450-dependent metabolism *in vivo* (Augustine & Zemaitis, 1986; Moochhala & Renton, 1986).

It induced dose-dependent malonaldehyde production in rat renal microsomes (Inselmann *et al.*, 1988). It bound with high affinity to cyclophilin, a low-molecular-weight cytosolic protein that occurs ubiquitously in eukaryotic cells and is thought to be a regulator of T- and B-cell activation (Harding & Handschumacher, 1988; Quesniaux *et al.*, 1988).

Ciclosporin inhibited T-lymphocyte proliferation (Borel *et al.*, 1977) but did not affect protein kinase C. It inhibited the augmentation of ornithine decarboxylase levels in mouse skin induced by phorbol ester (Elder *et al.*, 1988) and interfered with intracellular calcium metabolism (for reviews, see Aszalos, 1988; Bijsterbosch *et al.*, 1988).

(iii) *Effects on reproduction and prenatal toxicity*

In routine studies to evaluate the safety of ciclosporin, oral administration at 1.5, 5 or 15 mg/kg bw to male and female rats daily from before mating (males, 12 weeks; females, two weeks) until weaning had no adverse effect on reproduction. In rats administered ciclosporin at 10-300 mg/kg bw orally from day 6 to 15 of gestation, there was no embryotoxic effect at doses up to 17 mg/kg bw. At 30 mg/kg bw, which was clearly toxic to the mother, high rates of embryolethality (90%)

occurred, average fetal weights were lower than those of controls and skeletal retardations were seen frequently, but there was no increase in the frequency of minor or major anomalies. At higher doses, embryolethality was 100%. In a similarly designed study in rabbits, using doses of 10-300 mg/kg bw, no adverse effect was observed up to 30 mg/kg. At 100 mg/kg and above, maternal toxicity was seen, with an increased frequency of resorptions; however, no major or minor anomaly was found. In a peri-/postnatal study in rats at three dose levels (5, 15, and 45 mg/kg bw), a distinct increase in pre-/perinatal and early postnatal mortality of offspring was observed at the highest dose level (Ryffel et al., 1983).

Two further studies confirm the toxic effects of ciclosporin on rat fetuses after daily exposure during late gestational stages at a maternally toxic dose (25 mg/kg). Fetal kidneys that could be examined showed evidence of ciclosporin-induced proximal tubular-cell damage (Brown et al., 1985; Mason et al., 1985).

When ciclosporin was administered subcutaneously for 14 days at daily doses of 10, 20 and 40 mg/kg bw to sexually mature male rats, dose-dependent changes in body and reproductive organ weights were noted. Histological examination of the testis showed degenerative changes, and sperm counts and motility were decreased in all three treated groups. Rats treated with the two highest doses were infertile (Seethalakshmi et al., 1987). This effect was reversible after withdrawal of the drug (Seethalakshmi et al., 1988).

(iv) *Genetic and related effects*

Ciclosporin did not induce mutation in *Salmonella typhimurium* in either the presence or absence of an exogenous metabolic system (Matter et al., 1982).

It did not induce mutations at the *hprt* locus of Chinese hamster V79 cells in the presence or absence of an exogenous metabolic system (Zwanenburg et al., 1988). It induced sister chromatid exchange in human peripheral lymphocytes *in vitro* (Yuzawa et al., 1986, 1987).

At doses up to 1000-3000 mg/kg, ciclosporin did not induce chromosomal aberrations or micronuclei in bone-marrow cells of CD-1 mice or Chinese hamsters *in vivo*, or unscheduled DNA synthesis [dose unspecified] or dominant lethal mutations in CD-1 mice (Matter et al., 1982).

(b) *Humans*

(i) *Pharmacokinetics*

The kinetics of ciclosporin has been reviewed (Bowers et al., 1986; Grevel, 1986a,b; Lemaire et al., 1986; Vine & Bowers, 1987; Grevel, 1988; McMillan, 1989). In studies on the kinetics of ciclosporin, radioimmunoassay and liquid chromatography have generally been used. If not indicated otherwise, the data given below are from studies in which high-performance liquid chromatography analysis was used, which is the most specific for ciclosporin.

Absorption of orally administered ciclosporin is variable and low: the oral bioavailability was 35 ± 11% in heart transplant patients (Venkataramanan *et al.*, 1986), 36 ± 17% in adult uraemic patients (Grevel *et al.*, 1989) and 27 ± 20% in 41 renal transplant recipients; it was < 10% in 17% of these subjects (Ptachcinski *et al.*, 1985). Peak blood ciclosporin concentrations were reached between 1 and 8 h after oral dosing (Beveridge *et al.*, 1981; Ptachcinski *et al.*, 1985; Venkataramanan *et al.*, 1986).

Ciclosporin is rapidly and widely distributed; distribution half-times after intravenous administration have been reported to be 0.1 ± 0.03 h (Follath *et al.*, 1983) and 0.3-0.5 h (Yee *et al.*, 1984). The steady-state apparent volume of distribution is large, and means of 2.7-5.1 l/kg have been calculated (Follath *et al.*, 1983; Yee *et al.*, 1984; Ptachcinski *et al.*, 1985; Venkataramanan *et al.*, 1986; Clardy *et al.*, 1988). Concentrations of ciclosporin in rejected kidney were higher than preoperative values in the blood of three patients (Kahn *et al.*, 1986; Rosano *et al.*, 1986). High concentrations of ciclosporin and its metabolites are found in, e.g., fat, gall-bladder, liver, gastrointestinal tract and pancreas (Atkinson *et al.*, 1983a; Kahan *et al.*, 1983a; Ried *et al.*, 1983).

After the distribution phase, two further first-order disappearance phases may be discerned, with half-times of approximately 1 and 16 h, respectively (Follath *et al.*, 1983). Even in a case of acute overdose of ciclosporin (5000 mg), saturation of clearance was not observed (Schroeder *et al.*, 1986). Clearance of ciclosporin from the blood is rapid: in bone-marrow transplant recipients with normal liver and kidney function, clearance of 12.8 ± 1.6 ml/min per kg was reported; in those with elevated serum bilirubin but normal renal function, it was 9.8 ± 2.1 ml/min per kg. In another study, however, no relationship was noted between the disappearance of ciclosporin from the blood and the degree of impairment of hepatic function in patients with primary biliary cirrhosis (Robson *et al.*, 1984). In renal and heart transplant recipients, average clearance values of 6.5 and 5.7 ml/min per kg were reported (Ptachcinski *et al.*, 1985; Venkataramanan *et al.*, 1986), while in patients with renal failure clearance was 369 ml/kg per h [6.15 ml/min per kg] (Follath *et al.*, 1983). In healthy subjects, a value of 51 ml/h per kg [8.5 ml/min per kg] was reported (Grevel *et al.*, 1986); in this study, however, the radioimmunological assay method was used, which provides an underestimate of clearance (Grevel *et al.*, 1989).

After administration of tritiated ciclosporin to two patients, 6% of the dose was recovered in the urine (Maurer *et al.*, 1984; Maurer, 1985; Lemaire *et al.*, 1986). In healthy volunteers, approximately 0.1-0.2% of a dose was excreted in the urine as unchanged ciclosporin (Beveridge *et al.*, 1981; Maurer & Lemaire, 1986).

More ciclosporin and ciclosporin metabolites were detected in the bile than in urine after intravenous and oral administrations (Kahan *et al.*, 1983b; Venkataramanan *et al.*, 1985). Unchanged ciclosporin is a minor component in the bile (mean, 0.29% of an oral dose) (Venkataramanan *et al.*, 1985).

The concentration of ciclosporin in blood cells is approximately double that in the plasma (Follath *et al.*, 1983). The majority of ciclosporin and/or its metabolites in serum is bound to different lipoprotein fractions (Mraz *et al.*, 1983; Gurecki *et al.*, 1985). After treatment of pregnant women with ciclosporin, it was detected in cord blood at concentrations somewhat lower than those in maternal blood (Lewis *et al.*, 1983; Venkataramanan *et al.*, 1988; Rose *et al.*, 1989). Ciclosporin has also been detected in breast milk (Lewis *et al.*, 1983).

The first study of the metabolism of ciclosporin in humans was performed by Maurer *et al.* (1984), who isolated and identified nine ether-extractable metabolites from the urine of two patients who had received a single oral dose of 300 mg ^{3}H-ciclosporin. All identified metabolites retained the intact cyclic peptide structure; the sites on the molecule that are changed by metabolism are indicated in Figure 1. The primary metabolites were products of hydroxylation; the secondary metabolites identified were products of oxidation or demethylation of oxidized primary metabolites or of a cyclization reaction. Similar oxidized ciclosporin metabolites have been identified in the blood and bile of patients treated with ciclosporin (Hartman *et al.*, 1985; Rosano *et al.*, 1986; Lensmayer *et al.*, 1987a,b; Wallemacq *et al.*, 1989a,b; Wang *et al.*, 1989). Twenty-seven ciclosporin metabolites were identified in human bile; these included a vicinal dihydrodiol and a demethylated vicinal dihydrodiol, suggesting that an epoxide is the intermediate (Wallemacq *et al.*, 1989a).

In addition to metabolites generated by oxidation, demethylation and cyclization reactions, three further metabolites have been isolated in which the double bond in amino acid **1** (**AA1** in Fig. 1) is probably saturated (Wang *et al.*, 1989). This metabolite and metabolites **1, 8, 17** and **203-218** (Fig. 1) were reported to be the major metabolites of ciclosporin in human bile (Hartman *et al.*, 1985; Maurer, 1985; Wang *et al.*, 1989; Maurer & Lemaire, 1986). A sulfate conjugate of ciclosporin was also identified in human bile and plasma (Henricsson *et al.*, 1989). Metabolite **17** was the main metabolite in human blood, and metabolites **1, 8** and **21** were the other major ones (Maurer, 1985; Maurer & Lemaire, 1986; Rosano *et al.*, 1986). Metabolite **17** was the main metabolite detected in kidney (Rosano *et al.*, 1986).

A cytochrome P450 isolated from human liver catalysed the formation of mono- and dihydroxylated and demethylated metabolites from ciclosporin (Combalbert *et al.*, 1989). This cytochrome is encoded by the gene P450IIIA3, as is nifedipine oxidase; it is induced by treatment with rifampicin (Kronbach et al., 1988; Combalbert et al., 1989).

(ii) *Immunosuppressive action*

The pharmacological effects of ciclosporin on the human immune system have been reviewed (Thomson, 1983; Shevach, 1985; Drugge & Handschumacher, 1988; Kerman, 1988; Kahan, 1989; Lorber, 1989). The ratio of T-helper cells to T-suppressor cells was decreased in renal transplant recipients during treatment with ciclosporin and prednisolone (Kerman et al., 1987). Production of α-interferon, γ-interferon and interleukin-2 by isolated leukocytes was decreased in renal and heart transplant patients receiving ciclosporin and prednisolone, as compared to healthy volunteers (Dupont et al., 1985).

Many studies have been published on the immunosuppressive effects of ciclosporin since the detection (Borel et al., 1977) of its biological and clinical significance in the early 1970s (for review, see Feutren & Bach, 1987). Its immunosuppressive effects have been demonstrated experimentally to lead to tolerance of tissue grafts (Morris et al., 1980; Pennock et al., 1981; Bain et al., 1988; Chisholm & Bevan, 1988; Finsen et al., 1988; Kimura et al., 1988; Lear et al., 1988; White & Lim, 1988; for reviews, see Lorber, 1986; Tutschka, 1986; Hopt et al., 1988; Kahan et al., 1988a,b) and to affect a variety of experimental autoimmune diseases, such as uveitis (Nordmann et al., 1986; Dinning et al., 1987; Mahlberg et al., 1987; Caspi et al, 1988a,b; Kaswan et al., 1988), myasthenia gravis (for review see Feutren & Bach, 1987; for a tabular summary, see Gunn et al., 1988), mercuric chloride-induced glomerulonephritis (Aten et al., 1988), allergic encephalomyelitis (Polman et al., 1988) and serum sickness nephritis (Shigematsu & Koyama, 1988).

Ciclosporin is preferentially active on proliferating T cells (White et al., 1979) and selectively inhibits T-helper cell function (Caspi et al., 1988a,b) while sparing T-suppressor cell activities (Kupiec-Weglinski et al., 1984; Bucy, 1988). It inhibits the production of interleukin-2 (Larsson, 1980; Bunjes et al., 1981; Caspi et al., 1988b; Tracey et al., 1988) from T-helper cells and of interleukin-1 from splenic adherent cells (Bunjes et al., 1981). Ciclosporin metabolites also suppressed concanavalin A-stimulated human peripheral blood mononuclear cell proliferation (Cheung et al., 1988).

Ciclosporin was bound to a low-affinity site ($K_D = 3\text{-}6 \times 10^{-7}$ M) on human splenic T-lymphocytes *in vitro*, while B-lymphocytes showed both a high-affinity ($K_D = 2 \times 10^{-9}$ M) and a low-affinity binding site (LeGrue et al., 1983).

Ciclosporin depressed the synthesis of γ-interferon by human thymocytes and T-lymphocytes *in vitro* (Reem et al., 1983; McKenna et al., 1989), as well as the synthesis of lymphotoxin and tumour necrosis factor by lymphocytes activated in mixed-lymphocyte culture or by concanavalin A (McKenna et al., 1989; Szturm et *al.*, 1989). Ciclosporin reduced T-cell growth factor (interleukin-2) gene transcription in a cloned human leukaemic T-cell line (Krönke *et al.*, 1984) and binding of radiolabelled human recombinant interleukin-2 to high-affinity receptors in human T-lymphocytes (Povlsen *et al.*, 1989). Ciclosporin also inhibited the release of γ-interferon from alloactivated human peripheral blood mononuclear cells (Bishop & Hall, 1988).

(iii) *Adverse effects*

The adverse effects of ciclosporin therapy have been reviewed (Kahan *et al.*, 1985; Bennett & Norman, 1986; Myers, 1986; Keown *et al.*, 1987; Mihatsch *et al.*, 1988a,b; Racusen & Solez, 1988; Schachter, 1988; Weidle & Vlasses, 1988; Dieperink, 1989; Mihatsch *et al.*, 1989; Reynolds, 1989; Steinmuller, 1989).

The first report on the use of ciclosporin in the treatment of renal allograft rejection (Calne *et al.*, 1978) documented nephrotoxicity, hepatotoxicity and hirsutism as side-effects of the therapy. Nephrotoxicity has since been amply documented as the most prevalent and serious complication of ciclosporin therapy, in recipients of kidney transplants (Calne *et al.*, 1979; Klintmalm *et al.*, 1981a,b; Merion *et al.*, 1984) and in other transplant recipients (Powles *et al.*, 1980; Klintmalm *et al.*, 1981b; Shulman *et al.*, 1981; Atkinson *et al.*, 1983b; Hows *et al.*, 1983; Myers *et al.*, 1984). Morphological changes related to ciclosporin administration include diffuse interstitial fibrosis (associated with oligo- or anuria), tubular toxicity, peritubular capillary congestion and a combination of the last two. These two changes have been associated with acute renal damage; acutely impaired renal function was not, however, necessarily accompanied by microscopic changes. Arteriolopathy and interstitial fibrosis with tubular atropy, or a combination of the two, have been attributed to chronic ciclosporin toxicity (Mihatsch *et al.*, 1988a,b, 1989). Mechanisms of the renal toxicity of ciclosporin have been reviewed (Bennett *et al.*, 1988; Dieperink *et al.*, 1988; Grace, 1988; Neild, 1988; Benigni *et al.*, 1989).

Mild functional disturbances of the liver have been reported in 20-40% of treated patients (Klintmalm *et al.*, 1981a; Kahan *et al.*, 1985).

Other side-effects reported include gastrointestinal disturbances, hirsutism, acne, gingival hyperplasia, neurotoxicity, altered blood coagulability, hypertension, electrolyte changes and gout. Anaphylactoid reactions have occurred following intravenous administration of preparations containing ciclosporin (Kahan *et al.*, 1985; Bennett & Norman, 1986; Weidle & Vlasses, 1988; Lin *et al.*, 1989; Reynolds, 1989).

(iii) *Effects on reproduction and prenatal toxicity*

In two of three published reports of babies born to mothers treated throughout pregnancy with ciclosporin (Lewis *et al.*, 1983; Klintmalm *et al.*, 1984; Endler *et al.*,

1987), growth was retarded. However, whether this effect was due to the drug or to the general condition of the mother is uncertain.

(iv) *Genetic and related effects*

A group of 25 kidney transplant patients received daily oral treatment with ciclosporin at 12-14 mg/kg bw (reduced to 4 mg/kg) combined with variable doses of prednisolone for over one year (Fukuda *et al.*, 1987). In an extension of this study (Fukuda *et al.*, 1988), the number of patients was increased to 40. More patients receiving ciclosporin had chromosomal aberrations in their peripheral lymphocytes (68% and 48% in the two studies, respectively) than did 50 healthy individuals (0%) or 50 haemodialysis patients (2%). [The Working Group noted the poor reporting of the studies and that cells were cultured for 72 h.]

Unscheduled DNA synthesis was reported to be elevated in the lymphocytes of kidney transplant patients treated with ciclosporin [dose and length of treatment unspecified] in comparison with those from healthy individuals (Petitjean *et al.*, 1986). [The Working Group noted the incomplete reporting of the study.]

3.3 Case reports and epidemiological studies of carcinogenicity to humans

(*a*) *Case reports*

Numerous case reports have been published of neoplasms occurring in organ transplant recipients who received only ciclosporin, without azathioprine or cytotoxic agents. The majority of these neoplasms were lymphomas, commonly of the gastrointestinal tract (Thiru *et al.*, 1981; Beveridge *et al.*, 1984; Bencini *et al.*, 1985; Bloom *et al.*, 1985; Castro *et al.*, 1985; Thompson *et al.*, 1985; Walker *et al.*, 1989), but Kaposi's sarcoma and skin cancers have also been reported (Thompson *et al.*, 1985; Gorg *et al.*, 1986; Arico *et al.*, 1987; Cockburn, 1987; Bencini *et al.*, 1988; Civati *et al.*, 1988). Malignancies at other sites have also been seen (Maung *et al.*, 1985; Thompson *et al.*, 1985). Regression of lymphomas when the drug was discontinued has sometimes been reported (Bencini *et al.*, 1988).

In the most recent report from a registry of organ transplant recipients who developed tumours (Penn & Brunson, 1988), 412 tumours had been recorded in ciclosporin-treated patients. Of these, the most frequently reported were lymphoma (29%), skin cancer (22%) and Kaposi's sarcoma (11%). [The Working Group noted that the size of the underlying population was unknown; but, given the low incidence of Kaposi's sarcoma in the general population, the number of cases in this registry is strikingly large.]

Cockburn and Krupp (1989) described the occurrence of 186 neoplasms in organ transplant recipients treated with ciclosporin and reported to the drug manufacturer. The most frequent malignancies were lymphomas and leukaemias

(55 cases) and Kaposi's sarcoma (26 cases). The lymphomas were found predominantly in the gastrointestinal tract.

(b) Cohort studies

Anderson *et al.* (1978) reported that among 143 cardiac transplant recipients treated with ciclosporin and other immunosuppressive agents, six developed lymphomas.

Calne *et al.* (1979) followed up 34 organ transplant recipients treated with ciclosporin, six of whom had also received a cyclophosphamide derivative; three lymphomas developed—two in patients treated with ciclosporin only and one in a patient treated with both drugs.

Starzl *et al.* (1984) reported lymphoproliferative lesions (15 lymphomas, two other lesions) that occurred during follow-up in eight of 315 renal transplant, four of 129 heart transplant, three of 48 liver transplant and two of six heart-lung transplant patients treated, in general, with ciclosporin alone. In seven renal transplant patients with these lesions who were operated on for bowel perforation, discontinuation of ciclosporin treatment resulted in tumour regression, as determined by a second laparotomy.

Bencini *et al.* (1986) followed 67 renal transplant recipients treated with ciclosporin for 1-17 months (mean, 3.2 months); one developed a squamous epithelioma and one, skin nodules thought to be a lymphoma.

Sheil *et al.* (1987) reported three-year results of a trial of ciclosporin in renal transplant patients. One malignant melanoma and one adenocarcinoma of the remaining kidney were observed among 140 renal transplant patients receiving long-term treatment with ciclosporin alone, while no tumour was reported among a further 140 patients who received treatment with ciclosporin alone for three months followed by treatment with azathioprine.

Smith *et al.* (1989) reported that lymphomas developed in two of 712 organ transplant patients who received azathioprine, none of 160 treated with ciclosporin and seven of 132 who received both.

Cockburn and Krupp (1989) followed up 4040 organ transplant recipients treated with ciclosporin and compared observed with expected numbers based on population rates. Increased risks were noted for lymphoma (relative risk, 27.5; 11 cases observed), skin cancers (6.8; 11) and urinary-tract cancers (5.9; 11). [The Working Group noted that it was not clear that the only immunosuppressive treatment received was ciclosporin.]

Table 1 summarizes the studies in which lymphomas were reported in transplant patients who had received ciclosporin but not azathioprine or cytotoxic drugs. The Working Group estimated upper limits for the expected values (not

Table 1. Non-Hodgkin's lymphomas in organ transplant patients treated with ciclosporin (without azathioprine or cytotoxic drugs)

No. of patients	Maximal follow-up (years)	Non-Hodgkin's lymphomas		Reference
		Expected[a]	Observed	
28	1.5	0.02	2	Calne et al. (1979)
498	4	1.0	11	Starzl et al. (1984)
67	1.5	0.05	0	Bencini et al. (1986)
120	5[b]	0.3	0	Sheil et al. (1987)
160	5	0.4	0	Smith et al. (1989)
873 (total)		1.8	13	

[a]As estimated by the Working Group
[b]Mean, as given in paper

provided in the original papers), on the basis of assumptions adverse to a causal relationship, as follows:

(i) When the total period of follow-up was not given, the time of observation of every patient was equivalent to the maximal observation time of the relevant study.

(ii) The incidence rate for any age group below 70 years was the highest published in the Connecticut Tumor Registry (higher than in any UK or Australian registry), i.e., 50/100 000 per year (Muir et al., 1987).

(iii) All patients followed up received only ciclosporin. In fact, it is known that some had received other agents, but only patients with lymphomas who had not received other agents were included in the count of observed cases.

Even with the above assumptions, the occurrence of lymphomas was remarkably high.

[The Working Group noted that in many studies no information on dose, survival or follow-up time was given for any group, and it was difficult to compare rates. As is clear from estimates of expected numbers made by the Working Group, however, the incidence of lymphoma in the cohort studies is remarkably high. In addition, Kaposi's sarcoma has figured prominently in case reports. It is also noteworthy that lymphomas regressed following discontinuation of ciclosporin in two studies. A higher incidence of lymphomas was noted when ciclosporin was used in combination with other imunosuppressive agents, as was a frequent practice soon after its introduction (Anderson *et al.*, 1978; Calne *et al.*, 1979; Kinlen, 1982; Beveridge *et al.*, 1984). This is consistent with other evidence that the intensity of immunosuppression has an important influence on lymphoma incidence.]

4. Summary of Data Reported and Evaluation

4.1 Exposure data

Ciclosporin has been used as an immunosuppressive agent since the mid-1980s.

4.2 Experimental carcinogenicity data

Ciclosporin was tested for carcinogenicity by oral administration in two studies in mice and in one study in rats. In one study in mice, it accelerated the development of leukaemias; tumours were not induced in a chronic bioassay. In rats, negative results were obtained in a study with limited sensitivity.

Ciclosporin enhanced the development of lymphomas induced in two strains of male mice by single whole-body irradiation or *N*-methyl-*N*-nitrosourea. In grafted macaques, ciclosporin increased the incidence of lymphomas, a neoplasm that occurs extremely infrequently in this species of monkeys. When given in combination with various other immunosuppressive regimens, ciclosporin induced a substantial increase in the incidence of lymphomas when compared to immunosuppressive regimens excluding ciclosporin. This drug also enhanced the incidence of intestinal adenocarcinomas induced in male rats by *N*-methyl-*N*-nitrosourea.

4.3 Human carcinogenicity data

In case reports, both lymphomas and Kaposi's sarcoma have been associated frequently with exposure to ciclosporin. Four cohort studies recorded a high incidence of lymphoma in organ transplant recipients; in two of these, ciclosporin was given without azathioprine or cytotoxic drugs. In several cases, there has been well-documented regression of lymphoma following withdrawal of the drug.

4.4 Other relevant data

Ciclosporin induced dose-dependent changes in reproductive organ weights in male rats and caused sterility at high doses. Fetal mortality was observed in rats and rabbits when the drug was administered during the second half of gestation at maternally toxic doses. No other sign of embryo- or fetotoxicity was noted.

Ciclosporin is rapidly absorbed and widely distributed in humans and in experimental animals. It is extensively metabolized by the cytochrome P450 system. Adverse effects include nephro- and hepatotoxicity. The compound is immunosuppressive, resulting in tolerance to tissue grafts; its main effect is on the early proliferation of T-cells.

In a single study, ciclosporin was reported to increase the incidence of chromosomal aberrations in the lymphocytes of kidney transplant patients.

Ciclosporin did not induce dominant lethal mutations in mice, chromosomal aberrations in the bone marrow of Chinese hamsters or micronuclei in the bone marrow of Chinese hamsters or mice *in vivo*. It induced sister chromatid exchange in human peripheral lymphocytes *in vitro* but did not induce gene mutations in Chinese hamster cells. Ciclosporin did not induce mutations in *Salmonella typhimurium*. (See Appendix 1.)

4.5 Evaluation[1]

There is *sufficient evidence* for the carcinogenicity of ciclosporin in humans.

There is *limited evidence* for the carcinogenicity of ciclosporin in experimental animals.

Overall evaluation

Ciclosporin *is carcinogenic to humans (Group 1)*.

5. References

Anderson, J.L., Fowks, R.E., Bieber, C.P. & Stinson, E.B. (1978) Idiopathic cardiomyopathy, age, and suppressor-cell dysfunction as risk determinants of lymphoma after cardiac transplantation. *Lancet*, ii, 1174-1177

Arico, M., Bosco, M. & Galeone, A. (1987) Manifestazioni cutanee in trapiantati renali. Due case di sarcoma di Kaposi. [Cutaneous manifestations in renal transplant patients. Two cases of Kaposi's sarcoma (Ital.).] *G. ital. Dermatol. Venerol.*, 122, 637-642

Aszalos, A. (1988) Cyclosporin: some aspects of its mode of action. A review. *J. Med.*, 19, 297-316

Aten, J., Bosman, C.B., De Heer, E., Hoedemaeker, P.J. & Weening J.J. (1988) Cyclosporin A induces long-term unresponsiveness in mercuric chloride-induced autoimmune glomerulonephritis. *Clin. exp. Immunol.*, 73, 307-311

---

[1]For description of the italicized terms, see Preamble, pp. 26–29.

Atkinson, K., Boland, J., Britton, K. & Biggs, J. (1983a) Blood and tissue distribution of cyclosporine in humans and mice. *Transplant. Proc.*, *15*, 2430-2433

Atkinson, K., Biggs, J.C., Hayes, J., Ralston, M., Dodds, A.J., Concannon, A.J. & Naidoo, D. (1983b) Cyclosporin A associated nephrotoxicity in the first 100 days after allogeneic bone marrow transplantation: three distinct syndromes. *Br. J. Haematol.*, *54*, 59-67

Augustine, J.A. & Zemaitis M.A. (1986) The effects of cyclosporin A (CsA) on hepatic microsomal drug metabolism in the rat. *Drug Metab. Dispos.*, *14*, 73-78

Awni, W.M. & Maloney, J.A. (1988) Optimized high-performance liquid chromatographic method for the analysis of cyclosporine and three of its metabolites in blood and urine. *J. Chromatogr.*, *425*, 233-236

Awni, W.M. & Sawchuk, R.J. (1985) The pharmacokinetics of cyclosporine. I. Single dose and constant rate infusion studies in the rabbit. *Drug Metab. Dispos.*, *13*, 127-132

Bäckman, L., Brandt, I., Ringdén, O. & Dallner, G. (1987) Distribution of ^{3}H-cyclosporine A in mice by autoradiography. *Transplant. Proc.*, *19*, 1236-1239

Bäckman, L., Brandt, I., Dallner, G. & Ringdén, O. (1988) Tissue distribution of [^{3}H]cyclosporine A in mice. *Transplant. Proc.*, *20* (*Suppl. 2*), 684-691

Bain, J.R., Mackinnon, S.E., Hudson, A.R., Falk, R.E., Falk, J.A. & Hunter, D.A. (1988) The peripheral nerve allograft: a dose-response curve in the rat immunosuppressed with cyclosporin A. *Plastic Reconstr. Surg.*, *82*, 447-457

Barnhart, E. (1989) *Physicians' Desk Reference*, 43rd ed., Oradell, NJ, Medical Economics, pp. 1892-1894

Belitsky, P., Ghose, T., Givner, M., Rowden, G. & Pope, B. (1986) Tissue distribution of cyclosporine A in the mouse: a clue to toxicity? *Clin. Nephrol.*, *25* (*Suppl. 1*), S27-S29

Bencini, P.L., Montagnino, G., Crosti, C. & Sula, F. (1985) Squamous-cell epithelioma and cyclosporine treatment. *Br. J. Dermatol.*, *113*, 373-374

Bencini, P.L., Montagnino, G., DeVecchi, A., Crosti, C. & Tarantino, A. (1986) Cutaneous lesions in 67 cyclosporin-treated renal transplant recipients. *Dermatologica*, *172*, 24-30

Bencini, P.L., Marchesi, L., Cainelli, T. & Crosti, C. (1988) Kaposi's sarcoma in kidney transplant recipients treated with cyclosporin. *Br. J. Dermatol.*, *118*, 709-714

Benigni, A., Chiabrando, C., Piccinelli, A., Perico, N., Gavinelli, M., Furci, L., Patino, O., Abbate, M., Bertani, T. & Remuzzi G. (1988) Increased urinary excretion of thromboxane B_2 and 2,3-dinor-TxB_2 in cyclosporin A nephrotoxicity. *Kidney int.*, *34*, 164-174

Benigni, A., Perico, N. & Remuzzi, G. (1989) Abnormalities of arachidonate metabolism in experimental ciclosporin nephrotoxicity. *Am. J. Nephrol.*, *9* (*Suppl. 1*), 72-77

Bennett, W.M. & Norman, D.J. (1986) Action and toxicity of cyclosporine. *Ann. Rev. Med.*, *37*, 215-224

Bennett, W.M., Elzinga, L. & Kelley, V. (1988) Pathophysiology of cyclosporine nephrotoxicity: role of eicosanoids. *Transplant. Proc.*, *20*, 628-633

Bertault-Peres, P., Bonfils, C., Fabre, G., Just, S., Cano, J.-P. & Maurel, P. (1987) Metabolism of cyclosporin A. II. Implication of the macrolide antibiotic inducible cytochrome P-450 3c from rabbit liver microsomes. *Drug Metab. Dispos.*, *15*, 391-398

Betschart, J.M., Virji, M.A. & Shinozuka, H. (1988) Cyclosporine A-induced alterations in rat hepatic glycogen metabolism. *Transplant. Proc.*, 20 (Suppl. 3), 880-884

Beveridge, T., Gratwohl, A., Michot, F., Niederberger, W., Nuesch, E., Nussbaumer, K., Schaub, P. & Speck, B. (1981) Cyclosporin A: pharmacokinetics after a single dose in man and serum levels after multiple dosing in recipients of allogeneic bone-arrow grafts. *Curr. Ther. Res.*, 30, 5-18

Beveridge, T., Krupp, P. & McKibbin, C. (1984) Lymphomas and lymphoproliferative lesions developing under cyclosporin therapy. *Lancet*, i, 788

Bieber, C.P., Pennock, J.L. & Reitz, B.A. (1982) Lymphoma in cyclosporin A-treated nonhuman primate allograft recipients. In: Rosenberg, S. & Kaplan, H., eds, *Malignant Lymphomas*, London, Academic Press, pp. 219-229

Bijsterbosch, M.K., Mclaughlin, J.B., Holman, M. & Klaus, G.G.B. (1988) Activation and proliferation signals in mouse B cells. IX. Protein kinase C activators synergize with non-mitogenic anti-immunoglobulin antibodies to drive B cells into G1. *Immunology*, 64, 163-168

Billich, A. & Zocher, R. (1987) Enzymatic synthesis of cyclosporin A. *J. biol. Chem.*, 262, 17258-17259

Birckel, P., Jehl, F., Jaegle, M.L. & Minck, R. (1988) Méthode de dosage de la cyclosporine A et de son principal métabolite par chromatographie liquid haute performance. Comparaison avec la méthode radioimmunologique. [Method for the determination of cyclosporin A and its main metabolite by high-performance liquid chromatography. Comparison with radioimmunoassay (Fr.).] *Thérapie*, 43, 111-116

Bishop, A.G. & Hall, B.M. (1988) Effects of immunosuppressive drugs on functions of activated T lymphocytes. *Transplantation*, 45, 967-972

Bloom, R.E., Brennan, J.K., Sullivan, J.L., Chiganti, R.S.K., Dinsmore, R. & O'Reilly, R. (1985) Lymphoma of host origin in a marrow transplant recipient in remission of acute myeloid leukemia and receiving cyclosporin A. *Am. J. Hematol.*, 18, 73-83

Boland, J., Atkinson, K., Britton, K., Darveniza, P., Johnson, S. & Biggs, J. (1984) Tissue distribution and toxicity of cyclosporin A in the mouse. *Pathology*, 16, 117-123

Borel, J.F., Feurer, C., Magnée, C. & Stähelin, H. (1977) Effects of the new anti-lymphocytic peptide cyclosporin A in animals. *Immunology*, 32, 1017-1025

Bowers, L.M., Canafax, D.M., Singh, J., Seifedlin, R., Simmons, R.L. & Najarian, J.S. (1986) Studies of cyclosporine blood levels: analysis, clinical utility, pharmacokinetics, metabolites, and chronopharmacology. *Transplant. Proc.*, 18 (Suppl. 5), 137-143

Brown, P.A.J., Gray, E.S., Whitting, P.H. & Thomson, A.W. (1985) Effects of cyclosporin A on fetal development in the rat. *Biol. Neonate*, 48, 172-180

Brunner, L.J., Vadiei, K. & Luke, D.R. (1988) Cyclosporine disposition in the hyperlipidemic rat model. *Res. Commun. chem. Pathol. Pharmacol.*, 59, 339-348

Bucy, R.P. (1988) The effects of immunosuppressive pharmacological agents on the induction of cytotoxic and suppressor T lymphocytes in vitro. *Immunopharmacology*, 15, 65-72

Bunjes, D., Hardt, C., Röllinghoff, M. & Wagner, H. (1981) Cyclosporin A mediates immunosuppression of primary cytotoxic T cell responses by impairing the release of interleukin 1 and interleukin 2. *Eur. J. Immunol.*, *11*, 657-661

Burke, M.D. & Whiting, P.H. (1986) The role of drug metabolism in cyclosporine A nephrotoxicity. *Clin. Nephrol.*, *25 (Suppl. 1)*, S111-S116

Buss, W.C., Stepanek, J. & Bennett, W.M. (1988) Proposed mechanism of cyclosporine toxicity: inhibition of protein synthesis. *Transplant. Proc.*, *20 (Suppl. 3)*, 863-867

Calne, R.Y., White, D.J.G., Thiru, S., Evans, D.B., McMaster, P., Dunn, D.C., Craddock, G.N., Pentlow, B.D. & Rolles, K. (1978) Cyclosporin in patients receiving renal allografts from cadaver donors. *Lancet*, *ii*, 1323-1327

Calne, R.Y., Rolles, K., White, D.J.G., Thiru, S., Evans, D.B., McMaster, P., Dunn, D.C., Craddock, G.N., Henderson, R.G., Aziz, S. & Lewis, P. (1979) Cyclosporin A initially as the only immunosuppressant in 34 recipients of cadaveric organs: 32 kidneys, 2 pancreases, and 2 livers. *Lancet*, *ii*, 1033-1036

Caspi, R.R., McAllister, C.G., Gery, I., Borel, J., Hiestand, P. & Nussenblatt, R.B. (1988a) In vitro effects of cyclosporines A and G on activation of an autoimmune T cell line. *Transplant. Proc.*, *20 (Suppl. 2)*, 110-114

Caspi, R.R., McAllister, C.G., Gery, I. & Nussenblatt, R.B. (1988b) Differential effects of cyclosporins A and G on functional activation of a T-helper-lymphocyte line mediating experimental autoimmune uveoretinitis. *Cell. Immunol.*, *113*, 350-360

Castro, C.J., Klimo, P. & Worth, A. (1985) Unifocal aggressive lymphoma in the gastrointestinal tract in a renal transplant patient treated with cyclosporin A and prednisone. *Cancer*, *55*, 1665-1667

Cheung, F., Wong, P.Y., Cole, E., Cohen, Z. & Levy, G.A. (1988) Generation and characterization of cyclosporine metabolites produced in a hepatic microsomal system. *Transplant. Proc.*, *20 (Suppl. 2)*, 633-636

Chisholm, P.M. & Bevan, D.J. (1988) T Cell activation in the presence of cyclosporine in three in vivo allograft models. *Transplantation*, *46 (Suppl.)*, 80S-85S

Christians, U., Schlitt, H.J., Bleck, J.S., Schiebel, H.M., Kownatzki, R., Maurer, G., Strohmeyer, S.S., Schottmann, R., Wonigeit, K., Pichlmayr, R. & Sewing, K.-F. (1988a) Measurement of cyclosporine and 18 metabolites in blood, bile and urine by high-performance liquid chromatography. *Transplant. Proc.*, *20 (Suppl. 2)*, 609-613

Christians, U., Zimmer, K.-C., Wonigeit, K., Maurer, G. & Sewing, K.-F. (1988b) Liquid-chromatographic measurement of cyclosporin A and its metabolites in blood, bile, and urine. *Clin. Chem.*, *34*, 34-39

Civati, G., Busnach, G., Brando, B., Broggi, M.L., Brunati, C., Casadei, G.P. & Minetti, L. (1988) Occurrence of Kaposi's sarcoma in renal transplant recipients with low doses of cyclosporine. *Transplant. Proc.*, *20*, 924-928

Clardy, C.W., Schroeder, T.J., Myre, S.A., Wadhwa, N.K., Pesce, A.J., First, M.R., McEnery, P.T., Balistreri, W.F., Harris, R.E. & Melvin, D.B. (1988) Clinical variablity of cyclosporine pharmacokinetics in adult and pediatric patients after renal, cardiac, hepatic, and bone marrow transplants. *Clin. Chem.*, *34*, 2012-2015

Cockburn, I. (1987) Assessment of the risks of malignancy and lymphomas developing in patients using Sandimmune. *Transplant. Proc., 19*, 1804-1807

Cockburn, I.T.R. & Krupp, P. (1989) The risk of neoplasms in patients treated with cyclosporine A. *J. Autoimmunol., 2*, 723-731

Coffman, T.M., Carr, D.R., Yarger, W.E. & Klotman, P.E. (1987) Evidence that renal prostaglandin and thromboxane production is stimulated in chronic cyclosporine nephrotoxicity. *Transplantation, 43*, 282-285

Combalbert, J., Fabre, I., Fabre, G., Dalet, I., Derancourt, J., Cano, J.P. & Maurel, P. (1989) Metabolism of cyclosporin A. IV. Purification and identification of the rifampicin-inducible human liver cytochrome P450 (cyclosporin A oxidase) as a product of P450IIIA gene subfamily. *Drug Metab. Dispos., 17*, 197-207

Demetris, A.J., Nalesnik, M.A., Kunz, H.W., Gill, T.J. & Shinozuka, H. (1984) Sequential analyses of the development of lymphoproliferative disorders in rats receiving cyclosporine. *Transplantation, 38*, 239-246

Dieperink, H. (1989) Cyclosporin A nephrotoxicity. *Dan. med. Bull., 36*, 235-248

Dieperink, H., Starklint, H., Kemp, E. & Leyssac, P.P. (1988) Comparative pathophysiology and histopathology of cyclosporine nephrotoxicity. *Transplant. Proc., 3 (Suppl. 3)*, 785-791

Dinning, W.J., Nussenblatt, R.B., Kuwabara, T. & Leake, W. (1987) The induction of tolerance by cyclosporine-G in experimental autoimmune uveitis in the Lewis rat. *J. ocul. Pharmacol., 3*, 135-140

Donatsch, P., Abisch, E., Homberger, M., Traber, R., Trapp, M. & Voges, R. (1981) A radioimmunoassay to measure cyclosporin A in plasma and serum samples. *J. Immunoassay, 2*, 19-32

Drugge, R.J. & Handschumacher, R.E. (1988) Cyclosporine—mechanism of action. *Transplant. Proc., 2 (Suppl. 2)*, 301-309

D'Souza, M.J., Gourdikian, K.B. & Mujukian, A.L. (1988) Comparison of cyclosporine A and G pharmacokinetics. *Drug Metab. Dispos., 16*, 895-897

Duncan, J.I., Thomson, A.W., Aldridge, R.D., Simpson, J.G. & Whiting, P.H. (1986) Cyclosporine-induced renal structural damage: influence of dosage, strain, age and sex with reference to the rat and guinea pig. *Clin. Nephrol., 25 (Suppl. 1)*, S14-S17

Dupont, E., Huygen, K., Schandene, L., Vandercruys, M., Palfliet, K. & Wybran, J. (1985) Influence of in vivo immunosuppressive drugs on production of lymphokines. *Transplantation, 39*, 143-147

Elder, J.T., Gupta, A.K., Fisher, G.J. & Voorhees, J.J. (1988) Cyclosporine inhibits ornithine decarboxylase gene expression and acute inflammation in response to phorbol ester treatment of hairless mouse skin. *Transplant. Proc., 20 (Suppl. 4)*, 95-104

Endler, E., Derfler, K. & Schaller, A. (1987) Schwangerschaft und Geburt nach Nierentransplantation unter Cyclosporin A. [Pregnancy and delivery in kidney transplant recipients on cyclosporin A (Ger.).] *Geburtsh. Frauenheilk., 47*, 660-663

Feutren, G. & Bach, J.F. (1987) Cyclosporine et maladies auto-immunes. Première partie: bases expérimentales. [Ciclosporin and autoimmune diseases. Part 1: experimental basis (Fr.).] *Rev. Méd. interne, 8*, 91-98

Finsen, B., Poulsen, P.H. & Zimmer, J. (1988) Xenografting of fetal mouse hippocampal tissue to the brain of adult rats: effects of cyclosporin A treatment. *Exp. Brain Res.*, 70, 117-133

Follath, W., Wenk, M., Vozeh, S., Thiel, G., Brunner, F., Loertscher, R., Lemaire, M., Nussbaumer, K., Niederberger, W. & Wood, A. (1983) Intravenous cyclosporine kinetics in renal failure. *Clin. Pharmacol. Ther.*, 34, 638-643

Friedman, A.L., Kahng, K.U., Monaco, D.O., Rosen, B.D. & Wait, R.B. (1988) Cyclosporine nephrotoxicity in conscious sheep. *Transplant. Proc.*, 20 (Suppl. 3), 595-602

Fukuda, M., Aikawa, I., Ohmori, Y., Yoshimura, N., Nakai, I., Matui, S. & Oka, T. (1987) Chromosome aberrations in kidney transplant recipients. *Transplant. Proc.*, 19, 2245-2247

Fukuda, M., Ohmori, Y., Aikawa, I., Yoshimura, N. & Oka, T. (1988) Mutagenicity of cyclosporine in vivo. *Transplant. Proc.*, 20 (Suppl. 3), 929-930

Gillum, D.M., Truong, L., Tasby, J., Migliore, P. & Suki, W.N. (1988) Chronic cyclosporine nephrotoxicity. A rodent model. *Transplantation*, 46, 285-292

Gnutzmann, K.H., Hering, K. & Gutsche, H.-U. (1986) Effect of cyclosporine on the diluting capacity of the rat kidney. *Clin. Nephrol.*, 25 (Suppl. 1), S51-S56

Gorg, K., Gorg, C., Havemann, K. & Lange, H. (1986) Hodgkinsche Erkrankung nach Niertransplantion unter Cyclosporin A. [Hodgkin's disease after kidney transplantation and cyclosporin A (Ger.).] *Klin. Wochenschr.*, 64, 663-665

Grace, A.A. (1988) Cyclosporine A nephrotoxicity—the role of thromboxane A_2. *Prostagland. Leukotr. essent. fatty Acids*, 32, 157-164

Gratwohl, A., Riederer, I., Graf, E. & Speck, B. (1986) Cyclosporine toxicity in rabbits. *Lab. Anim.*, 20, 213-220

Grevel, J. (1986a) Absorption of cyclosporine A after oral dosing. *Transplant. Proc.*, 6 (Suppl. 5), 9-15

Grevel, J. (1986b) Pharmacokinetics, metabolism and interactions of ciclosporin. *Contr. Nephrol.*, 51, 23-30

Grevel, J. (1988) Significance of cyclosporine pharmacokinetics. *Transplant. Proc.*, 20 (Suppl. 2), 428-434

Grevel, J., Nuesch, E., Abisch, E. & Kutz, K. (1986) Pharmacokinetics of oral cyclosporin A (Sansimmun) in healthy subjects. *Eur. J. clin. Pharmacol.*, 31, 211-216

Grevel, J., Reynolds, K.L., Rutzky, L.P. & Kahan, B.D. (1989) Influence of demographic factors on cyclosporine pharmacokinetics in adult uremic patients. *J. clin. Pharmacol.*, 29, 261-266

de Groen, P.C. (1988) Hypothesis. Cyclosporine, low-density lipoprotein, and cholesterol. *Mayo Clin. Proc.*, 63, 1012-1021

Gunn, H.C., Hiestand, P.C. & Hanglow, A.C. (1988) Ciclosporin treatment in experimental autoimmune myasthenia gravis. *Monogr. Allergy*, 25, 96-107

Gurecki, J., Warty, V. & Sanghvi, A. (1985) The transport of cyclosporine in association with plasma lipoprotiens in heart and liver transplant patients. *Transplant. Proc.*, 17, 1997-2002

Hahn, H.-J., Dunger, A., Laube, F., Besch, W., Radloff, E., Kauert, C. & Kotzke, G. (1986) Reversibility of the acute toxic effect of cyclosporin A on pancreatic B cells of Wistar rats. *Diabetologia*, 29, 489-494

Hamaguchi, K., Nakamura, M., Ono, J. & Takaki, R. (1988) Ultrastructural and functional studies of pancreatic B cells in Wistar rats treated with immunotherapeutic doses of cyclosporin. *Diabetes Res. clin. Pract.*, 5, 135-143

Harding, M.W. & Handschumacher, R.E. (1988) Cyclophilin, a primary molecular target for cyclosporine. *Transplantation*, 46 (Suppl.), S29-S35

Hartman, N.R., Trimble, L.A., Vederas, J.C. & Jardine, I. (1985) An acid metabolite of cyclosporine. *Biochem. biophys. Res. Commun.*, 133, 964-971

Hassan, M.M.A. & Al-Yahya, M.A. (1987) Cyclosporine. *Anal. Profiles Drug Subs.*, 16, 145-205

Hattori, A., Perera, M.I.R., Witkowsky, L.A., Kunz, H.W., Gill, T.J., III & Shinozuka, H. (1986) Accelerated development of spontaneous thymic lymphomas in male AKR mice receiving cyclosporine. *Transplantation*, 41, 784-787

Hattori, A., Kunz, H.W., Gill, T.J., III, Pan, S.F. & Shinozuka, H. (1988) Diversity of promoting action of cyclosporine on the induction of murine lymphoid tumours. *Carcinogenesis*, 9, 1091-1094

Henricsson, S., Lindholm, A. & Johansson, A. (1989) Identification of a sulfate conjugate of cyclosporin. *Transplant. Proc.*, 21, 837-838

Hopt, U.T., Erath, F., Schareck, W., Greger, B. & Mellert, J. (1988) Effect of cyclosporine A on local inflammation in rejecting allografts. *Transplant. Proc.*, 20 (Suppl. 2), 163-169

Hows, J.M., Chipping, P.M., Fairhead, S., Smith, J., Baughan, A. & Gordon-Smith, E.C. (1983) Nephrotoxicity in bone marrow transplant recipients treated with cyclosporin A. *Br. J. Haematol.*, 54, 69-78

Humes, H.D. & Jackson, N.M. (1988) Cyclosporine effects on isolated membranes, proximal tubule cells, and interstitium of the kidney. *Transplant Proc.*, 20 (Suppl. 3), 748-758

Inselmann, G., Blank, M. & Baumann, H. (1988) Cyclosporine A induced lipid peroxidation in microsomes and effect on active and passive glucose transport by brush border membrane vesicles of rat kidney. *Res. Commun. chem. Pathol. Pharmacol.*, 62, 207-220

Jackson, N.M., Hsu, C.-H., Visscher, G.E., Venkatachalam, M.A. & Humes, H.D. (1987) Alterations in renal structure and function in a rat model of cyclosporine nephrotoxicity. *J. Pharmacol. exp. Ther.*, 242, 749-756

Jackson, N.M., O'Connor, R.P. & Humes, H.D. (1988) Interactions of cyclosporine with renal proximal tubule cells and cellular membranes. *Transplantation*, 46, 109-114

Johnson, F.E., Awed, E.M., Doerr, D.E., LaRegina, M.C., Tolman, K.C., Stoutenger, W.A. & Herbold, D.R. (1984) Effect of cyclosporine on carcinogenesis induced in rats by *N*-methyl-*N*'-nitro-*N*-nitrosoguanidine. *J. surg. Res.*, 37, 180-188

Kahan, B.D. (1989) Pharmacokinetics and pharmacodynamics of cyclosporine. *Transplant. Proc.*, 21 (Suppl. 1), 9-15

Kahan, B.D., Van Buren, C.T., Boileau, M., Ried, M., Payne, W.D., Flechner, S. & Newburger, J. (1983a) Cyclosporine A tissue levels in a cadaveric renal allograft recipient. *Transplantation*, 35, 96-99

Kahan, B.D., Ried, M. & Newburger, J. (1983b) Pharmacokinetics of cyclosporine in human renal transplantation. *Transplant. Proc.*, *15*, 446-453

Kahan, B.D., Van Buren, C.T., Flechner, S.M., Jarowenko, M., Yasumura, T., Rogers, A.J., Yoshimura, N., LeGrue, S., Drath, D. & Kerman, R.H. (1985) Clinical and experimental studies with cyclosporine in renal transplantation. *Surgery*, *97*, 125-140

Kahan, B.D., Didlake, R., Kim, E.E., Yoshimura, N., Kondo, E. & Stepkowski, S. (1988a) Important role of cyclosporine for the induction of immunologic tolerance in adult hosts. *Transplant. Proc.*, *20 (Suppl. 2)*, 438-450

Kahan, B.D., Didlake, R., Kim, E.E., Yoshimura, N., Kondo, E. & Stepkowski, S. (1988b) Important role of cyclosporine for the induction of immunologic tolerance in adult hosts. *Transplant. Proc.*, *20 (Suppl. 3)*, 23-35

Kahn, G.C., Shaw, L.M. & Kane, M.D. (1986) Routine monitoring of cyclosporine in whole blood and kidney tissue using high performance liquid chromatography. *J. anal. Toxicol.*, *10*, 28-34

Kaskel, F.J., Devarajan, P., Arbeit, L.A. & Moore, L.C. (1988) Effects of cyclosporine on renal hemodynamics and autoregulation in rats. *Transplant. Proc.*, *20 (Suppl. 3)*, 603-609

Kaswan, R.L., Kaplan, H.J. & Martin, C.L. (1988) Topically applied cyclosporin for modulation of induced immunogenic uveitis in rabbits. *Am. J. vet. Res.*, *49*, 1757-1759

Keown, P.A., Stiller, C.R. & Wallace, A.C. (1987) Effect of cyclosporine on the kidney. *J. Pediatr.*, *111*, 1029-1033

Kerman, R.H. (1988) Effect of cyclosporine immunusuppression in humans. *Transplant. Proc.*, *20*, 143-152

Kerman, R.H., Flechner, S.M., van Buren, C.T., Lorber, M.I. & Kahan, B.D. (1987) Immunoregulatory mechanisms in cyclosporine-treated renal allograft recipients. *Transplantation*, *43*, 205-210

Kimura, K., Money, S.R. & Jaffe, B.M. (1988) The effects of cyclosporine on varying segments of small-bowel grafts in the rat. *Surgery*, *104*, 64-69

Kinlen, L.J. (1982) Immunosuppressive therapy and cancer. *Cancer Surv.*, *1*, 565-583

Klintmalm, G.B.G., Iwatsuki, S. & Starzl, T.E. (1981a) Cyclosporin A hepatotoxicity in 66 renal allograft recipients. *Transplantation*, *32*, 488-489

Klintmalm, G.B.G., Iwatsuki, S. & Starzl, T.E. (1981b) Nephrotoxicity of cyclosporin A in liver and kidney transplant patients. *Lancet*, *i*, 470-471

Klintmalm, G., Althoff, P., Appleby, G. & Segerbrandt, E. (1984) Renal function in a newborn baby delivered of a renal transplant patient taking cyclosporine. *Transplantation*, *38*, 198-199

Kobel, H. & Traber, R. (1982) Directed biosynthesis of cyclosporins. *Eur. J. appl. Microbiol. Biotechnol.*, *14*, 237-240

Kobel, H., Loosli, H.R. & Voges, R. (1983) Contribution to knowledge of the biosynthesis of cyclosporin A. *Experientia*, *39*, 873-876

Kronbach, T., Fischer, V. & Meyer, U.A. (1988) Cyclosporine metabolism in human liver: identification of a cytochrome P-450III gene family as the major cyclosporine metabolizing enzyme explains interactions of cyclosporine with other drugs. *Clin. Pharmacol. Ther.*, *43*, 630-635

Krönke, M., Leonard, W.J., Depper, J.M., Arya, S.K., Wong-Staal, F., Gallo, R.C., Waldmann, T.A. & Greene, W.C. (1984) Cyclosporin A inhibits T-cell growth factor gene expression at the level of mRNA transcription. *Proc. natl Acad. Sci. USA*, *81*, 5214-5218

Kumar, M.S.A., White, A.G., Alex, G., Antos, M.S., Philips, E.M. & Abouna, G.M. (1988) Correlation of blood levels and tissue levels of cyclosporine with the histologic features of cyclosporine toxicity. *Transplant. Proc.*, *20 (Suppl. 2)*, 407-413

Kupiec-Weglinski, J.W., Filho, M.A., Strom, T.B. & Tilney, N.L. (1984) Sparing of suppressor cells: a critical action of cyclosporine. *Transplantation*, *38*, 97-101

Larsson, E.-L. (1980) Cyclosporin A and dexamethasone suppress T cell responses by selectively acting at distinct sites of the triggering process. *J. Immunol.*, *124*, 2828-2833

Lear, P.A., Watson, A.J., Crane, P.W., Farthing, M.J.G. & Wood, R.F.M. (1988) Autonomic function limits mucosal transport in cyclosporine-treated small intestinal transplants. *Transplant. Proc.*, *20 (Suppl. 3)*, 436-442

LeGrue, S., Friedman, A.W. & Kahan, B.D. (1983) Binding of cyclosporine by human lymphocytes and phospholipid vesicles. *J. Immunol.*, *131*, 712-718

Lemaire, M. & Tillement, J.P. (1982) Role of lipoproteins and erythrocytes in the in vitro binding and distribution of cyclosporin A in the blood. *J. Pharm. Pharmacol.*, *34*, 715-718

Lemaire, M., Maurer, G. & Wood, A.J. (1986) Pharmacokinetics and metabolism. *Prog. Allergy*, *38*, 93-107

Lensmayer, G.L., Wiebe, D.A. & Carlson, I.H. (1987a) Identification and analysis of nine metabolites of cyclosporine in whole blood by liquid chromatography. 1. Purification of analytical standards and optimization of the assay. *Clin. Chem.*, *33*, 1841-1850

Lensmayer, G.L., Wiebe, D.A. & Carlson, I.H. (1987b) Identification and analysis of nine metabolites of cyclosporine in whole blood by liquid chromatography. 2. Comparison of patients' results. *Clin. Chem.*, *33*, 1851-1855

Levy-Marchal, C., Tarr, A., Lokiec, F. & Czernichow, P. (1988) Plasma and tissue cyclosporine A concentrations in developing rats. *Transplant. Proc.*, *20 (Suppl. 2)*, 696-702

Lewis, G.L., Lamont, C.A.R., Lee, H.A. & Slapak, M. (1983) Successful pregnancy in a renal transplant recipient taking cyclosporin A. *Br. med. J.*, *286*, 603

Lin, C.Y., Shann, T.Y., Lui, W.Y. & Peng, F.K. (1989) Combined measurements of urinary neopterin, beta-2-microglobulin and serum gamma-interferon for early detection of renal graft rejection following change from cyclosporin A to immunosuppressive combination therapy. *Transplant. Proc.*, *21*, 1874-1877

Lorber, M.I. (1986) Cyclosporine action in blockade of cellular immune responses. *Year Immunol.*, *2*, 279-288

Lorber, M.I. (1989) The mechanism of ciclosporin immunosuppression. *Year Immunol.*, *4*, 253-263

Mahlberg, K., Uusitalo, H., Uusitalo, R., Palkama, A. & Tallberg, T. (1987) Suppression of experimental autoimmune uveitis in guinea pigs by ethylenediamine tetra-acetic acid, corticosteroids, and cyclosporin. *J. ocul. Pharmacol.*, *3*, 199-210

Mason, R.J., Thomson, A.W., Whiting, P.H., Gray E.S., Brown, P.A.J., Catte, G.R.D. & Simpson, J.G. (1985) Cyclosporine-induced fetotoxicity in the rat. *Transplantation, 39*, 9-12

Matter, B.E., Donatsch, P., Racine, R.R., Schmid, B. & Suter, W. (1982) Genotoxicity of cyclosporin A, a new immunosuppressive agent. *Mutat. Res., 105*, 257-264

Maung, R., Pinto, A., Robertson, A., Stuart, G.L.E., Klassen, J.K. & Hons, R.B. (1985) Development of ovarian carcinoma in a cyclosporin A immunosuppressed patient. *Obstet. Gynecol., 66 (Suppl.)*, 895-925

Maurer, G. (1985) Metabolism of cyclosporine. *Transplant. Proc., 17 (Suppl. 1)*, 19-26

Maurer, G. & Lemaire, M. (1986) Biotransformation and distribution in blood of cyclosporine and its metabolites. *Transplant. Proc., 17 (Suppl. 5)*, 25-34

Maurer, G., Loosli, H.R., Schreier, E. & Keller, B. (1984) Disposition of cyclosporine in several animal species and man. I. Structural elucidation of its metabolites. *Drug Metab. Dispos., 12*, 120-126

McKenna, R.M., Szturm, K., Jeffrey, J.R. & Rush, D.N. (1989) Inhibition of cytokine production by cyclosporine A and G. *Transplantation, 47*, 343-348

McMillan, M.A. (1989) Clinical pharmacokinetics of cyclosporin. *Pharmacol. Ther., 42*, 135-156

Merion, R.M., White, D.J.G., Thiru, S., Evans, D.B. & Calne, R.Y. (1984) Cyclosporine: five years' experience in cadaveric renal transplantation. *New Engl. J. Med., 310*, 148-154

Mihatsch, M.J., Thiel, G. & Ryffel, B. (1988a) Cyclosporine nephrotoxicity. *Adv. Nephrol., 17*, 303-320

Mihatsch, M.J., Thiel, G. & Ryffel, B. (1988b) Histopathology of cyclosporine nephrotoxicity. *Transplant. Proc., 20 (Suppl. 3)*, 759-771

Mihatsch, M.J., Thiel, G. & Ryffel, B. (1989) Cyclosporin A: action and side-effects. *Toxicol. Lett., 46*, 125-139

Monaco, D.O., Wait, R.B., Friedman, A.L. & Kahng, K.U. (1988) Effects of chronic cyclosporine therapy on renal vascular reactivity in the isolated perfused rabbit kidney. *Transplant. Proc., 20 (Suppl. 3)*, 578-583

Moochhala, S.M. & Renton, K.W. (1986) Inhibition of hepatic microsomal drug metabolism by the immunosuppressive agent cyclosporin A. *Biochem. Pharmacol., 35*, 1499-1503

Morris, P.J., Finch, D.R., Garvey, J.F., Poole, M.D. & Millard, P.R. (1980) Suppression of rejection of allogeneic islet tissue in the rat. *Diabetes, 29 (Suppl. 1)*, 107-112

Movsowitz, C., Epstein, S., Fallon, M., Ismail, F. & Thomas, S. (1988) Cyclosporin-A *in vivo* produces severe osteopenia in the rat: effect of dose and duration of administration. *Endocrinology, 123*, 2571-2577

Mraz, W., Zink, R.A., Graf, A., Preis, D., Illner, W.D., Land, W., Siebert, W. & Zottlein, H. (1983) Distribution and transfer of cyclosporine among the various human lipoprotein classes. *Transplant. Proc., 15*, 2426-2429

Muir, C., Waterhouse, J., Mack, T., Powell, J. & Whelan, S., eds (1987) *Cancer Incidence in Five Continents* (IARC Scientific Publications No. 88), Lyon, IARC, pp. 330-337, 644-651, 714-719, 732-737, 750-753

Myers, B.D. (1986) Cyclosporine nephrotoxicity. *Kidney int., 30*, 964-974

Myers, B.D., Ross, J., Newton, L., Luetscher, J. & Perlroth, M. (1984) Cyclosporine-associated chronic nephropathy. *New Engl. J. Med.*, 311, 699-705

Nagelkerke, J.F., Tijdens, R.B., Schwarz, E.P., Winters, M.F.G., Paul, L.C. & Mulder, G.J. (1987) The covalent binding of cyclosporin A to rat liver macromolecules in vivo and in vitro: the role of cytochrome P-450. *Toxicology*, 47, 277-284

Neild, G.H. (1988) Vasodilatory prostaglandins and cyclosporin nephrotoxicity. *Prostagland. Leukotr. essent. fatty Acids*, 33, 207-212

Niederberger, W., Lemaire, M., Maurer, G., Nussbaumer, K. & Wagner, O. (1983) Distribution and binding of cyclosporine in blood and tissues. *Transplant. Proc.*, 15 (Suppl. 1), 2419-2421

Nooter, K., Meershoek, B., Spaans, W., Sonneveld, P., Oostrum, R. & Deurloo, J. (1984a) Blood and tissue distribution of cyclosporin A after a single oral dose in the rat. *Experientia*, 40, 559-561

Nooter, K., Schultz, F. & Sonneveld, P. (1984b) Evidence for a possible dose-dependent pharmacokinetics of cyclosporin-A in the rat. *Res. Commun. chem. Pathol. Pharmacol.*, 43, 407-415

Nordmann, J.P., De Kozak, Y., Le Hoang, P. & Faure, J.P. (1986) Cyclosporine therapy of guinea pig autoimmune uveoretinitis induced with autologous retina. *J. ocul. Pharmacol.*, 2, 325-333

Paller, M.S. (1988a) The prostaglandin E_1 analog misoprostol reverses acute cyclosporine nephrotoxicity. *Transplant. Proc.*, 20 (Suppl. 3), 634-637

Paller, M.S. (1988b) Effects of the prostaglandin E_1 analog misoprostol on cyclosporine nephrotoxicity. *Transplantation*, 45, 1126-1131

Pell, M.A., Rosano, T.G., Brayman, K.L., Freed, B.M., Shaw, L.M. & Lempert, N. (1988) Predominance of native cyclosporin over metabolites in rat blood and tissue. *Transplant. Proc.*, 20 (Suppl. 2), 674-679

Penn, I. & Brunson, M.E. (1988) Cancers after cyclosporine therapy. *Transplant. Proc.*, 20 (Suppl.), 885-892

Pennock, J.L., Reitz, B.A., Bieber, C.P., Aziz, S., Oyer, P.E., Strober, S., Hoppe, R., Kaplan, H.S., Stinson, E.B. & Shumway, N.E. (1981) Survival of primates following orthotopic cardiac transplantation treated with total lymphoid irradiation and chemical immune suppression. *Transplantation*, 32, 467-473

Perera, M.I.R., Kunz, H.W., Gill, T.J., III & Shinozuka, H. (1986) Enhancement of induction of intestinal adenocarcinomas by cyclosporine in rats given a single dose of N-methyl-N-nitrosourea. *Transplantation*, 42, 297-302

Perico, N., Benigni, A., Zoja, C., Delaini, F. & Remuzzi, G. (1986a) Functional significance of exaggerated renal thromboxane A_2 synthesis induced by cyclosporin A. *Am. J. Physiol.*, 251, F581-F587

Perico, N., Zoja, C., Benigni, A., Ghilardi, F., Gualandris, L. & Remuzzi, G. (1986b) Effect of short-term cyclosporine administration in rats on renin-angiotensin and thromboxane A_2: possible relevance to the reduction in glomerular filtration rate. *J. Pharmacol. exp. Ther.*, 239, 229-235

Petitjean, P., Schmitt, M., Kempf, C., Cessler, U., Jahn, H. & Kempf, J. (1986) DNA repair synthesis in peripheral blood lymphocytes from kidney transplant patients treated with cyclosporine or with azathioprine, associated with corticosteroids. *Transplant Proc.*, *18*, 1330-1331

Pfaller, W., Kotanko, P. & Bazzanella, A. (1986) Morphological and biochemical observations in rat nephron epithelia following cyclosporine A (CsA) treatment. *Clin. Nephrol.*, *25 (Suppl. 1)*, S105-S110

Polman, C.H., Matthaei, I., de Groot, C.J.A., Koetsier, J.C., Sminia, T. & Dijkstra, C.D. (1988) Low-dose cyclosporin A induces relapsing remitting experimental allergic encephalomyelitis in the Lewis rat. *J. Neuroimmunol.*, *17*, 209-216

Povlsen, J.V., Moller, B.K., Christiansen, B.S. & Petersen, C.M. (1989) Cyclosporin A mediated immunosuppression in vitro: effect on high affinity interleukin-2 receptor expression and -turnover. *Tissue Antigens*, *33*, 4-14

Powles, R.L., Clink, H.M., Spence, D., Morgenstern, G., Watson, J.G., Selby, P.J., Woods, M., Barret, A., Jameson, B., Sloane, J., Lawler, S.D., Kay, H.E.M., Lawson, D., McElwain, T.J. & Alexander, P. (1980) Cyclosporin A to prevent graft-versus-host disease in man after allogeneic bone-marrow transplantation. *Lancet*, *ii*, 327-329

Ptachcinski, R.J., Venkataramanan, R., Rosenthal, J.T., Burckart, G.J., Taylor, R.J. & Hakala, T.R. (1985) Cyclosporine kinetics in renal transplantation. *Clin. Pharmacol.*, *38*, 296-300

Quesniaux, V.F.J., Schreier, M.H., Wenger, R.M., Hiestand, P.C., Harding, M.W. & Van Regenmortel, M.H.V. (1988) Molecular characteristics of cyclophilin-cyclosporine interaction. *Transplantation*, *46 (Suppl.)*, 23S-28S

Racusen, L.C. & Solez, K. (1988) Cyclosporine nephrotoxicity. *Int. Rev. exp. Pathol.*, *30*, 107-157

Reem, G.H., Cook, L.A. & Vilcek, J. (1983) Gamma interferon synthesis by human thymocytes and T lymphocytes inhibited by cyclosporin. *Science*, *221*, 63-65

Reynolds, J.E.F., ed. (1989) *Martindale. The Extra Pharmacopoeia*, 29th ed., London, The Pharmaceutical Press, pp. 614-619

Ried, M., Gibbons, S., Kwok, D., van Buren, C.T., Flechner, S. & Kahan, B.D. (1983) Cyclosporine levels in human tissues of patients treated for one week to one year. *Transplant. Proc.*, *15*, 218-221

Robson, S., Neuberger, J., Keller, H.P., Abisch, E., Niederberger, W., von Graffenried, B. & Williams, R. (1984) Pharmacokinetic study of cyclosporin A (Sandimmun) in patients with primary biliary cirrhosis. *Br. J. clin. Pharmacol.*, *18*, 627-631

Rogers, T.S., Elzinga, L., Bennett, W.M. & Kelley, V.E. (1988) Selective enhancement of thromboxane in macrophages and kidneys in cyclosporine-induced nephrotoxicity. *Transplantation*, *45*, 153-156

Rosano, T.G., Freed, B.M., Pell, M.A. & Lempert, N. (1986) Cyclosporine metabolites in human blood and renal tissue. *Transplant. Proc.*, *18 (Suppl. 5)*, 35-40

Rose, M.L., Dominguez, M., Leaver, N., Lachno, R. & Yacoub, M.H. (1989) Analysis of T cell subpopulations and cyclosporine levels in the blood of two neonates born to immunosuppressed heart-lung transplant recipients. *Transplantation*, *48*, 223-226

Rüegger, A., Kuhn, M., Lichti, H., Loosli, H.R., Hugenin, R., Quinquerez, C. & von Wartburg, A. (1976) Cyclosporin A, ein immunosuppressiv wirksamer Peptidmetabolit aus Trichoderma polysporum (Link ex Pers.) Rifai. [Cyclosporin A, an immunosuppressive active peptide metabolite from Trichoderma polysporum (Link ex Pers.) Rifai (Ger.).] *Helv. chim. Acta*, 59, 1075-1092

Ryffel, B. & Mihatsch, M.J. (1986) Cyclosporine nephrotoxicity. *Toxicol. Pathol.*, 14, 73-82

Ryffel, B., Donatsch, P., Madörin, M., Matter, B.E., Rüttimann, G., Schön, H., Stoll, R. & Wilson, J. (1983) Toxicological evaluation of cyclosporin A. *Arch. Toxicol.*, 53, 107-141

Ryffel, B., Donatsch, P., Hiestand, P. & Mihatsch, M.J. (1986) PGE_2 reduces nephrotoxicity and immunosuppression of cyclosporine in rats. *Clin. Nephrol.*, 25 (Suppl. 1), S95-S99

Sabbatini, M., Esposito, C., Uccello, F., De Nicola, L., Alba, M., Conte, G., Dal Canton, A. & Andreucci, V.E. (1988) Acute effects of cyclosporine on glomerular dynamics—micropuncture study in the rat. *Transplant. Proc.*, 20 (Suppl. 3), 544-548

Sangalli, L., Bortolotti, A., Jiritano, L. & Bonati, M. (1988) Cyclosporine pharmacokinetics in rats and interspecies comparison in dogs, rabbits, rats, and humans. *Drug Metab. Dispos.*, 16, 749-753

Schachter, M. (1988) Cyclosporine A and hypertension. *J. Hypertens.*, 6, 511-516

Schroeder, T.J., Wadhwa, N.K., Pesce, A.J. & First, M.R. (1986) An acute overdose of cyclosporin. *Transplantation*, 41, 406-409

Seethalakshmi, L., Menon, M., Malhotra R.K. & Diamond, D.A. (1987) Effect of cyclosporine A on male reproduction in rats. *J. Urol.*, 138, 991-995

Seethalakshmi, L., Diamond, D.A., Malhotra, R.K., Mazanitis, S.G., Kumar, S. & Menon, M. (1988) Cyclosporine-induced testicular dysfunction: a separation of the nephrotoxic component and an assessment of a 60-day recovery period. *Transplant. Proc.*, 20 (Suppl. 3), 1005-1010

Shah, A.K., Sawchuk, R.J., Gratwohl, A., Baldomero, H. & Speck, B. (1988) Subcutaneous absorption of cyclosporine in rabbits. *Transplant. Proc.*, 20 (Suppl. 2), 710-714

Sheil, A.G.R., Flavel, S., Disney, A.P.S., Mathew, T.H. & Hall, B.M. (1987) Cancer incidence in renal transplant patients treated with azathioprine or cyclosporine. *Transplant. Proc.*, 19, 2214-2216

Shevach, E.M. (1985) The effects of cyclosporin A on the immune system. *Ann. Rev. Immunol.*, 3, 397-423

Shigematsu, H. & Koyama, A. (1988) Suppressive effect of cyclosporin A on the induction of chronic serum sickness nephritis in the rat. *Acta pathol. jpn.*, 38, 11-19

Shinozuka, H., Hattori, A., Gill, T.J., III & Kunz, H.W. (1988) Experimental models of malignancies after cyclosporine therapy. *Transplant. Proc.*, 20, 893-899

Shulman, H., Striker, G., Deeg, H.J., Kennedy, M., Storb, R. & Thomas, E.D. (1981) Nephrotoxicity of cyclosporin A after allogeneic marrow transplantation. Glomerular and tubular injury. *New Engl. J. Med.*, 305, 1392-1395

Sikka, S.C., Koyle, M.A., Swerdloff, R.S. & Rajfer, J. (1988) Reversibility of cyclosporine-induced hypoandrogenism in rats. *Transplantation*, 45, 784-787

Smeesters, C., Chaland, P., Giroux, L., Moutquin, J.M., Etienne, P., Douglas, F., Corman, J., St-Louis, G. & Daloze, P. (1988a) Prevention of acute cyclosporine A nephrotoxicity by a thromboxane synthetase inhibitor. *Transplant. Proc.*, *20 (Suppl. 3)*, 658-664

Smeesters, C., Chaland, P., Giroux, L., Moutquin, J.M., Etienne, P., Douglas, F., Corman, J., St-Louis, G. & Daloze, P. (1988b) Prevention of acute cyclosporine A nephrotoxicity by a thromboxane synthetase inhibitor. *Transplant. Proc.*, *20 (Suppl. 2)*, 663-669

Smith, J.L., Wilkinson, A.H., Hunsicker, L.G., Tobacman, J., Kapelanski, D.P., Johnson, M., Wright, F.H., Behrendt, D.M. & Corry, R.J. (1989) Increased frequency of posttransplant lymphomas in patients treated with cyclosporin, azathioprine and prednisone. *Transplant. Proc.*, *21*,

Stanley Nahman, N., Cosio, F.G., Mahan, J.D., Henry, M.L. & Ferguson, R.M. (1988) Cyclosporine nephrotoxicity in spontaneously hypertensive rats. *Transplantation*, *45*, 768-772

Starklint, H., Dieperink, H., Kemp, E. & Leyssac, P.P. (1988a) Ultrastructural study of collapsed proximal tubules in perfusion/fixed kidneys of Sprague-Dawley rats treated with cyclosporine. *Transplant. Proc.*, *20 (Suppl. 3)*, 740-747

Starklint, H., Dieperink, H., Kemp, E. & Leyssac, P.P. (1988b) Subcapsular intersititial fibrosis in kidneys of rats treated with cyclosporine for 16 weeks. *Transplant. Proc.*, *20 (Suppl. 3)*, 816-820

Starzl, T.E., Nalesnik, M.A., Porter, K.A., Ho, M., Iwatsuki, S., Griffith, B.P., Rosenthal, J.T., Hakala, T.R., Shaw, B.W., Hardesty, R.L., Atchison, R.W. & Jaffe, R. (1984) Reversibility of lymphomas and lymphoproliferative lesions developing under cyclosporin-steroid therapy. *Lancet*, *i*, 583-587

Steinmuller, D.R. (1989) Cyclosporine nephrotoxicity. *Cleveland clin. med. J.*, *56*, 89-95

Stone, B., Warty, V., Dindzans, V. & Van Thiel, D. (1988) The mechanism of cyclosporine-induced cholestasis in the rat. *Transplant. Proc.*, *20 (Suppl. 3)*, 841-844

Sullivan, B.A., Hak, L.J. & Finn, W.F. (1985) Cyclosporine nephrotoxicity: studies in laboratory animals. *Transplant. Proc.*, *17 (Suppl. 1)*, 145-154

Szturm, K., Jeffery, J.R., Rush, D.N. & McKenna, R.M. (1989) Cyclosporin A and G inhibition of cytokine production. *Transplant. Proc.*, *21*, 857

Tejani, A., Lancman, I., Pomrantz, A., Khawar, M. & Chen, C. (1988) Nephrotoxicity of cyclosporine A and cyclosporine G in a rat model. *Transplantation*, *45*, 184-187

Thiru, S., Calne, R.Y. & Nagington, J. (1981) Lymphoma in renal allograft patients treated with cyclosporin-A as one of the immunosuppressive agents. *Transplant. Proc.*, *13*, 359-364

Thompson, J.F., Allen, R., Morris, P.J. & Wood, R. (1985) Skin cancer in renal transplant patients treated with cyclosporin. *Lancet*, *i*, 158-159

Thomson, A.W. (1983) Immunobiology of cyclosporin A—a review. *Aust. J. exp. biol. med. Sci.*, *61*, 147-172

Thomson, A.W., Whiting, P.H., Blair, J.T., Davidson, R.J.L. & Simpson, J.G. (1981) Pathological changes developing in the rat during a 3-week course of high dosage cyclosporin A and their reversal following drug withdrawal. *Transplantation*, *32*, 271-277

Tracey, D.E., Hardee, M.M., Richard, K.A. & Paslay, J.W. (1988) Pharmacological inhibition of interleukin-1 activity on T cells by hydrocortisone, cyclosporine, prostaglandins, and cyclic nucleotides. *Immunopharmacology*, 15, 47-62

Tutschka, P.J. (1986) Induction of tolerance with cyclosporin A. In: Meryman, H.T., ed., *Transplantation: Approaches to Graft Rejection*, New York, Alan R. Liss, pp. 209-226

Ueda, C.T., Lemaire, M., Gsell, G. & Nussbaumer, K. (1983) Intestinal lymphatic absorption of cyclosporin A following oral administration in an olive oil solution in rats. *Biopharm. Drug Dispos.*, 4, 113-124

US Pharmacopeial Convention, Inc. (1989) *US Pharmacopeia*, 22nd rev., Easton, PA, pp. 371-373

Venkataramanan, R., Starzl, T.E., Yang, S., Burckart, G.J., Ptachcinski, R.J., Shaw, B.W., Iwatsuki, S., van Thiel, D.H., Sanghi, A. & Seltman, H. (1985) Biliary excretion of cyclosporine in liver transplant patients. *Transplant. Proc.*, 17, 286-289

Venkataramanan, R., Burckart, G.J., Ptachcinski, R.J., Lee, A., Hardesty, R.E. & Griffith, B.T. (1986) Cyclosporine pharmacokinetics in heart transplant patients. *Transplant. Proc.*, 18, 768-770

Venkateramanan, R., Koneru, B., Wang, C.C., Burckart, G.J., Caritis, S.N. & Starzl, T.E. (1988) Cyclosporine and its metabolites in mother and baby. *Transplantation*, 46, 468-469

Verani, R. (1986) Cyclosporine nephrotoxicity in the Fischer rat. *Clin. Nephrol.*, 25 (*Suppl. 1*), S9-S13

Vernillet, L., Keller, H.P., Le Bigot, J.F. & Humbert, H. (1989) Determination of cyclosporin in plasma: specific radioimmunoassay with a monoclonal antibody and liquid chromatography compared. *Clin. Chem.*, 35, 608-611

Vine, W. & Bowers, L.D. (1987) Cyclosporine: structure, pharmacokinetics, and therapeutic drug monitoring. *Crit. Rev. clin. Lab. Sci.*, 25, 275-311

Wagner, O., Schreier, E., Heitz, F. & Maurer, G. (1987) Tissue distribution, disposition, and metabolism of cyclosporine in rats. *Drug Metab. Dispos.*, 15, 377-383

Walker, R.J., Horvath, J.S., Tiller, D.J. & Duggin, G.G. (1989) Malignant lymphoma in a renal transplant patient on cyclosporin A therapy. *Aust. N.Z. J. Med.*, 19, 154-155

Wallemacq, P.E., Lhoest, G. & Dumont, P. (1989a) Isolation, purification and structure elucidation of cyclosporin A metabolites in rabbit and man. *Biomed. environ. Mass Spectrom.*, 18, 48-56

Wallemacq, P.E., Lhoest, G., Latinne, D. & Bruyere, M. (1989b) Isolation, characterization and in vitro activity of human cyclosporin A metabolites. *Transplant. Proc.*, 21, 906-910

Wang, C.P., Hartman, N.R., Venkataramanan, R., Jardine, I., Lin, F.T., Knapp, J., Starzl, T.E. & Burckart, G.J. (1989) Isolation of 10 cyclosporine metabolites from human bile. *Drug Metab. Dispos.*, 17, 292-296

Weidle, P.J. & Vlasses, P.H. (1988) Systemic hypertension associated with cyclosporine: a review. *Drug Intell. clin. Pharmacol.*, 22, 443-451

White, D.J.G. & Lim, S.M.L. (1988) The induction of tolerance by cyclosporine. *Transplantation*, 46 (*Suppl.*), 118S-121S

White, D.J.G., Plumb, A.M., Pawelec, G. & Brons, G. (1979) Cyclosporin A: an immunosuppressive agent preferentially active against proliferating T cells. *Transplantation*, 27, 55-58

Whiting, P.H. & Simpson, J.G. (1988) Lithium clearance measurements as an indication of cyclosporin A nephrotoxicity in the rat. *Clin. Sci.*, 74, 173-178

Whiting, P.H., Thomson, A.W., Blair, J.T. & Simpson, J.G. (1982) Experimental cyclosporin A nephrotoxicity. *Br. J. exp. Pathol.*, 63, 88-94

Whiting, P.H., Thomson, A.W. & Simpson, J.G. (1986) Cyclosporine and renal enzyme excretion. *Clin. Nephrol.*, 25 (Suppl. 1), S100-S104

Windholz, M., ed. (1983) *The Merck Index*, 10th ed., Rahway, NJ, Merck & Co., p. 396

Wolf, B.A., Daft, M.C., Koenig, J.W., Flye, M.W., Turk, J.W. & Scott, M.G. (1989) Measurement of cyclosporine concentrations in whole blood: HPLC and radioimmunoassay with a specific monoclonal antibody and ^{3}H- or ^{125}I-labeled ligand compared. *Clin. Chem.*, 35, 1209-124

Wood, A.J. & Lemaire, M. (1985) Pharmacologic aspects of cyclosporine therapy: pharmacokinetics. *Transplant. Proc.*, 17 (suppl. 1), 27-32

Wood, A.J., Maurer, G., Niederberger, W. & Beveridge, T. (1983) Cyclosporine: pharmacokinetics, metabolism, and drug interactions. *Transplant. Proc.*, 15 (Suppl. 1), 2409-2412

Yee, G.C., Kennedy, M.S., Storb, R. & Thomas, E.D. (1984) Pharmacokinetics of intravenous cyclosporine in bone marrow transplant recipients. *Transplantation*, 38, 511-513

Yuzawa, K., Kondo, I., Fukao, K., Iwasaki, Y. & Hamaguchi, H. (1986) Mutagenicity of cyclosporine. *Transplantation*, 42, 61-63

Yuzawa, K., Fukao, K., Iwasaki, Y. & Hamaguchi, H. (1987) Mutagenicity of cyclosporine against human cells. *Transplant. Proc.*, 19, 1218-1220

Zwanenburg, T.S.B., Suter, W. & Matter, B.E. (1988) Absence of genotoxic potential for cyclosporine in experimental systems. *Transplant. Proc.*, 20 (Suppl. 2), 435-437

PREDNIMUSTINE

1. Chemical and Physical Data

1.1 Synonyms

Chem. Abstr. Services Reg. No.: 29069-24-7

Chem. Abstr. Name: Pregna-1,4-diene-3,20-dione, 21-(4-{4-[bis(2-chloroethyl)amino]phenyl}-1-oxybutoxy)-11,17-dihydroxy-(11β)-

Synonyms: Prednisolone, 21-(4-{*para*[bis(2-chloroethyl)-αβ-amino]phenyl}-butyrate); 11β,17,21-trihydroxypregna-1,4-diene-3,20-dione-21-(1-{*para*-[bis-(2-chloroethyl)amino]phenyl}butyrate); Leo 1031; NSC 134087

1.2 Structural and molecular formulae and molecular weight

$C_{35}H_{45}Cl_2NO_6$ Mol. wt: 646.66

1.3 Chemical and physical properties of the pure substance

From Windholz (1983), unless otherwise specified

(a) *Description*: Crystals from methanol-water
(b) *Melting-point*: 163-164 °C
(c) *Optical rotation*: $[\alpha]_D^{24} = +92.9°$ (c = 1.06 in chloroform)

(d) *Solubility*: Practically insoluble in water; soluble in ethanol, acetone, chloroform and methanol (Reynolds, 1989)

1.4 Technical products and impurities

Trade names: Mostarine; Sterecyt; Stéréocyt

2. Production, Occurrence, Use and Analysis

2.1 Production and occurrence

Prednimustine can be produced by the esterification of chlorambucil with prednisolone (Fex *et al.*, 1970). It is synthesized in Sweden.

Prednimustine is not known to occur naturally.

2.2 Use

Prednimustine is a cytostatic agent. It has been used in the treatment of various malignancies, including chronic lymphatic leukaemia and non-Hodgkin's lymphomas, at daily oral doses of 140-200 mg for three to five days or continuously at 20-30 mg per day (Reynolds, 1989; Szanto *et al.*, 1989). It has also been tested for use in the treatment of breast cancer (Loeber *et al.*, 1983; Rankin *et al.*, 1987).

2.3 Analysis

Prednimustine has been quantified in plasma by high-performance liquid chromatography (Newell *et al.*, 1979). It has also been quantified after hydrolysis to chlorambucil, by gas chromatography-mass spectrometry (Jakhammer *et al.*, 1977) and high-performance liquid chromatography (Workman *et al.*, 1987).

3. Biological Data Relevant to the Evaluation of Carcinogenic Risk to Humans

3.1 Carcinogenicity studies in animals

(a) *Oral administration*

Rat: Four groups of 30 female Sprague-Dawley rats, 100 days of age, received prednimustine [purity unspecified] at 12 mg/kg bw in a vehicle consisting of carboxymethylcellulose, Tween 80 and glucose in water by gavage once, twice, 4.5 or nine times per month for 18 months. The last group had significantly reduced survival. A group of 120 female rats received the vehicle alone by gavage nine times per month for 18 months. A significant increase ($p < 0.01$; Peto test: Peto *et al.*, 1980) in the incidence of squamous-cell carcinomas of the external auditory canal was observed (controls, 0/30; once per month, 0/30; twice per month, 1/30; 4.5 times per month, 2/30; nine times per month, 2/30). No increase in the incidence of other tumours was observed (Berger *et al.*, 1985, 1986).

(b) *Carcinogenicity of metabolites*

Chlorambucil has been evaluated in the *IARC Monographs* (IARC, 1975, 1981, 1987).

3.2 Other relevant data

(a) *Experimental systems*

(i) *Absorption, distribution, excretion and metabolism*

Following a subcutaneous injection of radiolabelled prednimustine at 20 mg/kg bw to female Wistar rats, radioactivity appeared gradually in blood plasma over 48 h. The levels of chlorambucil and phenylacetic mustard in plasma were below 5 μM. Radioactivity levels in all tissues studied were lower than those in plasma; in the small intestine, activity peaked at 2-4 h after administration. No or little radioactivity was detected in bone marrow (Newell *et al.*, 1981).

When radiolabelled prednimustine was injected intravenously to baboons, low urinary and biliary excretion was observed. The radioactivity in blood and kidney decreased with time, but it was stable in the liver over the observation period of 6 h. In muscle, prostate, lung, spleen and seminal vesicles, however, radioactivity levels rose after 4 and 6 h (Kirdani *et al.*, 1978).

Prednimustine is hydrolysed completely *in vitro* by rat plasma esterases to chlorambucil and prednisolone (Wilkinson *et al.*, 1978). A cholesterol ester of chlorambucil, originating from prednimustine by acyltransferase-catalysed transesterification, was detected when prednimustine was incubated with human, rat or dog plasma *in vitro*. The same ester was identified in plasma of dogs after intravenous injection *in vivo* (Gunnarsson *et al.*, 1984).

(ii) *Toxic effects*

In an acute lethality study, survival of Wistar rats given prednimustine at 128 mg/kg bw subcutaneously was 70% after 21 days. The drug was less toxic than chlorambucil and less toxic than chlorambucil and prednisolone given in combination (Harrap *et al.*, 1977).

In subacute toxicity experiments, the mortality caused by daily oral administrations of prednimustine for four weeks to Sprague-Dawley rats was low compared to that induced by chlorambucil and prednisolone given together. Mortality in prednimustine-treated animals was about 10% at dose levels of 32 and 64 mg/kg bw. Dose-related lymphopenia was observed, and spleen and adrenal weights were reduced (Fredholm *et al.*, 1978).

No symptom of toxicity was observed during a life-time carcinogenicity study with prednimustine given to Sprague-Dawley rats at 12 mg/kg bw one to nine times per month for 18 months (Berger *et al.*, 1986).

Prednimustine caused a dose-dependent decrease in survival in Chinese hamster V79-4 cells; it was at least three times as toxic as chlorambucil throughout the dose range (Hartley-Asp *et al.*, 1986). Dose-dependent cell death was also observed in the hormone-sensitive S49 mouse lymphoma cell line after incubation for 24 h with prednimustine at 10^{-8} M up to 5×10^{-7} M prednimustine (Harrap *et al.*, 1977).

(iii) *Effects on reproduction and prenatal toxicity*

No data were available to the Working Group.

(iv) *Genetic and related effects*

No data were available to the Working Group.

(b) *Humans*

(i) *Pharmacokinetics*

When prednimustine was given orally at doses up to 200 mg, no unchanged drug could be detected in blood (Newell *et al.*, 1979; Ehrsson *et al.*, 1983; Gaver *et al.*, 1983; Newell *et al.*, 1983; Oppitz *et al.*, 1989) or in urine (Kirdani *et al.*, 1978). When prednimustine was given orally at 20 mg, no chlorambucil or phenylacetic mustard was detected in the circulation (Newell *et al.*, 1979, 1983); however, when a higher dose (100 or 200 mg) was given, chlorambucil was detected in blood (Ehrsson *et al.*, 1983; Oppitz *et al.*, 1989). After a dose of 200 mg, phenylacetic mustard was also identified in the circulation (Oppitz *et al.*, 1989), and, after an oral dose of 100 mg, free prednisolone was detected (Sayed *et al.*, 1981). The concentrations of chlorambucil and its metabolites and of prednisolone detected in the circulation after an oral dose of prednimustine were lower than those after equimolar doses of chlorambucil and prednisolone given separately (Sayed *et al.*, 1981; Ehrsson *et al.*, 1983; Oppitz *et al.*, 1989). After a single oral dose of prednimustine, the peak values of chlorambucil and phenylacetic acid mustard in the serum were reached later and the disappearance half-time was longer than after administration of chlorambucil and prednisolone separately (Ehrsson *et al.*, 1983; Oppitz *et al.*, 1989). Three to six hours after a single oral dose of 40 mg/m^2 radiolabelled prednimustine, 50% of the plasma radioactivity could be extracted into organic solvents; the extractable proportion decreased with time and was <10% after 12-18 h. The terminal half-time of ten days for prednimustine-derived radioactivity in plasma could be attributed to these covalently bound metabolites (Gaver et al., 1983).

When a trace amount of double-labelled prednimustine (^{14}C in the bischloroethyl group, ^{3}H at positions 6 and 7 of the steroid part) was administered intravenously, ^{14}C and ^{3}H in the urine cochromatographed partially during the first hour after the injection but were fully separated thereafter, indicating that intact prednimustine is excreted in the urine only immediately after injection (Kirdani et al., 1978).

(ii) *Adverse effects*

Leukopenia and thrombocytopenia seem to be dose-dependent and may limit the dose that can be used. Nausea and vomiting are frequent (Könyves et al., 1975; Loeber et al., 1983; Rankin et al., 1987; Szanto et al., 1989).

(iii) *Effects on reproduction and prenatal toxicity*

No data were available to the Working Group.

(iv) *Genetic and related effects*

No adequate studies were available to the Working Group.

3.3 Case reports and epidemiological studies of carcinogenicity to humans

No data were available to the Working Group.

4. Summary of Data Reported and Evaluation

4.1 Exposure data

Prednimustine has been used as a cytostatic drug, mainly for the treatment of malignancies of lymphatic tissue.

4.2 Experimental carcinogenicity data

Prednimustine given by oral administration to rats induced a low but significant increase in the incidence of squamous-cell carcinomas of the external auditory canal.

4.3 Human carcinogenicity data

No data were available to the Working Group.

4.4 Other relevant data

In humans, prednimustine causes leukopenia and thrombocytopenia; in experimental animals, it causes lymphopenia. It is hydrolysed to chlorambucil and prednisolone *in vivo*. (See Appendix 1.)

4.5 Evaluation[1]

There is *inadequate evidence* for the carcinogenicity of prednimustine in experimental animals.

No data were available from studies in humans on the carcinogenicity of prednimustine.

Overall evaluation

Prednimustine *is not classifiable as to its carcinogenicity to humans (Group 3)*.

5. References

Berger, M.R., Habs, M. & Schmähl, D. (1985) Comparative carcinogenic activity of prednimustine, chlorambucil, prednisolone and chlorambucil plus prednisone in Sprague-Dawley rats. *Arch. Geschwulstforsch.*, 55, 429-442

Berger, M.R., Habs, M. & Schmähl, D. (1986) Long-term toxicology effects of prednimustine in comparison with chlorambucil, prednisolone, and chlorambucil plus prednisolone in Sprague-Dawley rats. *Semin. Oncol.*, 13 (Suppl. 1), 8-13

Ehrsson, H., Wallin, I., Nilsson, S.-O. & Johansson, B. (1983) Pharmacokinetics of chlorambucil in man after administration of the free drug and its prednisolone ester (Prednimustine, Leo 1031). *Eur. J. clin. Pharmacol.*, 24, 251-253

Fex, H.J., Hogberg, K.B. & Könyves, I. (1970) Corticosteroid p-bis(2-chloroethyl)-aminophenylcarboxylates as antitumor agents. *Chem. Abstr.*, 73, 391

Fredholm, B., Gunnarsson, K., Jensen, G. & Müntzing, J. (1978) Mammary tumour inhibition and subacute toxicity in rats of prednimustine and of its molecular components chlorambucil and prednisolone. *Acta pharmacol. toxicol.*, 42, 159-163

Gaver, R.C., Deeb, G., Pittman, K.A., Issel, B.F., Mittelman, A. & Smyth, R.D. (1983) Disposition of orally administered ^{14}C-prednimustine. *Cancer Chemother. Pharmacol.*, 11, 139-143

Gunnarsson, P.O., Johansson, S.-Å. & Svensson, L. (1984) Cholesterol ester formation by transesterification of chlorambucil: a novel pathway in drug metabolism. *Xenobiotica*, 14, 569-574

Harrap, K.R., Riches, P.G., Gilby, E.D., Sellwood, S.M., Wilkinson, R. & Könyves, I. (1977) Studies on the toxicity and antitumour activity of prednimustine, a prednisolone ester of chlorambucil. *Eur. J. Cancer*, 13, 873-881

Hartley-Asp, B., Gunnarsson, P.O. & Liljekvist, J. (1986) Cytotoxicity and metabolism of prednimustine, chlorambucil and prednisolone in a Chinese hamster cell line. *Cancer Chemother. Pharmacol.*, 16, 85-90

---

[1]For description of the italicized terms, see Preamble, pp. 26–29.

IARC (1975) *IARC Monographs on the Evaluation of Carcinogenic Risk of Chemicals to Man*, Vol. 9, *Some Aziridines, N-, S-, and O-Mustards and Selenium*, Lyon, pp. 125-134

IARC (1981) *IARC Monographs on the Evaluation of the Carcinogenic Risk of Chemicals to Humans*, Vol. 26, *Some Antineoplastic and Immunosuppressive Agents*, Lyon, pp. 115-136

IARC (1987) *IARC Monographs on the Evaluation of Carcinogenic Risks to Humans*, Suppl. 7, *Overall Evaluations of Carcinogenicity: An Updating of* IARC Monographs *Volumes 1 to 42*, Lyon, pp. 144-145

Jakhammer, T., Olsson, A. & Svenson, L. (1977) Mass fragmentographic determination of prednimustine and chlorambucil in plasma. *Acta pharm. suec.*, 14, 485-496

Kirdani, R.Y., Murphy, G.P. & Sandberg, A.A. (1978) Some metabolic aspects of a nitrogen mustard of prednisolone. *Oncology*, 35, 47-53

Könyves, I., Nordenskjöld, B., Plym Forshell, G., de Schryver, A. & Westerberg-Larsson, H. (1975) Preliminary clinical and absorption studies with prednimustine in patients with mammary carcinoma. *Eur. J. Cancer*, 11, 841-844

Loeber, J., Mouridsen, H.T., Christiansen, I.E., Dombernowsky, P., Mattsson, W. & Roerth, M. (1983) A phase III trial comparing prednimustine (LEO 1031) to chlorambucil plus prednisolone in advanced breast cancer. *Cancer*, 52, 1570-1576

Newell, D.R., Hart, L.I. & Harrap, K.R. (1979) Estimation of chlorambucil, phenyl acetic mustard and prednimustine in human plasma by high-performance liquid chromatography. *J. Chromatogr.*, 164, 114-119

Newell, D.R., Shepherd, C.R. & Harrap, K.R. (1981) The pharmacokinetics of prednimustine and chlorambucil in the rat. *Cancer Chemother. Pharmacol.*, 6, 85-91

Newell, D.R., Calvert, A.H., Harrap, K.R. & McElvain, T.J. (1983) Studies on the pharmacokinetics of chlorambucil and prednimustine in man. *Br. J. clin. Pharmacol.*, 15, 253-258

Oppitz, M.M., Musch, E., Malek, M., Rueb, H.P., von Unruh, G.E. & Loos, U. (1989) Studies on the pharmacokinetics of chlorambucil and prednimustine in patients using a new high-performance liquid chromatographic assay. *Cancer Chemother. Pharmacol.*, 23, 208-212

Peto, R., Pike, M.C., Day, N.E., Gray, R.G., Lee, P.N., Parish, S., Peto, J., Richards, S. & Wahrendorf, J. (1980) Guidelines for simple sensitive significance tests for carcinogenic effects in long-term animal experiments. In: *Long-term and Short-term Screening Assays for Carcinogens: A Critical Appraisal* (*IARC Monographs on the Evaluation of the Carcinogenic Risk of Chemicals to Humans*, Suppl. 2), Lyon, IARC, pp. 311-426

Rankin, E.M., Harvey, C., Knoght, R.K. & Rubens, R.D. (1987) Phase II trial of prednimustine as first-line chemotherapy in patients with advanced breast cancer. *Cancer Treat. Rep.*, 71, 1107-1108

Reynolds, J.E.F., ed. (1989) *Martindale. The Extra Pharmacopoeia*, 29th ed., London, The Pharmaceutical Press, pp. 647-648

Sayed, A., Van Hove, W. & Vermeulen, A. (1981) Prednisolone plasma levels after oral administration of prednimustine®. *Oncology*, 38, 351-355

Szanto, I., Fleischmann, T. & Eckhardt, S. (1989) Prednimustine treatment in malignant lymphomas. *Oncology*, 46, 205-207

Wilkinsson, R., Gunnarsson, P.O., Plym-Forshell, G., Renshaw, J. & Harrap, K.R. (1978) The hydrolysis of prednimustine by enzymes from normal and tumour tissues. In: Davis, W. & Harrap, K.R., eds, *Advances in Tumour Prevention, Detection and Characterization*, Amsterdam, Excepta Medica, pp. 260-273

Windholz, M., ed. (1983) *The Merck Index*, 10th ed., Rahway, NJ, Merck & Co., pp. 1109-1110

Workman, P., Oppitz, M., Donaldson, J. & Lee, F.Y.F. (1987) High-performance liquid chromatography of chlorambucil analogues. *J. Chromatogr.*, 422, 315-321

THIOTEPA

This substance was considered by previous working groups, in April 1975 and March 1987, under the title tris(1-aziridinyl)phosphine sulphide (IARC, 1975, 1987). Since that time, new data have become available, and these have been incorporated into the monograph and taken into consideration in the present evaluation.

1. Chemical and Physical Data

1.1 Synonyms

Chem. Abstr. Services Reg. No.: 52-24-4

Chem. Abstr. Name: Aziridine, 1,1′1″-phosphinothioylidynetris

Synonyms: NSC-6396; phosphoric tri(ethyleneamide); TESPA; thiophosphamide; thiotriethylenephosphoramide; triaziridinylphosphine sulfide; $N,N'N''$-tri-1,2-ethanediylphosphorothioic triamide; $N,N'N''$-tri-1,2-ethanediylthiophosphoramide; tri(ethyleneimino)thiophosphoramide; *meta*-triethylenethiophosphoramide; $N,N'N''$-triethylenethiophosphoramide; *meta*-tris(aziridin-1-yl)phosphine sulfide; triethylenethiophosphorotriamide; tris-(1-aziridinyl)phosphine sulfide; tris(1-aziridinyl)phosphine sulphide; tris-(ethyleneimino)thiophosphate; TSPA; WR-45312

1.2 Structural and molecular formulae and molecular weight

$C_6H_{12}N_3PS$ Mol. wt: 189.23

1.3 Chemical and physical properties of the pure substance

From Windholz (1983) and Barnhart (1989), unless otherwise indicated

(a) *Description*: White, crystalline solid; fine white crystalline flakes from pentane or ether

(b) *Melting-point*: 51.5°C; 52-57°C (Reynolds, 1989)

(c) *Solubility*: 1:8 in water; 19 g/100 ml water at 25°C; soluble in ethanol, diethyl ether, benzene and chloroform

(d) *Stability*: At temperatures above 2-8°C, thiotepa polymerizes and becomes inactive. The bulk drug is stable (up to two years) at 2-8°C, is unstable in acid and is sensitive to light. Aqueous solutions of 10 mg/ml are stable for five days at 2-8°C. Thiotepa is stable in alkaline solution.

1.4 Technical products and impurities

Trade names: Ledertepa, Onco Thiotepa, Tespamin; Thio-TEPA; Tifosyl

Thiotepa is available in vials containing 15 mg thiotepa, 80 mg sodium chloride and 50 mg sodium bicarbonate; when reconstituted, the pH is 7.6 (Barnhart, 1989).

2. Production, Occurrence, Use and Analysis

2.1 Production and occurrence

Thiotepa has been prepared by the addition of trichlorophosphine sulfide to aziridine and triethylamine (Kuh & Seeger, 1954) and by the addition of aziridine to phosphorus oxychloride (Bestian, 1950). Thiotepa is synthesized in Japan.

Thiotepa is not known to occur naturally.

2.2 Use

Thiotepa is a cytostatic agent. It has been used in the treatment of lymphomas and a variety of solid tumours, such as those of breast and ovary; it has also been used in cases of urinary bladder malignancies, meningeal carcinomatosis and various soft-tissue tumours (Wright *et al.*, 1958; Hollister & Coleman, 1980; Hagen *et al.*, 1987; Reynolds, 1989). Thiotepa is administered intramuscularly, intravenously and intrathecally; other parenteral routes (e.g., intratumoral injections) have also been used. It has been used as instillations in cases of urinary bladder carcinoma (Hollister & Coleman, 1980). Thiotepa has been used recently at high doses in combination chemotherapy with cyclophosphamide in patients with refractory malignancies treated with autologous bone transplantation (Henner *et al.*, 1987; Lazarus *et al.*, 1987; Williams *et al.*, 1987; Ackland *et al.*, 1988; Eder *et al.*, 1988; Williams *et al.*, 1989).

The initial dosage of thiotepa has generally been 5-40 mg [3-23 mg/m^2] at one- to four-weekly intervals (Wright *et al.*, 1958; Cohen *et al.*, 1986; Hagen *et al.*, 1987); doses up to 75 mg/m^2 have been used in children (Heideman *et al.*, 1989). The dosage is generally adjusted on the basis of changes in leukocyte counts. High-dose therapy has involved daily doses in excess of 1100 mg/m^2 (Lazarus *et al.*, 1987).

2.3 Analysis

Thiotepa has been determined in pharmaceutical preparations by colorimetric titration (US Pharmacopeial Convention, Inc., 1989) and in biological fluids by chromatography (Egorin *et al.*, 1985; Hagen *et al.*, 1985; McDermott *et al.*, 1985) and high-performance liquid chromatography (Sano *et al.*, 1988).

3. Biological Data Relevant to the Evaluation of Carcinogenic Risk to Humans

3.1 Carcinogenicity studies in animals

The carcinogenicity of antineoplastic drugs, including thiotepa, in animals has been reviewed (Berger, 1986).

(a) Intraperitoneal administration

Mouse: In a screening assay based on the accelerated induction of lung tumours in a strain highly susceptible to development of this neoplasm, three groups of ten male and ten female strain A/He mice, six to eight weeks of age, received intraperitoneal injections of thiotepa (purity, 95-99%) in 0.1 ml of purified tricaprylin three times per week for four weeks (total doses, 19, 47 and 94 mg/kg bw). A group of 80 males and 80 females received 24 injections of 0.1 ml of tricaprylin alone. All mice were killed 24 weeks after the first injection. The incidences of lung tumours in treated mice were 16/20, 10/20 and 11/20 in the groups receiving the high, mid and low doses, respectively, compared to 28% and 20% in male and female controls. The numbers of lung adenomas per mouse were significantly higher in the high-dose (1.50; $p < 0.001$) and mid-dose (0.74; $p < 0.05$) groups in comparison to male (0.24) and female (0.20) controls (Stoner *et al.*, 1973).

Groups of 35 male and 35 female B6C3F1 mice, six weeks of age, received intraperitoneal injections of thiotepa (purity, 98.0 ± 1.0%) at 1.15 or 2.3 mg/kg bw three times a week for up to 52 weeks and were observed for an additional 34 weeks. Two groups of 15 males and 15 females were untreated or received injections of phosphate-buffered saline vehicle only and served as matched controls. Pooled vehicle controls were also used, by adding 15 animals of each sex taken from a bioassay on another chemical. By 43 weeks, all high-dose females had died, and, by 56 weeks, all high-dose males had died. At weeks 86-87, 15/35 low-dose males, 17/35 low-dose females, 7/15 vehicle-control males and 12/15 vehicle-control females were still alive, at which time the study was terminated. Because of early deaths, statistical analyses were based only on time-adjusted incidences of tumours, eliminating those mice that had died before week 52. The incidences of malignant lymphoma and lymphocytic leukaemia combined were significantly greater in high-dose animals (32/32 females, 26/28 males; $p < 0.001$, Cochrane-Armitage test, Fisher's exact test) in comparison with vehicle and pooled controls (0/14 and 0/29 females; 1/8 and 1/18 males) (National Cancer Institute, 1978). [The Working Group noted the poor survival among the high-dose animals and that the study design involved controls pooled from different studies.]

Rat: Groups of 35-39 male and 31-35 female Sprague-Dawley rats, aged 35, 42 or 58 days, received intraperitoneal injections of thiotepa (purity, 98.0 ± 1.0%) at 0.7, 1.4 or 2.8 mg/kg bw three times a week for up to 52 weeks and were observed for additional periods of time. Two groups of ten males and ten females were untreated or received injections of buffered saline alone at 2.5 ml/kg bw and served as controls. A lower-dose group was started 69 weeks after the beginning of the original study, together with two additional control groups. Pooled vehicle controls were also used, by adding ten rats of each sex from bioassays on other chemicals. All high-dose males had died by week 19 and all high-dose females by week 21. Treatment of mid-dose groups was terminated at week 34, and animals were observed until weeks 78-81, at which time all of them had died. All other groups were observed until weeks 82-87. Because of early deaths, statistical analyses were based only on time-adjusted incidences of tumours, eliminating those rats that had died before week 52. Malignant lymphomas, lymphocytic leukaemia and granulocytic leukaemia were observed in 6/34 low-dose (pooled controls, 0/29; $p = 0.020$) and 6/16 mid-dose (pooled controls, 0/30; $p < 0.001$) males. Uterine adenocarcinomas were found in 7/21 mid-dose females (pooled controls, 0/28; $p = 0.001$) and 2/29 low-dose females but not in corresponding lower-dose controls. The incidence of adenocarcinomas of the mammary gland was significantly increased in mid-dose females (8/24; pooled controls, 1/28; $p = 0.006$), but this tumour was also observed in one lower-dose pooled control and in 3/10 lower-dose untreated controls. The incidences of neuroepitheliomas or nasal carcinomas (three in low-dose males, two in low-dose females, two in mid-dose females) were not statistically significantly increased, although they did not occur among corresponding controls or among the 388 pooled vehicle controls (National Cancer Institute, 1978). [The Working Group noted the high mortality among high- and mid-dose groups, which necessitated the later inclusion of the lower dose-treated group, and that the study design included controls pooled from different studies.]

(b) *Intravenous administration*

Rat: A group of 48 male BR46 rats, 100 days of age, received weekly intravenous injections of thiotepa [purity and vehicle unspecified] at 1 mg/kg bw for 52 weeks. A group of 89 untreated males served as controls. Of the treated animals, 30 were still alive when the first tumour appeared, compared to 65 controls. Malignant tumours developed in 9/30 treated animals (two sarcomas of the abdominal cavity, one lymphosarcoma, one 'myelosis', one seminoma, one fibrosarcoma and one haemangioendothelioma of the salivary gland, one mammary sarcoma, one phaeochromocytoma) and in 4/65 controls (three mammary sarcomas, one phaeochromocytoma) ($p < 0.01$). Benign tumours occurred in 5/30 treated and 3/65 control animals (Schmähl & Osswald, 1970; Schmähl, 1975). [The Working Group noted the short latency of tumour induction.]

3.2 Other relevant data

(a) *Experimental systems*

(i) *Absorption, distribution, excretion and metabolism*

One hour after intraperitoneal injection of thiotepa at 9.3 mg/kg bw into Sprague-Dawley rats, radioactivity was found in plasma (5.4%), peritoneal fluid (26%), urine (1.9%), kidney (0.7%), liver (3.8%), lung (0.6%) and muscle (25.9%) (Litterst *et al.*, 1982). In another study, 5 min after intravenous or intraarterial injection of labelled thiotepa in Sprague-Dawley rats, slightly higher levels of radioactivity were found in plasma, heart, kidneys and lungs, compared to other organs; 94-98% of radioactivity administered intravenously was excreted in urine within 8.5 h. Most of the urinary radioactivity was associated with unchanged thiotepa; tris(1-aziridinyl)phosphine oxide (tepa) was responsible for about 30% of the radioactivity (Boone *et al.*, 1962).

In female mongrel dogs, 75-85% of an intravenous dose of labelled thiotepa was recovered in the urine; only 0.2-0.3% unchanged thiotepa was found (Mellett *et al.*, 1962). Following intravenous (at 3 mg/kg bw) or oral (at 6 mg/kg bw) administration of thiotepa to dogs, about 13% of the dose was excreted as tepa. The plasma level of tepa was about 1.2 µg/ml 2 h after intravenous injection of thiotepa. The authors concluded that 50% of the administered thiotepa was absorbed (Mellett & Woods (1960).

A biexponential decline in thiotepa concentration in plasma was seen during the first hours after intravenous injection of thiotepa at 5 mg/kg bw in

Swiss-Webster mice. The half-time was 0.21 min for the first phase and 9.62 min for the second (Egorin et al., 1984).

After an intravenous dose of thiotepa to rhesus monkeys, equilibrium with plasma levels in lumbar and ventricular cerebrospinal fluid was obtained rapidly. After intravenous administration, the total body clearance of thiotepa was about 35 ml/min (Strong et al., 1986).

The major urinary metabolite in rats, rabbits and dogs following a single intravenous injection of ^{32}P-thiotepa was tepa, which is also an alkylating agent. Most of the radioactivity in mouse urine, however, was recovered as inorganic phosphate. In mice and rats, a small proportion of radioactivity was detected in most tissues nine days after an intravenous injection of thiotepa; higher levels were detected in blood of rats (Craig et al., 1959).

After addition of thiotepa to sera from patients and healthy individuals, about 10% was bound to protein (Hagen & Nilsen, 1987).

(ii) *Toxic effects*

The LD_{50} of thiotepa in rats was about 9.5 mg/kg bw by intravenous injection and about 8.8 mg after intraarterial injection (Boone et al., 1962). The LD_{50} in mice was 400 mg/kg bw 24 h after an intraperitoneal injection. The acute lethality after 1 h and 24 h was markedly increased by intraperitoneal injection of 60 mg/kg bw pentobarbital shortly after the thiotepa injection (Munson et al., 1974). Pretreatment of mice with 40 mg/kg bw SKF525A also enhanced the acute lethality of thiotepa (Mellett & Woods, 1960).

Thiotepa caused a dose-dependent inhibition of the growth of P388 murine leukaemia cells in culture (Miller et al., 1988).

(iii) *Effects on reproduction and prenatal toxicity*

When rats were given thiotepa at 4 mg/kg bw by intraperitoneal injection on gestation day 12, teratogenic effects occurred in the offspring (Murphy et al., 1958). [The Working Group noted that the details given in the paper were insufficient to assess the significance of the effect.]

In an extensive study of the effects of thiotepa in pregnant mice, Tanimura (1968) demonstrated both dose-related and time-related effects. Prenatal mortality was most pronounced following intraperitoneal injection of 5-10 mg/kg bw on days 7.5 and 8.5 of gestation, and fetal growth was suppressed after injection on days 10.5-12.5 of gestation. The lowest single teratogenic dose was shown to be 1.0 mg/kg bw; the dose that caused 100% incidence of malformed fetuses was 10.0 mg/kg. The malformations observed were exencephaly, spina bifida, cleft palate, kinky tail and digit alterations.

(iv) *Genetic and related effects*

Thiotepa was mutagenic to *Salmonella typhimurium* TA1535 (Benedict *et al.*, 1977a) and TA100 (Pak *et al.*, 1979) but gave contradictory results in TA98 (Bruce & Heddle, 1979; Pak *et al.*, 1979) in the absence of an exogenous metabolic system. Rats perfused with thiotepa produced urine that was mutagenic to *S. typhimurium* (Pak *et al.*, 1979). In the host-mediated assay in mice, thiotepa was mutagenic to *S. typhimurium* TA1535 (Arni *et al.*, 1977) and G46 (Devi & Reddy, 1980).

Thiotepa induced forward mutations to 8-azaguanine resistance in *Aspergillus nidulans* (Bignami *et al.*, 1982) and chromosomal aberrations (Kihlman, 1975; Sturelid & Kihlman, 1975; Popa *et al.*, 1976) and sister chromatid exchange (Kihlman, 1975) in root meristem cells of *Vicia faba*. It induced sex-linked recessive lethal mutations in *Drosophila melanogaster* (Lüers & Röhrborn, 1965; Fahmy & Fahmy, 1970) and dominant lethal mutations in *Aedes aegypti* (Rodriguez & Rodriguez, 1985).

Thiotepa induced unscheduled DNA synthesis in unstimulated human peripheral lymphocytes (Titenko, 1983). It induced mutations at the *hprt* locus in Chinese hamster V79 cells (Paschin & Kozachenko, 1982), and, in a host-mediated assay with mice and mouse lymphoma L5178Y cells, it induced resistance to thymidine and methotrexate (Lee, 1973).

Thiotepa induced sister chromatid exchange in mouse cells (Andersen, 1983), a cloned hamster cell line (Banerjee & Benedict, 1979), Chinese hamster cells (Chebotarev & Selezneva, 1979; Chebotarev *et al.*, 1980; Selezneva *et al.*, 1982) and peripheral lymphocytes of rhesus monkeys (Kuzin *et al.*, 1987) and humans (Littlefield *et al.*, 1979; Mourelatos, 1979; Chebotarev & Listopad, 1980; Listopad & Chebotarev, 1982; Shcheglova & Chebotarev, 1983a). It induced chromosomal aberrations in a cloned hamster cell line (Benedict *et al.*, 1977b), in Chinese hamster CHO cells (Maier & Schmid, 1976; Sturelid, 1976), in peripheral lymphocytes of rabbits (Bochkov *et al.*, 1982) and in human peripheral lymphocytes *in vitro* (Hampel *et al.*, 1966; Bochkov & Kuleshov, 1972; Bochkov *et al.*, 1972; Chebotarev, 1974; Kirichenko, 1974; Kirichenko & Chebotarev, 1976; Yakovenko & Nazarenko, 1977; Bochkov *et al.*, 1979; Wolff & Arutyunyan, 1979; Yakovenko & Kagramanyan, 1982; Shcheglova & Chebotarev, 1983a). Thiotepa induced morphological transformation of C3H/10T½ cells (Benedict *et al.*, 1977b).

Thiotepa induced DNA cross-links in chick embryos (McCann *et al.*, 1971). It induced sister chromatid exchange (Shcheglova & Chebotarev, 1983b) and chromosomal aberrations (Malashenko & Surkova, 1974a,b, 1975; Sram, 1976; Leonard *et al.*, 1979; Malashenko & Surkova, 1979; Shcheglova & Chebotarev, 1983b) in bone marrow of mice treated *in vivo*. It induced micronuclei in the bone marrow of rats (Setnikar *et al.*, 1976) and mice (Maier & Schmid, 1976; Ioan *et al.*, 1977; Bruce & Heddle, 1979; Leonard *et al.*, 1979) and chromosomal aberrations in peripheral lymphocytes of rabbits (Bochkov et al., 1982) and rhesus monkeys (Kuzin et al., 1987) in vivo. Treatment of pregnant mice with thiotepa led to chromosomal aberrations in embryonic liver cells (Korogodina et al., 1979; Korogodina & S'yakste, 1981).

Thiotepa induced dominant lethal mutations (Machemer & Hess, 1971; Epstein et al., 1972; Setnikar et al., 1976; Sram, 1976; Semenov & Malashenko, 1981) and chromosomal aberrations in spermatogonia (Malashenko & Beskova, 1988) and spermatocytes [one dose] (Devi & Reddy, 1980; Meistrich et al., 1982) in mice in vivo. Treatment of male mice with thiotepa led to chromosomal aberrations in preimplantation embryos [one dose] (Malashenko et al., 1978a; Semenov & Malashenko, 1979). Thiotepa also induced sperm abnormalities (Bruce & Heddle, 1979) and heritable translocations [one dose] (Malashenko & Surkova, 1974b; Semenov & Malashenko, 1977; Malashenko et al., 1978b; Malashenko & Goetz, 1981) in mice in vivo. Thiotepa produced liver protein variants in F_1 fetuses derived from treated male mice [one dose] (Paschin & Ambrossieva, 1984).

(b) *Humans*

(i) *Pharmacokinetics*

Because of acid instability, absorption of thiotepa after oral administration is erratic and incomplete (Mellet et al., 1962). After an intravenous bolus injection of thiotepa at 12 mg/m^2, a biexponential disappearance from the plasma was observed; the second-phase half-time was 73.7 min (Egorin et al., 1985). Disappearance half-times of 1.3-2.1 h were reported in further studies (McDermott et al., 1985; Cohen et al., 1986; Hagen et al., 1987; Henner et al., 1987; Hagen et al., 1988; Heideman et al., 1989) after intravenous or intramuscular administration. At dose levels in excess of 25 mg/m^2 (Heideman et al., 1989), 180 mg/m^2 (Henner et al., 1987) and 4.8 mg/kg (Ackland et al., 1988), the plasma clearance of thiotepa was reported to decline with increasing dose. However, in one study with high doses (45-1215 mg/m^2), no dose-dependence of kinetics was reported (Lazarus et al., 1987). The volume of distribution of thiotepa has been reported to be approximately 50 l (Cohen et al., 1986; Henner et al., 1987; Hagen et al., 1988; Heidemann et al., 1989).

After an intravenous injection of thiotepa in paediatric patients, the cerebrospinal fluid:plasma ratio of thiotepa was 0.92 (Heideman et al., 1989). After intraventricular administration of thiotepa, the ratio of thiotepa concentrations in cerebral ventricular fluid:plasma was almost 1000 (Strong et al., 1986); in another, similar study, it was approximately 200 (Grochow et al., 1982). The urinary excretion of unchanged thiotepa is complete usually within 8 h of the injection, and less than 1.5% of the dose is excreted in the urine unchanged (Egorin et al., 1985; Hagen et al., 1985; Cohen et al., 1986; Hagen et al., 1987). Five minutes after an intravenous injection of thiotepa, tepa was observed in the blood; after 120 min, the concentration of tepa in the blood was higher than that of thiotepa. The proportion of thiotepa in urine was 1.5%, and that of tepa was 4.2%; other alkylating metabolites represented another 23.5% of the dose administered (Cohen *et al.*, 1986).

(ii) *Adverse effects*

The toxic effect of thiotepa that limits the dose that can be given is myelosuppression, characterized by granulocytopenia and thrombocytopenia; disturbances in hepatic and renal function, neurotoxicity, nausea and vomiting were uncommon at dose levels of approximately 75 mg/m^2 or less (Wright *et al.*, 1958; Heideman *et al.*, 1989). In high-dose therapy with autologous bone-marrow transplantantion, central nervous system disturbances, hepatic damage, infections, nausea, vomiting, diarrhoea, mucositis, skin rashes, haemorrhagic cystitis and cardiomyopathy may be severe (Lazarus *et al.*, 1987; Williams *et al.*, 1987, 1989). Severe myelosuppression has also been described after intravesicular instillations of thiotepa (Bruce & Edgcomb, 1967; Watkins *et al.*, 1967; Hollister & Coleman, 1980).

(iii) *Effects on reproduction and prenatal toxicity*

Use of thiotepa in the third trimester of pregnancy had no adverse effect on the progeny (Nicholson, 1968; Sweet & Kinzie, 1976). In a report of the effects of treatment of women with stage-II and stage-III Hodgkin's disease with radiotherapy and chemotherapy with TVPP (thiotepa, vinblastine, vincristine, procarbazine and prednisone), menstrual function ceased in two of four women aged 35-44 years but continued in all 30 women under 35 years of age. Ten of the women had a total of 12 babies, all with normal development (Lacher & Toner, 1986).

As reported in an abstract, transient azoospermia occurred in a man treated with thiotepa; the effect was reversed when the dose interval was increased from monthly to three-monthly dosing (Bayar *et al.* 1978).

(iv) *Genetic and related effects*

Five patients who received a total dose of thiotepa at 40-100 mg had 9.5 $\pm$ 1.07% aberrant cells in peripheral lymphocytes 24 h after the last treatment, compared with 1.4 $\pm$ 0.1% in a control group (Selezneva & Korman, 1973).

3.3 Case reports and epidemiological studies of carcinogenicity to humans

Many case reports have been made of cancer occurring following treatment with thiotepa (IARC, 1975; Nakanuma *et al.*, 1976; Anon., 1977; Hollister & Coleman, 1980; Sheibani *et al.*, 1980; Easton & Poon, 1983; Silberberg & Zarrabi,

1987). All report the occurrence of nonlymphocytic leukaemia, and usually thiotepa was the only chemotherapeutic agent administered.

No increased risk of second malignancies was found among 470 patients with colorectal cancer randomized to low-dose (four doses of 0.2 mg/kg bw) adjuvant therapy with thiotepa, followed for 3102 person-years (30 second noncolorectal malignancies observed, 31.4 expected; Boice et al., 1980). No increased risk of second malignancies was found among 90 patients with breast cancer randomized to adjuvant therapy with thiotepa for one year (at 0.8 mg/kg bw in divided doses followed by 0.2 mg/kg bw weekly maintenance); after an average follow-up of approximately five years, five nonskin, nonbreast cancers had occurred in 5819 person-years among 90 treated subjects compared with six in 4746 person-years among the 77 nonexposed patients (Kardinal & Donegan, 1980). [The Working Group considered these two studies to be too small to provide useful information.]

Kaldor et al. (1990) compared 114 cases of leukaemia that developed in patients previously diagnosed with ovarian cancer, with 342 controls with ovarian cancer who had survived as long as the cases and who were matched by age and year of diagnosis of ovarian cancer. Chemotherapy (without radiotherapy) was associated with a relative risk of 12 (95% confidence interval, 4.4-32) compared to treatment by surgery only. For nine cases and 11 controls, the only chemotherapy was thiotepa; 21 cases and 187 controls had had no chemotherapy. The matched relative risks were 8.3 and 9.7 in a lower- and a higher-dose group, and these were significantly different from 1.0 ($p < 0.01$). In the same study, four other alkylating agents known to be carcinogenic (melphalan, chlorambucil, cyclophosphamide and treosulphan; see IARC, 1987) were independently associated with significantly increased risks for leukaemia.

4. Summary of Data Reported and Evaluation

4.1 Exposure data

Thiotepa is a cytostatic agent that has been used in the treatment of malignant lymphomas and solid tumours, in a wide range of doses.

4.2 Experimental carcinogenicity data

Thiotepa was tested for carcinogenicity by intraperitoneal administration in mice and rats and by intravenous administration in male rats. In mice, it induced an increased incidence of lung tumours and lymphoproliferative malignancies in mice of each sex. In rats, intraperitoneal administration induced an increased incidence of lymphoproliferative malignancies in males and of uterine adenocarcinomas and mammary carcinomas in females. Intravenous administration to male rats induced tumours at a variety of sites.

4.3 Human carcinogenicity data

Several cases of leukaemia following treatment with thiotepa alone have been reported. One case-control study has shown a strong association between risk for leukaemia and treatment with thiotepa.

4.4 Other relevant data

In one study, there was no evidence that thiotepa therapy adversely affected subsequent fertility in women. Thiotepa is embryotoxic to mice and rats, and embryo- and fetolethality and gross structural abnormalities were induced during organogenesis after single intraperitoneal injections.

Thiotepa is converted to alkylating metabolites *in vivo*. It suppresses the bone marrow in humans.

In one study, increased frequencies of chromosomal aberrations were observed in peripheral lymphocytes of patients receiving thiotepa.

Thiotepa induced chromosomal aberrations in germ cells, sperm abnormalities and dominant lethal mutation in mice *in vivo*. It induced micronuclei in the bone marrow of rats and mice, chromosomal aberrations in bone-marrow cells and liver cells of mice and in peripheral lymphocytes of rabbits and rhesus monkeys and sister chromatid exchange in bone-marrow cells of mice *in vivo*. Thiotepa induced DNA damage in chick embryos. It induced chromosomal aberrations in cloned hamster cells, in Chinese hamster cells and in human cells, sister chromatid exchange in human, mouse, Chinese hamster and rabbit cells, gene mutations in Chinese hamster cells and unscheduled DNA synthesis in human peripheral lymphocytes *in vitro*. It induced cell transformation in mouse cells. Thiotepa induced sex-linked recessive lethal mutations in *Drosophila* and sister chromatid exchange and chromosomal aberrations in *Vicia faba*. It induced gene mutations in *Aspergillus nidulans* and *Salmonella typhimurium*. (See Appendix 1.)

4.5 Evaluation[1]

There is *sufficient evidence* for the carcinogenicity of thiotepa in humans.

There is *sufficient evidence* for the carcinogenicity of thiotepa in experimental animals.

---

[1]For description of the italicized terms, see Preamble, pp. 26–29.

Overall evaluation

Thiotepa *is carcinogenic to humans (Group 1)*.

5. References

Ackland, S.P., Choi, K.E., Ratain, M.J., Egorin, M.J., Williams, S.F., Sinkule, J.A. & Bitran, J.D. (1988) Human plasma pharmacokinetics of thiotepa following administration of high-dose thiotepa and cyclophosphamide. *J. clin. Oncol.*, 6, 1192-1196

Andersen, O. (1983) Effects of coal combustion products and metal compounds on sister chromatid exchange (SCE) in a macrophagelike cell line. *Environ. Health Perspect.*, 47, 239-253

Anon. (1977) Case records of the Massachusetts General Hospital. Case 28—1977. *New Engl. J. Med.*, 297, 102-106

Arni, P., Mantel, T., Deparade, E. & Müller, D. (1977) Intrasanguine host-mediated assay with *Salmonella typhimurium*. *Mutat. Res.*, 45, 291-307

Banerjee, A. & Benedict, W.F. (1979) Production of sister chromatid exchanges by various cancer chemotherapeutic agents. *Cancer Res.*, 39, 797-799

Barnhart, E. (1989) *Physician's Desk Reference*, 43rd ed., Oradell, NJ, Medical Economics, p. 1152

Bayar, H., Danielli, L. & Glazerman, M. (1978) Transient azoospermia in a male treated with thiotepa. *Arch. Androl.*, 1, 367

Benedict, W.F., Baker, M.S., Haroun, L., Choi, E. & Ames, B.N. (1977a) Mutagenicity of cancer chemotherapeutic agents in the *Salmonella*/microsome test. *Cancer Res.*, 37, 2209-2213

Benedict, W.F., Banerjee, A., Gardner, A. & Jones, P.A. (1977b) Induction of morphological transformation in mouse C3H10T½ clone 8 cells and chromosomal damage in hamster A(T1)Cl-3 cells by cancer chemotherapeutic agents. *Cancer Res.*, 37, 2202-2208

Berger, M.R. (1986) Carcinogenicity of alkylating cytostatic drugs in animals. In: Schmähl, D. & Kaldor, J.M., eds, *Carcinogenicity of Alkylating Cytostatic Drugs* (IARC Scientific Publications No. 78), Lyon, IARC, pp. 161-176

Bestian, H. (1950) Chemistry and pharmacology of a new antihistamine. *Med. Monatsschr.*, 4, 258-260

Bignami, M., Carere, A., Conti, G., Conti, L., Crebelli, R. & Fabrizi, M. (1982) Evaluation of 2 different genetic markers for the detection of frameshift and missense mutagens in *A. nidulans*. *Mutat. Res.*, 97, 293-302

Bochkov, N.P. & Kuleshov, N.P. (1972) Age sensitivity of human chromosomes to alkylating agents. *Mutat. Res.*, 14, 345-353

Bochkov, N.P., Yakovenko, K.N., Chebotarev, A.N., Funes Cravioto, F. & Zhurkov, V.S. (1972) Distribution of defective chromosomes in human cells after treatment with chemical mutagens *in vitro* and *in vivo*. *Sov. Genet.*, 8, 1595-1601

Bochkov, N.P., Yakovenko, K.N. & Nazarenko, S.A. (1979) Combined effect of alkylating compounds on human chromosomes. *Sov. Genet.*, *15*, 109-116

Bochkov, N.P., Stukalov, S.V. & Chebotarev, A.N. (1982) Comparison of the frequency of chromosomal aberrations induced by thiophosphamide in rabbit lymphocytes *in vitro* and *in vivo*. *Bull. exp. Biol. Med.*, *94*, 1118-1121

Boice, J.D., Greene, M.H., Keehn, R.J., Higgins, G.A. & Fraumeni, J.F., Jr (1980) Late effects of low-dose adjuvant chemotherapy in colorectal cancer. *J. natl Cancer Inst.*, *64*, 501-511

Boone, I.U., Rogers, B.S. & Williams, D.L. (1962) Toxicity, metabolism, and tissue distribution of carbon^{14}-labeled N,N′,N″-triethylenethiophosphoramide (Thio-TEPA) in rats. *Toxicol. appl. Pharmacol.*, *4*, 344-353

Bruce, D.W. & Edgcomb, J.H. (1967) Pancytopenia and generalized sepsis folowing treatment of cancer of the bladder with instillations of triethylene thiophosphoramide. *Urology*, *97*, 482-485

Bruce, W.R. & Heddle, J.A. (1979) The mutagenic activity of 61 agents as determined by the micronucleus, *Salmonella*, and sperm abnormality assays. *Can. J. genet. Cytol.*, *21*, 319-334

Chebotarev, A.N. (1974) Investigation of the temperature dependence of the cytogenetic action of thiophosphamide in various concentrations on human lymphocytes. *Sov. Genet.*, *10*, 1178-1182

Chebotarev, A.N. & Listopad, G.G. (1980) Effect of exposure time to BUdR on the number of sister chromatid exchanges in human cells. *Dokl. biol. Sci.*, *252*, 238-240

Chebotarev, A.N. & Selezneva, T.G. (1979) Induction of sister chromatid exchanges by thiophosphamide at different phases of the cell cycle of a culture of Chinese hamster cells. *Sov. Genet.*, *15*, 1235-1239

Chebotarev, A.N., Selezneva, T.G. & Ressner, P. (1980) Frequency of sister chromatid exchanges in the cell culture of Chinese hamster with prolonged action of thiophosphamide. *Sov. Genet.*, *16*, 1384-1388

Cohen, B.E., Egorin, M.J., Kohlhepp, E.A., Alsner, J. & Gutierrez, P.L. (1986) Human plasma pharmacokinetics and urinary excretion of thiotepa and its metabolites. *Cancer Treat. Rep.*, *70*, 859-864

Craig, A.W., Fox, B.W. & Jackson, H. (1959) Metabolic studies of ^{32}P-labelled triethylenethiophosphoramide. *Biochem. Pharmacol.*, *3*, 42-50

Devi, K.R. & Reddy, P.P. (1980) Evaluation of thiotepa for genetic damage in mice. *Indian J. exp. Biol.*, *20*, 866-867

Easton, D.J. & Poon, M.A. (1983) Acute nonlymphocytic leukaemia following bladder instillations with thiotepa. *Can. med. Assoc. J.*, *129*, 578-579

Eder, J.P., Antman, K., Elias, A., Shea, T.C., Teicher, B., Henner, W.D., Schryber, S.M., Holden, S., Finberg, R., Chritchlow, J., Flaherty, M., Mick, R., Schnipper, L.E. & Frei, E., III (1988) Cyclophosphamide and thiotepa with autologous bone marrow transplantation in patients with solid tumors. *J. natl Cancer Inst.*, *80*, 1221-1226

Egorin, M.J., Akman, S.R. & Gutierrez, L. (1984) Plasma pharmacokinetics and tissue distribution of thiotepa in mice. *Cancer Treat. Rep.*, *68*, 1265-1268

Egorin, M.J., Cohen, B.E., Kohlhepp, E. & Gutierrez, P. (1985) Gas-liquid chromatographic analysis of N,N',N''-triethylene thiophosporamide and N,N',N''-triethylene phosphoramide in biological samples. *J. Chromatogr., 343*, 196-202

Epstein, S.S., Arnold, E., Andrea, J., Bass, W. & Bishop, Y. (1972) Detection of chemical mutagens by the dominant lethal assay in the mouse. *Toxicol. appl. Pharmacol., 23*, 288-325

Fahmy, O.G. & Fahmy, M.J. (1970) Gene elimination in carcinogenesis: reinterpretation of the somatic mutation theory. *Cancer Res., 30*, 195-205

Grochow, L.B., Grossman, S., Garrett, S., Murray, K., Trump, M. & Colvin, M. (1982) Pharmacokinetics of intraventricular thio-tepa (TT) in patients with meningeal carcinomatosis. *Proc. Am. Soc. clin. Oncol., 1*, 19

Hagen, B. & Nilsen, O.G. (1987) The binding of thio-TEPA in human serum and to isolated serum protein fractions. *Cancer Chemother. Pharmacol., 20*, 319-323

Hagen, B., Walseth, F., Walstad, R.A. & Iversen, T. (1985) Gas chromatographic assay of triethylenethiophosphoramide in serum and urine. *J. Chromatogr., 345*, 173-177

Hagen, B., Walseth, F., Walstad, R.A., Iversen, T. & Nilsen, O.G. (1987) Single and repeated dose pharmacokinetics of thio-TEPA in patients treated for ovarian carcinoma. *Cancer Chemother. Pharmacol., 19*, 143-148

Hagen, B., Walstad, R.A. & Nilsen, O.G. (1988) Pharmacokinetics of thio-TEPA at two different doses. *Cancer Chemother. Pharmacol., 22*, 356-358

Hampel, K.E., Kober, B., Rösch, D., Gerhartz, J. & Meinig, K.-H. (1966) The action of cytostatic agents on the chromosomes of human leukocytes in vitro. *Blood, 27*, 816-823

Heideman, R.L., Cole, D.E., Balis, F., Sato, J., Reaman, G.H., Packer, R.J., Singher, L.J., Ettinger, L.J., Gillespie, A., Sam. J. & Poplack, D.G. (1989) Phase I and pharmacokinetic evaluation of thiotepa in the cerebrospinal fluid and plasma of pediatric patients: evidence for dose-dependent plamsa clearance of thiotepa. *Cancer Res., 49*, 736-741

Henner, W.D., Shea, T.C., Furiong, E.A., Flaherty, M.D., Eder, J.P., Elias, A., Begg, C. & Antman, K. (1987) Pharmacokinetics of continuous-infusion high-dose thiotepa. *Cancer Treat. Rep., 71*, 1043-1047

Hollister, D., Jr & Coleman, M. (1980) Hematologic effects of intravesicular thiotepa therapy for bladder carcinoma. *J. Am. med. Assoc., 18*, 2065-2067

IARC (1975) *IARC Monographs on the Evaluation of Carcinogenic Risk of Chemicals to Man*, Vol. 9, *Some aziridines, N-, S- and O-Mustards and Selenium*, Lyon, pp. 75-94

IARC (1987) *IARC Monographs on the Evaluation of Carcinogenic Risks to Humans*, Suppl. 7, *Overall Evaluation of Carcinogenicity: An Updating of* IARC Monographs *Volumes 1 to 42*, Lyon, pp. 368-369

Ioan, D., Petrescu, M. & Maximilian, C. (1977) The mutagenic effect of ^{131}I and of two cytostatics revealed by the micronucleus test (MT). *Rev. Roum. med.-Endocrinol., 15*, 119-122

Kaldor, J.M., Day, N.E., Petersson, F., Clarke, A., Pedersen, D., Mehnert, W., Bell, J., Høst, H., Prior, P., Karjalainen, S., Neal, F., Koch, M., Band, P., Choi, W., Kirn, V.P., Arslan, A., Zarén, B., Belch, A.R., Storm, H., Kittelmann, B., Fraser, P. & Stovall, P. (1990) Leukemia following chemotherapy for ovarian cancer. *New Engl. J. Med.*, *322*, 1-6

Kardinal, C.G. & Donegan, W.L. (1980) Second cancers after prolonged adjuvant Thiotepa for operable carcinoma of the breast. *Cancer*, *45*, 2042-2046

Kihlman, B.A. (1975) Sister chromatid exchanges in *Vicia faba*. II. Effects of thiotepa, caffeine and 8-ethoxycaffeine on the frequency of SCE's. *Chromosoma*, *51*, 11-18

Kirichenko, O.P. (1974) Dependence of the cytogenetic action of thiophosphamide on the duration of treatment of human cells. *Sov. Genet.*, *10*, 1172-1175

Kirichenko, O.P. & Chebotarev, A.N. (1976) Dependence of the cytogenetic action of various thiophosphamide and phosphemid concentrations on the time of contact with human lymphocytes. *Sov. Genet.*, *12*, 759-765

Korogodina, Yu.V. & Lil'p I.G. (1978) Mutability of somatic cells of mice of different lines. Communication II. *Cytol. Genet.*, *12*, 35-37

Korogodina, Yu.V. & S'yakste, T.G. (1981) Mice of the 101/H line as a possible model of human diseases with chromosomal instability. *Sov. Genet.*, *17*, 634-637

Korogodina, Yu.V., Gordeeva, E.V. & Lil'p, I.G. (1979) Chromosomal aberrations in embryonic liver and bone marrow cells of A/He and C57BL/6 mice induced by thiotepa. *Bull. exp. Biol. Med.*, *88*, 1182-1184

Kuh, E. & Seeger, D.R. (1954) Thiophosphoric acid derivatives. US Patent 2,670,347, 23 February, to American Cyanamid Co.

Kuzin, S.M., Stukalov, S.V. & Popandopulo, P.G. (1987) Quantitative comparison of the cytogenetic effect of thiophosphamide on monkey lymphocytes in vivo and in vitro. *Bull. exp. Biol. Med.*, *103*, 394-396

Lacher, M.J. & Toner, K. (1986) Pregnancies and menstrual function before and after combined radiation (RT) and chemotherapy (TVPP) for Hodgkin's disease. *Cancer Invest.*, *4*, 93-100

Lazarus, H.M., Reed, M.D., Spitzer, T.R., Rabaa, M.S. & Blumer, J.L. (1987) High-dose iv thiotepa and cryopreserved autologous bone marrow transplantation for therapy of refractory cancer. *Cancer Treat. Rep.*, *71*, 689-695

Lee, S.Y. (1973) Current status of the host-mediated L5178Y system for detecting chemical mutagens. *Environ. Health Perspect.*, *6*, 145-149

Leonard, A., Poncelet, F., Grutman, G., Carbonelle, E. & Fabry, L. (1979) Mutagenicity tests with griseofulvin. *Mutat. Res.*, *68*, 225-234

Listopad, G.G. & Chebotarev, A.N. (1982) Comparative effectiveness of the induction of sister chromatid exchanges by ethylenimine derivatives in a human leukocyte culture. *Cytol. Genet.*, *16*, 40-44

Litterst, C.L., Torres, I.J., Arnold, S., McGunagle, D., Furner, R., Sikic, B.I. & Guarino, A.M. (1982) Absorption of antineoplastic drugs following large-volume i.p. administration to rats. *Cancer Treat. Rep.*, *66*, 147-155

Littlefield, L.G., Colyer, S.P., Sayer, A.M. & Dufrain, R.J. (1979) Sister-chromatid exchanges in human lymphocytes exposed during G_0 to four classes of DNA-damaging chemicals. *Mutat. Res.*, 67, 259-269

Lüers, H. & Röhrborn, G. (1965) Chemische Konstitution und mutagene Wirkung. [Chemical structure and mutagenicity (Ger.).] *Mutat. Res.*, 2, 29-44

Machemer, L. & Hess, R. (1971) Comparative dominant lethal studies with phenylbutazone, thio-tepa and MMS in the mouse. *Experientia*, 27, 1050-1052

Maier, P. & Schmid, W. (1976) Ten model mutagens evaluated by the micronucleus test. *Mutat. Res.*, 40, 325-338

Malashenko, A.M. & Beskova, T.B. (1988) Induction of chromosome defects by thiophosphamide in spermatogonia of mice of inbred lines 101HY, PTS/Y, and CBA/LacY. *Sov. Genet.*, 24, 320-325

Malashenko, A.M. & Goetz, P. (1981) Cytogenetic analysis of translocations induced by the chemical mutagen thio-tepa in spermatids of male mice. *Folia biol.*, 27, 178-185

Malashenko, A.M. & Surkova, N.I. (1974a) The mutagenic effect of thio-tepa in laboratory mice. Communication I. Chromosome aberrations in somatic and germ cells of male mice. *Sov. Genet.*, 10, 51-58

Malashenko, A.M. & Surkova, N.I. (1974b) The mutagenic effect of thio-tepa in laboratory mice. Communication III. Comparison of the effects of different doses in the germ and somatic cells of male mice. *Sov. Genet.*, 10, 1004-1008

Malashenko, A.M. & Surkova, N.I. (1975) The mutagenic effect of thio-tepa in laboratory mice. Communication V. Influence of the genotype of females in the realization of dominant lethal mutations induced in spermatids of males. *Sov. Genet.*, 11, 210-214

Malashenko, A.M. & Surkova, N.I. (1979) A new line of WR mice, highly sensitive to the cytogenetic effect of thioTEPA. *Cytol. Genet.*, 13, 45-48

Malashenko, A.M., Semenov, K.K., Selezneva, G.P. & Surkova, N.I. (1978a) Investigation of the mutagenic effect of chemical compounds on laboratory mice. *Sov. Genet.*, 14, 35-42

Malashenko, A.M., Semenov, K.K., Selezneva, G.P. & Surkova, N.I. (1978b) Studies of mutagenic effect of chemical compounds in laboratory mice. *Genetika*, 14, 52-61

McCann, J.J., Lo, T.M. & Webster, D.A. (1971) Cross-linking of DNA by alkylating agents and effects on DNA function in the chick embryo. *Cancer Res.*, 31, 1573-1579

McDermott, B.J., Double, J.A., Bibby, M.C., Wilman, D.E.V., Loadman, P.M. & Turner, R.L. (1985) Gas chromatographic analysis of triethylenethiophosphoramide and triethylenephosphoramide in biological specimens. *J. Chromatogr.*, 338, 335-345

Meistrich, M.L., Finch, M., da Cunha, M.F., Hacker, U. & Au, W.W. (1982) Damaging effects of fourteen chemotherapeutic drugs on mouse testis cells. *Cancer Res.*, 42, 122-131

Mellett, L.B. & Woods, L.A. (1960) The comparative physiological disposition of thio-TEPA and TEPA in the dog. *Cancer Res.*, 20, 524-532

Mellet, I.B., Hodgson, P.E. & Woods, L.S. (1962) Absorption and fate of C14-labeled N,N',N"-triethylenethiophosphoramide (thio-TEPA) in humans and dogs. *J. Lab. clin. Med.*, 60, 818-825

Miller, B., Tenenholz, T., Egorin, M.J., Sosnovsky, G., Rao, N.U.M. & Gutierrez, P.L. (1988) Cellular pharmacology of N,N',N"-triethylenethiophosphoramide. *Cancer Lett.*, *41*, 157-168

Mourelatos, D.C. (1979) Enhancement by caffeine of sister-chromatid exchange frequency induced by antineoplastic agents in human lymphocytes. *Experientia*, *35*, 822-823

Munson, A.E., Rose, W.C. & Bradley, S.G. (1974) Synergistic lethal action of alkylating agents and sodium pentobarbital in the mouse. *Pharmacology*, *11*, 231-240

Murphy, M.L., Moro del, A. & Lacon, C. (1958) The comparative effects of five polyfunctional alkylating agents on the rat fetus, with additional notes on the chick embryo. *Ann. N.Y. Acad. Sci.*, *68*, 763-782

Nakanuma, Y., Saiki, S., Hisazumi, H. & Matsubara, F. (1976) An autopsy case of atypical leukemia occurred during thiotepa administration. *Jpn. J. clin. Hematol.*, *20*, 75-81

National Cancer Institute (1978) *Bioassay of Thiotepa for Possible Carcinogenicity* (Tech. Rep. Ser. No. 58; DHEW Publ. No. (NIH) 78-1308), Washington DC, US Government Printing Office

Nicholson, H.O. (1968) Cytotoxic drugs in pregnancy. *J. Obstet. Gynaecol. Br. Commonwealth.*, *75*, 307-312

Pak, K., Iwasaki, T., Miyakawa, M. & Yoshida, O. (1979) The mutagenic activity of anti-cancer drugs and the urine of rats given these drugs. *Urol. Res.*, *7*, 119-124

Paschin, Y.V. & Ambrossieva, E.D. (1984) Electrophoretic enzyme variants detected in F1 progeny of males treated by alkylating mutagen. *Mutat. Res.*, *125*, 71-74

Paschin, Y.V. & Kozachenko, V.I. (1982) The modifying effect of hexavalent chromate on the mutagenic activity of thio-tepa. *Mutat. Res.*, *103*, 367-370

Popa, N.E., Atramentova, L.A. & Shakhbazov, V.G. (1976) Investigation of the cytogenetic and electrophoretic effect in the combined action of thiotepa and β-indoleacetic acid on *Vicia faba* L. seedlings. *Cytol. Genet.*, *10*, 11-13

Reynolds, J.E.F., ed. (1989) *Martindale. The Extra Pharmacopoeia*, London, The Pharmaceutical Press, pp. 652-653

Rodriguez, P.H. & Rodriguez, K.A. (1985) Dominant lethal effects of thiotepa in male *Aedes aegypti* (diptera: culicidae). *J. med. Entomol.*, *22*, 343-344

Sano, A., Matsutani, S. & Takitani, S. (1988) High-performance liquid chromatography of the antitumour agent triethylenethiophosphoramide and its metabolite triethylenephosphoramide with sodium sulphide, taurine and o-phthalaldehyde as per-column fluorescent derivatization reagents. *J. Chromatogr.*, *458*, 295-301

Schmähl, D. (1975) Experimental investigations with anti-cancer drugs for carcinogenicity with special reference to immunedepression. In: Grundmann, E. & Gross, R., eds, *The Ambivalence of Cytostatic Therapy*, Berlin, Springer, pp. 18-28

Schmähl, D. & Osswald, H., (1970) Experimental studies on carcinogenic effects of anticancer chemotherapeutics and immunosuppressives. *Arzneimittel.-forsch.*, *20*, 1461-1467

Selezneva, T.G. & Korman, N.P. (1973) Analysis of chromosomes of somatic cells in patients treated with antitumor drugs. *Sov. Genet.*, *9*, 1575-1579

Selezneva, T.G., Shatalina, I. & Chebotarev, A.N. (1982) Correlation to the efficiency of the induction of sister chromatid exchanges with the chemical structure of the mutagen. *Sov. Genet.*, *18*, 210-215

Semenov, K.K. & Malashenko, A.M. (1977) The search for translocation-heterozygous female mice among the progeny of males treated with chemical mutagen (thio-tepa). *Cytol. Genet.*, *11*, 59-61

Semenov, K.K. & Malashenko, A.M. (1979) Assessment of the contribution of thiophosphamide-induced chromosomal aberrations to preimplantation embryonic mortality in mice. *Bull. exp. Biol. Med.*, *88*, 1074-1076

Semenov, K.K. & Malashenko, A.M. (1981) Appearance of dominant lethal mutations during early embryogenesis of the mouse. *Sov. Genet.*, *17*, 309-313

Setnikar, I., Magistretti, M.J. & Veronese, M. (1976) Mutagenicity studies on nifurpipone and nitrofurantoin. *Proc. Eur. Soc. Toxicol.*, *17*, 405-412

Shcheglova, E.G. & Chebotarev, A.N. (1983a) Comparison of level of sister chromatid exchanges and chromosomal aberrations induced by chemical mutagens *in vitro*. *Bull. exp. Biol. Med.*, *96*, 1604-1606

Shcheglova, E.G. & Chebotarev, A.N. (1983b) Correlation between level of sister chromatid exchanges and chromosomal aberrations induced by chemical mutagens *in vivo*. *Bull. exp. Biol. Med.*, *96*, 1734-1736

Sheibani, K., Bukowski, R.M., Tubbs, R.R., Savage, R.A., Sebek, B.A. & Hoffman, G.C. (1980) Acute nonlymphocytic leukemia in patients receiving chemotherapy for nonmalignant diseases. *Hum. Pathol.*, *11*, 175-179

Silberberg, J.M. & Zarrabi, M.H. (1987) Acute nonlymphocytic leukemia after thiotepa instillation into the bladder: report of 2 cases and review of the literature. *J. Urol.*, *138*, 402-403

Sram, R.J. (1976) Relationship between acute and chronic exposures in mutagenicity studies in mice. *Mutat. Res.*, *41*, 25-42

Stoner, G.D., Shimkin, M.B., Kniazeff, A.J., Weisburger, J.H., Weisburger, E.K. & Gori, G.B. (1973) Test for carcinogenicity of food additives and chemotherapeutic agents by the pulmonary tumor response in strain A mice. *Cancer Res.*, *33*, 3069-3085

Strong, J.M., Collins, J.M., Lester, C. & Poplack, D.G. (1986) Pharmaco-kinetics of intraventricular and intravenous N,N',N"-triethylenethiophosphoramide (thiotepa) in rhesus monkeys and humans. *Cancer Res.*, *46*, 6101-6104

Sturelid, S. (1976) Enhancement by caffeine of cell killing and chromosome damage in Chinese hamster cells treated with thiotepa. *Hereditas*, *84*, 157-162

Sturelid, S. & Kihlman, B.A. (1975) Enhancement by methylated oxypurines of the frequency of induced chromosomal aberrations. *Hereditas*, *80*, 233-246

Sweet, D.L. & Kinzie, J. (1976) Consequences of radiotherapy and antineoplastic therapy for the fetus. *J. reprod. Med.*, *17*, 241-246

Tanimura, T. (1968) Relationship of dosage and time of administration to teratogenic effects of thiotepa in mice. *Okajimas Fol. anat. jpn.*, *44*, 203-253

Titenko, N.V. (1983) Unscheduled synthesis induced by thiophosphamide in human lymphocytes. *Tsitol. Genet.*, *17*, 58-62

US Pharmacopeial Convention, Inc. (1989) *The US Pharmacopeia*, 22nd rev., Easton, PA, p. 796

Watkins, W.E., Kozak, J.A. & Flanagan, M.J. (1967) Severe pancytopenia associated with the use of intravesical thio-tepa. *J. Urol.*, *98*, 470-471

Williams, S.F., Bitran, J.D., Kaminer, L., Westbrook, C., Jacobs, R., Ashenhurst, J., Robin, E., Purl, S., Beschorner, J., Schroeder, C. & Golomb, H.M. (1987) A phase I-II study of bialkylator chemotherapy, high-dose thiotepa, and cyclophosphamide with autologous bone marrow reinfusion in patients with advanced cancer. *J. clin. Oncol.*, *5*, 260-265

Williams, S.F., Bitran, J.D., Hoffman, P.C., Robin, E., Fullem, L., Beschorner, J., Golick, J. & Golomb, H.M. (1989) High-dose, multiple-alkylator chemotherapy with autologous bone marrow reinfusion in patients with advanced non-small cell lung cancer. *Cancer*, *63*, 238-242

Windholz, M., ed. (1983) *The Merck Index*, 10th ed., Rahway, NJ, Merck & Co., pp. 1382-1383

Wolff, S. & Arutyunyan, R. (1979) The apparent decrease in thiotepa-induced chromosome aberrations in human lymphocytes caused by an effect of WR2721 on the cell cycle as found by the definitively determined division method. *Environ. Mutagenesis*, *1*, 5-13

Wright, J.C., Golomb, F.M. & Gumport, S.L. (1958) Summary of results with triethylene thiophosphoramide. *Ann. N.Y. Acad. Sci.*, *68*, 937-966

Yakovenko, K.N. & Kagramanyan, M.S. (1982) Effects of conditions of storage of lymphocytes on the frequency of chromosome aberrations induced by continuous and fractionated action of thiophosphamide. *Cytol. Genet.*, *16*, 55-59

Yakovenko, K.N. & Nazarenko, S.A. (1977) Combined action of thiophosphamide and dipin on chromosomes of human lymphocytes. *Cytol. Genet.*, *11*, 53-56

TRICHLORMETHINE (TRIMUSTINE HYDROCHLORIDE)

This substance was considered by a previous Working Group, in April 1975, under the title trichlorotriethylamine hydrochloride (IARC, 1975). Since that time, new data have become available, and these have been incorporated into the monograph and taken into consideration in the present evaluation.

1. Chemical and Physical Data

1.1 Synonyms

Chem. Abstr. Services Reg. No.: 817-09-4

Chem. Abstr. Name: Ethanamine-2-Chloro-*N,N*-bis(2-chloroethyl) hydrochloride

Synonyms: HN3[1]; HN3 hydrochloride NSC-30211; R-47; SK-100; tri(β-chloroethyl)amine hydrochloride; trichlorotriethylamine hydrochloride; 2,2′,2″-trichlorotriethylamine hydrochloride; trimustine[1]; tris(2-chloroethyl)amine hydrochloride; tris(β-chloroethyl)amine hydrochloride; tris(2-chloroethyl)amine monohydrochloride; tris(β-chloroethyl)amine monohydrochloride; tris-*N*-lost; TS-160

1.2 Structural and molecular formulae and molecular weight

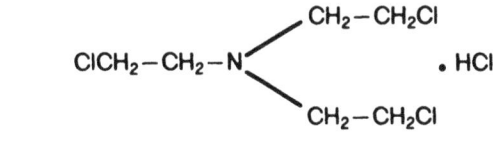

$C_6H_{12}Cl_3N \cdot HCl$ Mol. wt: 241.0

---

[1]This name is also used for the free base, trichlorotriethylamine.

1.3 Chemical and physical properties of the pure substance

From Reynolds (1982) and Windholz (1983)

(a) *Description*: Crystals
(b) *Melting-point*: 130-131°C
(c) *Solubility*: Very soluble in water; soluble in ethanol
(d) *Stability*: Aqueous solutions deteriorate rapidly.

1.4 Technical products and impurities

Trade names: Lekamin; Sinalost; Trillekamin; Trimitan

2. Production, Occurrence, Use and Analysis

2.1 Production and occurrence

Trichlormethine can be prepared by treating triethanolamine with thionyl chloride (Ward, 1935). No current manufacturer is known.

Trichlormethine is not known to occur naturally.

2.2 Use and therapy

Trichlormethine is a cytostatic agent. It was first used in the treatment of Hodgkin's disease and leukaemias in 1946 (Goodman *et al.*, 1946) and subsequently for other neoplastic diseases (Bratzel *et al.*, 1963; Bundesverband der pharmazeutischen Industrie, 1969). It was recognized in the 1977 and 1982 editions of *Martindale. The Extra Pharmacopoeia*, but not in the 1989 edition (Wade, 1977; Reynolds, 1982, 1989).

2.3 Analysis

A colorimetric method in which 4-(4'-nitrobenzyl)pyridine is used as the analytical reagent has been used to analyse for various alkylating agents. Trichlormethine may also be determined by thin-layer chromatography (Epstein *et al.*, 1955; Petering & Van Giessen, 1963; Sawicki & Sawicki, 1969).

3. Biological Data Relevant to the Evaluation of Carcinogenic Risk to Humans

3.1 Carcinogenicity studies in animals

The Working Group was aware of a short letter (Griffin *et al.*, 1950) in which experiments were described with mice and rats injected subcutaneously with trichlormethine.

Subcutaneous administration

Mouse: A group of 20 mice [age, strain and sex unspecified] received weekly subcutaneous injections of trichlormethine [purity unspecified] at 1 mg/kg bw in aqueous solution for ten weeks, after which time only four mice were alive and treatment was terminated. At survival times of 548-567 days, one of the four mice had a lung adenoma, one had a lung carcinoma and one had a lung carcinoma and a spindle-cell sarcoma at the site of injection. In a control group of 40 untreated mice killed between 14 and 18 months of age, six animals had lung adenomas, two had hepatomas and three had enlarged lymph nodes (Boyland & Horning, 1949). [The Working Group noted the very small number of surviving animals.]

Rat: Groups of ten male and ten female random-bred SPF Wistar rats, two months of age, received daily subcutaneous injections of trichlormethine [purity unspecified] at 0.1 or 0.25 mg/kg bw or weekly subcutaneous injections of 1 mg/kg bw in water for six months and were observed for one year after termination of treatment. Total doses were approximately 16.5, 40-42 and 24 mg/kg bw in the three treated groups, respectively. A control group of ten male and ten female rats received injections of 0.3 ml water only for six months. Survival was decreased in males receiving daily injections of trichlormethine. The incidences of sarcomas (mostly spindle-cell type) at the injection site were: males — low daily, 7/10 [$p < 0.0015$]; high daily, 8/10 [$p = 0.0004$]; weekly, 5/10 [$p = 0.016$]; females — low daily, 7/10 [$p < 0.0015$]; high daily, 7/9 [$p = 0.0007$]; weekly, 4/10 [$p = 0.04$]. In the group receiving 0.25 mg/kg bw daily, three males and one female had a mucus-secreting intestinal adenocarcinoma. Tumours were not seen in controls (Sýkora *et al.*, 1981).

3.2 Other relevant data

(a) *Experimental systems*

(i) *Absorption, distribution, excretion and metabolism*

No data were available to the Working Group.

(ii) *Toxic effects*

The LD_{50}s for mice, rats, rabbits and dogs after dermal application of trichlormethine were 7, 4.9, 19 and 1 mg/kg bw, respectively. After subcutaneous injections in saline, the LD_{50} for mice was 2.0 mg/kg bw. The LD_{50}s after intravenous injections were 0.7 mg/kg for rats and 2.5 mg/kg bw for rabbits (Anslow *et al.*, 1947).

Trichlormethine caused vomiting, anorexia and blood-containing faeces in dogs a few hours after a single intravenous injection of 1 mg/kg bw. Coma preceded death caused by anoxia as a consequence of peripheral circulatory failure (Houck *et al.*, 1947).

Decreased peripheral lymphocyte counts were observed in rabbits injected intravenously (Friederici, 1955) and in mice injected subcutaneously (Boyland & Horning, 1949) with trichlormethine.

This compound caused cross-links in membrane proteins and haemoglobin in human erythrocytes *in vitro* (Wildenauer & Weger, 1979; Ankel *et al.*, 1986); it alkylated nucleic acids *in vitro* (Szinicz *et al.*, 1981).

(iii) *Effects on reproduction and prenatal toxicity*

No data were available to the Working Group.

(iv) *Genetic and related effects*

Trichlormethine inhibited DNA synthesis and induced mutations at the *hprt* locus of Chinese hamster V79 cells (Slamenova *et al.*, 1983). It induced chromosomal aberrations in transplanted Walker rat carcinoma cells (Boyland *et al.*, 1948) and transplanted Ehrlich and Krebs tumour cells (Koller, 1969) following intraperitoneal injection into animals carrying these cells. [The Working Group noted that these early papers on transplanted tumour cells did not permit detailed evaluation.] A single intraperitoneal treatment with trichlormethine at 5 mg/kg induced dominant lethal mutations in mice (Sýkora & Gandalovicova, 1978).

(b) *Humans*

(i) *Pharmacokinetics*

No data were available to the Working Group.

(ii) *Adverse effects*

Lymphopenia, granulocytopenia, thrombocytopenia, anaemia, nausea and vomiting and thrombophlebitis in the vein receiving the infusion were reported after use of trichlormethine (Goodman *et al.*, 1946).

(iii) *Effects on reproduction and prenatal toxicity*

No data were available to the Working Group.

(iv) *Genetic and related effects*

No data were available to the Working Group.

3.3 Case reports and epidemiological studies of carcinogenicity to humans

No data were available to the Working Group.

4. Summary of Data Reported and Evaluation

4.1 Exposure data

Trichlormethine is a cytostatic agent that has been used since 1946 for the treatment of leukaemia and lymphoma.

4.2 Experimental carcinogenicity data

Trichlormethine was tested for carcinogenicity by subcutaneous injection in mice and rats. The study in mice was inadequate for evaluation. In rats, trichlormethine induced a high incidence of sarcomas (mostly spindle-cell type) in animals of each sex at the site of subcutaneous injection, as well as a few intestinal adenocarcinomas; neither tumour type was seen in controls.

4.3 Human carcinogenicity data

No data were available to the Working Group.

4.4 Other relevant data

In single studies, trichlormethine induced dominant lethal mutations in mice and gene mutations in Chinese hamster cells. (See Appendix 1.)

4.5 Evaluation[1]

There is *sufficient evidence* for the carcinogenicity of trichlormethine in experimental animals.

No data were available from studies in humans on the carcinogenicity of trichlormethine.

Overall evaluation

Trichlormethine *is possibly carcinogenic to humans (Group 2B)*.

5. References

Ankel, E.G., Ring, B.J., Lai, C.-S. & Holcenberg, J.S. (1986) The lack of effects of alkylating agents on mammalian cell membranes. *Int. J. Tissue React.*, *8*, 347-354

Anslow, W.P., Karnovsky, D.A., Jager, B.V. & Smith, H.W. (1947) The toxicity and pharmacological action of the nitrogen mustards and certain related compounds. *J. Pharmacol. exp. Ther.*, *91*, 224-235

Boyland, E. & Horning, E.S. (1949) The induction of tumours with nitrogen mustards. *Br. J. Cancer*, *3*, 118-123

Boyland, E., Clegg, J.W., Koller, P.C., Rhoden, E. & Warwick, O.H. (1948) The effects of chloroethylamines on tumours, with special reference to bronchogenic carcinomas. *Br. J. Cancer*, *2*, 17-29

---

[1] For description of the italicized terms, see Preamble, pp. 26–29.

Bratzel, R.P., Ross, R.B., Goodridge, T.H., Huntress, W.T., Flather, M.T. & Johnson, D.E. (1963) Survey of nitrogen mustards. *Cancer Chemother. Rep.*, 26, 1-322

Bundesverband der pharmazeutischen Industrie (1969) *Rote Liste* [Red List], Frankfurt

Epstein, J., Rosenthal, R.W. & Ess, R.J. (1955) Use of γ-(4-nitrobenzyl)pyridine as analytical reagent for ethyleneimines and alkylating agents. *Anal. Chem.*, 27, 1435-1439

Friederici, L. (1955) Der Einfluss von Sulfonamiden, Stickstoff-Lost, TEM und Aminopterin auf das Blut und die blutbildenden Organe des Kaninchens. [The influence of sulfonamides, nitrogen mustard, triethanomelamine and aminopterine on the blood and haematopoietic tissues of rabbits (Ger.).] *Folia haematol.*, 73, 49-74

Goodman, L.S., Wintrobe, M.M., Dameshek, W., Goodman, M.J., Gilman, M.A. & McLennan, M.T. (1946) Nitrogen mustard therapy. Use of methylbis(beta-chloroethyl)amine hydrochloride and tris(beta-chloroethyl)amine hydrochloride for Hodgkin's disease, lymphosarcoma, leukemia and certain allied and miscellaneous disorders. *J. Am. med. Assoc.*, 132, 126-132

Griffin, A.C., Brandt, E.L. & Tatum, E.L. (1950) Nitrogen mustards and cancer-inducing agents. *J. Am. med. Assoc.*, 144, 571

Houck, C.R., Crawford, B., Bannon, J.H. & Smith, H.W. (1947) Studies on the mechanism of death in dogs after systemic intoxication by the intravenous injection of methylbis(β-chloroethyl)amine or tris(β-chloroethyl)amine. *J. Pharmacol. exp. Ther.*, 90, 277-292

IARC (1975) *IARC Monographs on the Evaluation of the Carcinogenic Risk of Chemicals to Man, Vol 9, Some Aziridines, N-, S- and O-Mustards and Selenium*, Lyon, pp. 229-234

Koller, P.C. (1969) Mutagenic alkylating agents as growth inhibitors and carcinogens. *Mutat. Res.*, 8, 199-206

Petering, H.G. & Van Giessen, G.L. (1963) Colorimetric method for determination of uracil mustard and related alkylating agents. *J. pharm. Sci.*, 52, 1159-1162

Reynolds, J.E.F., ed. (1982) *Martindale. The Extra Pharmacopoeia*, 28th ed., London, The Pharmaceutical Press, p. 229

Reynolds, J.E.F., ed. (1989) *Martindale. The Extra Pharmacopoeia*, 29th ed., London, The Pharmaceutical Press, p. 653

Sawicki, E. & Sawicki, C.R. (1969) Analysis of alkylating agents: application to air pollution. *Ann. N.Y. Acad. Sci.*, 163, 895-921

Slamenova, D., Dusinska, M., Budayova, E. & Gabelova, A. (1983) The genetic effects of the cytostatic drug TS_{160} on Chinese hamster fibroblasts *in vitro*. *Mutat. Res.*, 116, 431-440

Sýkora, I. & Gandalovicova, D. (1978) Dominant-lethal assay of selected cytostatics. *Neoplasma*, 25, 523-533

Sýkora, I., Yortel, V., Marhan, O. & Dynterová, A. (1981) Carcinogenicity of trichloromethine hydrochloride (TS-160 Spofa) and morphological damage after its intraamniotic injection. *Neoplasma*, 28, 565-574

Szinicz, L., Albrecht, G.J. & Weger, N. (1981) Effect of various compounds on the reaction of tris(2-chloroethyl)amine with ribonucleic acid in vitro and on its toxicity in mice. *Arzneimittel.-forsch. (Drug Res.)*, 31, 1713-1717

Wade, A., ed. (1977) *Martindale. The Extra Pharmacopoeia*, 27th ed., London, The Pharmaceutical Press, p. 171

Ward, K. (1935) The chlorinated ethylamines—a new type of vesicant. *J. Am. chem. Soc.*, 57, 914-916

Wildenauer, D. & Weger, N. (1979) Reactions of the trifunctional nitrogen mustard tris(2-chloroethyl)amine (HN3) with human erythrocyte membranes in vitro. *Biochem. Pharmacol.*, 28, 2761-2769

Windholz, M., ed. (1983) *The Merck Index*, 10th ed., Rahway, NJ, Merck & Co., p. 1379

Witten, B., Magaha, E.P. & Williams, W.A. (1964) Chemical warfare. In: Kirk, R.E. & Othmer, D.F., eds, *Encyclopedia of Chemical Technology*, 2nd ed., Vol. 4, New York, John Wiley & Sons, pp. 871-875

ANTIMICROBIAL AGENTS

AMPICILLIN

1. Chemical and Physical Data

1.1 Synonyms

Chem. Abstr. Services Reg. No.: 69-53-4; 7177-48-2 (trihydrate); 69-52-3 (sodium salt)

Chem. Abstr. Name: 4-Thia-1-azabicyclo[3.2.0]heptane-2-carboxylic acid, 6-[(aminophenylacetyl)amino]-3,3-dimethyl-7-oxo-, {2S-[2α, 5α, 6β(S*)]}-

Synonyms: Anhydrous: (2S,5R,6R)-6-[(R)-2-Amino-2-phenylacetamido]-3,3-dimethyl-7-oxo-4-thia-1-azabicyclo[3.2.0]heptane-2-carboxylic acid; ampicillinum; ampicillinum anhydricum; anhydrous ampicillin; (6R)-6-(α-D-phenylglycylamino)penicillanic acid. Trihydrate: aminobenzylpenicillin (3H$_2$O); α-aminobenzyl-penicillin (3H$_2$O); ampicillinum trihydricum; (sodium salt) ampicillinnatrium; ampicillinum natricum

1.2 Structural and molecular formulae and molecular weight

$C_{16}H_9N_3O_4S$ Mol. wt: 349.40; 403.46 (3H$_2$O); 371.4 (sodium salt)

1.3 Chemical and physical properties of the pure substance

From Ivashkiv (1973), unless otherwise specified

(a) *Description*: White, crystalline powder; practically odourless; also occurs as trihydrate; pH of 10 g/ml aqueous solution, 3.5-6.0

(b) *Melting-point*: Ampicillin monohydrate melts with decomposition at 202°C; sodium ampicillin melts with decomposition at 205°C; sesquihydrate and anhydrous ampicillin decompose at 199-202°C. The melting range for ampicillin trihydrate with decomposition has been reported as 214.5-215°C and 202-204°C.

(c) *Optical rotation*: Ampicillin monohydrate, $[\alpha]_D^{21}$ +281° (c = 1 in H$_2$O); ampicillin sesquihydrate, $[\alpha]_D^{20}$ +283.1° (c in H$_2$O); sodium ampicillin $[\alpha]_D^{20}$ +209° (c = 0.2 in H$_2$O); anhydrous ampicillin $[\alpha]_D^{20}$ +287.9° (c = 1 in H$_2$O)

(d) *Solubility*: The solubilities of anhydrous ampicillin, ampicillin trihydrate and sodium ampicillin in various solvents are given in detail by Ivashkiv (1973).

(e) *Spectroscopy data*: Ultraviolet, infrared, nuclear magnetic resonance and mass spectra have been reported.

(f) *Stability*: Ampicillin powders are stable when stored in a closed system at 43% and 81% relative humidity at room temperature for six weeks. Ampicillin is also stable at 35°C in such closed systems for nine weeks. Stability decreases significantly in the presence of sugars (Reynolds, 1989).

(g) *Dissociation constant*: pK_a = 2.5, 7.3 (23°C)

1.4 Technical products and impurities

Trade names: A-Cillin; Adobacillin; Aletmicina; Alpen; Alpen-N; Amblosin; Amcill; Amcill-S; Amfipen; Ampen; Amperil; Ampibel; Ampi-Biopharma; Ampibiotic; Ampibronc Capsules; Ampicil; Ampicillat; Ampicilline; Ampiciman; Ampicin; Ampicur; Ampifen; Ampi-Framan; Ampigal; Ampikel; Ampilag; Ampilan; Ampiland; Ampilar; Ampilean; Ampilisa; Ampilux; Ampinebiot; Ampinova; Ampinoxi; Ampi-Oral; Ampiorus; Ampipenix; Ampi-Rol; Ampisint; Ampi-Tablinen; Ampitex; Ampivax; Ampi-Vial; Ampixilion; Ampi-Zoja; Amplibios; Amplicid; Amplimedix; Amplipen; Amplipenyl; Ampliscocil; Amplital; Amplizer; Anhypen; Anidropen; Antibiopen; Anticyl; Apo-Ampi; Argocillina; Austrapen; Bemicina; Benusel Oral; Binotal; Bio-ampi; Biocellina; Bionacillin; Biosan; Bonapicillin; Bristin; Britapen; Britcin; Cilleral; Cimexillin; Citicil; Cuxacillin; Cymbi; D-Amp; Deripen; Diancina; Doktacillin; Domicillin; DuraAmpicillin; Espectrosira; Espimin-Cilina; Eurocillin; Famicillin; Farmampil; Fidesbiotic; Fortapen; Fuerpen; Germicillina; Geycillina; Globipen Balsamico; Gobemcina; Gramcillina; Grampenil; Guicitrina; Helvecillin; Hostes; Iwacillin; Lampocillina; Lifeampil; Marisilan; Maxicilina; Medicillin-D; Morepen; Napicil; NC Cilin; Negmapen; Novoexpectro; Nuvapen; Omnipen; Omnipen-N; Overcillina; Panbiotic; Panestes; Pen-A; Pen Ampil; Penampil; Pen A/N; Penberin; Pen-Bristol;

Penbristol; Penbritin; Penbritine; Penbrock; Pénicline; Penimaster; Penimic; Penimul; Peninovel; Penisint B.G.; Penisintex; Penorsin; Penrite; Pensyn; Pentrex; Pentrexil; Pentrexyl; Pentrexyl-K; Petercillin; Pharcillin; Platocillina; Plumericin; Poenbiotico; Polycillin; Prestacilina; Principen; Principen/N; Quimetam; Racenacillin; Radiocillina; Resan; Rivocillin; Rosampline; Roscillin; Saicil; Semicillin; Sernabiotic; Servicilline; Sesquicillina; Sintopenyl; SK-Ampicillin; SK-Ampicillin-N; Spectracil; Sumipanto; Supen; Suractin; Synpenin; Synthecillin; Tauglicolcinna; Togram; Tokiocillin; Tolimal; Totaciclina; Totacillin; Totacillin N; Totalciclina; Totapen; Trafarbiot; Trifacilina; Ukapen; Ultrabion; Urebion Ampicillina; Valmingina; Viacilina-A; Vidopen

The following names have been used for multi-ingredient preparations containing ampicillin, ampicillin salts and ampicillin trihydrate: Ampicin-PRB; Ampiclox; Ampicyn; Flu-Amp; Magnapen; Nuvapen Reard; Orbecilina; Penbritin KS; Pentrex-F; Polycillin-PRB; Principen with Probenecid; Pro-Biosan; Unasyn

USP anhydrous ampicillin contains 900-1050 µg/mg ampicillin (calculated as the anhydrous base), and the trihydrate contains 845-988 µg/mg. Ampicillin is available in 125-, 200-, 250- and 500-mg tablets that contain 90-120% labelled active ingredient, in 125-, 250- and 500-mg capsules containing 90-120% labelled active ingredient, and as oral suspensions of 100, 125 and 250 mg/5 ml containing 90-120% of the labelled active ingredient and probenecid. The sodium salt of ampicillin is available for injection in vials of 0.125, 0.25, 0.5, 1, 2 and 10 g.

Impurities of ampicillin that occur during preparation of the product are D-(-)-α-phenylglycine and 6-aminopenicillanic acid. It has been reported that sodium ampicillin in aqueous solution undergoes a reaction to form oligomeric products (Van der Bijl *et al.*, 1988).

2. Production, Occurrence, Use and Analysis

2.1 Production and occurrence

Ampicillin is produced by the acylation of 6-aminopenicillanic acid with D-(-)-α-phenylglycine by either microbiological or chemical synthesis (Ivashkiv, 1973). It was first marketed in 1961 in the UK. It is synthesized in Austria, Brazil, Hungary, India, Italy, Japan, the Republic of Korea, Mexico, the Netherlands, Romania, Spain, Sweden, Turkey, the USA and Yugoslavia (Chemical Information Services, 1989-90).

In Sweden, ampicillin sales in 1988 were 0.05 defined daily doses per 1000 inhabitants (Apoteksbolaget, 1988, 1989). In 1988, over six million new prescriptions of ampicillin were issued in the USA (La Piana Simonsen, 1989).

Ampicillin is not known to occur naturally.

2.2 Use

Ampicillin is bactericidal and has a similar mode of action to that of benzylpenicillin, although it has a broader spectrum of activity, covering several additional gram-positive and gram-negative organisms. Ampicillin may have a synergistic action with aminoglycosides and with the β-lactamase inhibitors clavulanic acid and sulbactam (Foulds, 1986; Barnhart, 1989).

The clinical indications for ampicillin cover a variety of infections, including those of the respiratory and urinary tracts, gonorrhoea, meningitis, septicaemia and enteric infections.

Expressed in various formulations as ampicillin equivalents, the usual oral dosing is 0.25-1 g every 6 h. The disposition of ampicillin is altered in pregnancy, and therefore higher doses may be required for severe infections in pregnancy (Assael *et al.*, 1979). Children may be given half the adult dose. The usual doses of ampicillin given by injection are 500 mg every 4 or 6 h intramuscularly (painful), by slow (5 min) intravenous injection or by intravenous infusion. Intrapleural, intraperitoneal and intrathecal injections of ampicillin are used occasionally (Reynolds, 1989).

2.3 Analysis

Ampicillin can be analysed in pharmaceutical preparations by microbiological, iodometric, colorimetric, high-performance liquid chromatographic (US Food and Drug Administration, 1988) and fluorometric assays (Barbhaiya & Turner, 1976) and by gas chromatography-mass spectrometry (Wu *et al.*, 1977). Ampicillin can be analysed in biological fluids by high-performance liquid chromatography (Miyazaki *et al.*, 1983; Haginaka & Wakai, 1987; Abuirjeie & Abdel-Hamid, 1988).

3. Biological Data Relevant to the Evaluation of Carcinogenic Risk to Humans

3.1 Carcinogenicity studies in animals

Oral administration

Mouse: Groups of 50 male and 50 female B6C3F1 mice, seven to eight weeks of age, were administered ampicillin trihydrate (purity, 97%) by gavage at 0, 1500 or

3000 mg/kg bw in corn oil on five days per week for 103 weeks. The animals were maintained for a further one to two weeks, after which time they were killed. Weight gain was similar in all groups, and no significant difference in survival was observed in mice of either sex: at the end of the study period, 32/50, 21/50 and 20/50 males in the control, low-dose and high-dose groups, respectively, and 34/50, 27/50 and 28/50 females in the control, low-dose and high-dose groups, respectively, were still alive. In female mice, a slight increase in the incidence of benign lung tumours was observed (control, 1/50; low-dose, 0/50; high-dose, 4/50; $p = 0.049$, incidental tumour test). No increase in the incidence of any other neoplasm was recorded (National Toxicology Program, 1987; Dunnick *et al.*, 1989).

Rat: Groups of 50 male and 50 female Fischer 344/N rats, seven to eight weeks old, were administered ampicillin trihydrate (purity, 97%) by gavage at 0, 750 or 1500 mg/kg bw in corn oil on five days per week for 103 weeks. Animals were observed for a further one to two weeks, after which time they were killed. Mean body weights of treated males and females were similar to those of controls. At the end of the study, 31/50, 27/50 and 26/50 control, low-dose and high-dose males, respectively, and 32/50, 31/50 and 31/50 control, low-dose and high-dose females, respectively, were still alive. An increase in the incidence of mononuclear-cell leukaemia was observed in treated males: control, 5/50; low-dose, 14/50 ($p = 0.019$, life-table test); high-dose, 13/50 ($p = 0.029$, life-table test; $p = 0.024$, life-table test for trend). A dose-related increase in the incidence of combined benign and malignant phaeochromocytomas of the adrenal medulla was also observed in males: control, 13/50; low-dose, 16/50; high-dose, 23/49 ($p = 0.007$, incidental tumour test; $p = 0.007$, trend test for incidental tumours). The incidences of mammary gland fibroadenomas in females were: control, 16/50; low-dose, 25/50 ($p = 0.019$, incidental tumour test); high-dose, 19/50. No increase in the incidence of tumours at other sites was observed (National Toxicology Program, 1987; Dunnick *et al.*, 1989). [The Working Group noted the high frequency of spontaneous tumours and that the increase in the incidence of mammary gland fibroadenomas was not dose-related.]

3.2 Other relevant data

(a) *Experimental systems*

(i) *Absorption, distribution, excretion and metabolism*

Following intraperitoneal injection to rats, ampicillin was distributed throughout the major organ systems; the serum half-life was estimated to be 27 min (Fabre, 1977). Assay of serum collected after a single subcutaneous dose of sodium ampicillin at 10 mg/kg bw to guinea-pigs yielded ampicillin levels of approximately

10 μg/ml at 5 min, which fell rapidly to less than 0.2 μg/ml at 60 min (Young et al., 1987).

(ii) *Toxic effects*

The intraperitoneal LD_{50} for ampicillin was 3300 mg/kg bw for one-day-old rats and 4500 mg/kg bw for 83-day-old rats (Goldenthal, 1971). The oral LD_{50} in rats was 10 g/kg bw and that in mice, 15.2 g/kg bw (Khosid et al., 1975). Deaths occurred in 63, 45 and 100% of rabbits that received oral doses of ampicillin at 5, 15 and 50 mg/kg bw, respectively, for three consecutive days (Milhaud et al., 1976).

Ampicillin administered as a single oral or subcutaneous dose of up to 5000 mg/kg bw had no noticeable toxic effect in mice or rats. Intravenous administration of 2000 mg/kg bw to mice caused muscle tremors, slowed respiration and mild convulsions. No biochemical, haematological or histological abnormality was seen in rats administered ampicillin at 100 or 500 mg/kg bw for 12 weeks (Brown & Acred, 1961). Administration of 25 mg/l in the drinking-water to four-week-old rats for up to eight weeks resulted in an increase in body weight gain; no toxic effect was noted (King, 1975).

Nabata et al. (1988) reported that intravenous exposures of rats to ampicillin at 1200 mg/kg bw per day for 28 days were well tolerated. Intravenous administration of sulbactam:ampicillin (1:2) at 90-1800 mg/kg bw for 28 days caused caecal enlargement; deposition of glycogen-like droplets in the liver occurred at the higher dose levels.

The toxicity of ampicillin trihydrate has been studied in Fischer 344/N rats and B6C3F1 mice (National Toxicology Program, 1987). In 14-day studies of rats and mice administered ampicillin at 200-2400 mg/kg bw by gavage, dose-related clinical signs included diarrhoea and excessive salivation in the high-dose rats immediately after dosing. Diarrhoea of minimal severity was observed in high-dose mice given 2400 mg/kg. No dose-related gross pathology or histopathology was observed in either species.

In 13-week studies, doses of 180-3000 mg/kg bw were administered by gavage on five days per week to rats and mice. All rats given 300 mg/kg bw and one of ten male mice at either 2000 mg/kg or 3000 mg/kg had diarrhoea. No compound-related pathology or histopathology was observed grossly in either species.

In the two-year studies (see section 3.1), ampicillin at doses of 750 or 1500 mg/kg bw (rats) and 1500 or 3000 mg/kg bw (mice) was administered by gavage on five days per week for 103 weeks. Clinical signs observed in treated rats included diarrhoea, excessive urination and chromodacryorrhoea; those in treated mice included increased salivation and decreased activity. The incidence of C-cell hyperplasia of the thyroid gland was increased in low-dose male and high-dose female rats. High-dose male rats showed increased incidences of hyperkeratosis and acanthosis of the forestomach. In male and female mice, an increased incidence of forestomach lesions, including ulcers, inflammation, hyperkeratosis, acanthosis and evidence of fungal infection, was observed in exposed animals.

(iii) *Effects on reproduction and prenatal toxicity*

The absence of experimental details precluded assessment of the only study of prenatal toxicity (Korzhova *et al.*, 1981).

(iv) *Genetic and related effects*

Ampicillin induced lysogenic phage in *Staphylococcus aureus* (Manthey *et al.*, 1975). It did not induce a SOS response in *Escherichia coli* PQ37 (Venier *et al.*, 1989), and no differential toxicity was observed in *E. coli* in the absence (Green & Tweats, 1981) or presence of an exogenous metabolic system (Tweats *et al.*, 1981; De Flora *et al.*, 1984). In *Salmonella typhimurium* plate incorporation tests, ampicillin was not mutagenic in the presence or absence of an exogenous metabolic system (De Flora *et al.*, 1984; Mortelmans *et al.*, 1986; National Toxicology Program, 1987).

Treatment of *Vicia faba* seeds with a 0.5% solution of ampicillin led to chromosomal aberrations in root-tip meristem cells (Prasad, 1977).

Ampicillin did not induce mutation at the *tk* locus in L5178Y mouse lymphoma cells in the presence or absence of an exogenous metabolic system at concentrations up to 5000 µg/ml (National Toxicology Program, 1987). No increase in the frequency of sister chromatid exchange was observed in Chinese hamster CHO cells with concentrations of ampicillin up to 1500 µg/ml in the presence or absence of an exogenous metabolic system (National Toxicology Program, 1987). Ampicillin did not induce sister chromatid exchange in human lymphocytes *in vitro* (Jaju *et al.*, 1984). No chromosomal aberration was observed in Chinese hamster CHO cells treated with ampicillin at 0-1500 µg/ml in the presence or absence of an exogenous metabolic system (National Toxicology Program, 1987). Ampicillin did not induce chromosomal aberrations in human fibroblasts after 50 h of treatment with a concentration of 4000 µg/ml (Byarugaba *et al.*, 1975), but a dose of 28 µg/ml induced chromosomal aberrations in human peripheral lymphocytes *in vitro* (Jaju *et al.*, 1984). [The Working Group noted the low concentration used in this test, as compared to those of other reports.] It was reported in an abstract that ampicillin did not induce chromosomal aberrations in human lymphocytes *in vitro* at concentrations up to 10 mg/ml (Stemp *et al.*, 1988).

It was reported in an abstract that ampicillin at single- or double-dose oral regimens of 5 mg/kg did not induce micronuclei in rats treated *in vivo* (Stemp *et al.*, 1988).

(b) Humans

(i) *Pharmacokinetics*

The pharmacokinetics of ampicillin have been reviewed (Barza & Weinstein, 1976).

Ampicillin is relatively stable in the acid contents of the stomach; anhydrous or trihydrated ampicillin is absorbed incompletely from the gut after oral administration. Peak concentrations in plasma (2-6 mg/l after an oral dose of 500 mg) occur within 1-2 h. Ester prodrugs (pivampicillin, bacampicillin) and the condensation prodrug (hetacillin) of ampicillin are absorbed more readily than ampicillin (Jusko & Lewis, 1973; Loo *et al.*, 1974; Magni *et al.*, 1978; Pennington & Crooks, 1983). Ampicillin at 500 mg given by intramuscular injection as the sodium salt produced plasma peaks of 7-14 mg/l within about 1 h (Doluisio *et al.*, 1971).

Ampicillin is distributed widely, and therapeutic concentrations can be achieved in soft tissues, including ascitic, pleural and joint fluids (Lewis & Jusko, 1975). Bacampicillin produces higher tissue concentrations than ampicillin (Bronsveld *et al.*, 1978). Only 20% of ampicillin is bound to plasma proteins (Barza & Weinstein, 1976). It crosses the placenta (Hirsch *et al.*, 1974; Kraybill *et al.*, 1980), and detectable concentrations of ampicillin occur in the milk of nursing mothers (Chow & Jewesson, 1985).

Ampicillin is excreted *via* renal glomerular and tubular routes in the urine; its plasma half-time is usually 1-2 h (Sjövall, 1985) but is longer in elderly people (Triggs *et al.*, 1980). In patients with renal failure, the half-time was as long as 20 h (Hori *et al.*, 1983).

Healthy subjects metabolize about 20% of a given dose (250-500 mg) of ampicillin. Within 12 h, 7% of the total dose is excreted as metabolites in urine (Cole *et al.*, 1973; Haginaka & Wakai, 1987). Ampicillin is metabolized to 5R,6R-penicilloic acid and 5S,6R-penicilloic acid (Bird *et al.*, 1983) and to piperazine-2,5-dione after oral intake (Haginaka & Wakai, 1987). Other, unidentified metabolites have been reported (Masada *et al.*, 1979).

(ii) *Adverse effects*

Skin rashes (Almeyda & Levantine, 1972) are the most common side-effects of ampicillin treatment and are either urticarial or maculopapular. The allergic nature of the maculopapular rash is uncertain (Bierman *et al.*, 1972; Campbell & Soyka, 1977; Sokoloff, 1977; van Ketel, 1984). Non-allergic fever due to ampicillin occurs rarely (Mackowiak & LeMaistre, 1987). The overall incidence of skin reactions among a group of patients who received the drug between 1975 and 1982 was 59/1775 (3.3%) (Bigby *et al.*, 1986), although higher incidences have been reported. Unusually high incidences of skin rashes occur during treatment with ampicillin of glandular fever and lymphatic leukaemia (Cameron & Richmond, 1971; Lambert *et al.*, 1972).

Ampicillin commonly affects the gastrointestinal tract, at least in children (25-35%) (Feder, 1982). It has been reported to be one of the drugs most frequently associated with pseudomembranous colitis (Gorbach, 1987). Seizures have been reported after use of ampicillin in cases of underlying cerebral dysfunction (Serdaru *et al.*, 1982) or concomitant renal insufficiency resulting in high serum concentrations of ampicillin (Hodgman *et al.*, 1984).

(iii) *Effects on reproduction and prenatal toxicity*

In a study of 280 000 women belonging to a prepaid health plan in Seattle, WA (USA), all drug prescriptions and all pregnancy outcomes were monitored between July 1977 and December 1979. Among the liveborn babies of 6837 women, 80 (1.2%) had major congenital malformations. Four infants born to 309 women for whom ampicillin had been prescribed in the first trimester had major malformations [types not specified], giving a prevalence of 13 per 1000, which was not significantly different from the overall prevalence in the total population studied (12 per 1000) (Jick *et al.*, 1981).

In a second study of the same population covering January 1980 to June 1982, 6509 women had pregnancies ending in livebirths, and 105 (1.5%) of these had major congenital malformations. Three infants born to 409 women for whom ampicillin had been prescribed in the first trimester had major malformations [types not specified], giving a prevalence of seven per 1000, compared with an overall prevalence in the entire group of 15 per 1000 (Aselton *et al.*, 1985).

In a hospital study of Australian women, 7371 mothers had singleton pregnancies in 1978-81; 1060 of them had used amoxycillin or ampicillin [not recorded separately] at some time during pregnancy: 211 had been treated in the first trimester only and 73 in the first trimester and later. It was stated that there was no evidence of any association between use of these drugs and the incidence or type of congenital malformations, which were observed in 12 of the 284 (4.2%) exposed babies, compared with the nonexposed (297/6311, 4.7%). There was no association with use of these drugs and intrauterine growth retardation or perinatal death, but there was a significant ($p < 0.01$) difference in the rate of prematurity in the users (8.9%) compared with nonusers (6.5%), which was not due to age or differences in use of alcohol. There was also a significant ($p < 0.0001$) increase in the prevalence of low-birth-weight (<2.5 kg) babies among users (9.6%) compared with nonusers (6.6%), which was still significant ($p < 0.05$) when controlled for length of gestation (Colley *et al.* 1983). [The Working Group noted that the effects might have been due to underlying infection in the mothers.]

(iv) *Genetic and related effects*

No adequate study was available to the Working Group.

3.3 Case reports and epidemiological studies of carcinogenicity to humans

One case each of lymphoproliferative disease and Kaposi's sarcoma has been reported in association with use of ampicillin (Gordon & Luk, 1982; Brenner *et al.*, 1984).

Ampicillin was included in a hypothesis-generating cohort study designed to screen a large number (215) of drugs for possible carcinogenicity, which covered more than 140 000 subscribers enrolled in July 1969 to August 1973 in a prepaid medical care programme in northern California (USA). Computer records of persons to whom at least one drug prescription was dispensed were linked to cancer records from hospitals and the local cancer registry. Observed numbers of cancers were compared with expected numbers, standardized for age and sex, derived from the entire cohort. Three publications have summarized the screening findings for follow-up periods of up to seven years (Friedman & Ury, 1980), nine years (Friedman & Ury, 1983) and 15 years (Selby *et al.*, 1989). [The Working Group chose to omit mention of associations based on fewer than three cases.] Among 6706 persons who received ampicillin, an association was noted with subsequent skin cancer (four cases observed, 0.9 expected; $p < 0.05$) in the seven-year report. In the 15-year report, an association was noted with lung cancer (48 cases observed, 27.3 expected; $p < 0.002$). The latter association, although apparently not explained by cigarette smoking in an analysis of smoking habits carried out specifically for people taking ampicillin, was also seen for several other antibiotics. [The Working Group noted, as did the authors, that, since some 12 000 comparisons were made in this hypothesis-generating study, the associations should be verified independently. Data on duration of use were not provided.]

4. Summary of Data Reported and Evaluation

4.1 Exposure data

Ampicillin is a broad-spectrum antibiotic and has been used extensively to treat bacterial infections since 1961.

4.2 Experimental carcinogenicity data

Ampicillin was tested for carcinogenicity by oral administration in mice and rats. It increased the incidences of mononuclear-cell leukaemia and of phaeochromocytomas of the adrenal medulla in male rats. A slight increase in the incidence of benign lung tumours was observed in female mice.

4.3 Human carcinogenicity data

In a hypothesis-generating cohort study, use of ampicillin was associated with the occurrence of lung and skin cancers, but these findings could have been due to chance.

4.4 Other relevant data

Use of ampicillin during the first trimester of pregnancy has not been associated with an increase in the incidence of major congenital malformations.

Ampicillin increased the frequency of chromosomal aberrations in human lymphocytes but not in human fibroblasts *in vitro*. It did not induce chromosomal aberrations in Chinese hamster cells, mutations in mouse lymphoma cells or sister chromatid exchange in human lymphocytes or in Chinese hamster cells. Ampicillin induced chromosomal aberrations in *Vicia faba*. It was not mutagenic to *Salmonella typhimurium* and did not induce differential toxicity in *Escherichia coli* strains. (See Appendix 1.)

4.5 Evaluation[1]

There is *inadequate evidence* for the carcinogenicity of ampicillin in humans.

There is *limited evidence* for the carcinogenicity of ampicillin in experimental animals.

Overall evaluation

Ampicillin *is not classifiable as to its carcinogenicity to humans (Group 3)*.

5. References

Abuirjeie, M.A. & Abdel-Hamid, M.E. (1988) Simultaneous high-pressure liquid chromatographic analysis of ampicillin and cloxacillin in serum and urine. *J. clin. Pharmacol. Ther.*, *13*, 101-108

Almeyda, J. & Levantine, A. (1972) Drug reactions. XIX. Adverse cutaneous reactions to the penicillins—ampicillin rashes. *Br. J. Dermatol.*, *83*, 293-297

---

[1]For description of the italicized terms, see Preamble, pp. 26–29.

Apoteksbolaget (1988) *Svensk Läkemedelsstatistic* [Swedish Drugs Statistics], Stockholm, Pharmaceutical Association of Sweden

Apoteksbolaget (1989) *Outprint of the Drug Data Base (17 October 1989)*, Stockholm, Pharmaceutical Association of Sweden

Aselton, P., Jick, H., Milunsky, A., Hunter, J.R. & Stergachis, A. (1985) First trimester drug use and congenital disorders. *Obstet. Gynecol.*, 65, 451-455

Assael, B.M., Como, M.L., Miraglia, M., Pardi, G. & Sereni, F. (1979) Ampicillin kinetics in pregnancy. *Br. J. clin. Pharmacol.*, 8, 286-288

Barbhaiya, R.H. & Turner, P. (1976) Fluorimetric determination of ampicillin and cephalexin. *Br. J. Pharmacol.*, 58, 473P

Barnhart, E. (1989) *Physicians' Desk Reference*, 43rd ed., Oradell, NJ, Medical Economics, p. 303

Barza, M. & Weinstein, L. (1976) Pharmacokinetics of the penicillins in man. *Clin. Pharmacokinet.*, 1, 297-308

Bierman, C.W., Pierson, W.E., Zeitz, S.J., Hoffman, L.S. & Van Arsdel, P.P., Jr (1972) Reactions associated with ampicillin therapy. *J. Am. med. Assoc.*, 220, 1098-1100

Bigby, M., Jick, S., Jick, H. & Arndt, K. (1986) Drug-induced cutaneous reactions: a report from the Boston collaborative drug surveillance program on 15 438 consecutive inpatients, 1975 to 1982. *J. Am. med. Assoc.*, 256, 3358-3363

Bird, A.E., Cutmore, E.A., Jennings, K.R. & Marschall, A.C. (1983) Structure re-assignment of a metabolite of ampicillin and amoxycillin and epimerization of the penicilloic acids. *J. Pharm. Pharmacol.*, 35, 138-143

Brenner, S., Shohet, J. & Rozen, P. (1984) Kaposi's sarcoma appearing during ampicillin treatment. *Harefuah*, 106, 313-314

Bronsveld, W., Stam, J. & McLaren, D.M. (1978) Concentrations of ampicillin in pleural fluid and serum after single and repetitive doses of bacampicillin. *Scand. J. infect. Dis.*, Suppl. 14, 274-277

Brown, D. & Acred, P. (1961) 'Penbritin'—a new broad-spectrum antibiotic, preliminary pharmacology and chemotherapy. *Br. med. J*, ii, 197-198

Byarugaba, W., Rüdiger, H.W., Koske-Westphal, T., Wöhler, W. & Passarge, E. (1975) Toxicity of antibiotics on cultured human skin fibroblasts. *Humangenetik*, 18, 263-267

Cameron, S.J. & Richmond, J. (1971) Ampicillin hypersensitivity in lymphatic leukaemia. *Scott. med. J.*, 16, 425-427

Campbell, A.B. & Soyka, L.F. (1977) More comment on the ampicillin rash problem. *Pediatrics*, 59, 638-639

Chemical Information Services (1989-90) *Directory of World Chemical Producers*, Oceanside, NY

Chow, A.W. & Jewesson, P.J. (1985) Pharmacokinetics and safety of antimicrobial agents during pregnancy. *Rev. infect. Dis.*, 7, 287-313

Cole, M., Kenig, M.D. & Hewitt, V.A. (1973). Metabolism of penicillins to penicilloic acids and 6-aminopenicillanic acid in man and its significance in assessing penicillin absorption. *Antimicrobiol. Agents Chemother.*, 3, 463-468

Colley, D.P., Kay, J. & Gibson, G.T. (1983) Amoxycillin and ampicillin: a study of their use in pregnancy. *Aust. J. Pharm.*, *64*, 107-111

De Flora, S., Zanacchi, P., Camoirano, A., Bennicelli, C. & Badolati, G.S. (1984) Genotoxic activity and potency of 135 compounds in the Ames reversion test and in a bacterial DNA-repair test. *Mutat. Res.*, *133*, 161-198

Doluisio, J.T., LaPiana, J.C. & Dittert, L.W. (1971) Pharmacokinetics of ampicillin trihydrate, sodium ampicillin, and sodium dicloxacillin following intramuscular injection. *J. pharm. Sci.*, *60*, 715-719

Dunnick, J.K., Eustis, S.L., Huff, J.E. & Haseman, J.K. (1989) Two-year toxicity and carcinogenicity studies of ampicillin trihydrate and penicillin VK in rodents. *Fundam. appl. Toxicol.*, *12*, 252-257

Fabre, J. (1977) Pharmacocinetique tissulaire de la doxycycline comparée à celle d'autres antibiotiques chez le rat. [Tissue pharmacokinetics of doxycyline compared to those of other antibiotics in rats (Fr.).] *Nouv. Presse méd.*, *9*, 71-76

Feder, H.M. (1982) Comparative tolerability of ampicillin, amoxicillin, and trimethoprim-sulfamathoxazole suspensions in children with otitis media. *Antimicrob. Agents Chemother.*, *21*, 426-427

Foulds, G. (1986) Pharmacokinetics of sulbactam/ampicillin in humans: a review. *Rev. infect. Dis.*, *8 (Suppl. 5)*, S503-S511

Friedman, G.D. & Ury, H.K. (1980) Initial screening for carcinogenicity of commonly used drugs. *J. natl Cancer Inst.*, *65*, 723-733

Friedman, G.D. & Ury, H.K. (1983) Screening for possible drug carcinogenicity: second report of findings. *J. natl Cancer Inst.*, *71*, 1165-1175

Goldenthal, E. (1971) A compilation of LD50 values in newborn and adult animals. *Toxicol. appl. Pharmacol.*, *18*, 185-207

Gorbach, S.L. (1987) Bacterial diarrhoea and its treatment. *Lancet*, *ii*, 1378-1382

Gordon, M. & Luk, S.C. (1982) Atypical lymphoproliferative reaction to antibiotic therapy. *J. Am. Geriatr. Soc.*, *30*, 707-709

Green, M.H.L. & Tweats, D.J. (1981) An *Escherichia coli* differential killing test for carcinogens based on a *uvrA recA lexA* triple mutant. In: Stich, H.F. & San, R.H.C., eds, *Short-term Tests for Chemical Carcinogens*, New York, Springer, pp. 290-295

Haginaka, J. & Wakai, J. (1987) Liquid chromatogaphic determination of ampicillin and its metabolites in human urine by postcolumn alkaline degration. *J. pharm. Pharmacol.*, *39*, 5-8

Hirsch, H.A., Dreher, E., Perrochet, A. & Schmid, E. (1974) Transfer of ampicillin to the fetus and amniotic fluid during continuous infusion (steady state) and by repeated single intravenous injections to the mother. *Infection*, *2*, 207-212

Hodgman, T., Dasta, J.F., Armstrong, D.K., Visconti, J.A. & Reilley, T.E. (1984) Ampicillin-associated seizures. *South. med. J.*, *77*, 1323-1325

Hori, R., Okumura, K., Kamiya, A., Nihira, H. & Nakano, H. (1983) Ampicillin and cephalexin in renal insufficiency. *Clin. Pharmacol. Ther.*, *34*, 792-798

Ivashkiv, E. (1973) Ampicillin. *Anal. Profiles Drug Subst.*, *2*, 1-61

Jaju, M., Jaju, M. & Ahuja, Y.R. (1984) Evaluation of genotoxicity of ampicillin and carbenicillin on human lymphocytes *in vitro*: chromosome aberrations, mitotic index, cell cycle kinetics, satellite associations of acrocentric chromosomes and sister chromatid exchanges. *Hum. Toxicol.*, 3, 173-191

Jick, H., Holmes, L.B., Hunter, J.R., Madsen, S. & Stergachis, A. (1981) First trimester drug use and congenital disorders. *J. Am. med. Assoc.*, 246, 343-346

Jusko, W.J. & Lewis, G.P. (1973) Comparison of ampicillin and hetacillin pharmacokinetics in man. *J. pharm. Sci.*, 62, 69-76

van Ketel, W.G. (1984) Immunological investigations in patients with drug-induced skin eruptions. *Br. J. Dermatol.*, 110, 112-113

Khosid, G., Shteinberg, G., Balabanova, E., Baru, R., Chruagulova, N., Lapchinskaya, A., Lysenko, T., Shtegel'man, L. & Vil'shanskaya, F. (1975) Toxicological characteristics of ampicillin. *Antibiotiki (Moscow)*, 20, 653-657

King, J. (1975) The response of growing rats to a diet supplemented with the antibiotic ampicillin. *Lab. Anim.*, 9, 211-214

Korzhova, V.V., Lisitsyna, N.T. & Mikhailova, E.G. (1981) Effect of ampicillin and oxacillin on fetal and neonatal development. *Bull. exp. Biol. Med.*, 91, 169-171

Kraybill, E.N., Chaney, N.E. & McCarthy, L.R. (1980) Transplacental ampicillin: inhibitory concentrations in neonatal serum. *Am. J. Obstet. Gynecol.*, 138, 793-796

Lambert, H.P., Nye, F.J. & Stern, H. (1972) Letter. *Br. med. J.*, i, 688

La Piana Simonsen, L. (1989) Top 200 drugs of 1988. Branded new Rxs rise 4.0% and total Rxs move up 1.2%. *Pharm. Times*, 55, 40-48

Lewis, G.P. & Jusko, W.J. (1975) Pharmacokinetics of ampicillin in cirrhosis. *Clin. Pharmacol. Ther.*, 18, 475-484

Loo, J.C.K., Foltz, E.L., Wallick, M.S. & Kwan, K.C. (1974) Pharmacokinetics of pivampicillin and ampicillin in man. *Clin. Pharmacol. Ther.*, 16, 35-43

Mackowiak, P.A. & LeMaistre, C.F. (1987) Drug fever: a critical appraisal of conventional concepts. *Ann. intern. Med.*, 106, 728-733

Magni, L., Sjövall, J. & Syvälahti, E. (1978) Comparative clinical pharmacology of bacampicillin and high oral doses of ampicillin. *Infection*, 6, 283-287

Manthey, J., Pulverer, G. & Pillich, J. (1975) Chemische Induktion einer Lysogenie bei *Staphylococcus aureus*. [Chemical induction of lysogeny of *Staphylococcus aureus* (Ger.)]. *Zbl. Bakt. Hyg., I. Abt. Orig. A*, 231, 369-373

Masada, M., Nakagawa, T. & Uno, T. (1979) A new metabolite of ampicillin in man. *Chem. pharm. Bull.*, 27, 2877-2878

Milhaud, G., Renault, L., Vaissaire, J. & Maire, C. (1976) Sensibilité du lapin à l'ampicilline. [Sensitivity of rabbits to ampicillin (Fr.).] *Rec. méd. vét.*, 152, 843-847

Miyazaki, K., Ohtani, K., Sunada, K. & Arita, T. (1983) Determination of ampicillin, amoxicillin, cephalexin, and cephradine in plasma by high-performance liquid chromatography using fluorometric detection. *J. Chromatogr.*, 276, 478-482

Mortelmans, K., Haworth, S.S., Lawlor, T., Speck, W., Tainer, B. & Zeiger, E. (1986) *Salmonella* mutagenicity tests: II. Results from the testing of 270 chemicals. *Environ. Mutagenesis*, 8 (Suppl. 7), 1-119

Nabata, H., Iigima, M., Yamada, S., Munehasu, S., Suzuki, M. & Tachibana, M. (1988) Acute, subacute and chronic toxicity tests, and general pharmacological tests of Sulbactam-Ampicillin. *Chemotherapy*, 36, 58-65

National Toxicology Program (1987) *Toxicology and Carcinogenesis Studies of Ampicillin Trihydrate (CAS No. 7177-48-2) in F344/N Rats and B6C3F$_1$ Mice (Gavage Studies)* (NTP Technical Report 318), Research Triangle Park, NC, pp. 17-18, 139-143

Pennington, C.R. & Crooks, J. (1983) Antibiotics. I: New antibiotics and advances in antibiotic treatment. *Br. med. J.*, 286, 1732-1735

Prasad, A.B. (1977), Action of monofunctional alkylating agents and antibiotics on *Vicia faba* chromosomes. *Proc. Indian natl Sci. Acad.*, 43 (Part B), 19-25

Reynolds, J.E.F., ed. (1989) *Martindale. The Extra Pharmacopoeia*, 29th ed., London, The Pharmaceutical Press, pp. 116-122

Selby, J.V., Friedman, G.D. & Fireman, B.H. (1989) Screening prescription drugs for possible carcinogenicity: 11 to 15 years of follow-up. *Cancer Res.*, 49, 5736-5747

Serdaru, M., Diquet, B. & Lhermitte, F. (1982) Generalised seizures and ampicillin. *Lancet*, ii, 617-618

Sjövall, J. (1985) Renal excretion of intravenously infused amoxycillin and ampicillin. *Br. J. clin. Pharmacol.*, 19, 191-201

Sokoloff, B. (1977) Ampicillin rashes. *Pediatrics*, 59, 637-638

Stemp, G., Pascoe, S. & Gatehouse, D. (1988) *In vitro* and *in vivo* cytogenetic studies upon three β-lactam antibiotics (penicillin VK, ampicillin and carbenicillin). *Mutagenesis*, 3, 449

Triggs, E.J., Johnson, J.M. & Learoyd, B. (1980) Absorption and distribution of ampicillin in the elderly. *Eur. J. clin. Pharmacol.*, 18, 195-198

Tweats, D.J., Green, M.H.L. & Muriel, W.J. (1981) A differential killing assay for mutagens and carcinogens based on an improved repair-deficient strain of *Escherichia coli*. *Carcinogenesis*, 2, 189-194

US Food and Drug Administration (1988) *21 CFR Ch. I (4-1-88 Edition)*, 440.9a, Washington DC, US Government Printing Office, pp. 405-407

Van der Bijl, P., Seifart, H.I., Parkin, D.P. & Mattheyse, F.J. (1988) Oligomeric substances in ampicillin preparations. A comparison of Penbritin, Famicillin and Petercillin. *S. Afr. med. J.*, 73, 453-455

Venier, P., Monzini, R., Zordan, M., Clonfero, E., Paleologo, M. & Levis, A.G. (1989) Induction of SOS response in *Escherichia coli* strain PQ37 by 16 chemical compounds and human urine extracts. *Mutagenesis*, 4, 51-57

Wu, H.-L., Masada, M. & Uno, T. (1977) Gas chromatographic and gas chromatographic-mass spectrometric analysis of ampicillin. *J. Chromatogr.*, 137, 127-133

Young, J.D., Hurst, W.J., White, W.J. & Lang, C.M. (1987) An evaluation of ampicillin pharmacokinetics and toxicity in guinea pigs. *Lab. Anim. Sci.*, 37, 652-656

CHLORAMPHENICOL

This substance was considered by previous working groups, in October 1975 and March 1987 (IARC, 1976, 1987a,b). Since that time, new data have become available, and these have been incorporated into the monograph and taken into consideration in the present evaluation.

1. Chemical and Physical Data

1.1 Synonyms

Chem. Abstr. Services Reg. No.: 56-75-7

Chem. Abstr. Name: Acetamide, 2,2-dichloro-*N*-[2-hydroxy-1-(hydroxymethyl)-2-(4-nitrophenyl)ethyl]-[R-(R*,R*)]-

Synonyms: 2,2-Dichloro-*N*-[(αR,βR)-β-hydroxy-α-hydroxymethyl-4-nitrophenethyl]acetamide; D-(-)-threo-2-dichloroacetamido-1-*para*-nitrophenyl-1,3-propanediol; D-threo-*N*-dichloroacetyl-1-*para*-nitrophenyl-2-amino-1,3-propanediol; D-threo-(-)-2,2-dichloro-*N*-[β-hydroxy-α-(hydroxymethyl)-*para*-nitrophenethyl]acetamide; D-threo-*N*-(1,1'-dihydroxy-1-*para*-nitrophenylisopropyl)dichloroacetamide; D-(-)-threo-*para*-nitrophenyl-1-dichloroacetamido-2-propanediol-(1,3)

1.2 Structural and molecular formulae and molecular weight

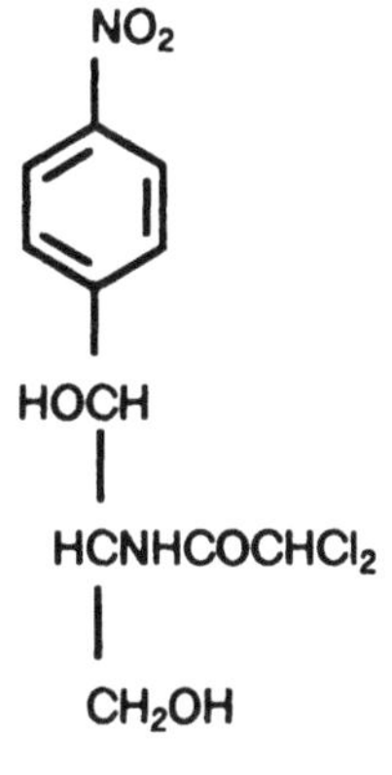

NO$_2$

HOCH

HCNHCOCHCl$_2$

CH$_2$OH

C$_{11}$H$_{12}$Cl$_2$N$_2$O$_5$ Mol. wt: 323.14

1.3 Chemical and physical properties of the pure substance

Data from Szulczewski and Eng (1975) and Al-Badr and El-Obeid (1986), unless otherwise specified

(a) *Description*: White to greyish-white or yellowish-white fine crystalline powder or fine crystals, needles or elongated plates. Of the four possible stereoisomers, only the αR,βR (or D-*threo*) form is active (Anon., 1979).

(b) *Melting-point*: 149-153°C (sublimes in high vacuum)

(c) *Optical rotation*: $[\alpha]_D^{27} = +18.6°$ (4.86% in ethanol)

(d) *Solubility*: 1:400 in water at 25°C; aqueous solutions are neutral; 1:6 in propylene glycol at 25°C; very soluble in methanol, ethanol, butanol, ethyl acetate, acetone; fairly soluble in diethyl ether (Windholz, 1983)

(e) *Spectroscopy data*: Ultraviolet, infrared, nuclear magnetic resonance and mass spectra have been reported.

(f) *Stability*: Stable in the solid state as a bulk drug and when present in solid dosage forms. Reasonable precautions taken to prevent excessive exposure to light or moisture are adequate to prevent significant decomposition over an extended period. In solution, chloramphenicol undergoes a number of degradative changes related to pH, temperature, photolysis and microbiological effects.

(g) *Reactivity*: The nitro group is readily reduced to the amine.

1.4 Technical products and impurities

Trade names: Ak-Chlor; Alcon Opulets Chloramphenicol; Amphicol; Antibiopto; Aquamycetin; Arcomicetina; Biomicin; Bioticaps; Cafenolo; Cébénicol; Chemicetina; Chemyzin; Chlomin; Chloramex; Chloramol; Chloratets; Chlorcol; Chlorofair; Chloromycetin; Chloroptic; Chlorsig; Cloramffen; Cloramplast; Clorbiotina; Clorfenicol Wolner; Clorofenicina; Cloromicetin; Cloromisol; Cloromoin; Cloroptic; Cutispray No. 4; Doctamicina; Econochlor; Espectro Medical; Farmicetina; Fenicol; Globenicol; Hortfenicol; I-Chlor; Iprobiot; Isopto Fenicol; Kamaver; Kemicetina; Kemicetine; Kloramfenikol Minims; Labamicol; Lennacol; Leukomycin; Levomicetina; Lomecitina; Micoclorina; Micodry; Minims Chloramphenicol; Mycetin; Mychel; Nevimycin; Normofenicol; Novochlorocap; Ocu-Chlor; Oftalent; Oleomycetin; Opclor; Ophtaphénicol; Ophthochlor; Paidomicetina; Pantofenicol; Pantovernil; Paraxin; Paraxin Succinat A; Pentamycetin; Plastodermo; Quemicetina; Ranphenicol; Rivomycine; Septicol; Sificetina; Sintomicetina; Sno Phenicol; Solnicol Ercé; Solu-Paraxin; Sopamycetin; Spersanicol; Succicaf; Synthomycetine; Thilocanfol; Tifomycine; Tramina; Troymycetin; Vernacetin

Many fixed combinations also contain chloramphenicol.

Chloramphenicol is often formulated as the cinnamate, palmitate (1.7 g equivalent to 1.0 g chloramphenicol) or sodium succinate salt (US Pharmacopeial Convention, 1975; Reynolds, 1989). Preparations are available as capsules (50, 100 and 250 mg; USP grade contains 90-120% of the labelled amount of active ingredient), ear drops (solution in propylene glycol), eye drops (0.5% solution or sterile, dry mixture of chloramphenicol and suitable buffers containing 90-130% of the labelled amount of chloramphenicol; US Pharmacopeial Convention, Inc., 1975) and eye ointment (1% chloramphenicol; USP grade contains 90-130% of the labelled amount of active ingredient); and as the palmitate in a suspension for oral administration (USP 5 ml, 30 mg/ml, containing 90-120% of the labelled amount of active ingredient) and the succinate in vials of 1 g for injection (USP grade containing 90-115% of the labelled amount of active ingredient).

2. Production, Occurrence, Use and Analysis

2.1 Production and occurrence

Chloramphenicol is an antibiotic produced by *Streptomyces venezuelae* (Ehrlich *et al.*, 1947). The crystalline antibiotic substance was isolated by Bartz in 1948 (Goodman & Gilman, 1970), and, in 1949, its structural determination (Rebstock *et al.*, 1949) and chemical synthesis (Controulis *et al.*, 1949) were reported.

Chloramphenical can be synthesized by condensation of *para*-nitrobenzoyl chloride with ethyl malonate to give *para*-nitroacetophenone, followed by bromination in acetic acid to form *para*-nitro-α-bromoacetophenone, and reaction of this with hexamethylene tetramine, followed by hydrolysis to give *para*-nitro-α-aminoacetophenone; subsequent acetylation of the amine group and condensation with formaldehyde give a hydroxymethyl group *alpha* to the amine group. Treatment with aluminium isopropylate reduces the keto group to a secondary alcohol, and, after deacetylation, condensation of the amine group with methyl dichloroacetate gives chloramphenicol (Anon., 1969). Chemical syntheses of chloramphenicol usually include a resolution step to separate stereoisomers.

In Japan, production by a fermentation process has also been described. The process resulted from the discovery and isolation of a new strain of microbe and does not require separation of stereoisomers (Anon., 1972).

Chloramphenicol is synthesized in Brazil, China, Czechoslovakia, the Federal Republic of Germany, Hungary, Italy, India, Israel, Japan, Mexico, Romania, South Africa, Spain and the USSR and has also been produced in France, Switzerland, the UK and the USA. Commercial production of chloramphenicol in the USA was first reported in 1948 (US Tariff Commission, 1949; Chemical Information Services, 1989-90).

In Sweden, 584 780 packages of chloramphenicol were sold in 1988 (Apoteksbolaget, 1988, 1989). In Finland, sales of chloramphenicol in 1987 were 0.01 defined daily doses per 1000 inhabitants (Finnish Committee on Drug Information and Statistics, 1988).

Chloramphenicol can be isolated from *Streptomyces venezuelae* in soil.

2.2 Use

Chloramphenicol is an antimicrobial agent recommended for serious infections in which the location of the infection, susceptibility of the pathogen or poor response to other therapy indicate restricted antimicrobial options. It has been used since the 1950s for a wide range of microbial infections, including typhoid fever and other forms of salmonellosis, and central nervous system, anaerobic and ocular infections (Bartlett, 1982; Sande & Mandell, 1985).

The usual dosage of chloramphenicol is 50 mg/kg daily in divided doses up to two to four weeks (Bartlett, 1982; Sande & Mandell, 1985). In certain indications, e.g. cystic fibrosis, treatment has been continued for years (Harley *et al.*, 1970).

An allowed daily intake (ADI) could not be set for chloramphenicol because of the dose-independence of chloramphenicol-induced aplastic anaemia (FAO/-WHO, 1969; FAO/WHO Expert Committee on Food Additives, 1988).

Chloramphenicol is believed to have been widely used as a veterinary antibiotic, despite legal controls in many countries, and there have been a few reports of residual amounts in various animal products (Allen, 1985). In countries in which its veterinary use is permitted, food regulations require withdrawal periods so as to avoid residues in the final product (FAO/WHO, 1969; FAO/WHO Expert Committee on Food Additives, 1988).

2.3 Analysis

Methods for the analysis of chloramphenicol have been reviewed (Wenk *et al.*, 1984; Al-Badr & El-Obeid, 1986). The compound has been determined in serum by high-performance liquid chromatography (Ryan *et al.*, 1984; Sood *et al.*, 1987; Meatherall & Ford, 1988) and enzyme immunoassay (Schwartz *et al.*, 1988).

Chloramphenicol has been analysed in pharmaceutical preparations using microbiological turbidimetric and spectrophotometric assays (US Food and Drug Administration, 1988; US Pharmacopeial Convention, Inc., 1989).

Analytical methods for chloramphenicol residues in meat, milk and eggs have been reviewed (Allen, 1985). The methods include high-performance liquid chromatography (Schmidt *et al.*, 1985) and radioimmunoassay (Arnold *et al.*, 1984; Arnold & Somogyi, 1985; Hock & Liemann, 1985).

3. Biological Data Relevant to the Evaluation of Carcinogenic Risk to Humans

3.1 Carcinogenicity studies in animals

(a) Oral administration

Mouse: In a study reported in an abstract, groups of 50 male and 50 female BALB/c mice, six weeks of age, were administered chloramphenicol [purity unspecified] at 0, 500 or 2000 mg/l in drinking-water for 104 weeks, at which time all survivors were killed. The incidences of lymphomas in mice of each sex (combined) were 3% in controls, 6% in low-dose animals and 12% in high-dose animals ($p < 0.05$). The incidences of other types of tumour were similar in treated and control animals (Sanguineti *et al.*, 1983). [The Working Group noted the incomplete reporting of the study.]

As reported in the same abstract, groups of 50 male and 50 female C57Bl/6N mice, six weeks of age, were administered chloramphenicol [purity unspecified] at 0, 500 or 2000 mg/l in drinking-water for 104 weeks, at which time all survivors were killed. The incidences of lymphomas in mice of each sex (combined) were 8% in controls, 22% in low-dose animals ($p < 0.05$) and 23% in high-dose animals ($p < 0.01$). The incidences of malignant liver-cell tumours in mice of each sex (combined) were: control, 0; low-dose, 2/90; and high-dose, 11/91 ($p < 0.01$) (Sanguineti *et al.*, 1983). [The Working Group noted the incomplete reporting of the study.]

(b) Intraperitoneal administration

Mouse: Two groups of 45 male BALB/c × AF_1 mice, six to eight weeks of age, received four intraperitoneal injections of 0.25 ml acetone in distilled water. After a 20-week rest period, one group received daily intraperitoneal injections of chloramphenicol [purity unspecified] at 0.25 ml (2.5 mg) in 0.9% saline solution on five days per week for five weeks. The mice were killed on day 350. Controls received injections of saline solution only. No increase in the incidence of tumours was observed (Robin *et al.*, 1981). [The Working Group noted the short duration of treatment and observation.]

(c) Administration with known carcinogens

Mouse: Two groups of 45 male BALB/c × AF_1 mice, six to eight weeks of age, received intraperitoneal injections every two weeks of four doses of 0.5 mg busulphan (1,4-butanediol dimethanesulfonate) in 0.25 ml acetone. After a 20-week rest period (on day 183 of the experiment), one group received chloramphenicol [purity unspecified] at 2.5 mg on five days per week for five weeks. On day 350 of the experiment, all surviving mice were killed. The incidence of lymphomas was 13/37 in the combined treatment group compared with 4/35 in a group treated with busulphan alone (p = 0.02, Fisher's exact test) (Robin *et al.*, 1981). [The Working Group noted the short duration of the experiment.]

3.2 Other relevant data

(a) Experimental systems

(i) *Absorption, distribution, excretion and metabolism*

In dogs, chloramphenicol was readily absorbed after oral administration of 50 mg/kg bw, giving plasma levels of 16.5 µg/ml 2 h after dosing (Watson, 1972, 1977a). Similar findings were made in rabbits (Cid *et al.*, 1983).

Five minutes after intravenous administration of ^{14}C-chloramphenicol to newborn pigs at 0.52 mg/kg bw, most tissues had higher levels of ^{14}C label than the blood; however, levels of chloramphenicol in bone marrow did not reach those noted in serum (Appelgren *et al.*, 1982).

Chloramphenicol and its metabolites were excreted in the urine of rats after oral dosing; up to 70% of an oral dose may be excreted in this way (Glazko *et al.*, 1949). About 0.4% of an intramuscular dose of 40 mg/kg to rats was detected in the bile within 4 h (Kunii *et al.*, 1983). In newborn pigs, most of an intravenous dose of chloramphenicol was excreted in the urine (Appelgren *et al.*, 1982). Following intravenous administration to goats, 69% of the dose was excreted in the urine within 12 h (Javed *et al.*, 1984).

Chloramphenicol was detected in the milk of goats and cattle after parenteral administration (Roy *et al.*, 1986); however, after oral administration [dose unspecified] to cattle, no chloramphenicol was detected in milk (De Corte-Baeten & Debackere, 1976).

In addition to free chloramphenicol and the glucuronide, the oxamic acid, alcohol, base, acetylarylamine and arylamine metabolites have been found in the urine of rats given intramuscular doses of ^{3}H-chloramphenicol (the 1R,2R-isomer). On the basis of recovered radioactivity, the major metabolites were assumed to be chloramphenicol base (~26%) and the acetylarylamine derivative (~20%) (Bories *et al.*, 1983).

In dogs, chloramphenicol base and chloramphenicol glucuronide conjugate were reported to be the major metabolites (Glazko *et al.*, 1950). Chloramphenicol, the glucuronide conjugate and the oxamic acid, acetylarylamine, arylamine and base derivatives were found in the urine of goats given intramuscular injections of chloramphenicol (Bories *et al.*, 1983).

The glucuronide is the main metabolic product in isolated rat hepatocytes exposed to chloramphenicol (Siliciano *et al.*, 1978). A study using perfused rat liver

and rat liver microsomes indicated that the arylamine derivative may undergo
N-oxidation to form nitrosochloramphenicol (Ascherl et al., 1985).

(ii) *Toxic effects*

The intravenous and intraperitoneal LD_{50}s for single doses of chloramphenicol in albino mice were 200 and 1320 mg/kg bw, respectively. The intravenous LD_{50} in rats was 170 mg/kg bw. Lethal amounts of chloramphenicol given orally or parenterally produced respiratory failure (Gruhzit et al., 1949). In rats treated with chloramphenicol at 50 and 100 mg/kg bw, the lipid content of the liver increased and the activities of aspartate and alanine aminotransferases in serum were elevated (Mandal et al., 1982).

After three groups of ten three-month-old Swiss mice were given daily intraperitoneal injections of chloramphenicol at 20, 40 or 100 mg/kg bw for three months, splenomegaly, hepatomegaly, lymph adenopathy and hypertrophy of the thymus occurred in a dose-dependent fashion (German & Loc, 1962).

Chloramphenicol caused decreased entry into S-phase in dividing bone-marrow cells of mice treated *in vivo* (Benes et al., 1980). The drug had a deleterious effect on bone-marrow recovery in mice after X-irradiation (Benes et al., 1980; Vacha et al., 1981) and after busulfan treatment in one study (Morley et al., 1976) but not another (Pazdernik & Corbett, 1980). Bone-marrow damage has been described in cats and dogs after 14-21 days' treatment with chloramphenicol (Penny et al., 1967; Watson, 1977b; Watson & Middleton, 1978; Watson, 1980). Effects included vacuolation of the myeloid and erythroid precursors and bone-marrow hypoplasia in cats, and suppression of erythropoiesis and a reduced rate of granulocyte formation but not bone-marrow vacuolation in dogs.

Chloramphenicol caused dose-related inhibition of erythroid and granulocytic colony forming units obtained from LAF_1 mice (Yunis, 1977).

Chloramphenicol and nitrosochloramphenicol inhibited DNA synthesis in rat bone-marrow cells *in vitro*. This effect was reversible with chloramphenicol but not with the nitroso compound. Similarly, the nitroso compound but not chloramphenicol bound irreversibly to bone-marrow cells (Gross et al., 1982). In another study *in vitro*, chloramphenicol and nitrosochloramphenicol had no effect on mouse haematopoietic precursor cells (Pazdernik & Corbett, 1979).

Several studies have demonstrated an effect of chloramphenicol on mitochondrial protein synthesis. *In vitro*, chloramphenicol inhibited mitochondrial protein synthesis in rat liver and rabbit bone marrow (Summ et al., 1976; Abou-Khalil et al., 1980). Nitrosochloramphenicol inhibited rat mitochondrial DNA polymerase *in vitro*, whereas the arylamine derivative and chloramphenicol itself did not (Lim et al., 1984).

(iii) *Effects on reproduction and prenatal toxicity*

High oral doses of chloramphenicol of 500-2000 mg/kg to rats and mice and of 500 and 1000 mg/kg to rabbits produced high incidences of embryonic and fetal deaths and fetal growth retardation in all three species. Teratogenic effects—predominantly umbilical hernia—were observed only in rats. The pregnant animals showed no toxic sign, except that those given the highest dose gained significantly less weight than controls (Fritz & Hess, 1971).

Groups of eight pregnant albino mice were given chloramphenicol orally at 25, 50, 100, or 200 mg/kg bw in 10 ml distilled water over the third stage of pregnancy for seven days. Animals were allowed to give birth, and the young were tested for conditioned avoidance response, electroshock seizure threshold and performance in open-field tests. Dose-related effects were seen in all three elements of the test: progeny of chloramphenicol-treated dams had reduced learning ability, higher brain seizure threshold and poorer performance in the open-field test (Al-Hachim & Al-Baker, 1974).

Chloramphenicol was also investigated for its effects on avoidance learning in rats. Four groups of 15 pregnant Wistar rats each were treated as follows: chloramphenicol was given subcutaneously at 50 mg/kg bw on days 7-21 of gestation; chloramphenicol was given subcutaneously at 50 and 100 mg/kg bw to pups for the first three days after birth; and the fourth group served as controls. No adverse effect on pregnancy or postnatal weight gain was seen, but when the animals were 60 days old, they had significant impairment of avoidance learning (Bertolini & Poggioli, 1981).

(iv) *Genetic and related effects*

The genetic toxicology of chloramphenicol has been reviewed (Rosenkranz, 1988).

Chloramphenicol did not induce lysogenic phage in *Staphylococcus aureus* (Manthey *et al.*, 1975). It did not induce differential toxicity in *Escherichia coli* (Slater *et al.*, 1971; Shimizu & Rosenberg, 1973; Longnecker *et al.*, 1974; Venturini & Monti-Bragadin, 1978; Mitchell *et al.*, 1980; Leifer *et al.*, 1981), *Salmonella typhimurium* (Nader *et al.*, 1981; Pall & Hunter, 1985), *Proteus mirabilis* (Adler *et al.*, 1976) or *Bacillus subtilis* (Kada *et al.*, 1972; Suter & Jaeger, 1982), although a contradictory positive result was obtained in the *rec* assay with *E. coli* (Suter & Jaeger, 1982). Chloramphenicol gave negative results in the SOS chromotest in *E. coli* (Mamber *et al.*, 1986). It induced breaks in DNA of *E. coli* B/r and *S. typhimurium* TA1976 (Jackson *et al.*, 1977). It did not induce mutations in *E. coli* (Hemmerly & Demerec, 1955) and was not mutagenic in plate incorporation assays with *S. typhimurium* in the presence or absence of an exogenous metabolic system (Brem *et al.*, 1974; McCann *et al.*, 1975; Mortelmans *et al.*, 1986). In a liquid pre-incubation assay, chloramphenicol did not induce reversions in *E. coli*; it did, however, induce forward mutations to azetidine-2-carboxylic acid resistance in the same bacterial strain. In the same assay system, chloramphenicol was weakly mutagenic to *S. typhimurium* TA98 in the presence or absence of an exogenous metabolic system (Mitchell *et al.*, 1980).

Chloramphenicol induced petite mutations in haploid strains of *Saccharomyces cerevisiae* (Weislogel & Butow, 1970; Williamson *et al.*, 1971) but not in diploid strains (Carnevali *et al.*, 1971).

Treatment of *Arabidopsis* seeds with chloramphenicol did not induce lethal mutations (Müller, 1965). Chloramphenicol induced chromosome breakage in root-tip meristem cells of germinating barley (Yoshida *et al.*, 1972) and *Vicia faba* seeds (Prasad, 1977). It did not induce micronuclei in pollen tetrads of *Tradescantia paludosa* (Ma *et al.*, 1984).

Chloramphenicol did not induce sex-linked recessive lethal mutations in *Drosophila melanogaster* treated either by injection (Clark, 1963) or by feeding (Nasrat *et al.*, 1977).

It inhibited DNA synthesis in human lymphoblastoid cell lines (Yunis *et al.*, 1973), in rat bone-marrow cells (Gross *et al.*, 1982) and in mouse Ehrlich ascites cells (Freeman *et al.*, 1977). DNA strand breaks were induced in human lymphocytes by chloramphenicol at 2.0 mM (Yunis *et al.*, 1987) but not at 0.8 mM in a human lymphoblastoid cell line, in human lymphocytes or in human bone-marrow cells (Isildar *et al.*, 1988). Chloramphenicol did not induce unscheduled DNA synthesis in Syrian hamster embryo cells in the presence or absence of an exogenous metabolic system (Suzuki, 1987).

The drug induced mutations at the *tk* locus of L5178Y mouse lymphoma cells in the presence and absence of an exogenous metabolic system (Mitchell *et al.*, 1988; Myhr & Caspary, 1988). It induced sister chromatid exchange in Syrian hamster embryo cells (Suzuki, 1987) but not in human leukocytes (Pant *et al.*, 1976). When human white blood cells were treated with low concentrations (10-40 µg/ml) of chloramphenicol, a concentration-dependent increase in the number of cells with chromosomal aberrations was observed (Mitus & Coleman, 1970). Chloramphenicol did not induce chromosomal aberrations in human lymphocytes (Jensen, 1972; Sasaki & Tonamura, 1973; Goh, 1979) or in human fibroblasts (Byarugaba *et al.*, 1975).

No morphological transformation was observed in Syrian hamster embryo cells after treatment with chloramphenicol at 100-1000 µg/ml (Suzuki, 1987). Chloramphenicol did not reproducibly enhance the transformation of Syrian hamster embryo cells by simian adenovirus SA7 (Hatch *et al.*, 1986).

Subcutaneous injections to C57Bl/10 mice of chloramphenicol at 320 mg/kg bw three times daily for three days led to inhibition of thymidine incorporation in bone-marrow cells (Benes *et al.*, 1980). Intramuscular injections of chloramphenicol (three times 1000 mg/kg bw) to Wistar rats did not induce chromosomal aberrations in bone-marrow cells (Jensen, 1972). At 50 mg/kg bw, the drug induced chromosomal aberrations in bone-marrow cells of mice [site of injection and number of animals tested unspecified] (Manna & Bardhan, 1972, 1977). Intramuscular injection of chloramphenicol at 50 mg/kg to Swiss albino mice [number of animals unspecified] induced chromosomal aberrations in mitotic and meiotic germ line cells (Roy & Manna, 1981).

Chloramphenicol did not induce dominant lethal mutations in mice when given twice at up to 15 000 mg/kg intraperitoneally (Epstein & Shafner, 1968; Ehling, 1971; Epstein *et al.*, 1972) but did when given at 500 mg/kg bw (Sram, 1972).

(b) Humans

(i) *Pharmacokinetics*

Chloramphenicol is readily absorbed from the gastrointestinal tract after oral administration of a crystalline powder of the active drug itself or a palmitate ester; the latter is hydrolysed in the small intestine to active chloramphenicol before absorption (Kauffman *et al.*, 1981). Esters of chloramphenicol—for example, the succinate—are converted to chloramphenicol *in vivo* (Salem *et al.*, 1981). Peak levels of 10-20 µg/ml appear 2-3 h after administration of chloramphenicol orally at 15 mg/kg bw (see Bartlett, 1982).

Chloramphenicol is also well absorbed by infants and neonates after oral administration. Serum (peak) concentrations of 20-24 µg/ml were noted after oral doses of 40 mg/kg bw to neonates. Infants given 26 mg/kg bw were found to have peak concentrations of 14 µg/ml (Mulhall *et al.*, 1983).

Chloramphenicol is distributed extensively in humans, regardless of its route of administration. The compound has been found in heart, lung, kidney, liver, spleen, pleural fluid, seminal fluid, ascitic fluid and saliva (Gray, 1955; Ambrose, 1984). It penetrates the blood-brain barrier, and its concentrations in cerebrospinal fluid can reach about 60% of that in plasma (Friedman *et al.*, 1979). The concentrations in brain tissue equal or even exceed those in plasma (Kramer *et al.*, 1969). Chloramphenicol easily crosses the placenta, and it is also excreted in breast milk (Havelka *et al.*, 1968).

Chloramphenicol has a half-time ranging from 1.6 to 4.6 h; using different techniques and in different adult patients, apparent volumes of distribution ranging from 0.2 to 3.1 l/kg have been measured (see Ambrose, 1984). The half-time is considerably longer in neonates (Rajchgot *et al.*, 1983): in one- to eight-day-old infants the half-life ranged from 10 to over 48 h, and in 11-day- to eight-week-old infants the range was 5-16 h (Glazer et al., 1980).

Six hours after an intravenous dose of 500 mg chloramphenicol succinate, the blood level was 4.5 µg/ml (2.8-6.9 µg/ml) in patients with chloramphenicol-induced bone-marrow depression, while in the control group the mean level was 1.2 µg/ml (0-2.3 µg/ml). Such findings suggest that patients susceptible to the effects of chloramphenicol on bone marrow may clear the drug from the blood more slowly than those who are not susceptible (Suhrland & Weisberger, 1969).

Chloramphenicol is excreted primarily in the urine (90%); up to 15% is excreted as the parent compound and the remainder as metabolites, including conjugated derivatives (Yunis, 1973; Burke et al., 1980; Ambrose, 1984). Glomerular excretion is thought to be the major mechanism of excretion (Glazko et al., 1949).

Approximately 48% of the chloramphenicol excreted in urine within 8 h of an oral dosing was the glucuronide conjugate; only 6% was excreted as the parent compound and 4% as the base derivative (Nagakawa et al., 1975; Baselt, 1982; Bories et al., 1983). The alcohol derivative has been detected in the urine of neonates (Dill et al., 1960).

Human liver microsomes have been shown to reduce the nitro group of chloramphenicol (Salem et al., 1981).

Chloramphenicol arylamide is formed by intestinal bacterial reduction of the NO_2 group to NH_2, which is acetylated and excreted in urine (Meissner & Smith, 1979). Oxamic acid (formed by oxidative dechlorination of the side chain) was identified as a major metabolite in one human volunteer (Corpet & Bories, 1987).

(ii) *Adverse effects*

The most important adverse effects of chloramphenicol involve the haematopoietic system (as reviewed by the FAO/WHO Expert Committee on Food Additives, 1988). Potentially fatal toxicity may develop in neonates exposed to excessive doses of chloramphenicol (Sande & Mandell, 1985). This so-called 'grey baby syndrome' may also occur in older children and in adults receiving doses resulting in serum concentrations of 40-200 µg/ml (see Bartlett, 1982). Other adverse effects include hypersensitivity reactions, gastrointestinal complaints and neurological complications after long-term treatment. Chloramphenicol can also precipitate haemolytic anaemia in subjects with glucose-6-phosphate dehydrogenase deficiency (Robertson et al., 1968).

Dose-dependent, reversible bone-marrow suppression affects primarily the erythroid series and occurs regularly when plasma concentrations of chloramphenicol are 25 µg/ml or higher (Scott et al., 1965; Yunis & Adamson, 1977). Another haematological side-effect is rare, unpredictable, non-dose-related aplastic anaemia, which often appears after the drug has been discontinued (Best, 1967).

The metabolite (or metabolites) responsible for the induction of aplastic anaemia in human beings is unknown, but nitrosochloramphenicol has been implicated (Nagai & Kanamuru, 1978; Yunis, 1988): it is known to be toxic to human bone-marrow cells *in vitro* and, moreover, is more toxic than chloramphenicol itself (Yunis *et al.*, 1980a,b). Metabolites of chloramphenicol, such as dehydrochloramphenicol, produced by intestinal bacteria, are more than 20-fold more cytotoxic than the parent drug (Yunis, 1988).

There have been many case reports of the occurrence of aplastic anaemia following administration of chloramphenicol by various routes (Rosenthal & Blackman, 1965; Nagao & Mauer, 1969; Carpenter, 1975; Yunis, 1978; Abrams *et al.*, 1980; Silver & Zuckerman, 1980; Flach, 1982; Fraunfelder *et al.*, 1982; Plaut & Best, 1982; Issaragrisil & Piankijagum, 1985; Korting & Kifle, 1985; Elberg & Hansen, 1986; von Muhlendahl, 1987). In many of these cases, large doses had been taken repeatedly over periods of many years before the onset of symptoms of aplastic anaemia. Case-control studies have also suggested an association between chloramphenicol use and aplastic anaemia (for review, see FAO/WHO Expert Committee on Food Additives, 1988). A widely discussed causal association between topical application of chloramphenicol eye-drops and aplastic anaemia (Wade, 1972; Carptenter, 1975; Fraunfelder *et al.*, 1982) has not been established.

(iii) *Effects on reproduction and prenatal toxicity*

In the Collaborative Perinatal Project, in which drug intake and pregnancy outcome were studied in a series of 50 282 women in 1959-65, 98 women had been exposed to choramphenicol during the first trimester of pregnancy. There were eight malformed children in the exposed group, giving a nonsignificant standardized relative risk (RR) of 1.17. A total of 348 women had had exposure at any time during pregnancy with no evidence of an increase in the incidence of congenital malformations (Heinonen *et al.*, 1977).

No adverse effect was reported in the children of 22 patients treated at various stages of pregnancy with chloramphenicol (Cunningham *et al.*, 1973).

(iv) *Genetic and related effects*

No adequate study was available to the Working Group.

3.3 Case reports and epidemiological studies

Numerous case reports have been published of leukaemia occurring following chloramphenicol-induced aplastic anaemia (Edwards, 1969; Seaman, 1969; Goh, 1971; Cohen & Huang, 1973; Meyer & Boxer, 1973; Hellriegel & Gross, 1974; Modan *et al.*, 1975; IARC, 1976; Ellims *et al.*, 1979; Witschel, 1986; IARC, 1987a); three case reports have been published of leukaemia following chloramphenicol therapy in the absence of interceding aplastic anaemia (Humphries, 1968; Popa & Iordacheanu, 1975; Aboul-Enein *et al.*, 1977).

Shu *et al.* (1987) reported a case-control study of 309 childhood leukaemia cases (under 15 years) notified to a population-based cancer registry in Shanghai, China, during 1974-86, and 618 age- and sex-matched population controls. Information was obtained from parents or guardians for lifetime use of selected drugs, including prescribed chloramphenicol and syntomycin (a racemic mixture of D- and L-chloramphenicol). The risk for all types of leukaemia combined showed a marked increase with accumulated use of chloramphenicol, yielding RRs of 1.7 (95% confidence interval, 1.2-2.5), 2.8 (1.5-5.1) and 9.7 (3.9-24.1) for one to five days', six to ten days' and more than ten days' treatment, respectively. The association was present in a subgroup in which first use had occurred more than five years prior to diagnosis and in one in which last use had been more than two years before diagnosis. Significant trends in risk with dose were observed both for acute lymphocytic leukaemia (56% of cases) and for acute nonlymphocytic leukaemia (30%). An association with leukaemia was also seen for use of syntomycin (RR, 1.9; 1.1-3.2). [The Working Group noted that interview was undertaken up to ten years after diagnosis, which adds to the possibility of differential recall between the parents of cases and controls. Little information was available with regard to use of other antibiotics, making it difficult to evaluate the possibility of bias.]

4. Summary of Data Reported and Evaluation

4.1 Exposure data

Chloramphenicol has been used widely as an antibiotic since the 1950s. Veterinary use of chloramphenicol has resulted in the occurrence of residues in animal-derived food.

4.2 Experimental carcinogenicity data

No adequate study was available to evaluate the carcinogenicity of chloramphenicol to experimental animals.

Intraperitoneal administration of chloramphenicol to mice enhanced the incidence of lymphomas induced by 1,4-butanediol dimethanesulfonate.

4.3 Human carcinogenicity data

Many case reports have described an unusual succession of leukaemia following chloramphenicol-induced aplastic anaemia and bone-marrow depression. Additional evidence for the association between use of chloramphenicol and leukaemia has come from a single large case-control study in China, which demonstrated a relationship with duration of exposure.

4.4 Other relevant data

Use of chloramphenicol during the first trimester of pregnancy has not been associated with an increase in the incidence of congenital malformations. Chloramphenicol caused embryo- and fetolethality in mice, rats and rabbits.

In humans, chloramphenicol causes aplastic anaemia. In both humans and animals administered chloramphenicol, reversible suppression of the bone marrow is frequent whenever the drug reaches relatively high plasma concentrations.

Chloramphenicol induced chromosomal aberrations in bone-marrow cells of mice but not of rats treated *in vivo*. It induced chromosomal aberrations in meiotic cells of male mice. Contradictory results were obtained in dominant lethal tests in mice. In human cells, chloramphenicol did not induce sister chromatid exchange or chromosomal aberrations but gave contradictory results for DNA damage. It induced sister chromatid exchange in Syrian hamster cells. Chloramphenicol induced gene mutations in mouse lymphoma cells but did not induce DNA damage in hamster cells. Chloramphenicol did not induce sex-linked recessive lethal mutations in *Drosophila*. It induced chromosomal aberrations in plants. In haploid yeast, chloramphenicol induced petite mutations. In most studies, chloramphenicol was not mutagenic to and did not cause DNA damage in *Salmonella typhimurium* or *Escherichia coli* and did not induce DNA damage in *Proteus mirabilis* or *Bacillus subtilis*. (See Appendix 1.)

4.5 Evaluation[1]

There is *limited evidence* for the carcinogenicity of chloramphenicol in humans.

There is *inadequate evidence* for the carcinogenicity of chloramphenicol in experimental animals.

In making the overall evaluation, the Working Group also took note of the following information. Chloramphenicol induces aplastic anaemia, and this condition is related to the occurrence of leukaemia.

Overall evaluation

Chloramphenicol *is probably carcinogenic to humans (Group 2A)*.

---

[1]For description of the italicized terms, see Preamble, pp. 26–29.

5. References

Abou-Khalil, S., Salem, Z. & Yunis, A.A. (1980) Mitochondrial metabolism in normal, myeloid, and erythroid hyperplastic rabbit bone-marrow: effect of chloramphenicol. *Am. J. Hematol.*, 8, 71-79

Aboul-Enein, M., El-Zayat, A., Hamza, M.R., El-Nawla, N.G. & Aboul-Nasr, L. (1977) Chloramphenicol as a possible leukaemogenic agent. *J. Egypt. public Health Assoc.*, 52, 1-5

Abrams, S.M., Degnan, T.J. & Vinciguerra, V. (1980) Marrow aplasia following topical application of chloramphenicol eye ointment. *Arch. intern. Med.*, 140, 576-577

Adler, B., Braun, R., Schöneich, J. & Böhme, H. (1976) Repair-defective mutants of *Proteus mirabilis* as a prescreening system for the detection of potential carcinogens. *Biol. Zentralbl.*, 95, 463-369

Al-Badr, A.A. & El-Obeid, H.A. (1986) Chloramphenicol. *Anal. Profiles Drug Subst.*, 15, 701-760

Albertini, S. & Gocke, E. (1988) Plasmid copy number and mutant frequencies in *S. typhimurium* TA102. *Environ. mol. Mutagenesis*, 12, 353-363

Al-Hachim, G.M. & Al-Baker, A. (1974) The prenatal effect of chloramphenicol on the postnatal development of mice. *Neuropharmacology*, 13, 233-237

Allen, E.H. (1985) Review of chromatographic methods for chloramphenicol residues in milk, eggs, and tissues of food-producing animals. *J. Assoc. off. anal. Chem.*, 68, 990-999

Ambrose, P.J. (1984) Clinical pharmacokinetics of chloramphenicol and chloramphenicol succinate. *Clin. Pharmacokinet.*, 9, 222-238

Anon. (1969) Leading world manufacturers of chloramphenicol. *Inf. Chim.*, March/April, pp. 47-52

Anon. (1972) New manufacturing process for chloramphenciol. *Chem. Econ. Eng. Rev.*, 4, 51

Anon. (1979) *Pharmaceutical Codex*, London, The Pharmaceutical Press, pp. 162-166

Apoteksbolaget (1988) *Svensk Läkemedelsstatistic* [Swedish Drugs Statistics], Stockholm, Pharmaceutical Association of Sweden

Apoteksbolaget (1989) *Outprint of the Drug Data Base (17 October 1989)*, Stockholm, Pharmaceutical Association of Sweden

Appelgren, L.-E., Eberhardson, B., Martin, K. & Slanina, P. (1982) The distribution and fate of ^{14}C-chloramphenicol in the new-born pig. *Acta pharmacol. toxicol.*, 51, 345-350

Arnold, D. & Somogyi, A. (1985) Trace analysis of chloramphenicol residues in eggs, milk, and meat: comparison of gas chromatography and radioimmunoassay. *J. Assoc. off. anal. Chem.*, 68, 984-990

Arnold, D., Berg, D., Boertz, A.K., Mallick, U. & Somogyi, A. (1984) Radioimmunologische Bestimmung von Chloramphenicol-Rückständen in Muskulatur, Milch und Eiern. [Radioimmunoassay of chloramphenicol residues in muscle, milk and eggs (Ger.).] *Arch. Lebensmittelhyg.*, 35, 121-148

Ascherl, M., Eyer, P. & Kampffmeyer, H. (1985) Formation and disposition of nitrosochloramphenicol in rat liver. *Biochem. Pharmacol.*, 34, 3755-3763

Bartlett, J.G. (1982) Chloramphenicol. *Med. Clin. North Am.*, 66, 91-102

Baselt, R.C. (1982) *Disposition of Toxic Drugs in Man*, 2nd ed., Davis, CA, Biochemical Publications, pp. 136-139

Benes, L., Rotreklova, E., Velcovsky, V. & Pospisil, M. (1980) Inhibition of bone marrow cell proliferation and DNA replication induced by chloramphenicol. *Folia biol.*, 26, 408-414

Bertolini, A. & Poggioli, R. (1981) Chloramphenicol administration during brain development: impairment of avoidance learning in adulthood. *Science*, 213, 238-239

Best, W.R. (1967) Chloramphenicol associated blood-dyscrasias. A review of cases submitted to the American Medical Association Registry. *J. Am. med. Assoc.*, 201, 181-188

Bories, G.F., Peleran, J.C., Wal, J.M. & Corpet, D.E. (1983) Simple and ion-pair high performance liquid chromatography as an improved analytical tool for chloramphenicol metabolic profiling. *Drug Metab. Dispos.*, 11, 249-254

Boyle, V.J. & Simpson, C.A. (1980) Bacterial DNA repair assay of selected compounds in pulp and paper mill effluents. *J. tech. Assoc. Pulp Paper Ind.*, 63, 127-130

Brem, H., Stein, A.B. & Rosenkranz, H.S (1974) The mutagenicity and DNA-modifying effect of haloalkanes. *Cancer Res.*, 34, 2576-2579

Burke, J.T., Wargin, W.A. & Blum, M.R. (1980) High-pressure liquid chromatographic assay for chloramphenicol, chloramphenicol-3-monosuccinate and chloramphenicol-1-monosuccinate. *J. pharm. Sci.*, 69, 909-912

Byarugaba, W., Rüdiger, H.W., Koske-Westphal, T., Wöhler, W. & Passarge, E. (1975) Toxicity of antibiotics on cultured human skin fibroblasts. *Humangenetik*, 28, 263-267

Carnevali, F., Leoni, L., Morpurgo, G. & Conti, G. (1971) Induction of cytoplasmic 'petite' mutation by antibacterial antibiotics. *Mutat. Res.*, 12, 357-363

Carpenter, G. (1975) Chloramphenicol eye-drops and marrow aplasia. *Lancet*, ii, 326-327

Chemical Information Services (1989-90) *Directory of World Chemical Producers, 1989/90*, Oceanside, NY

Cid, F., Mella, F., Gonzalez, X. & Gonzalez, R. (1983) Effects of anti-inflammatory drugs on the pharmacokinetics of chloramphenicol. *An. Real Acad. Farm.*, 49, 49-60

Clark, A.M. (1963) The effects of chloramphenicol, streptomycin and penicillin on the induction of mutations by X-rays in *Drosophila melanogaster*. *Z. Vererbungsl.*, 94, 121-125

Cohen, H.J. & Huang, A.T.-F. (1973) A marker chromosome abnormality—occurrence in chloramphenicol-associated acute leukemia. *Arch. intern. Med.*, 132, 440-443

Controulis, J., Rebstock, M.C. & Crooks, H.M., Jr (1949) Chloramphenicol (chloromycetin). V. Synthesis. *J. Am. chem. Soc.*, 71, 2463-2468

Corpet, D.E. & Bories, G.F. (1987) 3H-Chloramphenicol metabolism in human volunteer: oxamic acid as a new major metabolite. *Drug Metab. Dispos.*, 15, 925-927

Cunningham, F.G., Morris, G.B. & Mickal, A. (1973) Acute pyelonephritis of pregnancy: a clinical review. *Obstet. Gynecol.*, 42, 112-117

De Corte-Baeten, K. & Debackere, M. (1976) Excretion of chloramphenicol in the milk of lactating cows after oral and parenteral administration. *Dtsch. Tieraerztl. Wochenschr.*, *83*, 231-233

Dill, W.A., Thompson, E.M., Tisken, R.A. & Glazko, A.J. (1960) A new metabolite of chloramphenicol. *Nature*, *185*, 535-537

Edwards, L.D. (1969) Association between chloramphenicol hypoplastic anemia and acute myeloblastic leukemia: a case report. *Mil. Med.*, *134*, 1447-1449

Ehling, U.H. (1971) Comparison of radiation- and chemically-induced dominant lethal mutations in male mice. *Mutat. Res.*, *11*, 35-44

Ehrlich, J., Bartz, Q.R., Smith, R.M., Joslyn, D.A. & Burkholder, P.R. (1947) Chloromycetin, a new antibiotic from a soil actinomycete. *Science*, *106*, 417

Elberg, J.J. & Hansen W.H. (1986) Chloramphenicol eye drops and aplastic anaemia. *Ugeskr. Laeger.*, *148*, 2227-2228

Ellims, P.H., Van der Weyden, M.B., Brodie, G.N., Firkin, B.G., Whiteside, M.G. & Faragher, B.S. (1979) Erythroleukemia following drug induced hypoplastic anemia. *Cancer*, *44*, 2140-2146

Epstein, S.S. & Shafner, H. (1968) Chemical mutagens in the human environment. *Nature*, *219*, 385-387

Epstein, S.S., Arnold, E., Andrea, J., Bass, W. & Bishop, Y. (1972) Detection of chemical mutagens by the dominant lethal assay in the mouse. *Toxicol. appl. Pharmacol.*, *23*, 288-325

FAO/WHO (1969) *Specifications for the Identity and Purity of Food Additives and Their Toxicological Evaluation: Some Antibiotics* (World Health Organization Technical Report Series No. 430), Geneva, World Health Organization, pp. 41-43

FAO/WHO Expert Committee on Food Additives (1988) Chloramphenicol. In: *Toxicological Evaluation of Certain Veterinary Drug Residues in Food* (WHO Food Additives Series 23), Geneva, World Health Organization, pp. 1-71

Finnish Committee on Drug Information and Statistics (1988) *Suomen Lääketilasto 1987* [Finnish Statistics on Medicines 1987], Helsinki

Flach, A.J. (1982) Chloramphenicol and aplastic anemia. *Am. J. Ophthalmol.*, *93*, 664-665

Fraunfelder, F.T., Bagby, G.C. & Kelly, D.J. (1982) Fatal aplastic anemia following topical administration of ophthalmic chloramphenicol. *Am. J. Ophthalmol.*, *93*, 356-360

Freeman, K.B., Patel, H. & Haldar, D. (1977) Inhibition of deoxyribonucleic acid synthesis in Ehrlich ascites cells by chloramphenicol. *Mol. Pharmacol.*, *13*, 504-511

Friedman, C.A., Lovejoy, F.C, & Smith, A.L. (1979) Chloramphenicol disposition in infants and children. *J. Pediatr.*, *95*, 1071-1077

Fritz, H. & Hess, R. (1971) The effect of chloramphenicol on the prenatal development of rats, mice and rabbits. *Toxicol. appl. Pharmacol.*, *19*, 667-674

German, A. & Loc, T. (1962) Induction d'une tumeur transplantable chez des souris de lignée Swiss par injections répetées de chloramphenicol. [Induction of a transplantable tumour in Swiss mice by repeated injections of chloramphenicol (Fr.).] *Ann. Pharmacol. fr.*, *20*, 116-120

Glazer, J.P., Danish, M.A., Plotkin, S.A. & Yaffe, S.J. (1980) Disposition of chloramphenicol in low birth weight infants. *Pediatrics*, *66*, 573-578

Glazko, A.J., Wolf, L.M., Dill, W.A. & Bratton, A.C. (1949) Biochemical studies of chloramphenicol (chloromycetin). II. Tissue distribution and excretion studies. *J. Phamacol. exp. Ther.*, *96,*, 445-449

Glazko, A.J., Dill, W.A. & Rebstock, M.C. (1950) Biochemical studies on chloramphenicol (chloromycetin). III. Isolation and identification of metabolic products in urine. *J. biol. Chem.*, *183*, 679-691

Goh, K.O. (1971) Chloramphenicol, acute leukemia and chromosomal vacuolizations. *South. med. J.*, *64*, 815-9

Goh, K. (1979) Chloramphenicol and chromosomal morphology. *J. Med.*, *10*, 159-166

Goodman, L.S. & Gilman, A., eds (1970) *The Pharmacological Basis of Therapeutics*, 4th ed., London, MacMillan, pp. 1269-1274

Gray, J.D. (1955) The concentration of chloramphenicol in human tissues. *Can. med. Assoc. J.*, *72*, 778-779

Gross, B.J., Branchflower, R.V., Burke, T.R., Lees, D.E. & Pohl, L.R. (1982) Bone marrow toxicity *in vitro* of chloramphenicol and its metabolites. *Toxicol. appl. Pharmacol.*, *64*, 557-565

Gruhzit, O.M., Frisken, R.A., Reutner, T.F. & Martino, E. (1949) Chloramphenicol (chloromycetin), an antibiotic. Pharmacological and pathological studies in animals. *J. clin. Invest.*, *28*, 943-952

Harley, R.D., Huang, N.N., Macri, S.H. & Green, W.R. (1970) Optic neuritis and optic atrophy following chloramphenicol in cystic fibrosis patients. *Trans. Am. Acad. Ophthalmol. Otolaryngol.*, *74*, 1011-1031

Hatch, G.G., Anderson, T.M., Lubet, R.A., Kouri, R.E., Putman, D.L., Cameron, J.W., Nims, R.W., Most, B., Spalding, J.W., Tennant, R.W. & Schechtman, L.M. (1986) Chemical enhancement of SA7 virus transformation of hamster embryo cells: evaluation by interlaboratory testing of diverse chemicals. *Environ. Mutagenesis*, *8*, 515-531

Havelka, J., Hejzlar, M., Popov, V., Viktorinova, D. & Proxhazka, J. (1968) Excretion of chloramphenicol in human milk. *Chemotherapy*, *13*, 204-211

Heinonen, O.P., Slone, D. & Shapiro, S. (1977) *Birth Defects and Drugs in Pregnancy*, Littleton, MA, Publishing Sciences Group, pp. 297-301, 435

Hellgriegel, K.P. & Gross, R. (1974) Follow-up studies in chloramphenicol-induced aplastic anaemia. *Postgrad. med. J.*, *50* (Suppl. 5), 136-142

Hemmerly, J. & Demerec, M. (1955) XIII. Tests of chemicals for mutagenicity. *Cancer Res.*, *15* (Suppl. 3), 69-75

Hock, C. & Liemann, F. (1985) Die Entwicklung eines Radioimmunoassays zum Nachweis von Chloramphenicol und 3'-Chloramphenicol-Beta-D-Monoglucuronid. [The development of a radioimmunoassay for the detection of chloramphenicol and 3'-chloramphenicol-beta-D-monoglucuronide (Ger.).] *Arch. Lebensmittelhyg.*, *36*, 125-148

Humphries, K.R. (1968) Acute myelomonocytic leukaemia following chloramphenicol therapy. *N.Z. med. J.*, *68*, 248-249

IARC (1976) *IARC Monographs on the Evaluation of Carcinogenic Risk of Chemicals to Man*, Vol. 10, *Some Naturally Occurring Substances*, Lyon, pp. 85-98

IARC (1987a) *IARC Monographs on the Evaluation of Carcinogenic Risks to Humans*, Suppl. 7, *Overall Evaluations of Carcinogenicity: An Updating of* IARC Monographs *Volumes 1 to 42*, Lyon, pp. 145-146

IARC (1987b) *IARC Monographs on the Evaluation of Carcinogenic Risks to Humans*, Suppl. 6, *Genetic and Related Effects: An Updating of Selected* IARC Monographs *from Volumes 1 to 42*, Lyon, pp. 142-144

Isildar, M., Jimenez, J.J., Arimura, G.K. & Yunis, A.A. (1988) DNA damage in intact cells induced by bacterial metabolites of chloramphenicol. *Am. J. Hematol.*, *28*, 40-46

Issaragrisil, S. & Piankijagum, A. (1985) Aplastic anemia following topical administration of ophthalmic chloramphenicol: report of a case and review of the literature. *J. med. Assoc. Thailand*, *88*, 309-312

Jackson, S.F., Wentzell, B.R., McCalla, D.R. & Freeman, K.B. (1977) Chloramphenicol damages bacterial DNA. *Biochem. biophys. Res. Commun.*, *78*, 151-157

Javed, I., Nawaz, M., Ahmed, M., Rehman, Z.U. & Shah, B.H. (1984) Pharmacokinetics, renal clearance and urinary excretion of chloramphenicol in goats. *Pak. Vet.*, *4*, 151-157

Jensen, M.K. (1972) Phenylbutazone, chloramphenicol and mammalian chromosomes. *Humangenetik*, *17*, 61-64

Kada, T., Tutikawa, K. & Sadaie, Y. (1972) *In vitro* and host-mediated 'rec-assay' procedures for screening chemical mutagens; and phloxine, a mutagenic red dye detected. *Mutat. Res.*, *16*, 163-174

Kauffman, R.E., Miceli, J.N., Strevel, L., Buckley, J.A., Done, A.K. & Dajani, A.S. (1981) Pharmacokinetics of chloramphenicol succinate in infants and children. *J. Pediatr.*, *98*, 315-320

Korting, G.W. & Kifle, H. (1985) Systemic side-effects from external application of chloramphenicol. *Hautarzt*, *36*, 181-183

Kramer, P.W., Griffith, R.S. & Campbell, R.L. (1969) Antibiotic penetration of the brain. A comparative study. *J. Neurosurg.*, *31*, 295-302

Kunii, O., Komatsu, T. & Nishiya, H. (1983) Biliary excretion of antibiotics in rats. *Jpn. J. exp. Med.*, *53*, 51-58

Leifer, Z., Hyman, J. & Rosenkranz, H.S. (1981), Determination of genotoxic activity using DNA polymerase-deficient and -proficient *E. coli*. In: Stich, H.F. & San, R.H.C., eds, *Short-term Tests for Chemical Carcinogens*, New York, Springer, pp. 127-139

Lim, L.O., Abou-Khalil, W.H. & Yunis, A.A. (1984) The effect of nitrochloramphenicol on mitochondrial DNA polymerase activity. *J. Lab. clin. Med.*, *104*, 213-222

Longnecker, D.S., Curphey, T.J., James, S.T., Daniel, D.S. & Jacobs, N.J. (1974) Trial of a bacterial screening system for rapid detection of mutagens and carcinogens. *Cancer Res.*, *34*, 1658-1663

Ma, T., Harris, M.M., Anderson, V.A., Ahmed, I., Mohammad, K., Bare, J.L. & Lin, G. (1984) *Tradescantia*-micronucleus (Trad-MCN) tests on 140 health-related agents. *Mutat. Res., 138*, 157-167

Mamber, S.W., Okasinski, W.G., Pinter, C.D. & Tunac, J.B. (1986) The *Escherichia coli* K-12 SOS chromotest agar spot test for simple, rapid detection of genotoxic agents. *Mutat. Res., 171*, 83-90

Mandal, B., Hazra, N. & Maity, C.R. (1982) Metabolic and enzymatic changes in rats following high doses of tetracycline, chloramphenicol and trimethoprim. *Ann. natl Acad. med. Sci., 18*, 146-156

Manna, G.K. & Bardhan, S. (1972) Effects of two antibiotics on the chromosomes and mitotic frequency in the bone marrow cells of mice. *Chromosomes Today, 4*, 277-281

Manna, G.K. & Bardhan, S. (1977) Some aspects of chloramphenicol-induced bone marrow chromosome aberrations in mice. *J. Cytol. Genet., 12*, 10-17

Manthey, J., Pulverer, G. & Pillich, J. (1975) Chemische Induktion einer Lysogenie bei Staphylococcus aureus. [Chemical induction of lysogeny of *Staphylococcus aureus* (Ger.).] *Zentralbl. Bakteriol. Hyg. I. Abt. Orig. A, 231*, 369-373

McCann, J., Choi, E., Yamasaki, E. & Ames, B.N. (1975) Detection of carcinogens as mutagens in the *Salmonella*/microsome test: assay of 300 chemicals. *Proc. natl Acad. Sci. USA, 72*, 5135-5139

Meatherall, R. & Ford, D. (1988) Isocratic liquid chromatographic determination of theophylline, acetaminophen, chloramphenicol, caffeine, anticonvulsants, and barbiturates in serum. *Ther. Drug Monit., 10*, 101-115

Meissner, H.C. & Smith, A.L. (1979) The current status of chloramphenicol. *Pediatrics, 64*, 348-356

Meyer, J.S. & Boxer, M. (1973) Leukemic cellular thrombi in pulmonary blood vessels. Subleukemic myelogenous leukemia following chloramphenicol-induced aplastic anemia. *Cancer, 32*, 712-721

Mitchell, I. de G. & Gilbert, P.J. (1985) An assessment of the importance of error-prone repair and point mutations to forward mutation to L-azatidine-2-carboxylic acid resistance in *Escherichia coli*. *Mutat. Res., 149*, 303-310

Mitchell, I. de G., Dixon, P.A., Gilbert, P.J. & White, D.J. (1980) Mutagenicity of antibiotics in microbial assays: problems of evaluation. *Mutat. Res., 79*, 91-105

Mitchell, A.D., Rudd, C.J. & Caspary, W.J. (1988) Evaluation of the L5178Y mouse lymphoma cell mutagenesis assay: intralaboratory results for sixty-three coded chemicals tested at SRI International. *Environ. mol. Mutagenesis, 12 (Suppl. 13)*, 37-101

Mitus, W.J. & Coleman, N. (1970) In vitro effect of chloramphenicol on chromosomes. *Blood, 35*, 689-694

Modan, B., Segal, S., Shani, M. & Sheba, C. (1975) Aplastic anemia in Israel: evaluation of the etiological role of chloramphenicol on a community-wide base. *Am. J. med. Sci., 270*, 441-445

Morley, A., Trainor, K. & Remes, J. (1976) Residual marrow damage: possible explanation for idiosyncrasy to chloramphenicol. *Br. J. Haematol., 32*, 525-537

Mortelmans, K., Haworth, S., Lawlor, T., Speck, W., Tainer, B. & Zeiger, E. (1986) *Salmonella* mutagenicity tests: II. Results from the testing of 270 chemicals. *Environ. Mutagenesis, 8 (Suppl. 7),* 1-119

von Muhlendahl, K.E. (1987) Agranulocytosis after chloramphenicol eyedrops. *Dtsch. med. Wochenschr., 112,* 158-159

Mulhall, A., de Louvois, J. & Hurley, R. (1983) Chloramphenicol toxicity in neonates: its incidence and prevention. *Br. med. J., 287,* 1424-1427

Müller, A.J. (1965) A survey of agents tested with regard to their ability to induce recessive lethals in *Arabidopsis. Arabidopsis Inf. Serv., 2,* 22-24

Myhr, B.C. & Caspary, W.J. (1988) Evaluation of the L5178Y mouse lymphoma cell mutagenesis assay: intralaboratory results for sixty-three coded chemicals tested at Litton Bionetics, Inc. *Environ. mol. Mutagenesis, 12 (Suppl. 13),* 103-194

Nader, C.J., Potter, J.D. & Weller, R.A. (1981) Diet and DNA-modifying activity in human fecal extracts. *Nutr. Rep. int., 23,* 113-117

Nagai, K. & Kanamaru, A. (1978) Drug-induced aplastic anemia: effect of chloramphenicol on hemopoietic stem cells. In: Hibino, S., Takaku, F. & Shakidi, N.T., eds, *Aplastic Anemia,* Tokyo, University Park Press, pp. 343-353

Nagakawa, T., Masada, M. & Uno, T. (1975) Gas chromatographic determination and gas chromatographic-mass spectrometric analysis of chloramphenicol, thiamphenicol and their metabolites. *J. Chromatogr., 111,* 355-364

Nagao, T. & Mauer, A.M. (1969) Concordance for drug-induced aplastic anemia in identical twins. *New Engl. J. Med., 281,* 7-11

Nasrat, G.E., Ahmed, K.A., Nafei, H.A. & Abdel-Rahman, A.H. (1977) Mutagenic action of certain therapeutic drugs on *Drosophila melanogaster. ZANCO (Iraq), Series A, 3,* 214-227

Nestmann, E.R., Matula, T.I., Douglas, G.R., Bora, K.C. & Kowbel, D.J. (1979) Detection of the mutagenic activity of lead chromate using a battery of microbial tests. *Mutat. Res., 66,* 357-365

Pall, M.L. & Hunter, B.J. (1985) Carcinogens induce tandem duplications in *Salmonella. Mutat. Res., 152,* 131-145

Pant, G.S., Kamada, N. & Tanaka, R. (1976) Sister chromatid exchanges in peripheral lymphocytes of atomic bomb survivors and of normal individuals exposed to radiation and chemical agents. *Hiroshima J. med. Sci., 25,* 99-105

Pazdernik, T.L. & Corbett, M.D. (1979) Effects of chloramphenicol reduction products on hemopoietic precursor cells *in vitro. Pharmacologist, 19,* 191-195

Pazdernik, T.L. & Corbett, M.D. (1980) Role of chloramphenicol reduction products in aplastic anemia. *Pharmacology, 20,* 87-94

Penny, R.H.C., Carlisle, C.H., Prescott, C.W. & Davidson, H.A. (1967) Effects of chloramphenicol on the haemopoietic system of the cat. *Br. vet. J., 123,* 145-153

Plaut, M.E. & Best, W.R. (1982) Aplastic anemia after parenteral chloramphenicol: warning renewed. *New Engl. J. Med., 306,* 1486

Popa, G. & Iordacheanu, L. (1975) Lymphoblastic leukemia caused by chloramphenicol. *Rev. med. chir. Soc. med. natl Iasi, 79,* 197-200

Prasad, A.B. (1977) Action of monofunctional alkylating agents and antibiotics on *Vicia faba* chromosomes. *Proc. Indian natl Sci. Acad.*, *43* (Part B), 19-25

Quéinnec, G., Babilé, R., Darré, R., Berland, H.M. & Espinasse, J. (1975) Induction d'anomalies chromosomiques par le furoxone ou le chloramphénicol. [Induction of chromosomal anomalies by furoxone or chloramphenicol (Fr.).] *Rev. Méd. vét.*, *126*, 1611-1626

Rajchgot, P., Prober, C., Soldin, S., Golas, C., Good, F., Harding, L. & MacLeod, S. (1983) Chloramphenicol pharmacokinetics in the newborn. *Dev. Pharmacol. Ther.*, *6*, 305-314

Rebstock, M.C., Crooks, H.M., Jr, Controulis, J. & Bartz, Q.R. (1949) Chloramphenicol (chloromycetin). IV. Chemical studies. *J. Am. chem. Soc.*, *71*, 2458-2462

Reynolds, J.E.F., ed. (1989) *Martindale. The Extra Pharmacopoeia*, 29th ed., London, The Pharmaceutical Press, pp. 186-192

Robertson, P.R., Wahab, M.F.A. & Raasch, F.O. (1968) Evaluation of chloramphenicol and ampicillin in salmonella enteric fever. *New Engl. J. Med.*, *278*, 171

Robin, E., Berman, M., Bhoopalam, N., Cohen, H. & Fried, W. (1981) Induction of lymphomas in mice by busulfan and chloramphenicol. *Cancer Res.*, *41*, 3478-3482

Rosenkranz, H.S. (1988) Chloramphenicol: magic bullet or double-edge sword? *Mutat. Res.*, *196*, 1-16

Rosenthal, R.L. & Blackman, A. (1965) Bone-marrow hypoplasia following use of chloramphenicol eye drops. *J. Am. med. Assoc.*, *191*, 136-137

Roy, P.P. & Manna, G.K. (1981) Effects of chloramphenicol on the meiotic chromosomes of male mice, *Mus musculus*. In: Manna, G.K. & Sinha, U., eds, *Perspectives in Cytology and Genetics*, Vol. 3, Delhi, Hindasia Publishers, pp. 577-582

Roy, B.K., Banerjee, N.C. & Pandy, S.N. (1986) Distribution of chloramphenicol in goat blood and milk after intravenous injection. *Indian J. Anim. Health*, *25*, 33-35

Russell, G.R., Nader, C.J. & Partick, E.J. (1980) Induction of DNA repair by some selenium compounds. *Cancer Lett.*, *10*, 75-81

Ryan, F.J., Austin, M.A. & Mathies, J.C. (1984) Simple and precise method for liquid chromatographic determination of chloramphenicol in serum using a phase separation extraction. *Ther. Drug Monit.*, *6*, 465-470

Salem, Z., Murray, T. & Yunis, A.A. (1981) The nitroreduction of chloramphenicol by human liver tissue. *J. Lab. clin. Med.*, *97*, 881-886

Sande, M.A. & Mandell, G.L. (1985) Antimicrobial agents. In: Gilman A.G., Goodman, L.S., Rall, T.W. & Murad, F., eds, *Goodman and Gilman's The Pharmacological Basis of Therapeutics*, 7th ed., New York, Macmillan, pp. 1179-1184

Sanguineti, M., Rossi, L., Ognio, E. & Santi, L. (1983) Tumori indotti in topi BALB/c e C57Bl/6N dopo somministrazione cronica di chloramphenicolo. [Tumours induced in BALB/c and C57Bl/6N mice following chronic administration of chloramphenicol (Ital.).] (Abstract No. 50). In: *1a Riunione Nazionale di Oncologia Sperimentale e Clinica, Parma, 23-25 novembre 1983* [1st National Meeting on Experimental and Clinical Oncology, Parma, 23-25 November 1983], Parma, Camera di Commercio, p. 45

Sasaki, M.S. & Tonomura, A. (1973) A high susceptibility of Fanconi's anemia to chromosome breakage by DNA cross-linking agents. *Cancer Res.*, *33*, 1829-1836

Schmidt, T., Tomberg, W. & Büning-Pfane, H. (1985) Nachweis von Chloramphenicol mittels elektrochemischer Detektion. [Measurement of chloramphenicol with electrochemical detection (Ger.).] *Z. Lebensmittel-untersuch.*, *180*, 53-54

Schwartz, J.G., Casto, D.T., Ayo, S., Carnahan, J.J. & Jorgensen, J.H. (1988) A commercial enzyme immunoassay method (EMIT^{TM}) compared with liquid chromatography and bioassay methods for measurement of chloramphenicol. *Clin. Chem.*, *34*, 1872-1875

Scott, J.L., Finegold, S.M., Belthin, G.A. & Lawrence, J.S. (1965) A controlled double blind study of the hematologic toxicity of chloramphenicol. *New Engl. J. Med.*, *272*, 1137-1142

Seaman, A.J. (1969) Sequels to chloramphenicol aplastic anemia: acute leukemia and paroxysmal nocturnal hemoglobinuria. *Northwest Med.*, *68*, 831-834

Sekizawa, J. & Shibamoto, T. (1982) Genotoxicity of safrole-related chemicals in microbial test systems. *Mutat. Res.*, *101*, 127-140

Shimizu, M. & Rosenberg, B. (1973) A similar action to UV-irradiation and a preferential inhibition of DNA synthesis in E. coli by antitumor platinum compounds. *J. Antibiot.*, *26*, 243-245

Shu, X.O., Linet, M.S., Gao, R.N., Gao, Y.T., Brinton, L.A. & Jin, F. (1987) Chloramphenicol use and childhood leukemia in Shanghai. *Lancet*, *ii*, 934-937

Siliciano, R.F., Margolis, S. & Lietman, P.S. (1978) Chloramphenicol metabolism in isolated rat hepatocytes. *Biochem. Pharmacol.*, *27*, 2759-2762

Silver, B.J. & Zuckerman, K.S. (1980) Aplastic anaemia. Recent advances in pathogenesis and treatment. *Med. Clin. North Am.*, *64*, 607-627

Slater, E.E., Anderson, M.D. & Rosenkranz, H.S. (1971) Rapid detection of mutagens and carcinogens. *Cancer Res.*, *31*, 970-973

Sood, S.P., Green, V.I. & Bailey, C.L. (1987) Routine methods in toxicology and therapeutic drug monitoring by high performance liquid chromatography. II. A rapid microscale method for determination of chloramphenicol in blood and cerebrospinal fluid. *Ther. Drug Monit.*, *9*, 347-352

Sram, R.J. (1972) Effect of chloramphenicol and puromycin on the dominant lethals induced by TEPA in mice. *Folia biol.*, *18*, 367-373

Suhrland, L.G. & Weisberger, A.S. (1969) Delayed clearance of chloramphenicol from serum in patients with hematologic toxicity. *Blood*, *34*, 466-471

Summ, H.D., Draeger, E. & von Wasielowski, E. (1976) On the inhibitory effect of chloramphenicol on mitochondrial protein synthesis as a possible cause of its selective toxic side effects. *Arzneimittel-forsch.*, *26*, 28-32

Suter, W. & Jaeger, I. (1982) Comparative evaluation of different pairs of DNA repair-deficient and DNA repair-proficient bacterial tester strains for rapid detection of chemical mutagens and carcinogens. *Mutat. Res.*, *97*, 1-18

Suzuki, H. (1987) Assessment of the carcinogenic hazard of 6 substances used in dental practices. II. Morphological transformation, DNA damage and sister chromatid exchanges in cultured Syrian hamster embryo cells induced by formocresol, iodoform, zinc oxide, chloroform, chloramphenicol, tetracycline hydrochloride (Jpn.). *Shigaku*, *74*, 1385-1403

Szulczewski, D. & Eng, D. (1975) Chloramphenicol. *Anal. Profiles Drug Subst.*, *4*, 47-90

US Food and Drug Administration (1988) *Chloramphenicol* (21 CFR), Ch. 1, Washington DC, pp. 815-819

US Pharmacopeial Convention, Inc. (1975) *The US Pharmacopeia*, 19th rev., Easton, PA, pp. 77-79

US Pharmacopeial Convention, Inc. (1989) *The US Pharmacopeia*, 22nd rev., Easton, PA, pp. 271-275

US Tariff Commission (1949) *Synthetic Organic Chemicals, US Production and Sales 1948* (Second Series, Report No. 164), Washington DC, US Government Printing Office, p. 103

Vacha, J., Pspisil, M. & Velcovsky, V. (1981) The toxic effect of chloramphenicol on erythropoiesis in X-irradiated mice. *Chemotherapy*, 27, 131-138

Venturini, S. & Monti-Bragadin, C. (1978) Improvement in the sensitivity of DNA polymerase I-deficient *Escherichia coli* for detecting mutagens and carcinogens. *Appl. environ. Microbiol.*, 36, 794-797

Wade, A., ed. (1972) *Martindale. The Extra Pharmacopoeia*, 25th ed., London, The Pharmaceutical Press, pp. 230-233

Watson, A.D.J. (1972) Chloramphenicol plasma levels in the dog: a comparison of oral, subcutaneous and intramuscular administration. *J. small Anim. Pract.*, 13, 147-151

Watson, A.D.J. (1977a) Effect of concurrent drug therapy and of feeding of chloramphenicol levels after oral administration of chloramphenicol in dogs. *Res. vet. Sci.*, 22, 68-71

Watson, A.D.J. (1977b) Chloramphenicol toxicity in dogs. *Res. vet. Sci.*, 23, 66-69

Watson, A.D.J. (1980) Further observations on chloramphenicol toxicosis in cats. *Am. J. vet. Res.*, 41, 293-294

Watson, A.D.J. & Middleton, D.J. (1978) Chloramphenicol toxicosis in cats. *Am. J. vet. Res.*, 39, 1199-1203

Weislogel, P.O. & Butow, R.A. (1970) Low temperature and chloramphenicol induction of respiratory deficiency in a cold-sensitive mutant of *Saccharomyces cerevisiae*. *Proc. natl Acad. Sci. USA*, 67, 52-58

Wenk, M., Vozeh, S. & Follath, F. (1984) Serum level monitoring of antibacterial drugs—a review. *Clin. Pharmacokinet.*, 9, 475-492

Williamson, D.H., Maroudas, N.G. & Wilkie, D. (1971) Induction of the cytoplasmic petite mutation in *Saccharomyces cerevisiae* by the antibacterial antibiotics erythromycin and chloramphenicol. *Mol. Gen. Genet.*, 111, 209-223

Windholz, M., ed. (1983) *The Merck Index*, 10th ed., Rahway, NJ, Merck & Co., pp. 289-290

Witschel, H. (1986) Malignant lymphoma of the eyelids. *Ophthalmologica*, 193, 161-168

Yoshida, H., Yamamoto, K. & Yamaguchi, H. (1972) Fragmentation and nondisjunction of barley chromosomes after the treatment of chloramphenicol and cycloheximide. *Cytologia*, 37, 697-707

Yunis, A.A. (1977) Differential *in vitro* sensitivity of marrow erythroid and granulocytic colony forming cells to chloramphenicol. *Am. J. Hematol.*, 2, 355-363

Yunis, A.A. (1978) Drug-induced bone marrow aplasia. *Pesq. med. Biol.*, 11, 287-296

Yunis, A.A. (1988) Chloramphenicol: relation of structure to activity and toxicity. *Ann. Rev. Pharmacol. Toxicol.*, 28, 83-100

Yunis, A.A. & Adamson, J.W. (1977) Differential in vitro sensitivity of marrow erythroid and granulocytic colony forming cells to chloramphenicol. *Am. J. Hematol.*, *2*, 355-363

Yunis, A.A., Manyan, D.R. & Arimura, G.K. (1973) Comparative effect of chloramphenicol and thiamphenicol on DNA and mitochondrial protein synthesis in mammalian cells. *J. Lab. clin. Med.*, *81*, 713-718

Yunis, A.A., Miller, A.M., Salem, Z. & Arimura, G.K. (1980a) Chloramphenicol toxicity: pathogenetic mechanisms and the role of the p-NO_2 in aplastic anemia. *Clin. Toxicol.*, *17*, 359-373

Yunis, A.A., Miller, A.M., Salem, Z., Corbett, M.D. & Arimura, G.K. (1980b) Nitrosochloramphenicol: possible mediator in chloramphenicol-induced aplastic anemia. *J. Lab. clin. Med.*, *96*, 34-46

Yunis, A.A., Arimura, G.K. & Isildar, M. (1987) DNA damage induced by chloramphenicol and its nitroso derivative: damage in intact cells. *Am. J. Hematol.*, *24*, 77-84

NITROFURAL (NITROFURAZONE)

This substance was considered by a previous Working Group, in June 1974, under the title 5-nitro-2-furaldehyde semicarbazone (IARC, 1974). Since that time, new data have become available, and these have been incorporated into the monograph and taken into consideration in the present evaluation.

1. Chemical and Physical Data

1.1 Synonyms

Chem. Abstr. Services Reg. No.: 59-87-0

Chem. Abstr. Name: Hydrazinecarboxamide, 2-[(5-nitro-2-furanyl)methylene]-

Synonyms: 2-Furancarboxaldehyde; 5-nitrofuraldehyde semicarbazide; nitrofuraldehyde semicarbazone; 5-nitro-2-furaldehyde semicarbazone; 5-nitrofuran-2-aldehyde semicarbazone; 5-nitro-2-furancarboxaldehyde semicarbazone; 5-nitro-2-furfuraldehyde semicarbazone; 5-nitrofurfural semicarbazone; 5-nitro-2-furfural semicarbazone; (5-nitro-2-furfurylideneamino)urea; 1-(5-nitro-2-furfurylidene)semicarbazide

1.2 Structural and molecular formula and molecular weight

O_2N—furan—CH = NNHCONH$_2$

$C_8H_6N_4O_4$ Mol. wt: 198.14

1.3 Chemical and physical properties of the pure substance

From Windholz (1983) and Reynolds (1989)

(a) *Description*: Pale-yellow needles
(b) *Melting-point*: 236-240°C (decomposition)

(c) *Solubility*: Very slightly soluble (1:4200) in water at pH 6.0-6.5, soluble in alkaline solutions; slightly soluble in ethanol (1:590), propylene glycol (1:350), acetone (1:415), dimethylformamide (1:15) and polyethylene glycol (1:86); almost insoluble in chloroform (1:27000) and benzene (1:43500)

(d) *Spectroscopy data*: Infrared and ultraviolet spectra have been reported.

(e) *Stability*: Stable in solid state at less than 40°C when protected from light; darkens with prolonged exposure; discolours on contact with alkali

1.4 Technical products and impurities

Trade names: Acutol; Aldomycin; Alfucin; Amifur; Babrocid; Becafurazona; Becafurazone; Biofuracina; Biofurea; Chemofuran; Chixin; Cocafurin; Coxistat; Dermofural; Dymazone; Eldezol F-6; Fedacin; Flavazone; Fracine; Furacilin; Furacilinum; Furacillin; Furacin; Furacin-E; Furacine; Furacinetten; Furacin-HC; Furacoccid; Furacort; Furacycline; Furalcyn; Furaldon; Furalone; Furametral; Furan-ofteno; Furaplast; Furaseptyl; Furaskin; Furaziline; Furazin; Furazina; Furazol W; Furazone; Furesol; Furfurin; Furosem; Fuvacillin; Germex; Hemofuran; Ibiofural; Mammex; Mastofuran; Monafuracin; Nefco; NF-7; NFS; Nfz mix; Nifucin; Nifurid; Nifuzon; Nitrazone; Nitreofural; Nitrofurastan; Nitrofurazan; NSC-2100; Nitrozone; Otofural; Otofuran; Rivafurazon; Rivopon-S; Sanfuran; Spray-Dermis; Spray-foral; Vabrocid; Veterinary nitrofurazone; Yatrocin

Nitrofural has been reported to contain 3% 5-nitro-2-furaldehyde azine as an impurity (Morris *et al.*, 1969). It is available in the USA as creams, ointments, powders, solutions, sprays, suppositories and surgical dressings (Barnhart, 1989).

2. Production, Occurrence, Use and Analysis

2.1 Production and occurrence

The action of nitrofural as a topical antibacterial agent was first reported in the USA in 1944 (Dodd & Stillman, 1944), and the product was available for general use in 1945 (Miura & Reckendorf, 1967). Commercial production in the USA was first reported in 1955 (US Tariff Commission, 1956).

Nitrofural can be prepared by the reaction of 5-nitrofurfural with an aqueous solution of a mixture of semicarbazide hydrochloride (see IARC, 1987) and sodium acetate (Stillman & Scott, 1947). It can also be synthesized from the reaction of acetone semicarbazone or other semicarbazones with 5-nitrofurfuraldoxime (Gever & O'Keefe, 1960). It is synthesized in China, Hungary, India, Mexico and Spain (Chemical Information Services, 1989-90).

Nitrofural is not known to occur naturally.

2.2 Use

Nitrofural is a broad-spectrum bactericidal (Chamberlain, 1976). It also has antiprotozoal and antiparasitic activities (Reynolds, 1982).

Nitrofural is used locally for the treatment of wounds, burns, ulcers and skin infections; it has also been applied locally to the ear, eye and bladder. Nitrofural is used as a coccidiostatic and antibacterial agent in farm animals, administered in water or feed (Anon., 1979; Reynolds, 1989).

Oral administration has been restricted to the treatment of late-stage African trypanosomiasis that is refractory to melarsoprol. The dosage for adults is 500 mg three or four times daily for five to seven days. In addition, it has been given orally in doses of 100 mg four times daily for five to six days in the treatment of acute bacillary dysentery (Reynolds, 1982).

2.3 Analysis

Nitrofural has been analysed in pharmaceutical preparations by spectrophotometry (US Pharmacopieal Convention, Inc., 1980) and polarography (Mishra & Gode, 1985). The separation and identification of nitrofural in medicated feeds have been reviewed by Fishbein (1972). High-performance liquid chromatography methods for analysing nitrofural in medicated feeds have also been reported (Cieri, 1979; Thorpe, 1980).

3. Biological Data Relevant to the Evaluation of Carcinogenic Risk to Humans

3.1 Carcinogenicity studies in animals

(a) Oral administration

Mouse: Groups of 50 male and 50 female B6C3F$_1$ mice, seven to eight weeks of age, were administered nitrofural (99% pure) at 0, 150 or 310 mg/kg of diet for 103 weeks; all surviving animals were killed at 112 weeks. The average amount of nitrofural consumed per day was 14-16 mg/kg bw for low-dose male and female mice and 29-33 mg/kg bw for high-dose animals. Survival of high-dose males was lower than that of controls after week 88. At the end of the experiment, survival was: 39/50, 31/50 and 27/50 control, low-dose and high-dose males, and 39/50, 40/50 and 35/50 control, low-dose and high-dose females. Ovarian atrophy was found in 7/47 controls, 44/50 low-dose and 38/50 high-dose mice. Granulosa-cell tumours of the ovary developed in 4/50 low-dose and 9/50 high-dose females ($p = 0.03$, incidental tumour test for trend) compared with 1/47 controls. The incidence of benign mixed tumours of the ovary was 17/50 low-dose and 20/50 high-dose animals ($p < 0.001$, incidental tumour test for trend); no such tumour occurred among controls. No significant difference in the incidence of other types of tumour was observed among treated or control mice (National Toxicology Program, 1988; Kari et al., 1989).

Rat: A group of 30 female weanling Sprague-Dawley rats were administered nitrofural (pharmaceutical grade) at 1000 mg/kg of diet for 46 weeks (daily intake, 8-13 mg/rat), after which they were maintained on control diet for 20 weeks. A control group of 30 rats received control diet for 66 weeks. Of the treated females that lived 22 weeks or more, 22/29 developed mammary fibroadenomas, compared with 2/29 controls (Ertürk et al., 1970). [The Working Group noted that data on survival were not given.]

Groups of 50 male and 50 female Fischer 344/N rats, six to seven weeks of age, were administered nitrofural (99% pure) at 0, 310 or 620 mg/kg of diet for 103 weeks. The average amount of nitrofural consumed per day was 11-12 mg/kg bw for low-dose male and female rats and 24-26 mg/kg bw for high-dose animals. All surviving animals were killed at 111 weeks. Survival in high-dose males was lower than that in controls after week 92. At the end of the experiment, survival was: 33/50, 30/50 and 20/50 controls, low-dose and high-dose males, and 28/50, 37/50 and 31/50 controls, low-dose and high-dose females, respectively. Adenomas of the sebaceous glands of the skin were observed in high-dose males only (4/50 high-dose *versus* 0/50 control; $p = 0.067$, incidental tumour test). Mammary fibroadenomas occurred in 8/49 control, 36/50 low-dose ($p < 0.001$, incidental tumour test) and 36/50 high-dose females ($p < 0.001$, incidental tumour test; $p < 0.001$, incidental tumour test for trend); adenocarcinomas were also observed in one control and two high-dose females. Mononuclear-cell leukaemias occurred in 21/50 control males, 23/50 low-dose males and 6/50 high-dose males ($p = 0.04$, life-table test); 15/49 control females, 2/25 low-dose females ($p < 0.001$) and 2/50 high-dose females ($p < 0.001$ life-table test). Testicular interstitial-cell tumours occurred in 45/50 controls, 30/50 low-dose males ($p < 0.001$, incidental tumour test) and 28/50 high-dose males ($p < 0.001$, incidental tumour test; $p < 0.001$, incidental tumour test for trend) (National Toxicology Program, 1988; Kari et al., 1989).

(b) Transplacental administration

Mouse: A group of 20 pregnant ICR/Jcl mice, 10-12 weeks of age, received three subcutaneous injections of nitrofural [purity unspecified] at 75 μg/g bw suspended in 1% gelatin solution on days 13, 15 and 17 of gestation. Offspring were foster-nursed by untreated dams and were killed 32 weeks after birth. Treatment with nitrofural resulted in a marked reduction in the number of live births. At 32 weeks, 67/145 treated animals and 548/844 controls were still alive. The incidence of lung tumours was not significantly increased in nitrofural-treated mice as compared with gelatin-treated controls. All tumours reported were papillary adenomas of the lung (Nomura *et al.*, 1984). [The Working Group noted the short duration and limited reporting of the experiment; interlitter variation was not recorded.]

A group of newborn ICR/Jcl mice, exposed transplacentally as described above, received a subcutaneous injection of nitrofural [purity unspecified] at 75 μg/g bw suspended in 1% gelatin solution within 12 h of birth; three further injections were given on days 7, 14 and 21 after birth. A further group of mice received treatment with gelatin only, and another received no treatment. At 32 weeks, 61/176 treated animals and 548/844 controls were still alive. The number of tumour-bearing mice was 12/61 (19.7%; $p < 0.001$, χ^2 test with Yates' correction against gelatin controls) compared to 5/203 (2.5%) untreated controls. All tumours reported were papillary adenomas of the lung (Nomura *et al.*, 1984). [The Working Group noted the short duration and limited reporting of the experiment; interlitter variation was not recorded.]

3.2 Other relevant data

(a) *Experimental systems*

(i) *Absorption, distribution, excretion and metabolism*

Within 24 h after a single oral administration of 100 mg/kg bw ^{14}C-nitrofural to rats, about two-thirds of the radioactivity appeared in the urine, 26% in the faeces and approximately 1% in expired carbon dioxide; complete recovery of the administered dose was observed after 96 h, less than 15% of the label being recovered as unchanged parent compound (Tatsumi *et al.*, 1971). Major metabolites of nitrofural detected and identified in the urine of dosed rats included hydroxylaminofuraldehyde semicarbazone, aminofuraldehyde semicarbazone and 4-cyano-2-oxobutyraldehyde semicarbazone (Paul *et al.*, 1960). The reduced nitrofural metabolite, 4-cyano-2-oxobutyraldehyde semicarbazone, was detected in the urine of germ-free rats treated with the drug (Yeung *et al.*, 1983). Binding of ^{14}C label to liver protein, DNA, ribosomal RNA and kidney protein was demonstrated in rats after oral administration of ^{14}C-nitrofural (Tatsumi *et al.*, 1977).

Nitrofural is reduced by mouse liver homogenate and by several mammalian cell lines, most efficiently under gas mixtures containing 5% O_2 or less (Paul *et al.*, 1960; Olive & McCalla, 1975)

(ii) *Toxic effects*

Oral LD_{50} values of 590 mg/kg bw in rats and 460 mg/kg bw in mice have been reported (Miyaji, 1971). Mice and rats receiving 300 mg/kg bw or more orally showed hyperirritability, tremors and seizures and died from respiratory arrest (Krantz & Evans, 1945). In mice and rats, subcutaneous injection of large doses (3 g/kg bw) produced marked changes in the structure of the liver and kidney, but only slight hepatic changes were seen after lethal oral doses (45 mg/kg bw for four to six days) (Dodd, 1946).

Toxicity was studied by feeding diets containing nitrofural (99% pure) to groups of F344/N rats and B6C3F$_1$ mice for 14 days, 13 weeks or two years. In the 14-day studies, in which the doses ranged from 630 to 10 000 mg/kg of diet, nitrofural was more toxic to mice than to rats. In the 13-week studies, doses for rats ranged from 150 to 2500 mg/kg of diet and for mice from 70 to 1250 mg/kg of diet. At the higher doses, convulsive seizures and gonadal hypoplasia were observed in both species. Evidence of toxicity in rats also included degenerative arthropathy. In the two-year studies (see section 3.1), nitrofural caused testicular degeneration (atrophy of germinal epithelium and aspermatogenesis) in rats and degeneration of vertebral and knee articular cartilage in rats of each sex. In mice of each sex, nitrofural administration induced stimulus-sensitive convulsive seizures, primarily during the first year of study (National Toxicology Program, 1988; Kari *et al.*, 1989).

(iii) *Effects on reproduction and prenatal toxicity*

The gonadotoxicity of nitrofural in male mice has been recognized for more than three decades. Nissim (1957) showed that administration to mice in the diet at a dose equivalent to 375 mg/kg bw caused testicular atrophy. Similar degeneration was observed in rat testis following daily doses of 100 mg/kg bw by gastric intubation for seven days (Miyaji *et al.*, 1964).

In male Sprague-Dawley rats given nitrofural in the diet at a dosage equivalent to 64 mg/kg bw per day for 28 days, the mean weight of the testes was only 28% that of the controls. All stages of spermatogenesis were affected, but Sertoli cells and Leydig cells were not damaged (Hagenäs *et al.*, 1978).

After a single subcutaneous injection to ICR/Jcl mice of nitrofural at 300 mg/kg bw on day 10 of gestation, increased embryo- and fetomortality and decreased fetal weight were observed compared with controls. A significant ($p <$ 0.001) increase in the incidence of malformations was observed, predominantly affecting the limbs, digits and tail. After administration of nitrofural at 100 mg/kg bw subcutaneously on days 9-11, the only significant effect observed was a reduction in fetal weight (Nomura *et al.*, 1984).

Pregnant CD1 mice were given nitrofural in the diet at doses equivalent to 6.3-82 mg/kg bw from days 6-15 of gestation. No teratogenic effect was observed, but there was increased fetal death and reduced fetal weight at the highest dose (National Toxicology Program, 1988).

(iv) *Genetic and related effects*

The genetic toxicology of nitrofurans has been reviewed (Klemencic & Wang, 1978; McCalla, 1983).

Nitrofural inhibited DNA synthesis (Lu & McCalla, 1978) and caused prophage induction in *Escherichia coli* (McCalla & Voutsinos, 1974). It induced DNA strand breaks in *E. coli* (McCalla *et al.*, 1971; Tu & McCalla, 1975; Wentzell & McCalla, 1980) and in *Salmonella typhimurium* strain TA1975 (McCalla *et al.*, 1975). Nitrofural induced differential toxicity in *E. coli* (Yahagi *et al.*, 1974; Haveland-Smith *et al.*, 1979; Lu *et al.*, 1979) and *Bacillus subtilis* (Tanooka, 1977) but not *S. typhimurium* (Yahagi *et al.*, 1974).

Nitrofural induced mutations in *E. coli* (Zampieri & Greenberg, 1964; McCalla & Voutsinos, 1974; Yahagi *et al.*, 1974; McCalla *et al.*, 1975; Tanooka, 1977; Haveland-Smith *et al.*, 1979; Lu *et al.*, 1979; Ebringer & Bencova, 1980; Clarke & Shankel, 1989) in the absence of an exogenous metabolic system, but not in strains lacking nitroreductase activity (McCalla & Voutsinos, 1974; McCalla *et al.*, 1975). In the presence of a microsomal preparation from *Drosophila melanogaster*, nitrofural induced mutations in *E. coli* (Baars *et al.*, 1980). It was not mutagenic to *S. typhimurium* strains TA1535, TA1536, TA1537 or TA1538 (Yahagi *et al.*, 1974; McCalla *et al.*, 1975) but induced mutations in TA1535 in a fluctuation test (Green *et al.*, 1977) and in plate incorporation tests, only in the presence of an exogenous metabolic system (Zeiger *et al.*, 1987; National Toxicology Program, 1988). Nitrofural induced mutations in *S. typhimurium* TA100 and in TA98 in the presence and absence of an exogenous metabolic system (Yahagi *et al.*, 1976; Goodman *et al.*, 1977; Green *et al.*, 1977; Chin *et al.*, 1978; Rosin & Stich, 1978; Bruce & Heddle, 1979; Haveland-Smith *et al.*, 1979; Imamura *et al.*, 1983; Obaseiki-Ebor & Akerele, 1986; Ni *et al.*, 1987; Zeiger *et al.*, 1987; National Toxicology Program, 1988).

Nitrofural was mutagenic to *Neurospora crassa* (Ong, 1977) but not to *Aspergillus nidulans* (Bignami *et al.*, 1982).

Feeding of *Drosophila melanogaster* for three days with nitrofural at 5 mM did not induce sex-linked recessive lethal mutations (Kramers, 1982).

Nitrofural inhibited DNA synthesis in mouse L-929 cells (Olive, 1979a,b). It induced DNA strand breaks in human KB, Syrian hamster BHK-21 and mouse L-929 cells (Olive & McCalla, 1975; Olive, 1978). No unscheduled DNA synthesis was induced by nitrofural in either rat or mouse primary hepatocytes (Mori *et al.*, 1987) or in human fibroblasts (Tonomura & Sasaki, 1973).

Nitrofural induced mutations to 6-thioguanine resistance in Chinese hamster lung (V79) cells (Olive, 1981) but not in Chinese hamster ovary (CHO) cells

(Anderson & Phillips, 1985), either in the presence or absence of an exogenous metabolic system. It induced mutations at the *tk* locus of mouse L5178Y lymphoma cells (National Toxicology Program, 1988). Nitrofural induced sister chromatid exchange in CHO cells in the presence and absence of an exogenous metabolic system (National Toxicology Program, 1988). It induced chromosomal aberrations in Chinese hamster lung cells in the presence and absence of an exogenous metabolic system (Matsuoka *et al.*, 1979; Ishidate, 1988). In CHO cells, however, nitrofural induced chromosomal aberrations in the absence, but not in the presence, of an exogenous metabolic system (National Toxicology Program, 1988). Nitrofural did not induce chromosomal aberrations in human lymphocytes *in vitro* (Tonomura & Sasaki, 1973).

It was not active in micronucleus tests either in rats treated twice with 7.5-30 mg/kg bw intraperitoneally at 30 h and 6 h before they were killed (Goodman *et al.*, 1977) or in mice treated with 150 mg/kg bw intraperitoneally on five consecutive days (Bruce & Heddle, 1979). Nitrofural did not induce chromosomal aberrations in bone-marrow cells of rats either after a single intraperitoneal injection of 60 mg/kg bw (Goodman *et al.*, 1977) or after single oral doses of 40-400 mg/kg bw or five daily oral doses of 15-150 mg/kg bw (Anderson & Phillips, 1985).

Nitrofural did not induce sperm abnormalities in mice treated intraperitoneally with 15-150 mg/kg bw on five consecutive days (Bruce & Heddle, 1979).

(b) *Humans*

(i) *Pharmacokinetics*

Nitrofural is not significantly absorbed from skin or mucous membranes after local administration (Marion-Landais *et al.*, 1975; Harvey, 1985).

(ii) *Adverse effects*

Sensitization and generalized allergic skin reactions are known adverse effects of topically administered nitrofural. In a literature review of studies published in 1945-65, 176 (1.2%) cases of skin reactions were reported among 15 162 treated patients (Glascock *et al.*, 1969; Reynolds, 1989).

Nausea, vomiting, joint pains, headaches and polyneuritis are typical toxic effects after oral administration (Reynolds, 1989). Polyneuropathy is common among trypanosomiasis patients treated with nitrofural (Cancado *et al.*, 1964; Robertson & Knight, 1964; Spencer *et al.*, 1975).

Nitrofural has been reported to cause haemolytic anaemia in individuals with glucose-6-phosphate dehydrogenase deficiency (see Prankerd, 1962).

(iii) *Effects on reproduction and prenatal toxicity*

In the Collaborative Perinatal Project, in which drug intake and pregnancy outcome were studied in a series of 50 282 women in 1959-65, 234 women had been exposed to nitrofural administered topically during the first trimester of pregnancy. Fifteen malformed children were born in the exposed group, giving a standardized relative risk of 0.99 (Heinonen *et al.*, 1977).

(iv) *Genetic and related effects*

No data were available to the Working Group.

3.3 Case reports and epidemiological studies of carcinogenicity to humans

In a hypothesis-generating cohort study designed to screen a large number of drugs for possible carcinogenicity (described in detail in the monograph on ampicillin), 317 persons to whom at least one prescription for nitrofural had been dispensed during 1969-73 were followed up for up to 15 years (Selby *et al.*, 1989). No statistically significant association was noted with cancer at any site or at all sites combined. [The Working Group noted that the number of users was small and therefore the power of the study to detect carcinogenic effects was probably low. Data on duration of use were not provided.]

4. Summary of Data Reported and Evaluation

4.1 Exposure data

Nitrofural is an antibacterial agent used since 1945 mainly for the local treatment of skin infections. It has been used orally in the treatment of refractory African trypanosomiasis.

4.2 Experimental carcinogenicity data

Nitrofural was tested by oral administration in one study in mice and in two studies in rats, and by transplacental administration to mice. Oral administration to mice increased the incidence of granulosa-cell and benign mixed tumours of the ovary. In rats, an increased incidence of mammary fibroadenomas was observed in females in both studies. Two studies of transplacental administration of nitrofural to mice were inadequate for evaluation.

4.3 Human carcinogenicity data

In a hypothesis-generating cohort study, use of nitrofural was not associated with an increase in cancer incidence, but the power of the study was low.

4.4 Other relevant data

One study did not provide evidence that topical use of nitrofural during pregnancy is associated with birth defects. Nitrofural is gonadotoxic in male and female mice and in male rats and is teratogenic in mice.

In humans, nitrofural is poorly absorbed from skin and mucous membranes after local administration. The drug binds to liver protein and DNA as well as to kidney protein in rats treated *in vivo*.

Nitrofural did not induce chromosomal aberrations in rats, micronuclei in mice or rats or sperm abnormalities in mice. It induced sister chromatid exchange in Chinese hamster cells *in vitro*; contradictory results were obtained on the induction of chromosomal aberrations in mammalian cells. Nitrofural induced DNA strand breaks in human, hamster and mouse cells but did not induce unscheduled DNA synthesis in human, rat or mouse cells. Both positive and negative results were obtained in gene mutation assays in rodent cells. Nitrofural did not induce sex-linked recessive lethal mutations in *Drosophila*. It was mutagenic to *Neurospora* but not to *Aspergillus* and induced differential toxicity in *Escherichia coli* and *Bacillus subtilis* and mutations in *E. coli* and *Salmonella typhimurium*. (See Appendix 1.)

4.5 Evaluation[1]

There is *inadequate evidence* for the carcinogenicity of nitrofural in humans.

There is *limited evidence* for the carcinogenicity of nitrofural in experimental animals.

Overall evaluation

Nitrofural *is not classifiable as to its carcinogenicity to humans (Group 3)*.

5. References

Anderson, D. & Phillips, B.J. (1985) Nitrofurazone—genotoxicity studies in mammalian cells *in vitro* and *in vivo*. *Food. chem. Toxicol.*, 23, 1091-1098

Anon. (1979) *Pharmaceutical Codex*, 11th ed., London, The Pharmaceutical Press, p. 598

Baars, A.J., Blijleven, W.G.H., Mohn, G.R., Natarajan, A.T. & Breimer, D.D. (1980) Preliminary studies on the ability of *Drosophila* microsomal preparations to activate mutagens and carcinogens. *Mutat. Res.*, 72, 257-264

Barnhart, E. (1989) *Physicians' Desk Reference*, 43rd ed., Oradell, NJ, Medical Economics, p. 320

Bignami, M., Carere, A., Conti, G., Conti, L., Crebelli, R. & Fabrizi, M. (1982) Evaluation of 2 different genetic markers for the detection of frameshift and missense mutagens in *A. nidulans*. *Mutat. Res.*, 97, 293-302

---

[1]For description of the italicized terms, see Preamble, pp. 26–29.

Bruce, W.R. & Heddle, J.A. (1979) The mutagenic activity of 61 agents as determined by the micronucleus, *Salmonella*, and sperm abnormality assays. *Can. J. genet. Cytol.*, *21*, 319-334

Cancado, J.R., Marra, U.D. & Brener, Z. (1964) Clinical trial of 5-nitro-2-furaldehyde-semicarbazone (nitrofurazone) in chronic form of Chagas's disease. *Rev. Inst. Med. trop. Sao Paulo*, *6*, 12-16 [*Trop. Dis. Bull.*, *61*, 608]

Chamberlain, R.E. (1976) Chemotherapeutic properties of prominent nitrofurans. *J. antimicrob. Chemother.*, *2*, 325-332

Chemical Information Services (1989-90) *Directory of World Chemical Producers 1989/90*, Oceanside, NY

Chin, J.B., Sheinin, D.M.K. & Rauth, A.M. (1978) Screening for the mutagenicity of nitro-group containing hypoxic cell radiosensitizers using *Salmonella typhimurium* strains TA100 and TA98. *Mutat. Res.*, *58*, 1-10

Cieri, U.R. (1979) High pressure liquid chromatographic detection and estimation of furazolidone and nitrofurazone in animal feeds. *J. Assoc. off. anal. Chem.*, *62*, 168-170

Clarke, C.H. & Shankel, D.M. (1989) Antimutagenic specificity against spontaneous and nitrofurazone-induced mutations in *Escherichia coli* K12ND160. *Mutagenesis*, *4*, 31-34

Dodd, M.C. (1946) The chemotherapeutic properties of 5-nitro-2-furaldehyde semicarbazone (Furacin). *J. Pharmacol. exp. Ther.*, *86*, 311-323

Dodd, M.C. & Stillman, W.B. (1944) The *in vitro* bacteriostatic action of some simple furan derivatives. *J. Pharmacol. exp. Ther.*, *82*, 11-18

Ebringer, L. & Bencova, M. (1980) Mutagenicity of nitrofuran drugs in bacterial systems. *Folia microbiol.*, *25*, 388-396

Ertürk, E., Morris, J.E., Cohen, S.M., Price, J.M. & Bryan, G.T. (1970) Transplantable rat mammary tumors induced by 5-nitro-2-furaldehyde semicarbazone and by formic acid 2-[4-(5-nitro-2-furyl)-2-thiazolyl]hydrazide. *Cancer Res.*, *30*, 1409-1412

Fishbein, L. (1972) *Chromatography of Environmental Hazards*, Vol. 1, *Carcinogens, Mutagens and Teratogens*, Amsterdam, Elsevier

Gever, G. & O'Keefe, C.J. (1960) Azomethines of 5-nitro-2-formylfuran with hydrazine compounds. US Patent 2 927 110, 1 March

Glascock, H.W., Jr, MacLeod, P.F., Davis, J.B., Cuddihy, R.V. & Anzlowar, B.R. (1969) Is nitrofurazone a primary irritant or a potent sensitizer? A review of the literature, 1945-1965, and cases reported to the Medical Director. *Rev. Allergy appl. Immunol.*, *23*, 52-58

Goodman, D.R., Hakkinen, P.J., Nemenzo, J.H. & Vore, M. (1977) Mutagenic evaluation of nitrofuran derivatives in *Salmonella typhimurium*, by the micronucleus test, and by in vivo cytogenetics. *Mutat. Res.*, *48*, 295-306

Green, M.H.L., Rogers, A.M., Muriel, W.J., Ward, A.C., & McCalla, D.R. (1977) Use of a simplified fluctuation test to detect and characterize mutagenesis by nitrofurans. *Mutat. Res.*, *44*, 139-143

Hagenäs, L., Plöen, L. & Ritzen, E.M. (1978) The effect of nitrofurazone on the endocrine, secretory and spermatogenic functions of the rat testis. *Andrologia*, *10*, 107-126

Harvey, S.C. (1985) Antiseptics and disinfectants; fungicides; ectoparasiticides. In: Gilman, A., Goodman, L.S., Rall, T.W. & Murad, F., eds, *Goodman and Gilman's The Pharmacological Basis of Therapeutics*, 7th ed., New York, MacMillan, pp. 967-968

Haveland-Smith, R.B., Combes, R.D. & Bridges, B.A. (1979) Methodology for the testing of food dyes for genotoxic activity: experiments with Red 2G (C.I. 18050). *Mutat. Res.*, 64, 241-248

Heinonen, O.P., Slone, D. & Shapiro, S. (1977) *Birth Defects and Drugs in Pregnancy*, Littleton, MA, Publishing Sciences Group, pp. 296-313

IARC (1974) *IARC Monographs on the Evaluation of Carcinogenic Risk of Chemicals to Man*, Vol. 7, *Some Anti-thyroid and Related Substances, Nitrofurans and Industrial Chemicals*, Lyon, pp. 171-180

IARC (1987) *IARC Monographs on the Evaluation of Carcinogenic Risks to Humans*, Suppl. 7, *Overall Evaluations of Carcinogenicity: An Updating of IARC Monographs Volumes 1 to 42*, Lyon, p. 71

Imamura, A., Kurumi, Y., Danzuka, T., Kodama, M., Kawachi, T. & Nagao, M. (1983) Classification of compounds by cluster analysis of Ames test data. *Gann*, 74, 196-204

Ishidate, M., Jr, ed. (1988) *Data Book of Chromosomal Aberration Test In Vitro*, Amsterdam, Elsevier

Kari, F.W., Huff, J.E., Leininger, J., Haseman, J.K. & Eustis, S.L. (1989) Toxicity and carcinogenicity of nitrofurazone in F344/N rats and B6C3F$_1$ mice. *Chem. Toxicol.*, 27, 129-137

Klemencic, J.M. & Wang, C.Y. (1978) Mutagenicity of nitrofurans. In: Bryan, G.T., ed., *Carcinogenesis*, Vol. 4, *Nitrofurans*, New York, Raven Press, pp. 99-130

Kramers, P.G.N. (1982) Studies on the induction of sex-linked recessive lethal mutations in *Drosophila melanogaster* by nitroheterocyclic compounds. *Mutat. Res.*, 101, 209-236

Krantz, J.C. & Evans, W.E. (1945) A contribution to the pharmacology of 5-nitro-2-furaldehyde semicarbazone. *J. Pharmacol. exp. Ther.*, 85, 324-331

Lu, C. & McCalla, D.R. (1978) Action of some nitrofuran derivatives on glucose metabolism, ATP levels, and macromolecule synthesis in *Escherichia coli*. *Can. J. Microbiol.*, 24, 650-657

Lu, C., McCalla, D.R. & Bryant, D.W. (1979) Action of nitrofurans on *E. coli*. Mutation and induction and repair of daughter-strand gaps in DNA. *Mutat. Res.*, 67, 133-144

Marion-Landais, G., Heatis, J.P. & Herrett, R.J. (1975) Non-absorption of furazolidone from the vagina in women. *Curr. Ther. Res.*, 18, 510-512

Matsuoka, A., Hayashi, M. & Ishidate, M., Jr (1979) Chromosomal aberration tests on 29 chemicals combined with S9 mix *in vitro*. *Mutat. Res.*, 66, 277-290

McCalla, D.R. (1983) Mutagenicity of nitrofuran derivatives: review. *Environ. Mutagenesis*, 5, 745-765

McCalla, D.R. & Voutsinos, D. (1974) On the mutagenicity of nitrofurans. *Mutat. Res.*, 26, 3-16

McCalla, D.R., Reuvers, A. & Kaiser, C. (1971) Breakage of bacterial DNA by nitrofuran derivatives. *Cancer Res.*, 31, 2184-2188

McCalla, D.R., Voutsinos, D. & Olive, P.L. (1975) Mutagen screening with bacteria: niridazole and nitrofurans. *Mutat. Res., 31*, 31-37

Mishra, A.K. & Gode, K.D. (1985) Electrochemical reduction of nitrofurazone and its determination in pharmaceutical dosage forms by d.c. polarography. *Analyst, 110*, 1373-1376

Miura, K. & Reckendorf, H.K. (1967) The nitrofurans. In: Ellis, G.P. & West, G.B., eds, *Progress in Medicinal Chemistry*, Vol. 5, New York, Plenum, pp. 320-381

Miyaji, T. (1971) Acute and chronic toxicity of furylfuramide in rats and mice. *Tohoku J. exp. Med., 103*, 331-369

Miyaji, T., Miyamoto, M. & Ueda, Y. (1964) Inhibition of spermatogenesis and atrophy of the testis caused by nitrofuran compounds. *Acta pathol. jpn., 14*, 261-273

Mori, H., Sugie, S., Yoshimi, N., Kinouchi, T. & Ohnishi, Y. (1987) Genotoxicity of a variety of nitroarenes and other nitro compounds in DNA-repair tests with rat and mouse hepatocytes. *Mutat. Res., 190*, 159-167

Morris, J.E., Price, J.M., Lalich, J.J. & Stein, R.J. (1969) The carcinogenic activity of some 5-nitrofuran derivatives in the rat. *Cancer Res., 29*, 2145-2156

National Toxicology Program (1988) *Toxicology and Carcinogenesis Studies of Nitrofurazone (CAS No. 59-87-0) in F344/N Rats and B6C3F$_1$ Mice (Feed Studies)* (NTP Technical Report 337), Research Triangle Park, NC, pp. 18-19, 160-164

Ni, Y.-C., Heflich, R.H., Kadlubar, F.F. & Fu, P.P. (1987) Mutagenicity of nitrofurans in *Salmonella typhimurium* TA98, TA98NR and TA98/1,8-DNP$_6$. *Mutat. Res., 192*, 15-22

Nissim, J. A. (1957) Increased pituitary gonadotrophin activity after degeneration of seminiferous tubules produced by nitrofurazone. *Lancet, i*, 304-305

Nomura, T., Kimura, S., Kanzaki, T., Tanaka, H., Shibata, K., Nakajima, H., Isa, T., Kurokawa, N., Hatanaka, T., Kinuta, M., Masada, K. & Sakamoto, Y. (1984) Induction of tumors and malformations in mice after prenatal treatment with some antibiotic drugs. *Med. J. Osaka Univ., 35*, 13-17

Obaseiki-Ebor, E.E. & Akerele, J.O. (1986) Nitrofuran mutagenicity: induction of frameshift mutations. *Mutat. Res., 175*, 149-152

Olive, P.L. (1978) Nitrofurazone-induced DNA damage to tissues of mice. *Chem.-biol. Interactions, 20*, 323-331

Olive, P.L. (1979a) Inhibition of DNA synthesis by nitroheterocycles I. Correlation with half-wave reduction potential. *Br. J. Cancer, 40*, 89-93

Olive, P.L. (1979b) Inhibition of DNA synthesis by nitroheterocycles II. Mechanisms of cytotoxicity. *Br. J. Cancer, 40*, 94-104

Olive, P.L. (1981) Correlation between the half-wave reduction potentials of nitroheterocycles and their mutagenicity in Chinese hamster V79 spheroids. *Mutat. Res., 82*, 137-145

Olive, P.L. & McCalla, D.R. (1975) Damage to mammalian cell DNA by nitrofurans. *Cancer Res., 35*, 781-784

Ong, T.-M. (1977) Mutagenic activities of nitrofurans in *Neurospora crassa*. *Mutat. Res., 56*, 13-20

Paul, H.E., Ells, V.R., Kopko, F. & Bender, R.C. (1960) Metabolic degradation of the nitrofurans. *J. med. pharm. Chem.*, 2, 563-584

Prankerd, T.A.J. (1962) Hemolytic effects of drugs and chemical agents. *Clin. Pharmacol. Ther.*, 4, 334-350

Reynolds, J.E.F., ed. (1982) *Martindale. The Extra Pharmacopoeia*, 28th ed., London, The Pharmaceutical Press, pp. 499-500

Reynolds, J.E.F., ed. (1989) *Martindale. The Extra Pharmacopoeia*, 29th ed., London, The Pharmaceutical Press, p. 674

Robertson, D.H.H. & Knight, R.H. (1964) Observations on the polyneuropathy and the disordered pyruvate metabolism induced by nitrofurazone in cases of sleeping sickness due to *Trypanosoma rhodesiense*. *Acta trop.*, 21, 239-263 [*Trop. Dis. Bull.*, 62, 179]

Rosin, M.P. & Stich, H.F. (1978) The inhibitory effect of cysteine on the mutagenic activities of several carcinogens. *Mutat. Res.*, 54, 73-81

Selby, J.V., Friedman, G.D. & Fireman, B.H. (1989) Screening prescription drugs for possible carcinogenicity: 11 to 15 years of follow-up. *Cancer Res.*, 49, 5736-5747

Spencer, H.C., Jr, Gibson, J.J., Jr, Brodsky, R.E. & Schultz, M.G. (1975) Imported African trypanosomiasis in the United States. *Ann. intern. Med.*, 82, 633-638

Stillman, W.B. & Scott, A.B. (1947) Substituted nitrofurans. US Patent 2 416 234, 18 February

Tanooka, H. (1977) Development and applications of *Bacillus subtilis* test systems for mutagens, involving DNA-repair deficiency and suppressible auxotrophic mutations. *Mutat. Res.*, 42, 19-32

Tatsumi, K., Ou, T., Yoshimura, H. & Tsukamoto, H. (1971) Metabolism of drugs. LXXIII. The metabolic fate of nitrofuran derivatives. (3) Studies on enzymes in small intestinal mucosa of rat catalyzing degradation of nitrofuran derivatives. *Chem. pharm. Bull.*, 21, 622-628

Tatsumi, K., Kitamura, S. & Yoshimura, H. (1977) Binding of nitrofuran derivatives to nucleic acids and protein. *Chem. pharm. Bull.*, 25, 2948-2952

Thorpe, V.A. (1980) Sample preparation of carbadox, furazolidone and ethopabate in medicated feeds for high pressure liquid chromatography. *J. Assoc. off. anal. Chem.*, 63, 981-984

Tonomura, A. & Sasaki, M.S. (1973) Chromosome aberrations and DNA repair synthesis in cultured human cells exposed to nitrofurans. *Jpn. J. Genet.*, 48, 291-294

Tu, Y. & McCalla, D.R. (1975) Effect of activated nitrofurans on DNA. *Biochim. biophys. Acta*, 402, 142-149

US Pharmacopeial Convention, Inc. (1980) *US Pharmacopeia*, 20th rev., Rockville, MD, pp. 550-551

US Tariff Commission (1956) *Synthetic Organic Chemicals, US Production and Sales 1955* (Second Series, Report No. 198), Washington DC, US Government Printing Office, p. 112

Wentzell, B. & McCalla, D.R. (1980) Formation and excision of nitrofuran-DNA adducts in *Escherichia coli*. *Chem.-biol. Interactions*, 31, 133-150

Windholz, M., ed. (1983) *The Merck Index*, 10th ed., Rahway, NJ, Merck & Co., p. 947

Yahagi, T., Nagao, M., Hara, K., Matsushima, T., Sugimura, T. & Bryan, G.T. (1974) Relationships between the carcinogenic and mutagenic or DNA-modifying effects of nitrofuran derivatives, including 2-(2-furyl)-3-(5-nitro-2-furyl) acrylamide, a food additive. *Cancer Res.*, *34*, 2266-2273

Yahagi, T., Matsushima, T., Nagao, M., Seino, Y., Sugimura, T. & Bryan, G.T. (1976) Mutagenicities of nitrofuran derivatives on a bacterial tester strain with an R factor plasmid. *Mutat. Res.*, *40*, 9-14

Yeung, T.C., Sudlow, G., Koch, R.L. & Goldman, P. (1983) Reduction of nitroheterocyclic compounds by mammalian tissues in vivo. *Biochem. Pharmacol.*, *32*, 2259-2263

Zampieri, A. & Greenberg, J. (1964) Nitrofurazone as a mutagen in *Escherichia coli*. *Biochem. biophys. Res. Commun.*, *14*, 172-176

Zeiger, E., Anderson, B., Haworth, S., Lawlor, T., Mortelmans, K. & Speck, W. (1987) *Salmonella* mutagenicity tests: III. Results from the testing of 255 chemicals. *Environ. Mutagenesis*, *9 (Suppl. 9)*, 1-110

NITROFURANTOIN

1. Chemical and Physical Data

1.1 Synonyms

Chem. Abstr. Services Reg. No.: 67-20-9; 17140-81-7 (monohydrate); 54-87-5 (sodium salt)

Chem. Abstr. Name: 2,4-Imidazolidinedione, 1-{[(5-nitro-2-furanyl)methylene]amino}-

Synonyms: 1-[(5-Nitrofurfurylidene)amino]imidazolidine-2,4-dione; 1-[(5-nitrofurfurylidene)amino]hydantoin

1.2 Structural and molecular formulae and molecular weight

$C_8H_6N_4O_5$ Mol. wt: 238.16

1.3 Chemical and physical properties of the pure substance

From Cadwallader and Jun (1976) and Windholz (1983)

(a) *Description*: Pale orange-yellow needles from dilute acetic acid
(b) *Melting-point*: 270-272°C (decomposes)
(c) *Solubility*: Solubilities of nitrofurantoin in many aqueous media and organic solvents have been reported.
(d) *Spectroscopy data*: Ultraviolet, infrared and nuclear magnetic resonance spectra have been reported.
(e) *Stability*: Tablets and suspension stable for five years at room temperature in regular glass containers; crystals and solutions discoloured by alkali and by exposure to light

(f) *Dissociation constant*: pK_a = 7.2

1.4 Technical products and impurities

Trade names: Berkfurin; Chemiofuran; Chemiofurin; Cistofuran; Cyantin; Cystit; Dantafur; Fua-Med; Furadantin; Furadantina; Furadantine; Furadöine; Furadonine; Furandoninium; Furalan; Furantoin; Furantoina; Furatin; Furedan; Furil; Furobactina; Furophen; Gurachel; Ituran; Ivadantin; Microdoin; Micturol Simple; Nephronex; Nierofu; Nifuran; Nitrex; Nitrofor-50; Nitrofor-100; Nitrofurantonum; Nitrofurin; Novofuran; N-Toin; Orafuran; Parfuran; Phenurin; Sarodant; Trantoin; Trocurine; Urantoin; Urefuran; Uretoin; Uriston; Urizept; Urodil; Urodin; Urolisa; Urolong; Urosagen; UroTablinen; Uro-Tablinen; Urotoin; Uvamine; Welfurin; Zoofurin

Macrocrystalline products: Furadantin MC; Macrodantin; Uvamin retard

Nitrofurantoin is available as tablets (50 mg and 100 mg) and as a suspension (Barnhart, 1989; Reynolds, 1989). Impurities in the tablets include calcium pyrophosphate, magnesium stearate, starch and sucrose; and those in the suspension include carboxymethyl cellulose, sodium citric acid, glycerine, magnesium aluminium silicate, methylparaben, propylparaben, saccharin (see IARC, 1987a), sodium citrate and sorbitol. Nitrofurantoin is available from at least one manufacturer in macrocrystalline form (Cunha, 1988).

2. Production, Occurrence, Use and Analysis

2.1 Production and occurrence

Nitrofurantoin can be prepared from 1-aminohydantoin sulfate or hydrochloride and 5-nitro-2-furaldehyde diacetate in isopropyl alcohol (see IARC, 1987b) media (Cadwallader & Jun, 1976). It is synthesized in China, India, Italy, the Netherlands and Spain (Chemical Information Services, 1989-90). In Sweden, sales of nitrofurantoin in 1988 were 0.09 defined daily doses per 1000 inhabitants (Apoteksbolaget, 1988, 1989).

Nitrofurantoin is not known to occur naturally.

2.2 Use

Nitrofurantoin is used extensively in the treatment and prophylaxis of uncomplicated lower urinary-tract infections. The usual oral dose for adults is 50-100 mg four times daily, with meals and at bedtime. Treatment is usually continued for 14 days. The daily dose for children is 5-7 mg/kg given in four divided oral doses. The dosage is reduced if continued beyond 14 days or if used for prophylaxis (Reynolds, 1989). In long-term treatment, a dose as low as 1 mg/kg may be used (Lohr *et al.*, 1977). A single dose of 50-100 mg at bedtime may be sufficient to prevent recurrences (Stamey *et al.*, 1977).

2.3 Analysis

Analytical methods have been described for nitrofurantoin in pharmaceutical formulations using thin-layer chromatography (Cadwallader & Jun, 1976), high-performance liquid chromatography (US Pharmacopeial Convention, Inc., 1989), polarography (Surmann & Aswakun, 1985; Morales *et al.*, 1987) and electrochemical methods (Fogg & Ghawji, 1988). Methods for analysing the compound in plasma and urine include high-performance liquid chromatography (Vree *et al.*, 1979), polarography (Morales *et al.*, 1987) and electrochemical analysis (Mason & Sandmann, 1976).

3. Biological Data Relevant to the Evaluation of Carcinogenic Risk to Humans

3.1 Carcinogenicity studies in animals

(a) *Oral administration*

Mouse: Groups of 52-53 male and 54 female (C57Bl/6N × DBA/2N)F_1 (BDF$_1$) mice, nine weeks of age, were administered nitrofurantoin [purity and crystalline form unspecified] at 0, 750 or 3000 mg/kg of diet for 104 weeks, when the experiment was terminated. At that time, survival in males and females combined was 50.5%, 42.5% and 46.2% in control, low-dose and high-dose groups, respectively. Administration of the high dose significantly lowered body weights in mice of each sex in comparison with controls. In males, a reduced incidence of hepatic adenomas was observed: 6/53 controls, 1/52 low-dose and 0/52 high-dose mice ($p = 0.014$, Fisher's exact test). No increase in the incidence of tumours at any site was observed (Ito *et al.*, 1983).

Groups of 50 male and 50 female Swiss (Crl:CD^R-1(ICR)BR) mice, about 50 days of age, received nitrofurantoin (pharmaceutical grade macrocrystals) at 0, 50, 100 or 200 mg/kg of diet for 22 months. Increased mortality was observed in males treated with the high-dose. In males, the incidences of malignant lymphomas at all sites were: controls, 2/50; low-dose, 6/50; mid-dose, 4/49; and high-dose, 10/50 [$p = 0.014$, Fisher's exact test; $p = 0.012$, Cochran-Armitage trend test] (Butler *et al.*, 1990).

Groups of 50 male and 50 female B6C3F$_1$ mice, eight to nine weeks of age, were fed nitrofurantoin (pharmaceutical grade) at 0, 1300 or 2500 mg/kg of diet for 103 weeks. Survival at termination of the experiment was reduced in control females: controls, 19/50; low-dose, 37/50; and high-dose, 37/50. Mean body weights of male and female high-dose mice were 12% lower than those of controls. In females, ovarian atrophy was seen in 0/50 control, 48/50 low-dose and 49/50 high-dose animals. Controls had ovarian abscesses (18/50) and suppurative inflammation of the uterus (11/50). There was no significant increase in the incidence of any individual type of tumour; however, when tubular adenomas and benign mixed tumours of the ovary are combined, the incidence is significant: 0/50 controls, 0/50 low-dose and 9/50 high-dose ($p = 0.01$, incidental tumour test) (National Toxicology Program, 1989). [The Working Group noted the poor survival and the high incidence of ovarian abscesses in the controls.]

In a study of ovarian atrophy, three groups of female B6C3F$_1$ mice, five to six weeks of age, were given nitrofurantoin (pharmaceutical grade) at 0, 350 or 500 mg/kg bw daily in the diet for 64 weeks. Intermittent sacrifices were made at 4, 8, 13, 17 and 47 weeks; the numbers of mice still alive at 65 weeks were 20 controls, 19 low-dose and 18 high-dose animals. Treated animals gained significantly less weight than the controls. There was no increase in the incidence of neoplasms of the reproductive system [the only tissues reported]. By week 43, there was evidence of ovarian atrophy in treated females; by the end of the study, the incidences were: control, 0/20; low-dose, 18/19; and high-dose, 18/18 (Stitzel *et al.*, 1989). [The Working Group noted the short duration of the study and the small number of animals used.]

Rat: A group of weanling female Sprague-Dawley rats (36 animals alive at ten weeks), weighing 40-72 g, was administered nitrofurantoin ('pure'; identity and purity checked by infrared and ultraviolet absorption spectrophotometry, melting-point and paper chromatography) at 1870 mg/kg of diet for 16 weeks, after which time the dose was reduced to 1000 mg/kg of diet in weeks 16-75 due to impaired growth and premature mortality. The experiment was terminated at week 80. A group of untreated rats served as controls (30 alive at ten weeks). No increase in tumour incidence was observed (Cohen *et al.*, 1973). [The Working Group noted the short duration of the experiment and the small number of effective animals.]

Two groups of 11-12 weanling, germ-free female Sprague-Dawley rats, weighing 85-100 g, were fed nitrofurantoin (extracted from pharmaceutical grade, macrocrystalline nitrofurantoin) at 0 or 1880 mg/kg of diet for 104 weeks. The growth rate in treated rats was slightly retarded as compared with that in controls. The median survival time was 96 weeks for controls and 90 weeks for treated animals. The incidences of mammary fibroadenomas were 2/11 controls and 9/12 treated rats ($p < 0.01$, Fisher's exact test). No increase in the incidence of tumours at other sites was observed (Wang et al., 1984). [The Working Group noted the small number of animals used.]

Groups of 50 male and 50 female Fischer 344 rats, six to seven weeks of age, were given nitrofurantoin (pharmaceutical grade) at 0, 600 or 1300 mg/kg bw (females) and 0, 1300 or 2500 mg/kg (males) of diet for 103 weeks. Mean body weights were similar in control and treated animals. Survival at termination of the experiment was: males—control, 24/50; low-dose, 27/50; and high-dose, 26/50; females—control, 25/50; low-dose, 26/50; and high-dose, 31/50. Chronic tubular nephropathy was observed in all treated rats. In males, the incidence of mainly microscopic renal tubular adenomas was 3/50 controls, 11/50 low-dose [$p = 0.02$, Fisher's exact test] and 19/50 [$p < 0.001$; Fisher's exact test] high-dose animals [$p < 0.001$, Cochran-Armitage test for trend]. Renal tubular carcinomas were seen in two high-dose males. Osteosarcomas were seen in one low-dose and two high-dose males. Reductions in the incidences of a number of neoplasias were observed in males: preputial gland adenomas—control, 6/48; low-dose, 5/50; and high-dose, 0/47 ($p = 0.018$, incidental tumour test); preputial gland carcinomas—control, 6/48; low-dose, 6/50; and high-dose, 0/47 ($p = 0.028$, incidental tumour test); and interstitial-cell adenomas of the testis—control, 47/50; low-dose, 45/50; and high-dose, 21/50 ($p < 0.001$, incidental tumour test). No change in tumour incidence was observed in females (National Toxicology Program, 1989). [The Working Group was not convinced of the neoplastic nature of the microscopic kidney lesions.]

(b) *Transplacental administration*

Mouse: A group of 10 pregnant ICR/Jcl mice, 10-12 weeks of age, received three subcutaneous injections of nitrofurantoin [purity unspecified] at 75 μg/g bw suspended in a 1% gelatin solution on days 13, 15 and 17 of gestation. Groups of 22 gelatin-treated and 76 untreated dams served as controls. Offspring were foster-nursed by untreated dams and were sacrificed 32 weeks after birth. Survival was comparable in treated and untreated mice at 32 weeks. The incidence of papillary adenomas of the lung in the offspring of nitrofurantoin-treated dams was 10/78, that in gelatine controls, 5/203, and that in untreated controls, 29/478 (Nomura et al., 1984). [The Working Group noted that the distribution of tumours among litters was not given, that the sex of the offspring was not given and that the experiment was short.]

3.2 Other relevant data

(a) *Experimental systems*

(i) *Absorption, distribution, excretion and metabolism*

The pharmacokinetics of nitrofurantoin have been reviewed (Conklin, 1978).

After oral or parenteral administration, nitrofurantoin is rapidly absorbed and is excreted primarily unchanged in the urine and bile of rats (Paul et al., 1960; Buzard et al., 1961; Veronese et al., 1974; Wierzba et al., 1982) and mice (Maiti & Banerjee, 1978). After intravenous administration of nitrofurantoin to dogs at 1.5-24 mg/kg bw, up to 23% was recovered from the bile, while urinary excretion accounted for up to 36% (Conklin & Wagner, 1971). In male Sprague-Dawley rats, 16-30% of a total dose of nitrofurantoin was recovered in the urine (Olivard et al., 1976). After a single administration of nitrofurantoin at 25 mg/kg bw by gavage to female albino rats, 52% and 2.0% of the total dose were recovered in the urine and faeces, respectively (Paul et al., 1960). Excretion of nitrofurantoin in the urine of rats has been reported to be age-dependent (Braunlich et al., 1978; Wierzba et al., 1982).

Intravenous administration of nitrofurantoin at 1.5-24 mg/kg bw to adult male beagle dogs weighing 10-16 kg stimulated bile excretion, and nitrofurantoin was found in bile (at 6 mg/kg bw, 22.6 ± 4.7% total dose) and urine (24.1 ± 4.7%) (Conklin & Wagner, 1971). Nitrofurantoin is excreted in bile, reabsorbed and recirculated enterohepatically (Conklin et al., 1973). After intravenous administration of nitrofurantoin to rats, the plasma half-time was 25 min, and 50% was recovered in the urine as unchanged compound (Buzard et al., 1961). The small intestine was considered to be the main site of absorption (Maiti & Banerjee, 1978).

4-Hydroxyfurantoin has been isolated from the urine of rats treated with nitrofurantoin (Olivard et al., 1976; Streeter et al., 1988). Reductive metabolism of nitrofurantoin under anaerobic conditions has been described in both rodent tissue and bacteria. In the absence of oxygen, nitrofurantoin appears to be reduced irreversibly *via* nitroso and/or hydroxylamine forms (Mason & Holtzman, 1975a; Biaglow et al., 1977; Leskovac & Popovic, 1980).

Under aerobic conditions *in vitro*, reduction of nitrofurantoin stimulates consumption of oxygen and production of superoxide anion, free radicals and hydrogen peroxide in avian liver and in mammalian liver, lung, small intestine, kidney and gastrointestinal contents (Mason & Holtzman, 1975b; Biaglow et al., 1977; Aufrere et al., 1978; Sasame & Boyd, 1979; Leskovac & Popovic, 1980; Peterson et al., 1982).

Under anaerobic conditions, microsomal and soluble fractions from rat lung and liver mediated the covalent binding of ^{14}C-nitrofurantoin-derived radioactivity to macromolecules. Covalent binding of ^{14}C-nitrofurantoin activity was greatest in the kidney, liver, ileum, lung and heart of rats (Boyd et al., 1979).

(ii) *Toxic effects*

The LD_{50} of nitrofurantoin in mice was 150 mg/kg bw by intraperitoneal injection and 306 mg/kg bw by gavage (Åkerblom & Campbell, 1973).

Subcutaneous administration of nitrofurantoin to male rats caused severe pulmonary damage characterized by oedema, congestion and haemorrhage (Boyd et al., 1979). Male and female rats administered nitrofurantoin orally at 20, 50 or 100 mg/kg bw twice a day were reported to develop structural and functional changes in the sciatic nerve (Behar et al., 1965).

When nitrofurantoin was administered to female mice in the diet at 350 and 500 mg/kg bw and animals were examined after 4-64 weeks of treatment, a dose-related effect on body weight gain was seen as well as a reduction in uterus:brain and ovary:brain weight ratios. Histological examination revealed a dose-related decrease in the occurrence of old corpora lutea and an increase in the occurrence of intermediate and atretic follicles. The effects were more pronounced with higher dose and longer treatments. Oestrous cycles were lengthened in a dose-dependent fashion. Ovaries were atrophic and non-functioning at 43 weeks (Stitzel et al., 1989).

In a 90-day toxicity study involving the administration of nitrofurantoin in the diets of rats and mice, necrosis of ovarian follicular epithelial cells was the principal pathological finding (Maronpot, 1987).

Four of five male and four of five female mice fed nitrofurantoin at 10 000 mg/kg of diet died within 14 days. No rats receiving up to 20 000 mg/kg of diet for 14 days died; treatment-related signs included inactivity, rough coats, sunken eyes, bright yellow urine and/or yellow fur. Feeding of nitrofurantoin at 10 000 mg/kg of diet to female rats for 13 weeks caused normal-to-mild necrosis of ovarian follicles; the effect was seen in a smaller proportion of animals receiving lower doses. Minimal-to-mild degeneration of the germinal epithelium of the testis was observed in male mice fed nitrofurantoin at up to 5000 mg/kg of diet for 13 weeks. Similar treatment of male mice caused minimal-to-mild necrosis of the kidney epithelium (National Toxicology Program, 1989).

In two-year studies (see section 3.1), ovarian atrophy was observed in low- and high-dose female mice, and testicular aspermatogenesis, degeneration of the germinal epithelium and atypical cells and depletion of the epididymis were observed at increased incidences in high-dose male mice. Spindle-cell hyperplasia of the adrenal cortex occurred in treated female mice, and mineralization of the renal medulla and dilatation of the renal tubules were observed in high-dose mice. Ovarian abscesses were observed in control but not in treated mice. In the two-year study in rats, fibrous osteodystrophy and mineralization of the glandular stomach occurred in treated animals. Atypical cells of the epididymis and degeneration of the testis were observed in high-dose animals; and fibrinoid necrosis of arterioles and perivascular infiltration of mononuclear cells were observed in the testis (National Toxicology Program, 1989).

(iii) *Effects on reproduction and prenatal toxicity*

Nitrofurantoin has similar toxic effects on the testis as other nitrofurans (Cohen, 1978). Rats treated with nitrofurantoin at 10 or 85 mg/kg bw by gastric intubation daily for one month showed depression of spermatogenesis, mainly at the stage of primary spermatocytes; some effect on spermatogonia was also observed. Partial regeneration had occurred by 48 days after cessation of treatment. The gonadotoxic effects could be prevented by simultaneous administration of 'cystine' (Yunda *et al.*, 1974). [The Working Group assumed that cysteine was meant.]

Testicular and ovarian degeneration was observed in F344/N rats given nitrofurantoin in the diet at a dose equivalent to 110 mg/kg bw (males) and 60 mg/kg bw (females) for 13 weeks. Testicular degeneration was observed in B6C3F1 mice given nitrofurantoin in the diet at a dose equivalent to 285 mg/kg bw for 13 weeks (National Toxicology Program, 1989).

In routine safety evaluations of nitrofurantoin macrocrystals, including studies of fertility and perinatal-postnatal effects in rats and teratogenicity in rats and rabbits, no adverse effect was observed with daily doses of 10, 20 and 30 mg/kg bw administered orally. In the fertility test, however, male rats were treated with only 10 mg/kg bw; at this dose, no adverse effect on fertility or testicular histology was observed (Prytherch *et al.*, 1984).

After subcutaneous injection of nitrofurantoin to ICR/Jcl mice at 100 or 250 mg/kg bw on days 9-11 of gestation, no increase in embryo- or fetomortality was observed, but a decrease in fetal weight occurred in the high-dose group only. A significant ($p < 0.001$) increase in the incidence of malformations (cleft palate and syndactyly) was observed in the high-dose group only (Nomura *et al.*, 1984).

(iv) *Genetic and related effects*

The mutagenicity of nitrofurans has been reviewed (Klemencic & Wang, 1978; McCalla, 1983).

Nitrofurantoin inhibited DNA synthesis in *Escherichia coli* (Lu & McCalla, 1978). It induced DNA single-strand breaks in a nitroreductase-proficient but not in a nitroreductase-deficient strain of *E. coli* (McCalla *et al.*, 1971). It induced differential toxicity in *E. coli*, *Salmonella typhimurium* and *Bacillus subtilis* in the presence and absence of an exogenous metabolic system (McCalla & Voutsinos, 1974; Yahagi *et al.*, 1974; Ebringer & Bencova, 1980; McCarroll *et al.*, 1981a,b; Suter & Jaeger, 1982; De Flora *et al.*, 1984).

Nitrofurantoin was weakly mutagenic to *E. coli* in the presence and absence of an exogenous metabolic system (McCalla & Voutsinos, 1974; Yahagi *et al.*, 1974; Setnikar *et al.*, 1976; Lu *et al.*, 1979; Ebringer & Bencova, 1980; Obaseiki-Ebor & Akerele, 1986). It was mutagenic to *S. typhimurium* TA100 and TA98, in the presence and absence of an exogenous metabolic system (Rosenkranz & Speck, 1976; Wang & Lee, 1976; Goodman *et al.*, 1977; Chin *et al.*, 1978; De Flora, 1979; Shirai & Wang, 1980; Haworth *et al.*, 1983; De Flora *et al.*, 1984; Ni *et al.*, 1987), and to TA97 (Obaseiki-Ebor & Akerele, 1986) but not to TA1535, TA1536, TA1537 or TA1538 (Yahagi *et al.*, 1974; Haworth *et al.*, 1983; De Flora *et al.*, 1984). The strong responses in the *Salmonella* mutagenicity tests are due to the high activity of bacterial nitroreductases (Rosenkranz & Speck, 1976; Wang & Lee, 1976; Rosenkranz & Mermelstein, 1983; Ni *et al.*, 1987).

Urine of rats fed a diet containing 0.5% nitrofurantoin was mutagenic to *S. typhimurium* (Wang & Lee, 1976).

The urine of rats treated orally with nitrofurantoin at 500 or 1000 mg/kg bw induced mitotic gene conversion in *S. cerevisiae* D4-RDII (Siebert *et al.*, 1979). In a host-mediated assay with mice treated orally with nitrofurantoin at 0.3 mM/kg [72 mg/kg], no increase in the frequency of gene conversion was found in *S. cerevisiae* D4 (Setnikar *et al.*, 1976). Oral treatment of rats with nitrofurantoin at 500 mg/kg bw led to an increase in the frequency of gene conversion in *S. cerevisiae* D4-RDII (Siebert *et al.*, 1979).

Nitrofurantoin did not induce gene conversion in *Saccharomyces cerevisiae* D4 (Setnikar *et al.*, 1976). In strains D4-RDII and D7, it induced mitotic gene conversion (Siebert *et al.*, 1979; Callen, 1981). It induced non-disjunction and mitotic crossing-over in spot tests with diploid strains of *Aspergillus nidulans* (Bignami *et al.*, 1974).

Nitrofurantoin fed or injected to adult *Drosophila melanogaster* gave ambiguous results in the sex-linked recessive lethal test (Kramers, 1982; Zimmering *et al.*, 1985). It gave positive results in the wing spot test in *Drosophila*, producing large single spots (Graf *et al.*, 1989).

Nitrofurantoin inhibited DNA synthesis in mouse L-929 cells (Olive, 1979) and in diploid human fibroblasts (Hirsch-Kauffmann *et al.*, 1978). In Chinese hamster ovary (CHO K_1-BH_4 and CHO UV-5) cells, it induced mutations to 6-thioguanine resistance in the presence, but not in the absence, of an exogenous metabolic system (Gao *et al.*, 1989). Nitrofurantoin induced DNA strand breaks in mouse L cells (Olive & McCalla, 1977), in purified rat liver nuclei and in the human cell line HuF_{22} (Parodi *et al.*, 1983). It did not induce unscheduled DNA synthesis in human fibroblasts (Tonomura & Sasaki, 1973) or in rat primary hepatocytes (Williams *et al.*, 1989).

Nitrofurantoin induced sister chromatid exchange in Chinese hamster CHO cells (Shirai & Wang, 1980) but not in the human fibroblastic cell line HE 2144 (Sasaki *et al.*, 1980). It did not induce chromosomal aberrations in human lymphocytes *in vitro* (Tonomura & Sasaki, 1973) or in the human cell line HE 2144

(Sasaki *et al.*, 1980). It induced chromosomal aberrations in Chinese hamster lung (CHL) cells (Ishidate, 1988).

Intraperitoneal injection of nitrofurantoin at up to 112 mg/kg bw induced DNA strand breaks in liver (Russo *et al.*, 1982), kidney, lung and spleen cells of rats and in mouse bone-marrow cells (Parodi *et al.*, 1983). Intraperitoneal treatment at up to 64 mg/kg bw induced sister chromatid exchange in mouse bone-marrow cells *in vivo* (Parodi *et al.*, 1983).

Nitrofurantoin at 80 mg/kg bw intraperitoneally gave negative results in the mouse spot test (Gocke *et al.*, 1983) and, at up to 200 mg/kg intraperitoneally or 400 mg/kg orally, in the rat micronucleus test (Setnikar *et al.*, 1976; Goodman *et al.*, 1977). At five daily intraperitoneal doses of 8 or 40 mg/kg bw, nitrofurantoin did not induce chromosomal aberrations in spermatocytes of mice (Fonatsch, 1977). It also gave negative results in the dominant lethal test in mice after intraperitoneal administration of 16 and 80 mg/kg bw (Epstein *et al.*, 1972) and equivocal results after five daily oral doses of 17.5 mg/kg bw (Setnikar *et al.*, 1976).

(b) *Humans*

(i) *Pharmacokinetics*

Nitrofurantoin is readily absorbed from the gastrointestinal tract (Reynolds, 1989). The macrocrystalline form is dissolved and absorbed more slowly and produces lower serum concentrations than the microcrystalline form, and peak concentrations in the urine are achieved more slowy (Cunha, 1988; Reynolds, 1989).

After oral administration of nitrofurantoin at 50 mg to six healthy men, the bioavailability was $94 \pm 13\%$ on a full stomach and $87 \pm 13\%$ on a fasting stomach (Hoener & Patterson, 1981). About 60% of the nitrofurantoin was bound to plasma proteins. After a 45-min intravenous infusion, the plasma distribution followed an open two-compartment model, with a terminal half-time of approximately 1 h. After oral and intravenous infusion, 34 and 47% of the dose was excreted unchanged in the urine, respectively, and 1.2-1.4% was recovered as the reduced metabolite aminofurantoin.

Nitrofurantoin is reduced to aminofurantoin, thus following pathways similar to those known for other nitrofurans (Hoener & Patterson, 1981). Hydroxylation of the furan ring of nitrofurantoin has also been shown (Olivard *et al.*, 1976).

Recovery of the drug in the urine is related linearly to creatinine clearance (Sachs *et al.*, 1968).

After parenteral administration, nitrofurantoin crosses the human placenta (Perry & Leblanc, 1967; Kobyletzki, 1968).

(ii) *Adverse effects*

In a study of 757 courses of nitrofurantoin in hospitalized patients, the overall frequency of adverse reactions was 9.2%. Toxic reactions constituted 5.1% of adverse effects; the remainder were allergic (Koch-Weser *et al.*, 1971).

The most common gastrointestinal side-effects of nitrofurantoin are nausea, vomiting and anorexia. These symptoms usually occur during the first week of treatment and are dose-related. Abdominal pain, gastrointestinal bleeding and diarrhoea occur less frequently and without a clear dose-response (Koch-Weser *et al.*, 1971; Gleckman *et al.*, 1979).

Pulmonary infiltration may be caused by sensitivity to nitrofurantoin (Israel & Diamond, 1962). Acute pulmonary sensitivity reactions are manifested by fever, chills, cough, dyspnoea, and possible bronchospasm and chest pain associated with eosinophilia (Glueck & Janower, 1969). Subacute pulmonary reactions have been considered to be a separate syndrome (Gleckman *et al.*, 1979; D'Arcy, 1985), developing after one month of treatment with nitrofurantoin, and are characterized by persistent and progressive cough, dyspnoea and fever, together with interstitial pneumonitis (Sollaccio *et al.*, 1966; Sovijärvi *et al.*, 1977). The chronic nitrofurantoin pulmonary reaction is characterized histologically by nonspecific, diffuse interstitial pneumonitis and fibrosis (Rosenow *et al.*, 1968; Ruikka *et al.*, 1971; Castleman, 1974; Holmberg *et al.*, 1980).

Nitrofurantoin has been associated with adverse effects on the liver, including acute hepatocellular and cholestatic injury (Goldstein *et al.*, 1974), as well as rare cases resembling chronic active hepatitis (Klemola *et al.*, 1975; Black *et al.*, 1980; Sharp *et al.*, 1980).

Peripheral polyneuropathy is the most common neurological side-effect, although dizziness, vertigo, diplopia and cerebellar disturbance have also been reported (Graebner *et al.*, 1973).

Haemolytic anaemia is a well-documented complication of nitrofurantoin therapy in patients with glucose-6-phosphate dehydrogenase deficiency (Swanson & Cook, 1977). Haemolysis has also been reported in patients deficient in enolase and glutathione peroxidases (Steinberg *et al.*, 1970; Stefanini, 1972). In addition, there have been case reports of megaloblastic anaemia (Bass, 1963), agranulocytosis (Palva & Lehmola, 1973; Böttiger & Westerholm, 1977) and aplastic anaemia (Böttiger & Westerholm, 1977).

(iii) *Effects on reproduction and prenatal toxicity*

In the Collaborative Perinatal Project, in which drug intake and pregnancy outcome were studied in a series of 50 282 women in 1959-65, 83 women had been exposed to nitrofurantoin during the first trimester of pregnancy. Six malformed children were born in the exposed group, giving a standardized nonsignificant relative risk of 1.07 (Heinonen *et al.* 1977).

Hailey *et al.* (1983) reported on the use of nitrofurantoin during 91 pregnancies in 81 women in one practice in 1972-80. In 36% of women, treatment was given during the first trimester. In the 91 pregnancies, one fetal death and two malformed babies (all with exposure during the second or third trimester) were observed. There was no significant difference in the incidence of mortality, malformation, prematurity or low birth weight compared with the general population.

In a brief review of the management of urinary-tract infections in pregnancy, it was stated that, in over 5000 pregnancies treated with nitrofurantoin macrocrystals at 100 mg daily for ten days, the treatment did not produce adverse fetal or neonatal effects and there was no recorded case of neonatal haemolytic anaemia (Whalley, 1985).

(iv) *Genetic and related effects*

Urine of 12 patients was collected before and after treatment with nitrofurantoin at 100 mg. Increased mutagenic activity in *S. typhimurium* TA100 was found in samples taken after treatment (Wang *et al.*, 1977).

3.3 Case reports and epidemiological studies of carcinogenicity to humans

A single case report has been published of focal nodular hyperplasia of the liver in association with nitrofurantoin treatment in a six-year-old girl who had been treated for seven months (Anttinen *et al.*, 1982).

In a hypothesis-generating cohort study designed to screen a large number of drugs for possible carcinogenicity (described in detail in the monograph on ampicillin), 1305 persons to whom at least one prescription for nitrofurantoin had been dispensed during 1969-73 were followed for up to 15 years (Selby *et al.*, 1989). Increased risks were noted for cancer of the uterine corpus (six cases observed, 2.1 expected; $p < 0.05$) and for cancer of other female genital organs (three cases observed, 0.3 expected; $p < 0.05$) during follow-up of up to nine years (Friedman & Ury, 1980, 1983), and for cancers of the nervous system [other than brain] (three cases observed, 0.6 expected; $p < 0.05$) during follow-up of up to 15 years (Selby *et al.*, 1989). [The Working Group noted, as did the authors, that, since some 12 000 comparisons were made in this study, the associations should be verified independently. Data on duration of use were not provided.]

4. Summary of Data Reported and Evaluation

4.1 Exposure data

Nitrofurantoin has been used since 1972 in the treatment of urinary-tract infections.

4.2 Experimental carcinogenicity data

Nitrofurantoin was tested by oral administration to mice in four studies and to rats in three studies and by transplacental administration to mice in one study. Two of the studies in mice, including the transplacental study, were inadequate for evaluation. In one study in mice, an increase in the incidence of ovarian tubular adenomas and benign mixed tumours was observed. In two studies in other strains of mice, no such increase was observed, although in one study there was an increase in the incidence of malignant lymphomas in males. One study in rats was inadequate for evaluation. A further study in female rats demonstrated an increase in the incidence of mammary fibroadenomas. In the third study in rats, although a few rare tumours were observed, there was no significant increase in the incidence of malignant neoplasms.

4.3 Human carcinogenicity data

In a hypothesis-generating cohort study, use of nitrofurantoin was associated with the occurrence of cancers of the female genital tract and nervous system, but these findings could have been due to chance.

4.4 Other relevant data

Use of nitrofurantoin during pregnancy has not been associated with birth defects. The drug has gonadotoxic effects in male and female rats and mice and teratogenic effects in mice at high doses.

In humans, use of nitrofurantoin has been associated with pulmonary fibrosis, hepatocellular injury, aplastic anaemia and other blood dyscrasias.

Nitrofurantoin gave negative results in the mouse spot test and in the rat micronucleus test. It did not induce chromosomal aberrations in male germ cells or dominant lethal effects in mice. It induced DNA strand breaks in rats and mice and sister chromatid exchange and unscheduled DNA synthesis in bone-marrow cells of mice. Nitrofurantoin induced DNA strand breaks in mouse, rat and human cells *in vitro* and increased the frequency of sister chromatid exchange in Chinese hamster cells but not in human cells *in vitro*. Nitrofurantoin induced chromosomal aberrations in Chinese hamster cells but not in human cells *in vitro*. It did not induce unscheduled DNA synthesis in human fibroblasts or rat hepatocytes *in vitro*. It induced gene mutations in Chinese hamster cells. Nitrofurantoin gave ambiguous results in *Drosophila* in the sex-linked recessive lethal test but positive results in the wing spot test. It gave contradictory results in tests for mitotic gene conversion in *Saccharomyces cerevisiae*. Nitrofurantoin induced differential toxicity in *Escherichia coli*, *Salmonella typhimurium* and *Bacillus subtilis* and mutations in *E. coli* and *S. typhimurium*. (See Appendix 1.)

4.5 Evaluation[1]

There is *inadequate evidence* for the carcinogenicity of nitrofurantoin in humans.

There is *limited evidence* for the carcinogenicity of nitrofurantoin in experimental animals.

Overall evaluation

Nitrofurantoin *is not classifiable as to its carcinogenicity to humans (Group 3)*.

5. References

Åkerblom, E.B. & Campbell, D.E.S. (1973) Nitrofuryltriazole derivatives as potential urinary tract antibacterial agents. *J. med. Chem.*, 16, 312-317

Antinnen, H., Ahonen, A., Leinonen, A., Kallioinen, M. & Heikkinen, E.S. (1982) Diagnostic imaging of focal nodular hyperplasia of the liver developing during nitrofurantoin therapy. *Acta med. scand.*, 211, 227-232

Apoteksbolaget (1988) *Svensk Läkemedelsstatistik* [Swedish Drugs Statistics], Stockholm, Pharmaceutical Association of Sweden

Apoteksbolaget (1989) *Outprint of the Drug Data Base (17 October 1989)*, Stockholm, Pharmaceutical Association of Sweden

Aufrere, M.B., Hoener, B.-A. & Vore, M. (1978) Reductive metabolism of nitrofurantoin in the rat. *Drug Metab. Dispos.*, 6, 403-411

Barnhart, E. (1989) *Physicians' Desk Reference*, 43rd ed., Oradell, NJ, Medical Economics, pp. 1485-1486

---

[1]For description of the italicized terms, see Preamble, pp. 26–29.

Bass, B.H. (1963) Megaloblastic anemia due to nitrofurantoin. *Lancet, i*, 530-531

Behar, A., Rachmilewitz, E., Rahamimoff, R. & Denman, M. (1965) Experimental nitrofurantoin polyneuropathy in rats. *Arch. Neurol., 13*, 160-163

Biaglow, J.E., Jacobson, B.E. & Nygaard, O.F. (1977) Metabolic reduction of 4-nitroquinoline-N-oxide and other radical-producing drugs to oxygen-reactive intermediates. *Cancer Res., 37*, 3306-3313

Bignami, M., Morpurgo, G., Pagliani, R., Carere, A., Conti, G. & Di Giuseppe, G. (1974) Non-disjunction and crossing-over induced by pharmaceutical drugs in *Aspergillus nidulans*. *Mutat. Res., 26*, 159-170

Black, M., Rabin, L. & Schatz, N. (1980) Nitrofurantoin-induced chronic active hepatitis. *Ann. intern. Med., 92*, 62-64

Böttiger, L.E. & Westerholm, B. (1977) Adverse drug reactions during treatment of urinary tract infections. *Eur. J. clin. Pharmacol., 11*, 439-442

Boyd, M.R., Stiko, A.W. & Sasame, H.A. (1979) Metabolic activation of nitrofurantoin—possible implications for carcinogenesis. *Biochem. Pharmacol., 28*, 601-606

Braunlich, H., Bonow, A. & Schroter, S. (1978) Age-dependence of renal tubular reabsorption of nitrofurantoin. *Arch. int. Pharmacodyn. Ther., 232*, 92-101

Butler, W.H., Graham, T.C. & Sutton, M.L. (1990) Oncogenicity study of macrodantin in Swiss mice. *Food chem. Toxicol., 28*, 49-54

Buzard, J.A., Conklin, J.D., O'Keefe, E. & Paul, M.F. (1961) Studies on the absorption, distribution and elimination of nitrofurantoin in the rat. *J. Pharmacol. exp. Ther., 131*, 38-43

Cadwallader, D.E. & Jun, H.W. (1976) Nitrofurantoin. *Anal. Profiles Drug Subst., 5*, 346-373

Callen, D.F. (1981) Comparison of the genetic activity of AF-2 and nitrofurantoin in log and stationary phase cells of *Saccharomyces cerevisiae*. *Environ. Mutagenesis, 3*, 651-658

Castleman, B. (1974) Case 22-1974 Massachusetts General Hospital: weekly clinico-pathological exercises. *New Engl. J. Med., 290*, 1309-1314

Chemical Information Services (1989-90) *Directory of World Chemical Producers 1989/90*, Oceanside, NY

Chin, J.B., Sheinin, D.M.K. & Rauth, A.M. (1978) Screening for the mutagenicity of nitro-group containing hypoxic cell radiosensitizers using *Salmonella typhimurium* strains TA100 and TA98. *Mutat. Res., 58*, 1-10

Cohen, S.M. (1978) Toxicity and carcinogenicity of nitrofurans. *Carcinogenesis, 4*, 171-231

Cohen, S.M., Ertürk, E., Von Esch, A.M., Crovetti, A.J. & Bryan, G.T. (1973) Carcinogenicity of 5-nitrofurans, 5-nitroimidazoles, 4-nitrobenzenes, and related compounds. *J. natl Cancer Inst., 51*, 403-417

Conklin, J.D. (1978) The pharmacokinetics of nitrofurantoin and its related bioavailability. *Antibiot. Chemother., 25*, 233-252

Conklin, J.D. & Wagner, D.L. (1971) Excretion of nitrofurantoin in dog hepatic bile. *Br. J. Pharmacol., 43*, 140-150

Conklin, J.D., Sobers, R.J. & Wagner, D.L. (1973) Further studies on nitrofurantoin excretion in dog hepatic bile. *Br. J. Pharmacol., 48*, 273-277

Cunha, B.A. (1988) Nitrofurantoin—current concepts. *Urology*, 32, 67-71

D'Arcy, P. (1985) Nitrofurantoin. *Drug Intell. clin. Pharmacol.*, 19, 540-547

De Flora, S. (1979) Metabolic activation and deactivation of mutagens and carcinogens. *Ital. J. Biochem.*, 28, 81-103

De Flora, S., Zanacchi, P., Camoirano, A., Bennicelli, C. & Badolati, G.S. (1984) Genotoxic activity and potency of 135 compounds in the Ames reversion test and in a bacterial DNA-repair test. *Mutat. Res.*, 133, 161-198

Ebringer, L. & Bencova, M. (1980) Mutagenicity of nitrofuran drugs in bacterial systems. *Folia microbiol.*, 25, 388-396

Epstein, S.S., Arnold, E., Andrea, J., Bass, W. & Bishop, Y. (1972) Detection of chemical mutagens by the dominant lethal assay in the mouse. *Toxicol. appl. Pharmacol.*, 23, 288-325

Fogg, A.G. & Ghawji, A.B. (1988) Reductive amperometric determination of nitrofurantoin and acetazolamide at a sessile mercury drop electrode using flow injection analysis. *Analyst*, 113, 727-730

Fonatsch, C. (1977) Effect of nitrofurantoin on meiosis of the male mouse. *Hum. Genet.*, 39, 345-351

Friedman, G.D. & Ury, H.K. (1980) Initial screening for carcinogenicity of commonly used drugs. *J. natl Cancer Inst.*, 65, 723-733

Friedman, G.D. & Ury, H.K. (1983) Screening for possible drug carcinogenicity: second report of findings. *J. natl Cancer Inst.*, 71, 1165-1175

Gao, N., Ni, Y.-C., Thornton-Manning, J.R., Fu, P.P. & Heflich, R.H. (1989) Mutagenicity of nitrofurantoin and furazolidine in Chinese hamster ovary cell strains. *Mutat. Res.*, 225, 181-187

Gleckman, R., Alvarea, S. & Joubert, D.W. (1979) Drug therapy reviews: nitrofurantoin. *Am. J. Hosp. Pharm.*, 36, 342-351

Glueck, M.A. & Janower, M.L. (1969) Nitrofurantoin lung disease. Clues to pathogenesis. *Am. J. Roentgenol.*, 107, 818

Gocke, E., Wild, D., Eckhardt, K. & King, M.-T. (1983) Mutagenicity studies with the mouse spot test. *Mutat. Res.*, 117, 201-212

Goldstein, L.I., Ishak, K.G. & Burns, W. (1974) Hepatic injury associated with nitrofurantoin therapy. *Digest. Dis.*, 19, 987-998

Goodman, D.R., Hakkinen, P.J., Nemenzo, J.H. & Vore, M. (1977) Mutagenic evaluation of nitrofuran derivatives in *Salmonella typhimurium*, by the micronucleus test, and by in vivo cytogenetics. *Mutat. Res.*, 48, 295-306

Graebner, R.W., Herskowitz, A. & Augusta, G. (1973) Cerebellar toxic effects from nitrofurantoin. *Arch. Neurol.*, 29, 195-196

Graf, U., Frei, H., Kägi, A., Katz, A.J. & Würgler, F.E. (1989) Thirty compounds tested in the *Drosophila* wing spot test. *Mutat. Res.*, 222, 359-373

Hailey, F.J., Fort, H., Williams, J.C. & Hammers, B. (1983) Foetal safety of nitrofurantoin macrocrystals therapy during pregnancy: a retrospective analysis. *J. intern. Med. Res.*, 11, 364-369

Haworth, S., Lawlor, T., Mortelmans, K., Speck, W. & Zeiger, E. (1983) *Salmonella* mutagenicity test results for 250 chemicals. *Environ. Mutagenesis, Suppl. 1*, 3-142

Heinonen, O.P., Slone, D. & Shapiro, S. (1977) *Birth Defects and Drugs in Pregnancy*, Littleton, MA, Publishing Sciences Group, pp. 296-313

Hirsch-Kauffmann, M., Herrlich, P. & Schweiger, M. (1978) Nitrofurantoin damages DNA of human cells. *Klin. Wochenschr.*, 56, 405-407

Hoener, B.-A. & Patterson, S.E. (1981) Nitrofurantoin disposition. *Clin. Pharmacol. Ther.*, 29, 808-816

Holmberg, L., Boman, G., Böttiger, L.E., Eriksson, B., Spross, R. & Wessling, A. (1980) Adverse reactions to nitrofurantoin — analysis of 921 reports. *Am. J. Med.*, 69, 733-738

IARC (1987a) *IARC Monographs on the Evaluation of the Carcinogenic Risk of Chemicals to Humans*, Suppl. 7, *Overall Evaluation of Carcinogenicity: An Updating of* IARC Monographs *Volumes 1 to 42*, Lyon, pp. 334-339

IARC (1987b) *IARC Monographs on the Evaluation of the Carcinogenic Risk of Chemicals to Humans*, Suppl. 7, *Overall Evaluation of Carcinogenicity: An Updating of* IARC Monographs *Volumes 1 to 42*, Lyon, p. 65

Ishidate, M., Jr, ed. (1988) *Data Book of Chromosomal Aberration Test* In Vitro, Amsterdam, Elsevier

Israel, H.L. & Diamond, P. (1962) Recurrent pulmonary infiltration and pleural effusion due to nitrofurantoin sensitivity. *New Engl. J. Med.*, 266, 1024-1026

Ito, A., Naito, M., Naito, Y. & Watanabe, H. (1983) Tumorigenicity test of N-(5-nitro-2-furfurylidine)-1-aminohydantoin by dietary administration in BDF_1 mice. *Hiroshima J. med. Sci.*, 32, 99-

Klemencic, J.M. & Wang C.Y. (1978) Mutagenicity of nitrofurans. In: Bryan, G.T., ed., *Carcinogenesis*, Vol. 4, *Nitrofurans*, New York, Raven Press, pp. 99-130

Klemola, H., Penttilä, O., Runeberg, L. & Tallqvist, G. (1975) Anicteric liver damage during nitrofurantoin medication. *Scand. J. Gastroenterol.*, 10, 501-505

Kobyletzki, D.V. (1968) Studies on pharmacokinetics at the time of parturition and lactation. *Med. Welt*, 19, 2010-2019

Koch-Weser, J., Sidel, V.W., Dexter, M., Parish, C., Finer, D.C. & Kanarek, P. (1971) Adverse reactions to sulfisoxazole, sulfamethoxazole, and nitrofurantoin. Manifestations and specific reaction rates during 2118 courses of therapy. *Arch. intern. Med.*, 128, 399-404

Kramers, P.G.N. (1982) Studies on the induction of sex-linked recessive lethal mutations in *Drosophila melanogaster* by nitroheterocyclic compounds. *Mutat. Res.*, 101, 209-236

Leskovac, V. & Popovic, M. (1980) Mechanism of reduction of nitrofurantoin on liver microsomes. *Pharmacol. Res. Commun.*, 12, 13-27

Lohr, J.A., Nunley, D.H., Howards, S.S. & Ford, R.F. (1977) Prevention of recurrent urinary tract infections in girls. *Pediatrics*, 59, 562-565

Lu, C. & McCalla, D.R. (1978) Action of some nitrofuran derivatives on glucose metabolism, ATP levels, and macromolecule synthesis in *Escherichia coli*. *Can. J. Microbiol.*, 24, 650-657

Lu, C., McCalla, D.R. & Bryant, D.W. (1979) Action of nitrofurans on *E. coli*. Mutation and induction and repair of daughter-strand gaps in DNA. *Mutat. Res.*, 67, 133-144

Maiti, T.K. & Banerjee, S. (1978) Intestinal absorption of nitrofuratoin. *Indian J. exp. Biol.*, 16, 360-362

Maronpot, R.R. (1987) Ovarian toxicity and carcinogenicity in eight recent National Toxicology Program studies. *Environ. Health Perspect.*, 73, 125-130

Mason, R.P. & Holtzman, J.L. (1975a) The mechanism of microsomal and mitochondrial nitroreductase. Electron spin resonance evidence for nitroaromatic free radical intermediates. *Biochemistry*, 14, 1626-1632

Mason, R.P. & Holtzman, J.L. (1975b) The role of catalytic superoxide formation in the O_2 inhibition of nitroreductase. *Biochem. biophys. Res. Commun.*, 67, 1267-1274

Mason, W.D. & Sandmann, B. (1976) Determination of nitrofurantoin in urine by reduction at rotating platinum electrode. *J. pharm. Sci.*, 65, 599-601

McCalla, D.R. (1983) Mutagenicity of nitrofuran derivatives: review. *Environ. Mutagenesis*, 5, 745-765

McCalla, D.R. & Voutsinos, D. (1974) On the mutagenicity of nitrofurans. *Mutat. Res.*, 26, 3-16

McCalla, D.R., Reuvers, A. & Kaiser, C. (1971) Breakage of bacterial DNA by nitrofuran derivatives. *Cancer Res.*, 31, 2184-2188

McCarroll, N.E., Piper, C.E. & Keech, B.H. (1981a) An *E. coli* microsuspension assay for the detection of DNA damage induced by direct-acting agents and promutagens. *Environ. Mutagenesis*, 3, 429-444

McCarroll, N.E., Keech, B.H. & Piper, C.E. (1981b) A microsuspension adaptation of the *Bacillus subtilis* 'rec' assay. *Environ. Mutagenesis*, 3, 607-616

Morales, A., Richter, P. & Toral, I. (1987) Polarographic determination of nitrofurazone and furazolidone in pharmaceutical formations and urine. *Analyst*, 112, 971-973

National Toxicology Program (1989) *Toxicology and Carcinogenesis Studies of Nitrofurantoin (CAS No. 67-20-9) in F344/N Rats and B6C3F1 Mice (Feed Studies)* (NTP Technical Report No. 341), Research Triangle Park, NC

Ni, Y.-C., Heflich, R.H., Kadlubar, F.F. & Fu, P.P. (1987) Mutagenicity of nitrofurans in *Salmonella typhimurium* TA98, TA98NR and TA98/1,8-DNP_6. *Mutat. Res.*, 192, 15-22

Nomura, T., Kimura, S., Kanzaki, T., Tanaka, H., Shibata, K., Nakajima, H., Isa, T., Kurokawa, N., Hatanaka, T., Kinuta, M., Masada, K. & Sakamoto, Y. (1984) Induction of tumors and malformations in mice after prenatal treatment with some antibiotic drugs. *Med. J. Osaka Univ.*, 35, 13-17

Obaseiki-Ebor, E.E. & Akerele, J.O. (1986) Nitrofuran mutagenicity: induction of frameshift mutations. *Mutat. Res.*, 175, 149-152

Olivard, J., Rose, G.M., Klein, G.M. & Heotis, J.P. (1976) Metabolic and photochemical hydroxylation of 5-nitro-furancarboxaldehyde derivatives. *J. med. Chem.*, 19, 729-731

Olive, P.L. (1979) Inhibition of DNA synthesis by nitroheterocycles. I. Correlation with half-wave reduction potential. *Br. J. Cancer*, 40, 89-93

Olive, P.L. & McCalla, D.R. (1977) Cytotoxicity and DNA damage to mammalian cells by nitrofurans. *Chem.-biol. Interactions*, 16, 223-233

Palva, I.P. & Lehmola, U. (1973) Agranulocytosis caused by nitrofurantoin. *Acta med. scand.*, *194*, 575-576

Parodi, S., Pala, M., Russo, P., Balbi, C., Abelmoschi, M.L., Taningher, M., Zunino, A., Ottaggio, L., De Ferrari, M., Carbone, A. & Santi, L. (1983) Alkaline DNA fragmentation, DNA disentanglement evaluated viscosimetrically and sister chromatid exchanges, after treatment *in vivo* with nitrofurantoin. *Chem.-biol. Interactions*, *45*, 77-94

Paul, M.F., Paul, H.E., Bender, R.C., Kopko, F., Harrington, C.M., Ells, V.R. & Buzzard, J.A. (1960) Studies on the distribution and excretion of certain nitrofurans. *Antibiot. Chemother.*, *10*, 287-302

Perry, J.E. & Leblanc, A.L. (1967) Transfer of nitrofurantoin across the human placenta. *Tex. Rep. biol. Med.*, *25*, 265-269

Peterson, F.J., Combs, G.F., Jr, Holtzman, J.L. & Mason, R.B. (1982) Metabolic activation of oxygen by nitrofurantoin in the young chick. *Toxicol. appl. Pharmacol.*, *65*, 162-169

Prytherch, J.P., Sutton, M.L., Denine, E.P. (1984) General reproduction, perinatal-postnatal, and teratology studies of nitrofurantoin macrocrystals in rats and rabbits. *J. Toxicol. environ. Health*, *13*, 811-823

Reynolds, J.E.F., ed. (1989) *Martindale. The Extra Pharmacopoeia*, London, The Parmaceutical Press, pp. 272-274

Rosenkranz, H.S. & Mermelstein, R. (1983) Mutagenicity and genotoxicity of nitroarenes: all nitro-containing chemicals were not created equal. *Mutat. Res.*, *114*, 217-267

Rosenkranz, H.S. & Speck, W.T. (1976) Activation of nitrofurantoin to a mutagen by rat liver nitroreductase. *Biochem. Pharmacol.*, *25*, 1555-1556

Rosenow, E.C., DeRemee, R.A. & Dines, E.E. (1968) Chronic nitrofurantoin pulmonary reaction: report of five cases. *New Engl. J. Med.*, *279*, 1258-1262

Ruikka, L., Vaissali, T. & Saarimaa, H. (1971) Progressive pulmonary fibrosis during nitrofurantoin therapy: a case history with autopsy report. *Scand. J. respir. Dis.*, *52*, 162-166

Russo, P., Pala, M., Nicolo, G., Santi, L. & Parodi, S. (1982) DNA damage in liver of rats treated with nitrofurantoin. *Mutat. Res.*, *105*, 377-382

Sachs, J., Greer, T., Noell, P. & Kunin, C.M. (1968) Effect of renal function on urinary recovery of orally administered nitrofurantoin. *New Engl. J. Med.*, *278*, 1032-1035

Sasaki, M., Sugimura, K., Yoshida, M.A. & Abe, S. (1980) Cytogenetic effects of 60 chemicals on cultured human and Chinese hamster cells. *Kromosomo*, *II-20*, 574-584

Sasame, H.A. & Boyd, M.R. (1979) Superoxide and hydrogen peroxide production and NADPH oxidation stimulated by nitrofurantoin in lung microsomes: possible implications for toxicity. *Life Sci.*, *24*, 1091-1096

Selby, J.V., Friedman, G.D. & Fireman, B.H. (1989) Screening prescription drugs for possible carcinogenicity: 11 to 15 years of follow-up. *Cancer Res.*, *49*, 5736-5747

Setnikar, I., Magistretti, M.J. & Veronese, M. (1976) Mutagenicity studies on nifurpipone and nitrofurantoin. *Proc. Eur. Soc. Toxicol.*, *17*, 405-412

Sharp, J.R., Ishak, K.G., & Zimmerman, H.J. (1980) Chronic active hepatitis and severe hepatic necrosis associated with nitrofurantoin. *Ann. intern. Med.*, *92*, 119-120

Shirai, T. & Wang, C.Y. (1980) Enhancement of sister-chromatid exchange in Chinese hamster ovary cells by nitrofurans. *Mutat. Res.*, 79, 345-350

Siebert, D., Bayer, U. & Marquardt, H. (1979) The application of mitotic gene conversion in *Saccharomyces cerevisiae* in a pattern of four assays, *in vitro* and *in vivo*, for mutagenicity testing. *Mutat. Res.*, 67, 145-156

Sollaccio, P.A., Ribaudo, C.A. & Grace, W.J. (1966) Subacute pulmonary infiltration due to nitrofurantoin. *Ann. intern. Med.*, 65, 1284-1286

Sovijärvi, A.R.A., Lomola, M., Stenius, B. & Idänpään-Heikkilä, J. (1977) Nitrofurantoin-induced acute, subacute and chronic pulmonary reactions. *Scand. J. respir. Dis.*, 58, 41-50

Stamey, T.A., Condyt, M. & Mihara, G. (1977) Prophylactic efficacy of nitrofurantoin macrocrystals and trimethoprim-sulfamethoxazole in urinary infections. Biological effects on the vaginal and rectal flora. *New Engl. J. Med.*, 296, 780-783

Stefanini, M. (1972) Chronic hemolytic anemia associated with erythrocyte enolase deficiency exacerbated by ingestion of nitrofurantoin. *Am. J. clin. Pathol.*, 58, 408-414

Steinberg, M., Brauer, M.J. & Necheles, T.F. (1970) Acute hemolytic anemia associated with erythrocyte glutathione-peroxidase deficiency. *Arch. intern. Med.*, 125, 302-303

Stitzel, K.A., McConnell, R.F. & Kierckman, T.A. (1989) Effects of nitrofurantoin on the primary and secondary reproductive organs of female B6C3F1 mice. *Toxicol. Pathol.*, 17, 774-781

Streeter, A.J., Krueger, T.R. & Hoener, B.A. (1988) Oxidative metabolism of 5-nitrofurans. *Pharmacology*, 36, 283-288

Surmann, P. & Aswakun, P. (1985) Polarographische simultanbestimmung von Nitrofurantoin und Phenazopyridin in Tabletten. [Simultaneous polarographic determination of nitrofurantoin and phenazopyridin in tablets (Ger.).] *Arch. Pharm.*, 318, 14-21

Suter, W. & Jaeger, I. (1982) Comparative evaluation of different pairs of DNA repair-deficient and DNA repair-proficient bacterial tester strains for rapid detection of chemical mutagens and carcinogens. *Mutat. Res.*, 97, 1-18

Swanson, M. & Cook, R. (1977) *Drugs, Chemicals and Blood Dyscrasias*, Hamilton, IL, Drug Intelligence Publications, pp. 685-695

Tonomura, A. & Sasaki, M.S. (1973) Chromosome aberrations and DNA repair synthesis in cultured human cells exposed to nitrofurans. *Jpn. J. Genet.*, 48, 291-294

US Pharmacopeial Convention, Inc. (1989) *US Pharmacopeia*, 22nd rev., Easton, PA, pp. 947-950

Veronese, M., Salvaterra, M., Barzaghi, D. & Setnikar, I. (1974) Urinary excretion in the rat of nifurpipone (NP) and of nitrofurantoin (NTF) administered by different routes. *Arzneimittel-forsch.*, 24, 39-43

Vree, T.B., Hekster, Y.A., Baars, A.M., Damsma, J.E. & van der Kleijn, E. (1979) Determination of nitrourantoin (Furadantine) and hydroxymethylnitrofurantoin (Urfadyn) in plasma and urine of man by means of high-performance liquid chromatography. *J. Chromatogr.*, 162, 110-116

Wang, C.Y. & Lee, L.H. (1976) Mutagenic activity of carcinogenic and noncarcinogenic nitrofurans and of urine of rats fed these compounds. *Chem.-biol. Interactions*, *15*, 69-75

Wang, C.Y., Benson R.C., Jr & Bryan, G.T. (1977) Mutagenicity for *Salmonella typhimurium* of urine obtained from humans receiving nitrofurantoin. *J. natl Cancer Inst.*, *58*, 871-873

Wang, C.Y., Croft, W.A. & Bryan, G.T. (1984) Tumor production in germ-free rats fed 5-nitrofurans. *Cancer Lett.*, *21*, 303-308

Whalley, P.J. (1985) Management of urinary tract infection during pregnancy. In: Schroder, F.H., ed., *Recent Advances in the Treatment of Urinary Tract Infections* (Royal Society of Medicine Services International Congress and Symposium Series No. 97), London, Royal Society of Medicine Services Ltd, pp. 37-43

Wierzba, K., Wankowicz, B., Rogoyski, A., Porkopczyk, J., Piekarczyk, A., Kaminska, E. & Bozkowa, K. (1982) Experimental and clinical pharmacokinetics of nitrofurantoin in the early period of life. *Pädiat. Pädol.*, *17*, 293-299

Williams, G.M., Mori, H. & McQueen, C.A. (1989) Structure-activity relationships in the rat hepatocyte DNA-repair test for 300 chemicals. *Mutat. Res.*, *221*, 263-286

Windholz, M., ed. (1983) *The Merck Index*, 10th ed., Rahway, NJ, Merck & Co., pp. 6438-6439

Yahagi, T., Nagao, M., Hara, K., Matsushima, T., Sugimura, T. & Bryan, G.T. (1974) Relationships between the carcinogenic and mutagenic or DNA-modifying effects of nitrofuran derivatives, including 2-(2-furyl)-3-(5-nitro-2-furyl)acrylamide, a food additive. *Cancer Res.*, *34*, 2266-2273

Yunda, I.F., Melnik, A.M. & Kushniruk, Y.I. (1974) Experimental study of the gonadotoxic effect of nitrofurans and its prevention. *Int. Urol. Nephrol.*, *6*, 125-135

Zimmering, S., Mason, J.M., Valencia, R. & Woodruff, R.C. (1985) Chemical mutagenesis testing in *Drosophila*. II. Results of 20 coded compounds tested for the National Toxicology Program. *Environ. Mutagenesis*, *7*, 87-100

OTHER DRUGS

CIMETIDINE

1. Chemical and Physical Data

Cimetidine

1.1 Synonyms

Chem. Abstr. Services Reg. No.: 51481-61-9

Chem. Abstr. Name: Guanidine N-cyano-N'-methyl-N"-(2-{[(5-methyl-1H-imidazol-4-yl)methyl]thio}ethyl)-

Synonym: 2-Cyano-1-methyl-3-[2-(5-methylimidazo-4-ylmethylthio)ethyl]guanidine

1.2 Structural and molecular formula and molecular weight

$C_{10}H_{16}N_6S$ Mol. wt: 252.34

1.3 Chemical and physical properties of the pure substance

From Windholz (1983) and Bavin *et al.* (1984)

(a) *Description*: White to off-white crystalline powder
(b) *Melting point*: 141-143°C (base), 193°C dec (hydrochloride)
(c) *Solubility*: Soluble (1.14%) in water at 37°C; soluble in ethanol; very slightly soluble in chloroform; insoluble in diethyl ether. The hydrochloride is freely soluble in water; soluble in ethanol; very slightly soluble in chloroform; and practically insoluble in diethyl ether.

(d) *Spectroscopy data*: Ultraviolet, infrared, nuclear magnetic resonance and mass spectral data have been reported.

(e) *Stability*: Dry compound, stored in a closed container at room temperature, showed no decomposition after five years. Cimetidine hydrochloride is stable for 48 h at normal room temperature when diluted with most commonly used solutions for intravenous injection.

1.4 Technical products and impurities

Trade names: Acibilin; Aciloc; Acinil; Altramet; Cianosel; 'Cim'; Cimal; Cimegan; Cimet; Cimetid; Cimetidina; Cimetin; Cimetum; Cinamet; Cinulcus; Citimid; Citius; Climatidine; Dina; Duncamet; Duogastril; Duractin; Dyspamet; Edalene; Etidine; Eureceptor; Evicer; Fisiol; Fremet; Gasmetin; Gastrobitan; Gastro H2; Gastromet; Himetin; Itacem; Lucimet; Lucomet; Mansal; Nimus (Udine) Gadol; Notul; Novocimetine; Peptol; Prometidine; Regastric; SKF 92334; Stomakon; Tagacid; Tagama; Tagagel; Tagamet; Tametin; Temic; Tratul; Tratul Retard (SR); Ulcedine; Ulcenon; Ulcerdine; Ulcerfen; Ulcestop; Ulcidin; Ulcimet; Ulcodina; Ulcomedina; Ulhys; Vagolisal; Valmagen

Hydrochloride: Biomag; Brumetidina; Cimet; Notul

Cimetidine is available for oral administration as 200- or 300-mg tablets. The hydrochloride is available for oral administration as a 300 mg/5 ml solution and for parenteral administration as a 150 mg/ml liquid.

Impurities in tablets available in the USA include cellulose, D&C yellow #0, FD&C Blue #2, FD&C Red #40, FD&C yellow #6, hydroxypropyl methylcellulose, iron oxides (see IARC, 1987a), magnesium stearate, povidone, propylene glycol, sodium lauryl sulfate, sodium starch glycolate, starch and titanium dioxide (see IARC, 1989a). Impurities in the liquid (oral) preparation are ethanol (2.8%), FD&C Yellow #6, methylparaben, polyoxyethylene polyoxypropylene glycol, propylene glycol, propylparaben, saccharin sodium (see IARC, 1987b), sodium chloride, sodium phosphate, sorbitol and water. Solutions for intramuscular or intravenous injections contain phenol (0.5%; see IARC, 1989b) (Barnhart, 1989).

Single-dose, premixed plastic containers for intravenous administration are available (300 mg cimetidine, 0.45 g sodium chloride and no preservative) (Barnhart, 1989).

N-*Nitrosocimetidine*

1.1 Synonyms

Chem. Abstr. Services Reg. No.: 73785-50-7

Chem. Abstr. Name: Guanidine, *N*-cyano-*N'*-methyl-*N'*-nitroso-*N"*-(2-{[(5-methyl-1*H*-imidazol-4-yl)methyl]thio}ethyl)-

1.2 Structural and molecular formulae and molecular weight

$C_{10}H_{15}N_7OS$ Mol wt: 281.33

1.3 Chemical and physical properties of the pure substance

From Bavin *et al.* (1980) and Foster *et al.* (1980)

(a) *Description*: Pale-yellow crystals
(b) *Melting-point*: 112-113°C
(c) *Solubility*: Soluble in dimethylsulfoxide
(d) *Spectroscopy data*: Ultraviolet, nuclear magnetic resonance and field desorption mass spectra have been recorded.
(e) *Stability*: Unstable in alkaline solution

1.4 Technical products and impurities

N-Nitrosocimetidine has been synthesized for research purposes (Bavin *et al.*, 1980; Foster *et al.*, 1980). The *N*-methyl-*N'*-cyanoguanidine moiety of cimetidine can be converted to the corresponding *N*-nitroso derivative (*N*-nitrosocimetidine) by the action of acidic solutions of nitrite (Bavin *et al.*, 1980).

2. Production, Occurrence, Use and Analysis

2.1 Production and occurrence

Cimetidine is prepared from 2-methyl-3-hydroxymethyl-1*H*-imidazole *via* a multistep synthesis involving sequential additions of 2-mercaptoethylamine, dimethylcyanodithioimidocarbonate and methylamine and variations of this method (Durant *et al.*, 1974; Bavin *et al.*, 1984). The hydrochloride is prepared by addition of hydrochloric acid and ethyl acetate as an ethanolic suspension of cimetidine (Bavin *et al.*, 1984).

Cimetidine is synthesized in Brazil, Hungary, India, Italy, Mexico, the Republic of Korea, Spain, Taiwan and Yugoslavia (Chemical Information Services, 1989-90).

In Sweden, cimetidine sales in 1988 were 2.32 defined daily doses (1 g) per 1000 inhabitants (Apoteksbolaget, 1988, 1989). In Finland, cimetidine sales in 1987 were 0.15 defined daily doses per 1000 inhabitants (Finnish Committee on Drug Information and Statistics, 1987). In the USA, cimetidine was the sixth ranking prescription drug in 1988 (La Piana Simonsen, 1989).

Cimetidine is not known to occur as a natural product.

The intragastric formation of *N*-nitrosocimetidine has been proposed *via* reaction of cimetidine with nitrous acid (Elder *et al.*, 1979a,b).

2.2 Use

As a histamine H_2-receptor antagonist, cimetidine inhibits gastric acid secretion and reduces pepsin output; it may also inhibit other actions of histamine that are mediated *via* H_2-receptors. Its clinical indications include duodenal and gastric ulcers, oesophageal reflux, selected cases of persistent dyspepsia and pathological hypersecretory states such as the Zollinger-Ellison syndrome. Due to its capacity to inhibit acid secretion, it is also indicated for the prophylaxis of gastrointestinal haemorrhage in stress ulceration and in patients at risk of acid aspiration during general anaesthesia. Cimetidine may also be used to reduce malabsorption and fluid loss in patients with the short-bowel syndrome and to reduce the degradation of enzyme supplements given to patients with pancreatic insufficiency (Reynolds, 1989). Treatment of damage to the gastric mucosa by non-steroidal anti-inflammatory drugs (Friedman *et al.*, 1989) is a minor indication.

Cimetidine may be given orally (400 mg two to four times daily), by the nasogastric route or parenterally by intramuscular or slow intravenous injections (200 mg) as well as by intravenous infusion (400 mg in 1 h repeated every 4-6 h) (Reynolds, 1989). In maintenance therapy of duodenal ulcer, cimetidine has been administered daily for up to five years (Barnhart, 1989).

The use of cimetidine in children, in particular in neonates, is limited. In full-term neonates, the dosage adjustments are based on renal function, and the dose of 15-20 mg/kg daily is reduced in premature infants (Ziemniak *et al.* 1984). The dosage regimen in children aged 4-13 years is 30 mg/kg bw daily, divided into three or more doses (see Reynolds, 1989).

In elderly people, the standard dose of cimetidine can be reduced by about 30-50% without loss of effectiveness (see p. 248) (Redolfi *et al.*, 1979).

2.3 Analysis

Analysis of cimetidine and its metabolites in biological fluids by high-performance liquid chromatography has been described (Randolph *et al.*, 1977; Kunitani *et al.*, 1981; Ziemniak *et al.*, 1981; Lloyd & Martin, 1985; Chiou *et al.*,

CIMETIDINE 239

1986; Kaneniwa *et al.*, 1986; Strong & Spino, 1987; Rustum & Hoffman, 1988). Cimetidine can be analysed in pharmaceutical preparations by high-performance liquid chromatography, thin-layer chromatography and spectrophotometric methods (Bavin *et al.*, 1984; Lovering & Curran, 1985).

A method for the analysis of *N*-nitrosocimetidine in human gastric juice samples using reverse-phase high-performance liquid chromatography with an *N*-nitroso compound specific detector has been reported (Shuker & Tannenbaum, 1983).

3. Biological Data Relevant to the Evaluation of Carcinogenic Risk to Humans

3.1 Carcinogenicity studies in animals

Cimetidine

(a) Oral administration

Mouse: In a two-generation carcinogenicity study, groups of male BALB/c and female C57Bl/6 mice [numbers unspecified], seven to eight weeks of age, were given pharmaceutical-grade cimetidine at either what was stated to be a common human dose—0.113 mg/ml—or at 1.13 mg/ml in their drinking-water for two weeks. Treated mice were mated, and F_0 females were treated throughout gestation, lactation and the remainder of their lives. The hybrid progeny (F_1) were weaned at four weeks and were also dosed throughout their life. A group of 20 untreated female C57Bl/6 mice served as controls for the treated dams and were mated with untreated BALB/c males. A group of 51 male and 66 female untreated hybrid progeny served as controls for the F_1 generation. The average daily doses of cimetidine were 18.8 mg/kg bw and 190 mg/kg bw, and the average total doses were 15.5 g/kg bw and 155 g/kg bw in the low-dose and high-dose groups, respectively. All moribund mice were killed and subjected to complete necropsy, and all major organs, tissues and lesions were examined histologically. Among the treated C57Bl/6 dams, the effective numbers of animals were 15 at the low dose and 16 at the high dose, with mean survival times of 21-24 months; no significant difference in either survival rates or tumour incidence was observed in comparison with the control group. Among the progeny, the effective numbers of females ranged from 39 to 66 among the different groups, with mean survival times of 28.0-30.8 months; the effective numbers of males ranged from 50 to 79 among the different groups, with mean survival times of 23.5-27 months. In the cimetidine-treated progeny, a significant dose-related increase in the incidence of lymphoid neoplasms [site and histology unspecified] was observed in females (31/66, 30/65 and 41/59 in the control, low- and high-dose groups, respectively; $p = 0.008$, Fisher's exact test) (Anderson et al., 1985). [The Working Group noted the high incidence of this neoplasm in control animals.]

Rat: Groups of 65, 70 and 100 male and 65, 70 and 99 female SPF Wistar rats, 5.5 weeks of age, received clinical-grade cimetidine at 150, 378 or 950 mg/kg bw (which represent 30, 75 and 190 times the dose required for 50% inhibition of basal gastric acid secretion in the rat and are equivalent to 9, 22.6 and 57 times the recommended daily dose for a 60-kg human) in distilled water by gavage daily for two years. One control group of 84 males and 85 females received distilled water by gavage daily, and another group of 107 males and 108 females served as untreated controls. Interim kills were carried out at 6, 10 and 12 months after the start of the experiment, during which a total of 54/235 and 55/234 treated males and females and 32/191 and 32/193 control males and females were killed. The experiment was terminated at 105-106 weeks, at which time survival was: males—untreated controls, 58/107; water controls, 34/84; low-dose, 24/65; mid-dose, 14/70; and high-dose, 34/100; females—untreated controls, 71/108; water controls, 32/85; low-dose, 26/65; mid-dose, 18/70; and high-dose, 34/99. During the first year of the experiment, those rats that died did so mainly as a result of either reflux or direct administration of the dose into the trachea. All rats were necropsied, and major organs and tissues were examined histologically. An increased incidence of benign Leydig-cell tumours of the testis was observed among treated animals (low-dose, 15/65; mid-dose, 14/68; high-dose, 23/98) as compared to combined controls (35/191). The increase was significant in the low- and high-dose groups ($p < 0.025$ for both groups; Peto test: Peto et al., 1980). A slightly greater incidence of follicular-cell tumours (benign and malignant) of the thyroid gland was observed in high-dose males (4/98) as compared to control males (2/191) ($p = 0.049$, Peto exact test) (Leslie et al., 1981).

Dog: Eight male and four female beagle dogs, 7-9.5 months of age, received a daily oral administration of cimetidine in film-coated tablets at 144 mg/kg bw for 385 weeks. Four male and two female controls received placebo tablets. Multiple biopsies of gastric mucosa were taken at intervals of about six months from week 177 to week 363. Two cimetidine-treated and three control dogs died during the experiment. All animals were necropsied, and numerous samples from the stomach and other major organs and tissues were examined histologically. No increase in the incidence of either neoplasms or preneoplastic lesions was observed among the treated animals (Walker et al., 1987a). [The Working Group noted the small number of animals used and the high mortality].

(b) Administration with other compounds

Mouse: In the study described on p. 239, groups of male BALB/c and female C57Bl/6 mice were given sodium nitrite at either 0.184 or 1.84 mg/ml or cimetidine at 0.113 or 1.13 mg/ml with sodium nitrite at either 0.184 or 1.84 mg/ml in the drinking-water for two weeks. Treated mice were mated, and females were treated throughout gestation, lactation and for the remainder of their lives. The hybrid progeny were weaned at four weeks of age and dosed from that time throughout their lives. No increase in tumour incidence was seen in the dams. Among the progeny, there was a dose-related increase in the incidence of lung tumours in males: 30/52, 36/50 and 71/79 in the untreated control, low- and high-dose groups, respectively ($p < 0.01$, Cox exact test for trend) (Anderson *et al.*, 1985).

Rat: Two groups of 20 male Sprague-Dawley rats, weighing 250 g, were wounded surgically in the antro-fundic gastric mucosa. Seven days later, the groups received 1-1.4 ml of either sodium nitrate at 3.75 mg/ml and sodium nitrite at 0.75 mg/ml in deionized water (nitrate-nitrite solution) or commercial-grade cimetidine at 25 mg/kg bw in nitrate-nitrite solution, by gavage daily on six days per week for six months. A group of 50 males served as untreated controls. An interim kill of five rats from each group was carried out at six months, and all surviving rats were killed at 14-15 months. Including the five animals per group from the interim kill, 19 and 20 animals from the nitrate-nitrite and treated groups were necropsied, but samples for histological examination were taken only from the stomach and grossly visible lesions. No neoplasm was found (Elder *et al.*, 1982). [The Working Group noted the small number of animals used, the short duration of the study and the limited histological examination.]

Two groups of 25 Sprague-Dawley rats received weekly subcutaneous injections of either 1,2-dimethylhydrazine alone at 20 mg/kg bw for 16 weeks or concurrently with cimetidine at 100 mg/kg bw daily in the drinking-water for 26 weeks, at which time the experiment was terminated. One group of ten rats received cimetidine treatment only. No increase in the incidence of colonic tumours was observed in the combined cimetidine plus 1,2-dimethylhydrazine-treated group (15/22) over that in the group receiving 1,2-dimethylhydrazine alone (14/22); no such tumour occurred in rats given cimetidine alone (Nee *et al.*, 1984). [The Working Group noted the small number of animals used and the short duration of treatment.]

Two groups of 15 weanling male Sprague-Dawley rats received 1,2-dimethylhydrazine at 30 mg/kg bw in saline by gavage once a week for five weeks. Four days after the last treatment, the groups received either cimetidine at 500 mg/ml in the drinking-water or drinking-water alone, until the animals were killed, seven months after the beginning of the experiment. All animals were necropsied, and samples from the gastrointestinal tract and lymph nodes from the peritoneal cavity and lungs were examined histologically. The incidence of colonic carcinomas among survivors was significantly different ($p < 0.05$; Mann-Whitney non-parametric test) for the group receiving 1,2-dimethylhydrazine (4/13) compared with that receiving 1,2-dimethylhydrazine and cimetidine together (10/14) (Caignard *et al.*, 1984). [The Working Group noted the absence of a group treated with cimetidine only.]

N-*Nitrosocimetidine*

Because of the suspicion that *N*-nitrosocimetidine might be a carcinogenic derivative of cimetidine, it was tested in a number of studies. *N*-Nitroso compounds are often potent carcinogens, and so, in these studies, small numbers of animals were used. Since the studies would have detected a potent carcinogen, they are included to support the interpretation that *N*-nitrosocimetidine is, at least, not a strong carcinogen.

(*a*) *Oral administration*

Mouse: In the study described on p. 239, groups of male BALB/c and female C57Bl/6 mice were given *N*-nitrosocimetidine (purity, 98%) at either 0.113 or 1.13 mg/ml in the drinking-water for two weeks. Treated mice were mated, and females were treated throughout gestation, lactation and for the remainder of their lives. The hybrid progeny were weaned at four weeks of age and dosed from that time throughout their life. The average daily doses of *N*-nitrosocimetidine were 18.8 mg/kg bw and 190.0 mg/kg bw, and the average total doses were 15.5 g/kg bw and 155 g/kg bw in the low-dose and high-dose groups, respectively. No significant difference in either survival rates or the incidence of tumours was observed between treated and control groups (Anderson *et al.*, 1985).

Two groups of 20 female hybrid B6D2F$_1$ mice, eight weeks of age, were given four weekly intragastric administrations of olive oil, which was used as the vehicle for other compounds; one week after the last dose, they received either *N*-nitrosocimetidine at 1.13 mg/ml in the drinking-water or deionized water alone. All survivors were killed 14 months after the beginning of treatment. Papillomas of the forestomach occurred in 2/20 mice receiving *N*-nitrosocimetidine and in 0/19 controls (Anderson *et al.*, 1988). [The Working Group noted the small number of animals used.]

Groups of male BALB/CanNCr mice, six weeks of age, received intraperitoneal injections of saline solution once a week for ten weeks, after which time they were given *N*-nitrosocimetidine at 0, 1.0 or 1.8 mg/ml in the drinking-water. All survivors were killed at 14 months. The effective numbers of animals were 13 in the group receiving *N*-nitrosocimetidine and 15 in the control group. Lung neoplasms [type unspecified] were observed in 3/13 animals in each treated group and in 6/15 control mice (Anderson *et al.*, 1988). [The Working Group noted the small number of animals used and the short duration of the study.]

Rat: Groups of 20 male and 20 female outbred Sprague-Dawley rats, approximately 100 days old, received *N*-nitrosocimetidine at 50 or 500 mg/kg bw by gavage twice a week for one year. A group of 50 male and 50 female rats served as untreated controls. All animals were observed for life or were killed when moribund, and were necropsied. Samples from the forestomach, glandular stomach, duodenum and all other organs with gross lesions were examined histologically. Mean survival was 393 days in high-dose animals, 400 days in low-dose animals and 630 days in controls. No increase in the incidence of tumours and no gastric neoplasm were found in treated animals (Habs *et al.*, 1982a,b). [The Working Group noted the small number of animals used and the poor survival of treated animals.]

Two groups of 20 male Sprague-Dawley rats, weighing 250 g, were wounded surgically in the antro-fundic gastric mucosa. Seven days later, the groups received 1-1.4 ml of either sodium nitrate at 3.75 mg/ml and sodium nitrite at 0.75 mg/ml in deonized water (nitrate-nitrite solution) or *N*-nitrosocimetidine at 2.80 mg/ml in nitrate-nitrite solution, by gavage daily on six days per week for six months. A group of 50 males served as untreated controls. An interim kill of five rats from each group was carried out at six months, and all surviving rats were killed at 14-15 months. Including the five animals per group from the interim kill, 19, 16 and 9 animals from the respective groups were necropsied, but samples for histological examination were taken only from the stomach and grossly visible lesions. A gastric carcinoma at the site of wounding was found in one rat treated with *N*-nitrosocimetidine. No other neoplasm was found (Elder *et al.*, 1982). [The Working Group noted the small number of animals used.]

Groups of 20 male and 20 female Fischer 344 rats [age unspecified] received *N*-nitrosocimetidine at 20 ml (0.15 mg/ml) in deionized water daily as drinking fluid on five days per week for 106 weeks (total dose, 1.6 g/rat). Groups of 20 males and 20 females were untreated and served as controls. All survivors were killed at week 131, and all animals were necropsied and major organs and lesions examined histologically. At 90 weeks, survival was 19/20 males and 20/20 females in the treated group and 15/20 males and 17/20 females in controls. No increase in the incidence of tumours was observed (Lijinksy & Reuber, 1984). [The Working Group noted the small number of animals used.]

(b) Skin application

Mouse: Groups of 20 female Swiss mice [age unspecified] received twice-weekly 25-μl skin applications on the shaved interscapular skin of either *N*-nitrosocimetidine (reagent grade) at 2.2 or 5.6 mg/ml in acetone (total doses, 12 or

31 mg/mouse), or acetone alone for 110 weeks or were left untreated. Skin was the only tissue examined grossly and histologically. At week 100, survival among treated animals was 18/20 at the low dose and 13/20 at the high dose. A malignant lymphoma of the skin [site unspecified] was observed in one high-dose mouse (Lijinsky, 1982). [The Working Group noted that the tumour incidence among control groups was not specified and that survival was poor in the group given the high dose.]

3.2 Other relevant data

(a) *Experimental systems*

(i) *Absorption, distribution, excretion and metabolism*

The kinetics, absorption, distribution, metabolism and elimination of cimetidine in humans and experimental animals have been reviewed (Griffiths *et al.*, 1977).

In rats and dogs, cimetidine is rapidly absorbed; the concentration of unchanged cimetidine in plasma is greater than that of any metabolite, and the plasma half-time is about 1 h. The drug is excreted mainly unchanged in the urine. The principal metabolite in both rats and dogs is formed by oxidation of the side-chain sulfur to give the sulfoxide (Taylor, D.C. *et al.*, 1978).

In rats, detoxication of *N*-nitrosocimetidine involves denitrosation, primarily (but not exclusively) by haemoglobin sulfhydryl residues. The rates of degradation of *N*-nitrosocimetidine by isolated whole blood decreased in the order: rat > mouse ≈ guinea-pig > hamster ≈ human; the half-time of *N*-nitrosocimetidine at 37°C was ~2 min in hamster blood and 27 min in human blood. After intravenous administration to hamsters *in vivo*, the half-time of *N*-nitrosocimetidine was ≤5 min and degradation *via* denitrosation reached 100%. Additional denitrosating activity was found in the cytosol of several organs from rats and hamsters; this activity required reduced glutathione (Jensen, 1983; Jensen *et al.*, 1987).

The metabolic fate of *N*-nitrosocimetidine has been investigated, although it has not been shown to be formed in animals *in vivo*.

Radiolabelled *N*-nitrosocimetidine, but not cimetidine, methylated DNA in a variety of tissues in rats after oral administration (Gombar & Magee, 1982). In studies in which cimetidine was administered with an excess of nitrite by stomach tube to rats, no evidence could be obtained for the presence of O^6-methylguanine in DNA isolated from stomach, liver or intestine (large and small pooled) (Kyrtopoulos *et al.*, 1982). *N*-Nitrosocimetidine produced a low level of DNA alkylation (determined as 7-methylguanine) in the liver and other organs of hamsters after intravenous administration (Jensen *et al.*, 1987).

(ii) *Toxic effects*

The oral LD_{50}s of cimetidine were approximately 2.6 g/kg bw in mice, 5 g/kg bw in rats, 4 g/kg bw in hamsters and 2.60 g/kg bw in dogs. The intraperitoneal LD_{50}s were 470 mg/kg bw in mice, 650 mg/kg bw in rats and 880 mg/kg bw in hamsters (Crean *et al.*, 1981).

Daily oral administration of 160 mg/kg bw cimetidine to female Sprague-Dawley rats for two months increased total gastrin-cell numbers, gastrin-cell density of antral mucosa and parietal-cell density of fundic mucosa, as compared with controls (Del Tacca *et al.*, 1987). In contrast, in male Wistar/Lewis rats receiving cimetidine orally at 150-200 mg/kg bw daily for up to 12 months, it was not possible to demonstrate by autoradiography epithelial proliferation in either fundus or antrum as a consequence of treatment (Eastwood & Quimby, 1983).

In studies of up to 24 months' duration, rats receiving repeated doses of cimetidine at up to 950 mg/kg bw per day showed few adverse effects. Liver weight was consistently increased at the highest dose, and testis, prostate and seminal vesicle weights were reduced in a dose- and time-related manner (Brimblecombe *et al.*, 1985).

In a study of up to 12 months' duration, two dogs receiving cimetidine at 504 mg/kg bw per day orally exhibited degenerative changes in the liver, renal tubular nephrosis and elevated levels of serum transaminases. No such change was seen with doses of 366 mg/kg bw per day or less. Prostate weights were reduced in a dose- and time-related manner. In beagle dogs administered cimetidine at 144 mg/kg bw per day orally, no treatment-related effect was seen after four years, on the basis of haematology, clinical biochemistry, urinalysis, electrocardiography or clinical condition, and no treatment-associated change was observed in biopsies of gastric mucosa. After seven years of follow-up, no change of the stomach mucosa was seen during regular biopsy (Crean *et al.*, 1981; Brimblecombe *et al.*, 1985).

In-vivo and in-vitro studies suggest that cimetidine inhibits gastric acid secretion in rats and dogs by blocking histamine H_2-receptors in the gastric mucosa (Brimblecombe *et al.*, 1978). Cimetidine administered intraperitoneally to male Wistar rats at 20 mg/kg bw twice daily for seven days reduced the gastric mucosal concentrations of prostaglandin E_2 and 6-keto-prostaglandin F_{1a}, both 30 min and 24 h after the last injection (Arakawa *et al.*, 1988).

In rats, the oral LD_{50} of *N*-nitrosocimetidine did not differ from that of cimetidine itself. No tissue-specific toxic lesion could be attributed to the nitroso derivative (Ogiu *et al.*, 1986).

(iii) *Effects on reproduction and prenatal toxicity*

In routine safety evaluation studies on cimetidine, including fertility and peri- and postnatal studies in rats and teratology studies in mice, rats and rabbits, no adverse effect was reported with oral doses of up to 950 mg/kg bw (Brimblecombe *et al.*, 1978). [The Working Group noted the lack of detailed reporting.]

Cimetidine has been shown to possess weak antiandrogenic activity in rats, as shown by reduced weights of testis, prostate and seminal vesicles (Brimblecombe *et al.*, 1978; Pereira, 1987). Inhibition of dihydrotestosterone binding to the prostatic androgen receptor has been demonstrated (Sivelle *et al.*, 1982).

Differentiation of the genital organs of male fetuses is influenced by endogenous testosterone produced during prenatal development, and gonadal and sexual dysfunction have been reported in adult male rats after prenatal and neonatal exposure to cimetidine at daily doses of 17.1 and 137 mg/kg bw in drinking-water from day 12 of pregnancy until weaning on postnatal day 21 (Anand & Van Thiel, 1982; Parker *et al.*, 1984a,b). These results were not confirmed in other studies. Rats were administered cimetidine at 180 mg/kg bw daily in the drinking-water from day 12 of pregnancy until the end of lactation or during late lactation only, or a combination of drinking-water during pregnancy and early lactation and gavage treatment during late lactation. Several end-points, such as anogenital distance, serum testosterone, mating performance and sexual organ weights, were evaluated soon after littering or up to 148 days postnatally. Maternally administered cimetidine had no effect in male offspring on any parameter measured (Walker *et al.*, 1987b).

In another study, cimetidine was administered to rats in drinking-water from day 17 of gestation through day 7 of lactation. With the highest drug concentration tested (4 mg/ml), the daily dose ingested ranged from about 400 mg/kg bw before parturition to approximately 850 mg/kg bw afterwards. The developmental profile of serum dehydroepiandrosterone, androstenedione, testosterone and 5-α-dihydrotestosterone, when measured at 1, 4 and 18 weeks of age, was unaffected by perinatal exposure to cimetidine (Shapiro *et al.*, 1988).

The effects of maternally administered cimetidine during lactation on the development of drug metabolizing enzymes in BALB/c mouse pups have been investigated. When dams were administered cimetidine at 50 mg/kg bw per day intraperitoneally for six weeks after delivery, microsomal enzyme activity was inhibited in pups. Dams were less affected than pups (Kwanashie, 1989).

(iv) *Genetic and related effects*

Cimetidine did not induce differential toxicity in *Escherichia coli* (Pool *et al.*, 1979; De Flora, 1981).

Cimetidine was reported not to be mutagenic to *Salmonella typhimurium* (De Flora & Picciotto, 1980; O'Connor *et al.*, 1987). Cimetidine alone or in combination with sodium nitrite gave negative results in *S. typhimurium* in a host-mediated assay in mice (Baumeister, 1982).

No single-strand breakage, measured by the alkaline elution assay, was found in the DNA of a transformed mouse epithelial cell line after treatment with cimetidine at concentrations of up to 5 mM (Schwarz et al., 1980). In an alkaline elution assay with rat primary hepatocytes, the highest concentration of cimetidine hydrochloride (3 mM) induced a significant increase in the frequency of DNA strand breaks (Martelli et al., 1983). No such effect was observed in human hepatocytes (Martelli et al., 1986).

Cimetidine hydrochloride induced unscheduled DNA synthesis in cultures of rat primary hepatocytes (Martelli et al., 1983; Lefevre & Ashby, 1985), while the base was inactive (Lefevre & Ashby, 1985). In another study, cimetidine [form not specified] did not induce unscheduled DNA synthesis in rat hepatocytes (Williams et al., 1989). Human hepatocytes from four donors did not exhibit unscheduled DNA synthesis after treatment with cimetidine hydrochloride (Martelli et al., 1986). In an abstract, it was reported that cimetidine did not induce mutation to 6-thioguanine resistance, to trifluorothymidine resistance or to ouabain resistance in a human lymphoblastoid cell line (TK6) after 1-h treatment with concentrations of up to 1.2 mM, with a cell survival of 6% (Tatsumi et al., 1987).

Cimetidine did not induce sister chromatid exchange in human lymphocytes *in vitro* (Inoue et al., 1985).

When rats were given cimetidine orally at 250 mg/kg bw, no DNA damage was detected in cells of the gastric mucosa (Pino & Robbiano, 1983) or in liver cells (Brambilla et al., 1982); combination treatment with sodium nitrite also gave negative results.

N-Nitrosocimetidine and cimetidine treated with sodium nitrite in an acid environment like that of human gastric juice have consistently been shown to be directly mutagenic *in vitro*: either treatment induced differential toxicity and mutation in bacteria, inhibited DNA synthesis in human cells and induced DNA single-strand breaks, mutation, sister chromatid exchange, chromosomal damage and morphological transformation in mammalian cells. For a comprehensive tabulation of these data and their references, see Appendix 2.

(b) *Humans*

(i) *Pharmacokinetics*

The pharmacokinetics of cimetidine have been reviewed (Reynolds, 1989).

Cimetidine is readily absorbed from the gastrointestinal tract, and peak plasma concentrations are obtained about 1 h after administration on an empty stomach and about 2 h after administration with food (Somogyi & Gugler, 1983). The bioavailability of cimetidine is 60-70%, as a result of moderate first-pass metabolism. Twenty percent of cimetidine is bound to plasma proteins, and its elimination half-time from plasma is about 2 h; it is partially metabolized in the liver to the sulfoxide and to hydroxymethylcimetidine. After intravenous administration, 50-80% of the dose was excreted unchanged in the urine. After an oral dose, the corresponding figure was 40%. Cimetidine penetrates the blood-brain barrier with difficulty but easily crosses the placental barrier and is excreted into milk, where the concentrations may be higher than those in plasma. Dose-dependent kinetics of cimetidine have been observed in neonates (Lloyd et al., 1985).

A markedly reduced plasma clearance of cimetidine has been reported in elderly patients (Gugler & Somogyi, 1979; Redolfi et al., 1979). A decrease in non-renal clearance of cimetidine was reported in patients with liver cirrhosis (Gugler et al., 1982; Cello & Oie, 1983); in one study, this effect was limited to cirrhosis patients with a history of hepatic encephalopathy (Ziemniak et al., 1983). Renal failure may lead to elevated plasma levels of cimetidine (Larsson et al., 1982).

(ii) *Adverse effects*

The toxicity of cimetidine has been reviewed (Penston & Wormsley, 1986). Adverse effects are infrequent and are usually reversible following reduction of dosage or withdrawal of therapy. Diarrhoea, rashes and other allergic phenomena have been reported. Various symptoms of the central nervous system have been reported frequently, particularly at greater than therapeutic doses (Nelson, 1977; Illingworth & Jarvie, 1979; Schentag et al., 1979). Adverse haematological effects possibly associated with cimetidine are rare and include granulocytopenia or agranulocytosis, thrombocytopenia and pancytopenia (Penston & Wormsley, 1986).

Strongly reduced gastric acid secretion favours colonization of the stomach by bacteria, some of which can reduce nitrate to nitrite and catalyse nitrosation of amino precursors at neutral pH (Hill, 1986; Leaf et al., 1989). Since these conditions could lead to intragastric formation of nitroso compounds, gastric juice samples from patients before and after treatment with cimetidine have been analysed for total nitroso compounds or nitrite in several studies. Fasting gastric juice from 140 patients taking cimetidine for a variety of gastric or duodenal disorders (daily doses of 0.2-1.6 g for periods of one week to 45 months) and 267 subjects who had not taken the drug were analysed. Significantly higher mean levels of total nitroso compounds were found in the former group (Reed et al., 1981).

In a study of a group of 23 peptic ulcer patients after a six-week course of 1 g cimetidine per day, a statistically significant increase in nitrite and nitroso compound concentrations was found (Stockbrugger et al., 1982). In six volunteers who took 200 mg cimetidine three times a day and 400 mg a night for at least three weeks, increases in the level of gastric juice nitrite were found only rarely (Muscroft et al., 1981). In eight healthy subjects studied half-hourly or hourly for 24-h periods before, during and after cimetidine treatment (two weeks with 1 g per day), no significant difference in the level of intragastric nitrite or total nitroso compounds was found following cimetidine treatment (Milton-Thompson *et al.*, 1982).

Gastric juice and urine collected from 17 duodenal ulcer patients receiving 0.8 g cimetidine per day for four to six weeks were analysed for nitrosation capacity before, during and after treatment using the *N*-nitrosoproline test (Ohshima & Bartsch, 1981). Cimetidine treatment did not lead to a uniform or pronounced rise in gastric levels of total nitroso compounds or urinary *N*-nitrosoproline levels (Bartsch *et al.*, 1984).

The methods used for determining total nitroso compounds in gastric juice in all these studies have been criticized because of their lack of specificity (Pignatelli *et al.*, 1987); moreover, in none of the studies was *N*-nitrosocimetidine itself measured in the gastric juice samples.

Cimetidine inhibits cytochrome P450-dependent microsomal mixed-funciton oxidase (Pelkonen & Puuronen, 1980), elevating the plasma levels of other drugs, such as lignocaine, phenytoin, theophylline, warfarin and ciclosporin (Somogyi & Muirhead, 1987; Rodighiero, 1989).

(iii) *Effects on reproduction and prenatal toxicity*

A number of case reports have been published of cimetidine use in pregnancy, indicating no adverse effect (Corazza *et al.*, 1982; Meggs *et al.*, 1984) or abnormal outcome (Glade *et al.*, 1980; Say *et al.*, 1985); the significance of these reports cannot be assessed.

In a UK postmarketing surveillance study, 9928 patients given cimetidine in general practices were compared with 9351 age- and sex-matched unexposed people from the same practices; 98.8% of takers and 97.7% of controls were successfully followed up for at least one year (Colin-Jones *et al.*, 1983, 1985a,b). In the 20 exposed women and the 22 controls who became pregnant during the study year, there was no evidence of an adverse effect of cimetidine treatment.

Impotence, reduced sperm count and gynaecomastia have been reported in men treated with cimetidine. In one study, gynaecomastia was reported in 20/6240 men (3.2/1000), but in only 13 of these was cimetidine thought to be the likely cause. Impotence was reported in 12/6240 men (2/1000) taking cimetidine and in 3/5868 controls (0.5/1000); however, impotence and gynaecomastia were not reported in the same individuals (Colin-Jones *et al.*, 1985a,b). [The Working Group considered that, because of the method of ascertainment, underreporting was likely.] In other studies in which cimetidine was administered at doses larger than those normally used in ulcer therapy, these adverse effects were more common. In a study by Jensen *et al.* (1983), of patients with gastric hypersecretion (mostly Zollinger-Ellison syndrome) who were treated with high doses of cimetidine, 11/22 subjects developed one or more signs or symptoms of impotence, breast tenderness or gynaecomastia. The 11 affected subjects had received a mean daily dose of 5.3 g, compared with 3.0 g in the unaffected group. Spence and Celestin (1979), however, reported gynaecomastia in 5/25 (20%) male patients treated with 1.6 g cimetidine daily. In all the reported cases, the condition reversed rapidly after cessation of and sometimes during treatment.

Several well-controlled studies have shown no effect of cimetidine on sperm count (Wang *et al.*, 1982; Paulsen *et al.*, 1983; Bianchi Porro *et al.*, 1985), but one showed a small but significant reduction (Van Thiel *et al.*, 1979). No consistent effect on plasma levels of gonadotrophins or sex hormones was demonstrated in these studies.

(iv) *Genetic and related effects*

When gastric juice from patients who had received cimetidine at 200 mg 2 h earlier was incubated with sodium nitrite at 10 μg/ml, a significant increase in the number of revertants was seen in *S. typhimurium* TA100 in the absence of an exogenous metabolic system (DeFlora & Picciotto, 1980).

Gastric juice taken from 49 patients 1-3 h after intake of cimetidine at 400 mg was mutagenic when tested in *S. typhimurium* TA100; no mutagenic activity was seen in samples taken 12 h later (Morris *et al.*, 1984). When the mutagenicity of gastric juice from eight fasting patients under cimetidine treatment (400 mg twice daily) was tested before and after administration of the drug, using *S. typhimurium* TA98 and TA100, considerable variation in mutagenicity was seen between subjects, all samples being mutagenic even before therapy. No significant change in mutagenic activity was detected after therapy and there was no relation to duration of therapy, changes in gastric pH or ulcer healing (O'Connor *et al.*, 1987)

3.3 Case reports and epidemiological studies in humans

(*a*) *Case reports*

Numerous case reports of neoplasms following cimetidine use have been published (Welsh *et al.*, 1977; Murray *et al.*, 1978; Taylor, T.V. *et al.*, 1978; Buck *et al.*, 1979; Elder *et al.*, 1979a,b; Reed *et al.*, 1979; Taylor *et al.*, 1979; Hawker *et al.*, 1980; Kjærgaard *et al.*, 1980; Knigge *et al.*, 1980; Stoddard *et al.*, 1980; Scotcher *et al.*, 1981; Taylor *et al.*, 1981; Kaplinsky *et al.*, 1982; Eschar *et al.*, 1983; Porter *et al.*, 1984; Stockley & Kiff, 1987). The stomach has been the most frequently reported cancer site, followed by lymphomas of the gastrointestinal tract; less commonly, benign and malignant tumours at other sites have been reported (Kaplinsky *et al.*, 1982; Eschar *et al.*, 1983). Most of the cases were diagnosed within one year; the longest interval was five years (Stockley & Kiff, 1987). In certain of the reports, gastric carcinoma had arisen after oesophagitis or duodenal ulcer—conditions not thought to be associated with gastric carcinoma. In other reports, gastric ulcers diagnosed as benign on the basis of biopsy samples and appearance on gastroscopy have been followed by malignant changes.

(b) *Cohort studies*

A cohort of (initially) 9940 individuals who received cimetidine during 1977-79 in the UK and who were followed up for four years has been the subject of four papers (Colin-Jones *et al.*, 1982, 1983, 1985a,b). Also studied were (initially) 9366 controls matched for age, sex and general practice, who did not receive cimetidine, but these were followed up for only one year. For this reason, national rates were used as the standard for evaluation of mortality (incident cancers were evaluated only in the first year). A total of 330 deaths were due to neoplasms in cimetidine users (compared to 65.6 expected), most of the excess being gastric and lung cancers. The relative risks (RRs) declined markedly over the study period: for gastric cancer, the approximative RRs for men and women combined (and observed numbers) were 12.9 (45 deaths), 3.4 (12), 1.8 (6) and 2.3 (8) after one, two, three and four years follow-up, respectively. Some of the patients were known to have had cancer before cimetidine use was started, and, even among deaths after the first year, there were three such deaths from gastric cancer. For lung cancer, the RRs in the four periods were 2.8 (35 deaths), 2.0 (25), 1.4 (17) and 1.8 (22). In an approximately 5% sample of study participants, 45% of the exposed and 28% of unexposed subjects had smoked > 15 cigarettes per day five years previously. [The Working Group noted that cigarette smoking is associated with peptic ulcer as well as lung cancer and that smoking habits were not accounted for in the evaluation of lung cancer risk.]

A second cohort study concerned cancer incidence among 16 739 patients treated with cimetidine in Denmark in the period 1977-81 who were followed for up to eight years by linkage procedures with the central population and national cancer registers (Møller *et al.*, 1989). A total of 105 cases of gastric cancer were recorded, compared with 39.5 expected (RR, 2.6). The RR was greatest early in the follow-up period, declining markedly later. For sites with positive associations and for all other sites combined, the RRs and observed numbers of cases during the first year, during the second and third years and for more than three years of follow-up are shown in Table 1. The increased risks for gastric cancer were greater in persons with a diagnosis of gastric ulcer (19.3 (45 observed cases), 3.5 (16) and 3.2 (13) for the three time periods) than in those with duodenal ulcer (2.2, 1.1 and 1.1, with seven observed cases each). Increased incidences of gastric and certain other gastrointestinal malignancies were noted particularly in the first year of follow-up. The increased incidences of lymphatic and haematopoietic malignancies were due mainly to non-Hodgkin's lymphoma of the stomach and small intestine. The risk

Table 1. Relative risks (RRs) and numbers of cases observed after different periods in patients treated with cimetidine[a]

Site	<1 year		1–3 years		>3 years	
	RR	Obs	RR	Obs	RR	Obs
Stomach	9.4	57	2.3	27	1.7	21
Pancreas	4.7	21	1.5	15	1.7	14
Colon	2.1	23	1.8	38	1.3	26
Small intestine	10.5	4	3.9	3	3.4	2
Lymphatic and haematopoietic tissue	3.0	22	0.9	13	1.5	20
Lung	1.4	34	1.7	83	1.6	73
Other sites	1.1	91	1.4	218	1.1	169

[a]From Møller et al. (1989). RRs calculated by the Working Group for the two sexes combined

for lung cancer did not change appreciably over time. [The Working Group noted that no data on smoking status were provided.]

By record linkage, 3802 cimetidine users and an equal number of non-users matched by age, sex and general practitioner in Tayside, Scotland, were followed up for mortality during a period of four years (Beardon et al., 1988). Mortality due to neoplasms of the digestive organs and peritoneum was markedly increased in the cimetidine takers, with a RR of 2.7 (95% confidence interval, 1.6-4.7) based on 49 deaths. The largest excesses were seen for neoplasms of the oesophagus, stomach and pancreas. Mortality from all causes among cimetidine users was increased only during the first two years of follow-up [corresponding data by duration of follow-up were not presented for cancer]. There was no significant increase in mortality due to neoplasms of respiratory and intrathoracic organs (32 deaths; RR, 1.1; 95% confidence interval, 0.67-1.8) or other neoplasms.

[The Working Group noted, as did the authors of the relevant studies, that in the case reports and studies undiagnosed gastric and intra-abdominal neoplasms could have been responsible for the symptoms that led to use of cimetidine. This possibility is supported by the short interval between exposure and observation of increased RRs and by the decreasing risks for intra-abdominal cancer, particularly gastric cancer, with time. The maximal interval that follow-up studies have so far covered is only eight years.]

4. Summary of Data Reported and Evaluation

4.1 Exposure data

Cimetidine is a histamine H_2-receptor antagonist which inhibits gastric acid secretion. Since its introduction in the mid-1970s, it has been used widely by oral administration for the treatment of duodenal and gastric ulcers.

Although cimetidine can be nitrosated *in vitro* in the presence of nitrite under acidic conditions to form *N*-nitrosocimetidine, no study in experimental animals or in humans has demonstrated that this reaction occurs *in vivo*.

4.2 Experimental carcinogenicity data

Cimetidine was tested for carcinogenicity by oral administration in single studies in mice, rats and dogs. In the experiment in mice, dams were treated throughout life beginning two weeks prior to pregnancy, with no increase in tumour incidence. In female progeny that were exposed throughout life from conception, there was an increase in the incidence of lymphomas, although these tumours also occurred at relatively high rates in control animals. In rats, an increase in the incidence of benign Leydig-cell tumours of the testis was observed in the low- and high-dose groups but not in the mid-dose group. The study in dogs was inadequate for evaluation.

In a study in which mice were exposed from conception throughout life to a combination of cimetidine and sodium nitrite, males had an increased incidence of lung neoplasms, although these tumours also occurred at a high frequency in control animals.

N-Nitrosocimetidine was tested for carcinogenicity by oral administration in mice and rats and by skin application in mice. The experiments in rats and three of the studies in mice were inadequate for evaluation. In one study by oral administration in mice, there was no increase in the incidence of tumours.

4.3 Human carcinogenicity data

In a large number of case reports, cancer, particularly gastric cancer, was diagnosed at various intervals after the start of cimetidine therapy. These reports are difficult to interpret because gastric cancer is a common malignancy and cimetidine is a commonly used drug, and coincidence cannot be ruled out.

Three cohort studies showed increased incidences of gastric cancer but also of other gastrointestinal cancers among cimetidine users; however, as for the case reports, the association could well have been due to the drug being given for symptoms of pre-existing cancers. This interpretation is supported by a diminution of the association with increasing duration of follow-up. Two of the studies also showed an association between cimetidine use and lung cancer, but confounding with cigarette smoking could well have been the explanation.

4.4 Other relevant data

Cimetidine has been associated with reversible impotence and other anti-androgenic effects in men.

N-Nitrosocimetidine is rapidly converted to cimetidine *in vivo* in experimental animals.

Cimetidine did not induce single-strand breaks in DNA from rats treated *in vivo*, nor did it methylate DNA in a variety of tissues of rats *in vivo*. It did not induce single-strand breaks in the DNA of rat cells treated *in vitro*. Cimetidine was not mutagenic to and did not cause DNA damage in *Salmonella typhimurium* or *Escherichia coli*. Cimetidine hydrochloride induced single-strand breaks and unscheduled DNA synthesis in rat but not human cells *in vitro*. It did not cause sister chromatid exchange in human cells *in vitro*.

Cimetidine in combination with sodium nitrite did not induce DNA damage *in vivo* or methylate DNA in a variety of tissues of rats *in vivo*. Gastric juice from cimetidine-treated patients was mutagenic to bacteria when enriched with nitrite.

N-Nitrosocimetidine has not been demonstrated in gastric juice of humans; however, increased gastric concentrations of nitrite and total *N*-nitroso compounds have been reported in some studies of patients taking cimetidine. *N*-Nitrosocimetidine induced DNA damage, sister chromatid exchange, chromosomal aberrations and morphological transformation in mammalian cells *in vitro* and caused DNA damage and mutation in bacteria. Radiolabelled *N*-nitrosocimetidine methylated DNA in a variety of tissues of rats *in vivo*. (See Appendix 1.)

4.5 Evaluation[1]

There is *inadequate evidence* for the carcinogenicity of cimetidine in humans.

There is *inadequate evidence* for the carcinogenicity of cimetidine in experimental animals.

Overall evaluation

Cimetidine *is not classifiable as to its carcinogenicity to humans (Group 3)*.

---

[1]For description of the italicized terms, see Preamble, pp. 26–29.

5. References

Alldrick, A.J., Rowland, J.R. & Gangolli, S.D. (1984) Exposure of E. coli to nitrosocimetidine induces the adaptive response to alkylating agents. *Mutat. Res., 139*, 111-114

Anand, S. & Van Thiel, D.H. (1982) Prenatal and neonatal exposure to cimetidine results in gonadal and sexual dysfunction in adult males. *Science, 218*, 493-494

Anderson, L.M., Giner-Sorolla, A., Haller, I.M. & Budinger, J.M. (1985) Effects of cimetidine, nitrite, cimetidine plus nitrite and nitrosocimetidine on tumors in mice following transplacental plus lifetime exposure. *Cancer Res., 45*, 3561-3566

Anderson, L.M., Hagiwara, A., Giner-Sorolla, A., Koratch, R.M., Rehm, S., Riggs, C.W. & Rice, J.M. (1988) N-Nitrosocimetidine as a modifier of chemically-initiated tumours in mice. *Cancer Lett., 42*, 159-167

Apoteksbolaget (1988) *Svensk Läkemedelsstatistic* [Swedish Drugs Statistics], Stockholm, Pharmaceutical Association of Sweden

Apoteksbolaget (1989) *Outprint of the Drug Data Base (17 October 1989)*, Stockholm, Pharmaceutical Association of Sweden

Arakawa, T., Satoh, H., Fukuda, T., Sakuma, H., Nakamura, H. & Kobayashi, K. (1988) Gastric mucosal resistance and prosanoid levels after cimetidine treatment in rats. *Digestion, 41*, 1-8

Athanasiou, K. & Kyrtopoulos, S.A. (1981) Induction of sister chromatid exchanges and chromosome aberrations in cultured mammalian cells by N-nitrosocimetidine. *Cancer Lett., 14*, 71-75

Barnhart, E. (1989) *Physicians Desk Reference*, 43rd ed., Oradell, NJ, Medical Economics, p. 307

Barrows, L.R., Gombar, C.T. & Magee, P.N. (1982) Mutation, DNA labeling, and transformation of BHK-21/CL 13 cells by MNNG, and nitrosocimetidine. *Mutat. Res., 102*, 145-158

Bartsch, H., Ohshima, H., Muñoz, N., Crespi, M., Cassale, V., Ramazotti, V., Lambert, R., Minaire, Y., Forichon, J. & Walters, C.L. (1984) In-vivo nitrosation, precancerous lesions and cancers of the gastrointestinal tract. On-going studies and preliminary results. In: O'Neill, I.K., von Borstel, R.C., Miller, C.T., Long, J. & Bartsch, H., eds, *N-Nitroso Compounds: Occurrence, Biological Effects and Relevance to Human Cancer* (IARC Scientific Publications No. 57), Lyon, IARC, pp. 955-962

Baumeister, M. (1982) Experimental models for the biological detection of N-nitroso compounds formed from amines and nitrite. *Toxicol. Lett., 12*, 281-288

Bavin, P.M.G., Durant, G.J., Miles, P.D., Mitchell, R.C. & Pepper, E.S. (1980) Nitrosation of cimetidine — [N''-cyano-N-methyl-N''-(2-[(5-methylimidazol-4-yl)methylthio])ethylguanidine]. *Chem. Res., 5*, 212-213

Bavin, P.M.G., Post, A. & Zarembo, J.E. (1984) Cimetidine. *Anal. Profiles Drug Subst., 13*, 127-182

Beardon, P.H., Brown, S.V. & McDevitt, D.G. (1989) Gastrointestinal events in patients prescribed non-steroidal anti-inflammatory drugs: a controlled study using record linkage in Tayside. *Q. J. Med., 71*, 497-505

Bianchi Porro, G., Ragni, G., Ruspa, M., Petrillo, M. & Barattini, G. (1985) Long-term treatment with cimetidine does not essentially affect the hypothalamic-pituitary-gonadal axis in man. *Hepato-gastroenterology, 32*, 77-80

Brambilla, G., Cavanna, M., Maura, A., Pino, A., Robbiano, L., Carlo, P., Biassoni, F. & Ricci, R. (1982) Absence of DNA damage in liver of rats given high doses of cimetidine and sodium nitrite. *J. Pharmacol. exp. Ther., 221*, 222-227

Brimblecombe, R.W., Duncan, W.A., Durant, G.J., Emmett, C., Ganellin, C.R., Leslie, G.B. & Parsons, M.E. (1978) Characterisation and development of cimetidine as a histamine H_2 receptor antagonist. *Gastroenterology, 74*, 339-347

Brimblecombe, R.W., Leslie, G.B. & Walker, T.F. (1985) Toxicology of cimetidine. *Hum. Toxicol., 4*, 13-25

Buck, J.P., Murgatroyd, R.E., Boylston, A.W. & Baron, J.H. (1979) Perforation of gastric carcinoma (at site of previous benign ulcer) after withdrawal of cimetidine. *Lancet, i*, 42

Caignard, A., Martin, M., Reisser, D., Thomas, B. & Martin, F. (1984) Effects of cimetidine and indomethacin on the growth of dimethylhydrazine-induced or transplanted intestinal cancers in the rat. *Br. J. Cancer, 50*, 661-665

Cello, J.P. & Oie, S. (1983) Cimetidine disposition in patients with Laennec's cirrhosis during multiple dosing therapy. *Eur. J. clin. Pharmacol., 25*, 223-229

Chemical Information Services Ltd (1989-90) *Directory of World Chemical Producers*, Oceanside, NY

Chiou, R., Stubbs, R.J. & Bayne, W.F. (1986) Determination of cimetidine in plasma and urine by high-performance liquid chromatography. *J. Chromatogr., 377*, 441-446

Colin-Jones, D.G., Langman, M.J.S., Lawson, D.H. & Vessey, M.P. (1982) Cimetidine and gastric cancer: preliminary report from post-marketing surveillance study. *Br. med. J., 285*, 1311-1313

Colin-Jones, D.G., Langman, M.J.S., Lawson, D.H. & Vessey, M.P. (1983) Postmarketing surveillance of the safety of cimetidine: 12 months mortality report. *Br. med. J., 286*, 1713-1716

Colin-Jones, D.G., Langman, M.J.S., Lawson, D.H. & Vessey, M.P. (1985a) Postmarketing surveillance of the safety of cimetidine: mortality during second, third, and fourth years of follow up. *Br. med. J., 291*, 1084-1088

Colin-Jones, D.G., Langman, M.J.S., Lawson, D.H. & Vessey, M.P. (1985b) Post-marketing surveillance of the safety of cimetidine: twelve-month morbidity report. *Q. J. Med., 54*, 253-268

Corazza, G.R., Gasbarrini, G., DiNisio, Q. & Zulli, P. (1982) Cimetidine (Tagamet) in peptic ulcer therapy during pregnancy. *Clin. Trials J., 19*, 91-93

Crean, G.P., Leslie, G.B., Walker, T.F., Whitehead, S.M. & Roe, F.J.C. (1981) Safety evaluation of cimetidine: 54 month interim report on long-term study in dogs. *J. appl. Toxicol., 1*, 159-164

De Flora, S. (1981) Cimetidine, ranitidine, and their mutagenic nitroso derivatives. *Lancet, ii*, 993-994

De Flora, S. & Picciotto, A. (1980) Mutagenicity of cimetidine in nitrite-enriched human gastric juice. *Carcinogenesis, 1*, 925-930

Del Tacca, M., Gheraardi, G., Polloni, A., Bernardini, C. & Petrucci, A. (1987) The effects of prolonged administration of cimetidine or pirenzepine on gastric mucosal cell kinetics, serum gastrin levels and acid secretory responses in rats. *Int. J. Tissue React.*, 5, 419-426

Durant, G.J., Emmett, J.C. & Ganellin, C.R. (1974) FRG patent 2,344,779 (CA 80 146168j)

Eastwood, G.L. & Quimby, G.F. (1983) Effect of chronic cimetidine ingestion on fundic and antral epithelial proliferation in the rat. *Digest. Dis. Sci.*, 28, 61-64

Elder, J.B., Ganguli, P.C. & Gillespie, I.E. (1979a) Cimetidine and gastric cancer. *Lancet, i*, 1005-1006

Elder, J.B., Ganguli, P.C. & Gillespie, I.E. (1979b) Gastric cancer in patients who have taken cimetidine. *Lancet, i*, 245

Elder, J.B., Ganguli, P.C., Koffman, C.G., Wells, S. & Williams, G. (1982) Possible role of cimetidine and its nitrosation products in human stomach cancer. In: Magee, P.N., ed., *Nitrosamines in Human Cancer* (Banbury Report No. 12), Cold Spring Harbor, NY, CSH Press, pp. 335-349

Eshchar, J., Neuman, M.G., Pavlotzky, M. & Saibil, F.G. (1983) Zollinger-Ellison syndrome, prolonged cimetidine administration and nasopharyngeal carcinoma:—a coincidence? *Int. J. Tissue React.*, 5, 411-414

Finnish Committee on Drug Information and Statistics (1987) *Finnish Statistics on Medicine*, Helsinki, National Board of Health

Foster, A.B., Jarman, M., Manson, D. & Shulten, H.R. (1980) Structure and reactivity of nitrosocimetidine. *Cancer Lett.*, 9, 47-52

Friedman, H., Seckman, C.E., Schwartz, J.H., Lanza, E.L., Royer, G.L. & Stubbs, C.M. (1989) The effects of flurbiproten, aspirin, cimetidine, and antacids on the gastric and duodenal mucosa of normal volunteers. An endoscopic and photographic study. *J. clin. Pharmacol.*, 29, 559-562

Glade, G., Saccar, C.L. & Pereira, G. (1980) Cimetidine in pregnancy: apparant transient liver impairment in the newborn. *Am. J. Dis. Child.*, 134, 87-88

Gombar, C.T. & Magee, P.N. (1982) DNA-methylation by nitrosocimetidine and N-methyl-N'-nitro-N-nitrosoguanidine in the intact rat. *Chem.-biol Interactions*, 40, 149-157

Griffiths, R., Lee, R.M. & Taylor, D.C. (1977) Kinetics of cimetidine in man and experimental animals. In: Burland, W.L. & Simkins, M.A., eds, *Cimetidine: Proceedings of the Second International Symposium on Histamine H_2-Receptor Antagonists*, Amsterdam, Excerpta Medica, pp. 38-51

Gugler, R. & Somogyi, A. (1979) Reduced cimetidine clearance with age. *New Engl. J. Med.*, 301, 435

Gugler, R., Muller-Liebenau, B. & Somogyi, A. (1982) Altered disposition and availability of cimetidine in liver cirrhotic patients. *Br. J. clin. Pharmacol.*, 14, 421-429

Habs, M., Schmähl, D., Eisenbrand, G. & Preussmann, R. (1982a) Carcinogenesis studies with *N*-nitrosocimetidine. Part II: Oral administration to Sprague-Dawley rats. In: Magee, P.N., ed., *Nitrosamines in Human Cancer*, (Banbury Report No. 12), Cold Spring Harbor, NY, CSH Press, pp. 403-405

Habs, M., Eisenbrand, G., Habs, H. & Schmähl, D. (1982b) No evidence of carcinogenicity of N-nitrosocimetidine in rats. *Hepato-gastroenterology*, 29, 265-266

Hawker, P.C., Muscroft, T.J. & Keighley, M.R.B. (1980) Gastric cancer after cimetidine in patient with two negative pre-treatment biopsies. *Lancet*, i, 709-710

Henderson, E.E., Basilio, M. & Davis, R.M. (1981) Cellular DNA damage by nitrosocimetidine: a comparison with N-methyl-N'-nitroso-nitrosoguanidine and X-irradiation. *Chem.-biol. Interactions*, 38, 87-98

Hill, M.J. (1986) *Microbes and Human Carcinogenesis*, London, Edward Arnold

IARC (1987a) *IARC Monographs on the Evaluation of Carcinogenic Risks to Humans*, Suppl. 7, *Overall Evaluations of Carcinogenicity: An Updating of* IARC Monographs *Volumes 1 to 42*, Lyon, pp. 216-219

IARC (1987b) *IARC Monographs on the Evaluation of Carcinogenic Risks to Humans*, Suppl. 7, *Overall Evaluations of Carcinogenicity: An Updating of* IARC Monographs *Volumes 1 to 42*, Lyon, pp. 334-339

IARC (1989a) *IARC Monographs on the Evaluation of Carcinogenic Risks to Humans*, Vol. 47, *Some Organic Solvents, Resin Monomers and Related Compounds, Pigments and Occupational Exposures in Paint Manufacture and Painting*, Lyon, pp. 307-326

IARC (1989b) *IARC Monographs on the Evaluation of Carcinogenic Risks to Humans*, Vol. 47, *Some Organic Solvents, Resin Monomers and Related Compounds, Pigments and Occupational Exposures in Paint Manufacture and Painting*, Lyon, pp. 263-287

Ichinotsubo, D., MacKinnon, E.A., Liu, C., Rice, S. & Mower, H.F. (1981) Mutagenicity of nitrosated cimetidines. *Carcinogenesis*, 2, 261-264

Illingworth, R.N. & Jarvie, D.R. (1979) Absence of toxicity in cimetidine overdosage. *Br. med. J.*, i, 453-454

Inoue, K., Shibata, T., Kosaka, H., Uozumi, M., Tsuda, S. & Abe, T. (1985) Induction of sister-chromatid exchanges by N-nitrosocimetidine in cultured human lymphocytes and its inhibition by chemical compounds. *Mutat. Res.*, 156, 117-121

Jensen, D.E. (1983) Denitrosation as a determinant of nitrosocimetidine in vivo activity. *Cancer Res.*, 43, 5258-5267

Jensen, R.T., Collen, J., Pandol, S.J., Allende, H.D., Raufman, J.-P., Bissonnette, B.M., Duncan, W.C., Durgin, P.L., Gillin, J.C. & Gardner, J.D. (1983) Cimetidine-induced impotence and breast changes in patients with gastric hypersecretory states. *New Engl. J. Med.*, 308, 883-887

Jensen, D.E., Stelman, G.J. & Spiegel, A. (1987) Species differences in blood-mediated nitrosocimetidine denitrosation. *Cancer Res.*, 47, 353-359

Kaneniwa, N., Funaki, T., Furuta, S. & Watari, N. (1986) High-performance liquid chromatographic determination of cimetidine in rat plasma, urine and bile. *J. Chromatogr.*, 374, 430-434

Kaplinsky, N., Pines, A., Thaler, M. & Frankl, O. (1982) Breast tumor and polymyositis following cimetidine therapy—a possible association. *J. Rheumatol.*, 1, 156-157

Kjærgaard, J., Stadil, F. & Wulff, H.R. (1980) Cimetidin (Tagamet) og ventrikelcancer. [Cimetidine (Tagamet) and stomach cancer (Dan.).] *Ugeskr. Læg.*, 142, 2059-2060

Knigge, U., Dejgård, A. & Christiansen, P.M. (1980) Cancer ventriculi—og cimetidin. [Stomach cancer—and cimetidine (Dan.).] *Ugeskr. Læg.*, *142*, 2058-2059

Kunitani, M.G., Johnson, D.A., Upton, R.A. & Riegelman, S. (1981) Convenient and sensitive high-performance liquid chromatography assay for cimetidine in plasma or urine. *J. Chromatogr.*, *224*, 156-161

Kwanashie, H.O. (1989) Effects of maternally administered cimetidine during lactation on the development of drug metabolizing enzymes in mouse pups. *Biochem. Pharmacol.*, *38*, 204-206

Kyrtopoulos, S.A., Hadjiloucas, E. & Vrotsou, B. (1982) Nondetection of O^6-methylguanine in rat DNA following in vivo treatment with large doses of cimetidine alone or in combination with sodium nitrite. *Cancer Res.*, *42*, 1962-1966

La Piana Simonsen, L. (1989) Top 200 drugs of 1988. Branded new Rxs rise 4.0% and total Rxs move up 1.2%. *Pharm. Times*, *55*, 40-48

Larsson, R., Erlanson, G., Bodemar, G., Walan, A., Bertler, Å., Fransson, L. & Norlander, B. (1982) The pharmacokinetics of cimetidine and its sulphoxide metabolite in patients with normal and impaired renal function. *Br. J. clin. Pharmacol.*, *13*, 163-170

Leaf, C.D., Wishnok, J.S. & Tannenbaum, S.R. (1989) Mechanisms of endogenous nitrosation. *Cancer Surv.*, *8*, 323-334

Lefevre, P.A. & Ashby, J. (1985) Investigations into the reported ability of cimetidine to initiate UDS in rat hepatocyte primary cultures. *Environ. Mutagenesis*, *7*, 833-837

Leslie, G.B., Noakes, D.N., Pollitt, F.D., Roe, F.J.C. & Walker, T.F. (1981) A two-year study with cimetidine in the rat: assessment for chronic toxicity and carcinogenicity. *Toxicol. appl. Pharmacol.*, *61*, 119-137

Lijinsky, W. (1982) Carcinogenesis studies with nitrosocimetidine. In: Magee, P.N., ed., *Nitrosamines in Human Cancer* (Banbury Report No. 12), Cold Spring Harbor, NY, CSH Press, pp. 397-401

Lijinsky, W. & Reuber, M.D. (1984) Comparison of nitrosocimetidine with nitrosomethylnitroguanidine in chronic feeding tests in rats. *Cancer Res.*, *44*, 447-449

Lloyd, C.W. & Martin, W.J. (1985) Determination of cimetidine and metabolites in plasma by reversed-phase high-performance liquid chromatographic radial compression technique. *J. Chromatogr.*, *338*, 139-147

Lloyd, C.W., Martin, W.J. & Taylor, B.D. (1985) The pharmacokinetics of cimetidine and metabolites in a neonate. *Drug Intell. clin. Pharmacol.*, *19*, 203-205

Lovering, E.G. & Curran, N.M. (1985) High performance liquid chromatographic determination of cimetidine and related compounds (raw materials and tablets). *J. Chromatogr.*, *319*, 235-240

Martelli, A., Cavanna, M., Gambino, V., Robbiano, L. & Brambilla, G. (1983) Genotoxicity of cimetidine in primary cultures of rat hepatocytes. *Mutat. Res.*, *120*, 133-137

Martelli, A., Robbiano, L., Ghia, M., Giuliano, L., Angelini, G. & Brambilla, G. (1986) A study of the potential genotoxicity of cimetidine using human hepatocyte primary cultures: discrepancy from results obtained in rat hepatocytes. *Cancer Lett.*, *30*, 11-16

Meggs, W.J., Pescovitz, O.H., Metcalf, D., Loriaux, D.L., Cutler, G. & Kaliner, M. (1984) Progesterone sensitivity as a cause of recurrent anaphylaxis. *New Engl. J. Med.*, *311*, 1236-1238

Milton-Thompson, G.J., Ahmet, Z., Lightfoot, N.F., Hunt, R.H., Barnard, J., Brimblecombe, R.W., Moore, P.J., Bavin, P.M.G., Darrin, D.W. & Viney, N. (1982) Intragastric acidity, bacteria, nitrite, and N-nitroso compounds before, during, and after cimetidine treatment. *Lancet*, *ii*, 1091-1095

Møller, H., Lindvig, K., Klefter, R., Mosbech, J. & Jensen, O.M. (1989) Cancer occurrence in a cohort of patients treated with cimetidine. *Gut*, *30*, 1558-1562

Morris, D.L., Youngs, D., Muscroft, T.J., Cooper, J., Rajinski, C., Burdon, D.W. & Keighly, M.R.P. (1984) Mutagenicity in gastric juice. *Gut*, *25*, 723-727

Murray, C., Chapman, R., Isaacson, P. & Bamforth, J. (1978) Cimetidine and malignant gastric ulcers. *Lancet*, *i*, 1092

Muscroft, T.J., Burdon, D.W., Youngs, D.J. & Keighley, M.R.B. (1981) Cimetidine is unlikely to increase formation of intragastric N-nitroso-compounds in patients taking a normal diet. *Lancet*, *i*, 408-410

Nee, J., O'Higgins, N., Osborne, D.H. & Purdy, S. (1984) The role of histamine antagonists on the development of experimental cancer in the rat. *Irish J. med. Sci.*, *153*, 332-335

Nelson, P.G. (1977) Cimetidine and mental confusion. *Lancet*, *ii*, 928

O'Connor, H.J., Riley, S.E., Axon, A.T.R. & Garner, R.C. (1987) Effect of histamine H2-receptor antagonist therapy on the mutagenic activity of gastric juice. *Mutat. Res.*, *188*, 201-208

Ogiu, T., Hard, G.C., Magee, P.N. & Jensen, D.E. (1986) Comparison of the acute toxicity of N-nitrosocimetidine with three structurally related carcinogens in the rat. *Toxicol. Pathol.*, *4*, 395-403

Ohshima, H. & Bartsch, H. (1981) Quantitative estimation of endogenous nitrosation in humans by monitoring N-nitrosoproline excreted in the urine. *Cancer Res.*, *41*, 3658-3662

Parker, S., Schade, R.R., Pohl, C.R., Gavaler, J.S. & Van Thiel, D.H. (1984a) Prenatal and neonatal exposure of male rat pups to cimetidine but not ranitidine adversely affects subsequent adult sexual functioning. *Gastroenterology*, *86*, 675-680

Parker, S., Udani, M., Gavaler, J.S. & Van Thiel, D.H. (1984b) Pre- and neonatal exposure to cimetidine but not ranitidine adversely affects adult sexual functioning of male rats. *Neurobehav. Toxicol. Teratol.*, *6*, 313-318

Paulsen, C.A., Enzmann, G.D., Bremner, W.J., Perrin, B. & Rogers, B.J. (1983) Effects of cimetidine on reproductive function in men. In: Cohen, S., ed., *Update: H2-Receptor Antagonists, Proceedings of an International Symposium of the Royal Society of Medicine, London 24-26 August*, London, Biomedical Information Corp., pp. 169-178

Pelkonen, O. & Puurunen, J. (1980) The effect of cimetidine on *in vitro* and *in vivo* microsomal drug metabolism in the rat. *Biochem. Pharmacol.*, *29*, 3075-3080

Penston, J. & Wormsley, K.G. (1986) Adverse reactions and interactions with H_2-receptor antagonists. *Med. Toxicol.*, *1*, 192-216

Pereira, O.C.M. (1987) Some effects of cimetidine on the reproductive organs of rats. *Gen. Pharmacol.*, *18*, 197-199

Peto, R., Pike, M.C., Day, N.E., Gray, R.G., Lee, P.N., Parish, S., Peto, J., Richards, S. & Wahrendorf, J. (1980) Guidelines for simple sensitive significance tests for carcinogenic effects in long-term animal experiments. In: *Long-term and Short-term Screening Assays for Carcinogens: A Critical Appraisal (IARC Monographs on the Evaluation of the Carcinogenic Risk of Chemicals to Humans*, Suppl. 2), Lyon, IARC, pp. 311-426

Pignatelli, B., Richard, I., Bourgade, M.-C. & Bartsch, H. (1987) Improved group determination and total *N*-nitroso compounds in human gastric juice by chemical denitrosation and thermal energy analysis. *Analyst*, *112*, 945-949

Pino, A. & Robbiano, L. (1983) Absence of DNA fragmentation in gastric mucosa of rats treated with high doses of cimetidine and nitrite. *IRCS med. Sci.*, *11*, 172

Pool, B.L., Eisenbrand, G. & Schmähl, D. (1979) Biological activity of nitrosated cimetidine. *Toxicology*, *15*, 69-72

Porter, J.B., Janeway, C.M. & Hunter, J.R. (1984) Absence of a causal association between cimetidine and gastric cancer. *Gastroenterology*, *87*, 987-988

Randolph, W.C., Osborne, V.L., Walkenstein, S.S. & Intoccia, A.P. (1977) High-pressure liquid chromatographic analysis of cimetidine, a histamine H_2-receptor antagonist, in blood and urine. *J. pharm. Sci.*, *66*, 1148-1150

Redolfi, A., Borgogelli, E. & Lodola, E. (1979) Blood level of cimetidine in relation to age. *Eur. J. clin. Pharmacol.*, *15*, 257-261

Reed, P.I., Cassell, P.G. & Walters, C.L. (1979) Gastric cancer in patients who have taken cimetidine. *Lancet*, *i*, 1234-1235

Reed, P.I., Haines, K., Smith, P.L.R., House, F.R. & Walters, C.L. (1981) Effect of cimetidine on gastric juice N-nitrosamine concentration. *Lancet*, *ii*, 553-556

Reynolds, J.E.F., ed. (1989) *Martindale. The Extra Pharmacopoeia*, 29th ed., London, The Pharmaceutical Press, pp. 1082-1086

Rodighiero, V. (1989) Therapeutic drug monitoring of cyclosporin. Practical applications and limitations. *Clin. Pharmacokin.*, *16*, 27-37

Rustum, A.M. & Hoffman, N.E. (1988) Liquid chromatographic determination of cimetidine in whole blood and plasma by using short polymeric reverse phase column. *J. Assoc. off. anal. Chem.*, *71*, 519-522

Say, B., Barber, N. & Chambers, C. (1985) A case of MURCS association after exposure to cimetidine in utero. *Pediatr. Res.*, *19*, 329A

Schentag, J.J., Calleri, G., Rose, J.Q., Cerra, F.B., DeGlopper, E. & Bernhard, H. (1979) Pharmacokinetic and clinical studies in patients with cimetidine-associated mental confusion. *Lancet*, *i*, 177-178

Schwarz, M., Hummel, J. & Eisenbrand, G. (1980) Induction of DNA strand breaks by nitrosocimetidine. *Cancer Lett.*, *10*, 223-228

Scotcher, S., Sikora, K. & Freedman, L. (1981) Gastric cancer and cimetidine: does delay in diagnosis matter? *Lancet*, *ii*, 630-631

Shapiro, B.H., Hirst, S.A., Babalola, G.O. & Bitar, M.S. (1988) Prospective study on the sexual development of male and female rats perinatally exposed to maternally administered cimetidine. *Toxicol. Lett.*, 44, 315-329

Shuker, D.E.G. & Tannenbaum, S.R. (1983) Determination of nonvolatile *N*-nitroso compounds in biological fluids by liquid chromatography with postcolumn photohydrolysis detection. *Anal. Chem.*, 55, 2152-2155

Sivelle, P.C., Underwood, A.H. & Jelly, J.A. (1982) The effects of histamine H_2 receptor antagonists on androgen action in vivo and dihydrotestosterone binding to the rat prostate androgen receptor in vitro. *Biochem. Pharmacol.*, 31, 677-684

Somogyi, A. & Gugler, R. (1983) Clinical pharmacokinetics of cimetidine. *Clin. Pharmacokin.*, 8, 463-495

Somogyi, A. & Muirhead, M. (1987) Pharmacokinetic interactions of cimetidine. *Clin. Pharmacokin.*, 12, 321-366

Spence, R.W. & Celestin, L.R. (1979) Gynaecomastia associated with cimetidine. *Gut*, 20, 154-157

Stockbrugger, R.W., Cotton, P.B., Eugenides, N., Bartholomew, B.A., Hill, M.J. & Walters, C.L. (1982) Intragastric nitrites, nitrosamines, and bacterial overgrowth during cimetidine treatment. *Gut*, 23, 1048-1054

Stockley, I. & Kiff, E.S. (1987) Gastric carcinoma arising during five years treatment with cimetidine for duodenal ulceration. *Br. J. clin. Pract.*, 41, 578-579

Stoddard, J.C., Smith, J.A.R. & Johnson, A.G. (1980) Cimetidine, delay in diagnosis and carcinoma of the stomach. *Lancet*, ii, 199-200

Strong, H.A. & Spino, M. (1987) Highly sensitive determination of cimetidine and its metabolites in serum and urine by high-performance liquid chromatography. *J. Chromatogr.*, 422, 301-308

Tatsumi, K., Toyoda, M., Tachibana, A. & Takebe, H. (1987) Mutagenic activity of cimetidine and nitrosated cimetidine in human lymphoblastoid cells. *Mutat. Res.*, 182, 382

Taylor, D.C., Cresswell, P.R. & Bartlett, D.C. (1978) The metabolism and elimination of cimetidine, a histamine H_2-receptor antagonist, in the rat, dog and man. *Drug Metab. Dispos.*, 6, 21-30

Taylor, T.V., Menzies-Gow, N., Lovell, D. & La Brooy, S.J. (1978) Misleading response of malignant gastric ulcers to cimetidine. *Lancet*, i, 686-687

Taylor, T.V., Lee, D., Howatson, A.G., Anderson, J. & MacLeod, I.B. (1979) Gastric cancer in patients who have taken cimetidine. *Lancet*, i, 1235-1236

Taylor, T.V., Lee, D., Howatson, A.G., Anderson, J. & MacLeod, I.B. (1981) Gastric cancer and cimetidine. *J. R. Coll. Surg.*, 26, 34-35

Van Thiel, D.H., Gavaler, J.S., Smith, W.I. & Paul, G. (1979) Hypothalamic-pituitary-gonadal dysfunction in men using cimetidine. *New Engl. J. Med.*, 300, 1012-1015

Walker, T.F., Whitehead, S.M., Leslie, G.B., Crean, G.P. & Roe, F.J.C. (1987a) Safety evaluation of cimetidine: report at the termination of a seven-year study in dogs. *Hum. Toxicol.*, 6, 159-164

Walker, T.F., Bott, J.H. & Bond, B.C. (1987b) Cimetidine does not demasculinize male rat offspring exposed in utero. *Fundam. appl. Toxicol.*, *8*, 188-197

Wang, G., Lai, C.L., Lam, K.C. & Yeung, K.K. (1982) Effect of cimetidine on gonadal function in man. *Br. J. clin. Pharmacol.*, *13*, 791-794

Welsh, C.L., Craven, J.L. & Hopton, D. (1977) Cimetidine in alleviation of gastric cancer pain. *Br. med. J.*, *280*, 1413

Williams, G.M., Mori, H. & McQueen, C.A. (1989) Structure-activity relationships in the rat hepatocyte DNA-repair test for 300 chemicals. *Mutat. Res.*, *221*, 263-286

Windholz, M., ed. (1983) *The Merck Index*, 10th ed., Rahway, NJ, Merck & Co., p. 323

Ziemniak, J.A., Chiarmonte, D.A. & Schentag, J.J. (1981) Liquid-chromatographic determination of cimetidine, its known metabolites, and creatinine in serum and urine. *Clin. Chem.*, *27*, 272-275

Ziemniak, J.A., Bernhard, H. & Schentag, J.J. (1983) Hepatic encephalopathy and altered cimetidine kinetics. *Clin. Pharmacol. Ther.*, *34*, 375-382

Ziemniak, J.A., Wynn, R.J., Aranda, J.V., Zarowitz, B.J. & Schentag, J.J. (1984) The pharmacokinetics of metabolism of cimetidine in neonates. *Dev. Pharmacol. Ther.*, *7*, 30-38

DANTRON (CHRYSAZIN; 1,8-DIHYDROXYANTHRAQUINONE)

1. Chemical and Physical Data

1.1 Synonyms

Chem. Abstr. Services Reg. No.: 117-10-2 (replaces CAS Reg. No. 32073-07-7)
Chem. Abstr. Name: 9,10-Anthracenedione, 1,8-dihydroxy-
Synonyms: Antrapurol; danthron; dianthon; dihydroxyanthraquinone; 1,8-dihydroxy-9,10-anthraquinone; dioxyanthrachinonum; 1,8-dioxyanthraquinone

1.2 Structural and molecular formulae and molecular weight

$C_{14}H_8O_4$ Mol. wt: 240.23

1.3 Chemical and physical properties of the pure substance

(a) *Description*: Red or reddish-yellow needles or leaves (from ethanol) (Weast, 1985); orange crystalline powder (Anon., 1981)

(b) *Melting-point*: 193°C (Weast, 1985); 195°C (Anon., 1981)

(c) *Spectroscopy data*[1]: Infrared (Coblenz [5147]; Aldrich, prism [900D]; Aldrich, prism-FT [87D]), ultraviolet (Sadtler [4318]), proton nuclear

---

[1]Bracketed numbers are spectrum numbers in the relevant compilation.

magnetic resonance (Aldrich [91B]) and mass (Aldermaston [195]) spectral data have been reported (Sadtler Research Laboratories, 1980; Pouchert, 1981, 1983, 1985; Weast & Astle, 1985).

(d) *Solubility*: Very soluble in aqueous alkali hydroxides; soluble in acetone, chloroform, diethyl ether and ethanol; almost insoluble in water (Enviro Control, 1981; Weast, 1985)

1.4 Technical products and impurities

Trade Names: Altan; Antrapurol; Bancon; Benno; DanSunate D; Danthron; Diaquone; Dionone; Dorban; Dorbane; Duolax; Fructines-Vichy; Istin; Istizin; Julax; Laxanorm; Laxans; Laxanthreen; Laxenta; Laxipur; Laxipurin; Modane; Neokutin S; Pastomin; Prugol; Roydan; Scatron D; Solven; Unilax; Zwitsalax

The following trade names are those of multi-ingredient preparations containing dantron: Agarol Capsules; Coloxyl; Dorbanate; Dorbanex; Dorbantyl; Doss; Doxidan; Normax (Reynolds, 1989).

Dantron is available commercially at a purity of 95-99% (Aldrich Chemical Co., 1988; Lancaster Synthesis Ltd, 1988; Sigma Chemical Co., 1988).

2. Production, Occurrence, Use and Analysis

2.1 Production and occurrence

(a) *Production*

Dantron has been prepared by several processes, including the alkaline hydrolysis of 1,8-dinitroanthraquinone, the caustic fusion of 1,8-anthraquinonedisulfonic acid, the diazotization of 1,8-diaminoanthraquinone followed by hydrolysis of the bisdiazo compound, the acid hydrolysis of 1,8-dimethoxyanthraquinone in glacial acetic acid-sulfuric acid, the alkaline hydrolysis of 1,8-anthraquinonedisulfonic acid using calcium oxide, and the reaction of 1,8-dinitroanthraquinone with sodium formate or potassium formate (Michalowicz, 1981).

In 1987, US manufacturers voluntarily withdrew production of all human drug products containing dantron (Anon., 1987).

Dantron is synthesized in the Federal Republic of Germany, India, Japan, Poland, the UK and the USA (Chemical Information Services Ltd, 1989-90).

(b) *Natural occurrence*

Dantron has been isolated from dried leaves and stems of *Xyris semifuscata* harvested in Madagascar (Fournier *et al.*, 1975). Dantron is the basic structure of the aglycones of naturally occurring laxative glycosides, in, e.g., *Cassia* (senna), *Aloe*, *Rheum* and *Rhamnus* (cascara) species (Baars *et al.*, 1976; Reynolds, 1989).

Dantron has been identified in larvae of the elm-leaf beetle, *Pyrrhalta luteola*. The presence of a mixture of anthraquinones and anthrones was suggested to be a means of protection from predators, and these compounds appear to be biosynthesized by the insect (Howard *et al.*, 1982).

2.2 Use

Dantron has been widely used since the beginning of this century as a laxative and as an intermediate for dyes (Enviro Control, 1981; Michalowicz, 1981).

2.3 Analysis

Dantron can be determined in pharmaceutical preparations by high-performance liquid chromatography with ultraviolet detection (Wurster & Upadrashta, 1986) and by fluorimetry (Miller & Danielson, 1987). It has been determined in urine and faeces by gas chromatography with flame ionization detection (Baars *et al.*, 1976) and in urine by gas chromatography with mass spectrometry (Kok & Faber, 1981) and high-performance liquid chromatography with fluorimetry (Miller & Danielson, 1987).

3. Biological Data Relevant to the Evaluation of Carcinogenic Risk to Humans

3.1 Carcinogenicity studies in animals

(a) Oral administration

Mouse: A group of 20 male C3H/HeN mice, eight weeks of age, was fed dantron (commercial grade; no impurity detected on thin-layer chromatography) at 200 mg/kg diet for 540 days, at which time the experiment was terminated. A group of 20 untreated male mice served as controls. Hepatocellular adenomas were found in 9/17 treated and 5/19 control mice. Hepatocellular carcinomas were found in 4/17 treated mice (all also had adenomas), an incidence that was significantly different ($p < 0.05$; Fisher exact test) from that in controls (0/19). Adenomatous [polypoid] hyperplasia, occasionally associated with dysplastic changes, was observed in the caecum of 17/17 treated mice and in the remainder of the colon of 5/17 treated mice, but not in controls (Mori *et al.*, 1986).

Rat: A group of 18 male ACI rats, eight weeks of age, was fed dantron [purity unspecified] at 10 000 mg/kg diet for 16 months. A group of 15 untreated males served as controls. Twelve treated and 14 untreated rats survived more than one year. Nine tumours of the large intestine were found in 7/12 treated rats (three adenomas and four adenocarcinomas ($p < 0.02$) of the colon and two adenomas of the caecum). In addition, focal epithelial hyperplasia was observed frequently in the mucosa of the colon and caecum of treated rats with and without intestinal tumours. No intestinal tumour or hyperplastic lesion was found in the 14 controls (Mori et al., 1985).

(b) *Administration with known carcinogens*

Mouse: In a two-stage carcinogenesis experiment, a group of 20 female ICR/Ha Swiss mice, seven weeks of age, received a single skin application of 7,12-dimethylbenz[a]anthracene at 20 μg in 0.1 ml acetone, followed two weeks later by applications three times a week of commercial-grade dantron at 170 μg in 0.1 ml acetone. A control group of 20 female mice received only skin applications of dantron at 170 μg in 0.1 ml acetone three times a week. Median survival time of animals in both groups was greater than 490 days, when the experiment was terminated. No skin tumour was found in either group (Segal et al., 1971).

Rat: In a two-stage carcinogenicity study, groups of 30 male Sprague-Dawley rats, 50 days of age, received a single subcutaneous injection of 1,2-dimethyl-hydrazine (DMH) at 150 mg/kg bw. After one week they were fed dantron (purity, >97%) at 0, 600 or 2400 mg/kg diet; the average daily intakes were approximately 30 and 60 mg/kg bw. After 26 weeks, all animals were killed. Two additional groups of 30 male rats received either no treatment or were given the diet with the higher concentration of dantron alone. There was no significant difference in mean body weight gain between treated and control animals. In the rats treated with DMH plus dantron, the combined incidences of intestinal adenomas and adenocarcinomas were 4/30 in the low-dose and 2/30 in the high-dose group. The incidences of intestinal adenocarcinomas were 0/30 in untreated controls, 0/30 in the group treated with dantron alone and 2/30 in the group treated with DMH alone. The difference in tumour incidence between animals treated with DMH alone and DMH plus dantron was not significant (Sjöberg et al., 1988)

3.2 Other relevant data

(a) *Experimental systems*

(i) *Absorption, distribution, excretion and metabolism*

Male Wistar rats were given the sodium salt of dantron intravenously at 4.8, 22 or 58 μmol/kg [1.2, 5.3 or 14 mg/kg] bw or at 120 μmol/kg [28.8 mg/kg] bw by gastric tube. Metabolites identified in the bile and urine following administration by either route included the monosulfate, β-glucuronide and other unidentified metabolites. Following intravenous administration, about 80% of the dantron conjugates in bile were excreted after 1 h; the dose fractions found after 5 h represented about 20%, 30% and 40% of the low-, intermediate- and high-dose levels, respectively. The corresponding fractions in urine were 16%, 12% and 10%, giving rise to bile:urine excretion ratios of 1.3, 2.7 and 4.0, respectively. Only 30-50% of the dose could be accounted for by conjugates (Sund, 1987). Earlier studies also showed that after oral administration of dantron only 30-40% of the total dose administered could be recovered in faeces and urine, mostly during the first 24 h (Breimer & Baars, 1976).

In vitro, rat jejunum and colon transformed dantron into its monoglucuronide and monosulfate, the monoglucuronide being the major metabolite (Sund & Elvegård, 1988).

(ii) *Toxic effects*

The oral LD_{50} for dantron in male ARS/ICR mice was > 7 g/kg bw. Groups of four male and four female beagle dogs received either a vehicle capsule or a capsule containing dantron at 5 or 15 mg/kg bw daily for one year. No adverse effect was observed. The doses employed were reported to be several-fold higher than the usual clinical dose (Case *et al.*, 1977-78).

Apoptosis together with accumulation of lipofuscin pigment in gut wall was noted in guinea-pigs given dantron orally at 25 mg/kg bw (Walker *et al.*, 1988).

Male rats given dantron at 600 or 2400 mg/kg diet for 26 weeks (Sjöberg *et al.*, 1988) had enlarged lymph nodes in the mesocolon, which were brownish due to pigmentation of the accumulated mononuclear phagocytes. In kidney, pigment deposition was seen in the cortical region.

(iii) *Effects on reproduction and prenatal toxicity*

No data were available to the Working Group.

(iv) *Genetic and related effects*

Dantron was mutagenic to *Salmonella typhimurium* TA1537 in the presence and absence of an exogenous metabolic system (Brown & Brown, 1976; Liberman *et al.*, 1982). It was also mutagenic to TA2637 (Tikkanen *et al.*, 1983), TA102 (Levin *et al.*, 1984) and TA104 (Chesis *et al.*, 1984) in the presence of an exogenous metabolic system. In TA104, the results were not significantly changed by the addition of superoxide dismutase and catalase (Chesis *et al.*, 1984). In *S. typhimurium* TA100, TA1535, TA1538 and TA98, dantron was not mutagenic in the presence or absence of an exogenous metabolic system (Brown & Brown, 1976; Liberman *et al.*, 1982; Tikkanen *et al.*, 1983).

Dantron induced respiration-deficient mutants in yeast (Zetterberg & Swanbeck, 1971).

It induced unscheduled DNA synthesis in hepatocytes from mice (Mori *et al.*, 1984) and rats (Mori *et al.*, 1984; Kawai *et al.*, 1986) but not in another study with rat hepatocytes (Probst *et al.*, 1981). Dantron induced chromosomal aberrations in human peripheral lymphocytes *in vitro* in the absence of an exogenous metabolic system (Carballo *et al.*, 1981). In some studies, dantron inhibited gap-junctional intercellular communication in Chinese hamster V79 cells (Umeda *et al.*, 1980 [The Working Group noted that the way in which the data were presented precluded statistical analysis.]; Trosko *et al.*, 1982 [one dose]), but in other studies no such effect was found in Chinese hamster V79 cells (Kinsella, 1982; Zeilmaker & Yamasaki, 1986) or in human fibroblasts (Si *et al.*, 1988).

(b) Humans

(i) *Pharmacokinetics*

Following its administration within 24 h of the induction of labour in 12 women, dantron was found in maternal urine, neonatal urine and amniotic fluid. Most of the drug appeared as a glucuronide in both mothers and babies (Blair *et al.*, 1977).

(ii) *Adverse effects*

Liver damage was reported in a woman who had used a laxative containing dantron and dioctyl calcium sulfosuccinate for one year. The symptoms disappeared after discontinuation of the medication but reappeared upon resumption; none of the compounds given alone had any effect on the results of hepatic function tests (Tolman *et al.*, 1976).

A woman developed deep discoloration of the skin following ingestion of large amounts of a laxative containing dantron (Darke & Cooper, 1978). Such staining was also found in other studies, predominantly in elderly subjects, and was localized to the buttocks and thighs, with minor inflammatory symptoms (Bunney & Noble, 1974; Cox & Vickers, 1984). Contact of skin with faeces or urine containing the drug seems to be a prerequisite for discoloration. Inflammation, when present, may result from reduction of the parent compound in the colon to the diol derivative, which irritates both the gut and skin (Puschmann, 1983; Ippen, 1974), while the parent compound does not (Green *et al.*, 1988).

Melanosis coli, a state involving apoptosis and lipofuscin pigment accumulation in macrophages in colonic lamina propria, has been described in persons using anthraquinone laxatives (Bockus *et al.*, 1933; Speare, 1951; Wittoesch *et al.*, 1958; Steer & Colin-Jones, 1975; Badiali *et al.*, 1985; Walker *et al.*, 1988).

3.3 Case reports and epidemiological studies of carcinogenicity to humans

No data were available to the Working Group.

4. Summary of Data Reported and Evaluation

4.1 Exposure data

Dantron occurs naturally in several species of plants and in insects. It has been produced and widely used since the beginning of the century as a laxative and, to a lesser extent, as an intermediate for dyes. No data on occupational exposure levels were available.

4.2 Experimental carcinogenicity data

Dantron was tested for carcinogenicity by oral administration in single studies in male mice of one strain and in male rats of one strain. In mice, a small increase in the incidence of hepatocellular carcinomas and a large increase in adenomatous polypoid hyperplasia of the colon were observed; there was also an increased combined incidence of adenomas and adenocarcinomas of the colon and caecum. In rats, dantron increased the incidence of adenocarcinomas of the colon.

4.3 Human carcinogenicity data

No data were available to the Working Group.

4.4 Other relevant data

In one study, dantron caused chromosomal aberrations in human lymphocytes *in vitro*. It gave contradictory results with respect to the induction of unscheduled DNA synthesis in rodent cells and was mutagenic to yeast in one study and to *Salmonella typhimurium*. Dantron did not inhibit gap-junctional intercellular communication in human cells, but conflicting results were obtained in Chinese hamster cells. (See Appendix 1.)

4.5 Evaluation[1]

There is *sufficient evidence* for the carcinogenicity of dantron in experimental animals.

No data were available from studies in humans on the carcinogenicity of dantron.

---

[1]For definition of the italicized terms, see Preamble, pp. 26–29.

Overall evaluation

Dantron *is possibly carcinogenic to humans (Group 2B)*.

5. References

Aldrich Chemical Co. (1988) *1988-1989 Aldrich Catalog/Handbook of Fine Chemicals*, Milwaukee, WI, p. 552

Anon. (1981) *The Pharmaceutical Codex*, London, The Pharmaceutical Press, p. 244

Anon. (1987) Adria and Hoechst-Roussel Danthron-free OTC Laxatives. *FDC Reports Pink Sheet*, April 6, T&G-6-T&G-7

Baars, A.J., Vermeulen, R.J. & Breimer, D.D. (1976) Gas chromatographic determination of the laxative 1,8-dihydroxyanthraquinone in urine and faeces. *J. Chromatogr.*, 120, 217-220

Badiali, D., Marchezziano, A., Pallone, F., Paoluzi, P., Bausano, G., Iannoni, C., Materia, E., Anzini, F. & Corazziari, E. (1985) Melanosis of the rectum in patients with chronic constipation. *Dis. Colon Rectum*, 28, 241-245

Blair, A.W., Burdon, M., Powell, J., Gerrard, M. & Smith, R. (1977) Fetal exposure to 1:8 dihydroxyanthraquinone. *Biol. Neonate*, 31, 289-293

Bockus, H.L., Willard, J.H. & Bank, J. (1933) Melanosis coli. The etiologic significance of the anthracene laxatives: a report of forty-one cases. *J. Am. med. Assoc.*, 101, 1-6

Breimer, D.D. & Baars, A.J. (1976) Pharmacokinetics and metabolism of anthraquinone laxatives. *Pharmacology*, 14 (Suppl. 1), 30-47

Brown, J.P. & Brown R.J. (1976) Mutagenesis by 9,10-anthraquinone derivatives and related compounds in *Salmonella typhimurium*. *Mutat. Res.*, 40, 203-224

Bunney, M.H. & Noble, I.M. (1974) Red skin and Dorbanex. *Br. med. J.*, i, 731

Carballo, M.A., D'Aquino, M. & Aranda, E.I. (1981) Accion clastogenica de un compuesto antraquinonico en linfocitos humanos. [Mutagenic effect of an anthraquinone compound on human lymphocytes (Sp.).] *Medicina*, 41, 531-534

Case, M.T., Smith, J.K. & Nelson, R.A. (1977-78) Acute mouse and chronic dog toxicity studies of danthron, dioctyl sodium sulfosuccinate, foloxalkol and combinations. *Drug. chem. Toxicol.*, 1, 89-101

Chemical Information Services Ltd (1989-90) *Directory of World Chemical Producers*, Oceanside, NY

Chesis, P.L., Levin, D.E., Smith, M.T., Ernster, L. & Ames, B.N. (1984) Mutagenicity of quinones: pathways of metabolic activation and detoxification. *Proc. natl Acad. Sci. USA*, 81, 1696-1700

Cox, N.H. & Vickers, C.F.H. (1984) A cutaneous complication of Dorbanex therapy. *Clin. exp. Dermatol.*, 9, 624-626

Darke, C.S. & Cooper, R.G. (1978) Unusual case of skin discoloration. *Br. med. J.*, ii, 1188-1189

Enviro Control (1981) *Anthraquinone Dye Toxicological Profiles* (CSPC-Mono-82-2; US NTIS PB83-166033), Rockville, MD

Fournier, G., Ludwig Bercht, C.A., Paris, R.R. & Paris, M.R. (1975) 3-Methoxychrysazin, a new anthraquinone from *Xyris semifuscata*. *Phytochemistry, 14,* 2099

Green, P.G., Grattan, C.E.H., Kennedy, C.T.C. & Forbes, D.R. (1988) Patch testing with dithranol and its degradation products. *Contact Derm., 18,* 117-119

Howard, D.F., Phillips, D.W., Jones, T.H. & Blum, M.S. (1982) Anthraquinones and anthrones: occurrence and defensive function in a *Chrysomelid* beetle. *Naturwissenschaften, 69,* 91-92

Ippen, H. (1974) Red skin and Dorbanex. *Br. med. J., ii,* 345

Kawai, K., Mori, H., Sugie, S., Yoshimi, N., Inouie, T., Nakamuru, T., Nozawa, Y. & Matsushima, T. (1986) Genotoxicity in the hepatocyte/DNA repair test and toxicity to liver mitochondria of 1-hydroxyanthraquinone and several dihydroxyanthraquinones. *Cell Biol. Toxicol., 2,* 457-467

Kinsella, A.R. (1982) Elimination of metabolic co-operation and the induction of sister chromatid exchanges are not properties common to all promoting or co-carcinogenic agents. *Carcinogenesis, 3,* 499-403

Kok, R.M. & Faber, D.B. (1981) Qualitative and quantitative analysis of some synthetic, chemically acting laxatives in urine by gas chromatography-mass spectrometry. *J. Chromatogr., 222,* 389-398

Lancaster Synthesis Ltd. (1988) *Lancaster Organic Research Chemicals*, Windham, NH, p. 380

Levin, D.E., Hollstein, M., Christman, M.F. & Ames, B.N. (1984) Detection of oxidative mutagens with a new *Salmonella* tester strain (TA102). *Methods Enzymol., 105,* 249-254

Liberman, D.F., Fink, R.C., Schaefer, F.L., Mulcahy, R.J. & Stark, A.-A. (1982) Mutagenicity of anthraquinone and hydroxylated anthraquinones in the Ames/*Salmonella* microsome system. *Appl. environ. Microbiol., 43,* 1354-1359

Michalowicz, W.A. (1981) Preparation of hydroxyanthraquinones, US Patent 4,292,248 to American Color & Chemical Corp.

Miller, B.E. & Danielson, N.D. (1987) Fluorimetric determination of danthron in pharmaceutical tablets and in urine. *Anal. chim. Acta, 192,* 293-299

Mori, H., Kawai, K., Ohbayashi, F., Kuniyasu, T., Yamazaki, M., Hamasaki, T. & Williams, G.M. (1984) Genotoxicity of a variety of mycotoxins in the hepatocyte primary culture/DNA repair test using rat and mouse hepatocytes. *Cancer Res., 44,* 2918-2923

Mori, H., Sugie, S., Niwa, K., Takahashi, M. & Kawai, K. (1985) Induction of intestinal tumours in rats by chrysazin. *Br. J. Cancer, 52,* 781-783

Mori, H., Sugie, S., Niwa, K., Yoshimi, N., Tanaka, T. & Hirono, I. (1986) Carcinogenicity of chrysazin in large intestine and liver of mice. *Jpn. J. Cancer Res. (Gann), 77,* 871-876

Pouchert, C.J., ed. (1981) *The Aldrich Library of Infrared Spectra*, 3rd ed., Milwaukee, WI, Aldrich Chemical Co., p. 900

Pouchert, C.J., ed. (1983) *The Aldrich Library of NMR Spectra*, 2nd ed., Vol. 2, Milwaukee, WI, Aldrich Chemical Co., p. 91

Pouchert, C.J., ed. (1985) *The Aldrich Library of FT-IR Spectra*, Vol. 2, Milwaukee, WI, Aldrich Chemical Co., p. 87

Probst, G.S., McMahon, R.E., Hill, L.E., Thompson, C.Z., Epp, J.K. & Neal, S.B. (1981) Chemically-induced unscheduled DNA synthesis in primary rat hepatocyte cultures: a comparison with bacterial mutagenicity using 218 compounds. *Environ. Mutagenesis*, *3*, 11-32

Puschmann, M. (1983) The anthralin erythema: influence of concentration, duration of contact, oxidation products and corticosteroids. Clinical, reflection photometric, and microscopic examinations. *Z. Hautkr.*, *58*, 1646-1647

Reynolds, J.E.F., ed. (1989) *Martindale. The Extra Pharmacopeia*, 29th ed., London, The Pharmaceutical Press, pp. 1073-1112

Sadtler Research Laboratories (1980) *Standard Spectra Collection, 1980 Cumulative Index*, Philadelphia, PA

Segal, A., Katz, C. & Van Duuren, B.L. (1971) Structure and tumor-promoting activity of anthralin (1,8-dihydroxy-9-anthrone) and related compounds. *J. med. Chem.*, *14*, 1152-1154

Si, E.C.C., Pfeifer, R.W. & Yim, G.K.W. (1988) Anthralin, a non-phorbol tumor promoter, fails to inhibit metabolic cooperation in mutant human fibroblasts, but inhibits phytohemagglutinin-induced lymphocyte blastogenesis in vitro. *Toxicology*, *53*, 199-212

Sigma Chemical Co. (1988) *Biochemical and Organic Compounds for Research and Diagnostic Clinical Reagents*, St Louis, MO, p. 521

Sjöberg, P., Hedelin, U., Kronevi, T., Lydén-Skolowski, A., Magnusson, G., Montin, G., Olofsson, I.-M. & Lindquist, N.G. (1988) Pigmentation of kidneys and lymph nodes of mesocolon in rats fed diets containing the laxative danthron. *Toxicol. Lett.*, *44*, 299-306

Speare, G.S. (1951) Melanosis coli: experimental observations on its production and elimination in twenty-three cases. *Am. J. Surg.*, *82*, 631-637

Steer, H.W. & Colin-Jones, D.G. (1975) Melanosis coli: studies of the toxic effects of irritant purgatives. *J. Pathol.*, *115*, 199-205

Sund, R.B. (1987) Studies on laxatives: biliary and urinary excretion in rats given danthron by intravenous infusion or gastric intubation. *Pharmacol. Toxicol.*, *61*, 130-137

Sund, R.B. & Elvegård, S.-O. (1988) Anthraquinone laxatives: metabolism and transport of danthron and rhein in the rat small and large intestine in vitro. *Pharmacol.*, *36* (*Suppl. 1*), 144-151

Tikkanen, L., Matsushima, T. & Natori, S. (1983) Mutagenicity of anthraquinones in the Salmonella preincubation test. *Mutat. Res.*, *116*, 297-304

Tolman, K.G., Hammar, S. & Sannella, J.J. (1976) Possible hepatotoxicity of Doxidan®. *Ann. intern. Med.*, *84*, 290-292

Trosko, J.E., Jone, C., Aylsworth, C. & Tsushimoto, G. (1982) Elimination of metabolic cooperation is associated with the tumor promoters, oleic acid and anthralin. *Carcinogenesis*, *3*, 1101-1103

Umeda, M., Noda, K. & Ono, T. (1980) Inhibition of metabolic cooperation in Chinese hamster cells by various chemicals including tumor promoters. *Gann*, *71*, 614-620

Walker, N., Bennett, R.E. & Axelsen, R.A. (1988) Melanosis coli. A consequence of anthraquinone-induced apoptosis of colonic epithelial cells. *Am. J. Pathol.*, *131*, 465-476

Weast, R.C., ed. (1985) *CRC Handbook of Chemistry and Physics*, 66th ed., Boca Raton, FL, CRC Press, p. C-83

Weast, R.C. & Astle, M.J. (1985) *Handbook of Data on Organic Compounds*, Boca Raton, FL, CRC Press

Wittoesch, J.H., Jackman, R.J. & McDonald, J.R. (1958) Melanosis coli: general review and a study of 887 cases. *Dis. Colon Rectum*, *1*, 172-180

Wurster, D.E. & Upadrashta, S.M. (1986) Simultaneous quantitation of 1,8,9-anthracenetriol, 1,8-dihydroxy-9,10-anthraquinone, and 1,8,1',8'-tetrahydroxy-10,10'-dianthrone by reversed-phase high-performance liquid chromatography. *J. Chromatogr.*, *362*, 71-78

Zeilmaker, M. & Yamasaki, H. (1986) Inhibition of junctional intercellular communication as a possible short-term test to detect tumor-promoting agents: results with nine chemicals tested by dye transfer assay in Chinese hamster V79 cells. *Cancer Res.*, *46*, 6180-6186

Zetterberg, G. & Swanbeck, G. (1971) Studies on dithranol and diethanol-like compounds. *Acta dermatovenerol.*, *51*, 45-49

FUROSEMIDE (FRUSEMIDE)

1. Chemical and Physical Data

1.1 Synonyms

Chem. Abstr. Services Reg. No.: 54-31-9
Chem. Abstr. Name: 5-(Aminosulfonyl)-4-chloro-2-[(2-furanylmethyl)-amino]-benzoic acid
Synonym: Sulfamoylanthranilic acid, 4-chloro-*N*-furfuryl-5

1.2 Structural and molecular formulae and molecular weight

$C_{12}H_{11}ClN_2O_5S$ Mol. wt: 330.77

1.3 Chemical and physical properties of the pure substance

(a) *Description*: White, microcrystalline powder; crystals from aqueous ethanol (Reynolds, 1989)

(b) *Melting-point*: 206°C dec (Windholz, 1983)

(c) *Solubility*: Slightly soluble in water; soluble in aqueous solutions above pH 8; slightly soluble in chloroform, ethanol and diethyl ether; soluble in acetone, methanol and dimethylformamide (Windholz, 1983)

(d) *Spectroscopy data*: Ultraviolet and infrared spectra have been reported (Anon., 1979).

(e) *Stability*: Discolours on exposure to light (Barnhart, 1989); precipitates with calcium gluconate, ascorbic acid, tetracyclines, urea and adrenaline (Windholz, 1983)

(f) *Dissociation constant*: pK_a = 3.9 (Anon., 1979)

1.4 Technical products and impurities

Trade names: Aluzine; Aquamide; Aquasin; Arasemide; Discoid; Diural; Diuresal; Diurolasa; Dryptal; Durafurid; Errolon; Franyl; Frusetic; Furetic; Furix; Furo-basan; Fur-O-Ims; Furo-Puren; Furose; Furoside; Fusid; Hydrex; Hydro-rapid; Impugan; Lasiletten; Lasilix; Lasix; Laxur; Min-I-Jet Frusemide; Moilarorin; Neo-Renal; Nicorol; Novosemide; Odemase; Oedemex; Promedes; Puresis; Seguril; Sigasalur; SK-Furosemide; Uremide; Urex; Urex-M; Uritol

The following names have been used for multi-ingredient preparations containing furosemide: Diumide-K; Frumil; Frusene; Lasikal; Lasilactone; Lasipressin; Lasix + K; Lasoride

Furosemide is available as tablets (20 mg, 40 mg, 80 mg) with lactose, magnesium stearate, starch and talc (see IARC, 1987), and for injection in 2-, 4- and 10-ml ampoules containing furosemide at 10 mg/ml sterile solution in amber vials (water and sodium hydroxide). It is also available as an oral solution containing furosemide at 10 mg/ml and 11.5% alcohol, D & C Yellow #10, FD & C Yellow #6, glycerine, parabens, sodium hydroxide and sorbitol (Barnhart, 1989).

2. Production, Occurrence, Use and Analysis

2.1 Production and occurrence

Furosemide is prepared from 4,6-dichlorobenzoic acid-3-sulfonylchloride *via* a multistep synthesis involving the sequential addition of ammonia and 6-furfurylamine (Sturm *et al.*, 1962). It is synthesized in Brazil, Bulgaria, China, Hungary, Israel, Italy, Poland, Switzerland and the USA (Chemical Information Services, 1989-90).

Specific data on production of furosemide are not available, but the number of prescriptions for this drug in the USA increased from 16 million in 1973 to 23 million in 1981. The oral form (Lasix) alone was the eighth most frequently prescribed drug in the USA in 1985 (La Piana Simonsen, 1989). In Sweden, furosemide was sold at a level of 44.08 defined daily doses per 1000 inhabitants in 1988 (Apoteksbolaget, 1988, 1989). In Finland, furosemide sales were 13.87 defined daily doses (40 mg) per 1000 inhabitants in 1987 (Finnish Committee on Drug Information and Statistics, 1987).

Furosemide is not known to occur naturally.

2.2 Use

Furosemide is a potent, short-acting diuretic (Weiner & Mudge, 1985). It is used for the treatment of oedema of cardiac, hepatic or renal origin and in a variety of situations ranging from the control of hypertension to the symptomatic treatment of hypercalcaemia.

Furosemide has a steep dose-effect curve, and therapeutic doses range from 40 to 200 mg daily in adults (Weiner & Mudge, 1985). Treatment of oedema is usually started with an initial oral dose of 40 mg daily; in severe cases, a gradual increase up to 600 mg daily may be required. Intramuscular or slow intravenous injections of furosemide are also used, although the oral route is preferred. In the management of oliguria in acute or chronic renal failure, doses up to 6 g have been given in slow (less than 4 mg per min) intravenous infusions (see Reynolds, 1989).

The usual dose for children is 1-3 mg/kg bw daily given orally and 0.5-1.5 mg/kg bw by injection (Reynolds, 1989).

2.3 Analysis

Furosemide has been determined in biological fluids by high-performance liquid chromatography with detection by spectrofluorimetry (Uchino *et al.*, 1984; Sood *et al.*, 1987) and ultraviolet (Andreasen *et al.*, 1981) and mass spectrometry (Uchino *et al.*, 1984). Analysis of furosemide in pharmaceutical preparations by high-performance liquid chromatography and colorimetric complexation with copper has been reported (Mishra *et al.*, 1989; US Pharmacopeial Convention, Inc., 1989).

3. Biological Data Relevant to the Evaluation of Carcinogenic Risk to Humans

3.1 Carcinogenicity studies in animals

(a) Oral administration

Mouse: Groups of 50 male and 50 female B6C3F1 mice, eight weeks old, were fed furosemide (99% pure, USP grade) at 0, 700 or 1400 mg/kg of diet for 104 weeks. The average amounts of furosemide consumed per day were approximately 100 and 200 mg/kg bw for low- and high-dose groups, respectively. Mean body weights of treated and control mice were comparable. Final survival rates in males were:

control, 31/50; low-dose, 24/50; and high-dose, 26/50; and those in females were: control, 36/50; low-dose, 29/50; and high-dose, 18/50. Survival in high-dose females was significantly lower than that in controls ($p = 0.003$). All survivors were killed at weeks 105-107 then necropsied, and about 40 different tissues were examined microscopically. In female mice, a small but statistically significant increase in the incidence of mammary gland carcinomas was observed: control, 0/50; low-dose, 2/50; and high-dose, 5/48 ($p = 0.01$, logistic regression test for trend taking account of survival) (National Toxicology Program, 1989).

Rat: Groups of 50 male and 50 female F344/N rats, seven weeks old, were fed furosemide (99% pure; USP grade) at 0, 350 or 700 mg/kg of diet for 104 weeks. The average amounts of furosemide consumed per day were approximately 15 and 30 mg/kg bw for low- and high-dose groups, respectively. Mean body weights of treated and control mice were comparable. Survivors at 104-106 weeks in males were: controls, 17/50; low-dose, 17/50; and high-dose, 20/50; those in females were: controls, 35/50; low-dose, 31/50; and high-dose, 34/50. About 40 different tissues were examined microscopically. No statistically significant increase in the incidence of tumours at any site was reported; however, in males, meningiomas of the brain were observed in 3/50 low-dose rats *versus* 2/1928 in historical controls. The authors noted that these rare tumours occurred early in the study in low-dose animals (National Toxicology Program, 1989).

(b) Administration with known carcinogens

Rat: Four groups of 25 male Fischer 344 rats, five weeks of age, were given drinking water containing 0.01% or 0.05% *N*-nitrosobutyl-*N*-(4-hydroxybutyl)-amine (NBHBA) for four weeks, followed by no further treatment or administration of furosemide [purity unspecified] dissolved in 0.5% carboxymethyl cellulose by gavage three times per week for 32 weeks (total dose, 250 mg/kg bw). The experiment was terminated at 36 weeks. One group of 25 male rats was treated with furosemide alone. No treatment-related mortality was observed in any group, but body weights of furosemide-treated groups were significantly lower; almost all rats survived to the end of the experiment. Following sacrifice, all bladders were examined histologically. No significant difference in the incidence of bladder lesions (simple, papillary or nodular hyperplasia, papillomas or carcinomas) was seen in furosemide-treated *versus* other groups. Treatment with furosemide alone did not induce any lesion in the bladder (Shibata *et al.*, 1989). [The Working Group noted the short duration of the study and the limited pathological examination.]

3.2 Other relevant data

(a) *Experimental systems*

(i) *Absorption, distribution, excretion and metabolism*

After oral administration of furosemide to dogs, about 50% of the dose was absorbed (Yakatan *et al.*, 1979). In one study in male Sprague-Dawley rats, the bioavailability of oral furosemide was estimated to be 30% (Lee & Chiou, 1983).

The pharmacokinetics of the disappearance of furosemide from the blood is best described by two- or three-compartment open models, with dose-dependent variations in plasma protein binding (Hammarlund & Paalzow, 1982). In rats, furosemide is cleared from the plasma by the kidneys, is biotransformed by the liver or is excreted unchanged in the bile, with subsequent intestinal reabsorption (Kitani *et al.*, 1988). About 4% of furosemide administered intravenously to rats was recovered from the gut (Lee & Chiou, 1983). In contrast, biliary excretion of furosemide has been reported to be as high as 30% of doses of 50-100 mg/kg bw given to male Swiss mice (Spitznagle *et al.*, 1977). Glucuronidation of furosemide appears to take place in the kidney; removal of the liver did not affect clearance of furosemide in dogs (Lee & Chiou, 1983; Verbeeck *et al.*, 1981).

Covalent binding of furosemide to mouse liver proteins has been shown, and this was enhanced by administration of an inhibitor of epoxide hydrase, suggesting formation of an arene oxide intermediate involving the furan ring (Wirth *et al.*, 1976). *In vitro*, human liver microsomes can convert furosemide to metabolites that bind irreversibly to microsomal proteins (Dybing, 1977).

Formation of unidentified metabolites was demonstrated after incubation of furosemide with a 9000 × *g* supernatant fraction of washed stomach homogenates from rats. The apparent metabolism per gram of tissue was greater in the stomach than in the small intestine, large intestine or liver (Lee & Chiou, 1983).

(ii) *Toxic effects*

The oral LD_{50} for furosemide was approximately 2700 mg/kg bw in 60-day-old rats (Goldenthal, 1971), 2200 mg/kg bw in mice (Romanova & Rudzit, 1985) and 800 mg/kg bw in rabbits (Horioka *et al.*, 1982). The intravenous LD_{50} in rabbits was 800 mg/kg (Horioka *et al.*, 1982). Intraperitoneal injection of 400 mg/kg bw into male mice produced massive necrosis in both the midzonal and centrilobular areas of the liver; this damage was prevented by prior administration of cytochrome P450 inhibitors (Mitchell *et al.*, 1974).

Two of five male and three of five female rats that were fed diets containing furosemide at up to 46 g/kg for 14 days died before the end of the studies. Minimal-to-mild nephrosis was found in all rats that received furosemide at 1.3 or 46 g/kg and in one male receiving 5.1 g/kg. Microscopically, the toxic lesion was subcapsular or cortical and was characterized by tubular-cell regeneration;

mineralization was present at the corticomedullary junction. Dose-related nephrosis was also observed in mice in a 14-day study. In a 13-week study, male rats given a diet containing furosemide at 12.5 g/kg or more and females given a diet containing 15 g/kg had increased liver:body weight ratios; dose-related diuresis was also observed. Compound-related minimal-to-moderate nephrosis occurred in male rats given 5 or 10 g/kg and in females given 7.5 or 15 g/kg. Mineralization was observed at the corticomedullary junction in male rats given 0.625 g/kg or more. In mice, dose-related minimal-to-mild nephrosis was also observed in a 13-week study (National Toxicology Program, 1989).

In a two-year study (see section 3.1), nephropathy occurred with greater severity in dosed male rats than in non-dosed rats. In mice, compound-related nephropathy and dilatation of the renal pelvis occurred in males and females; and tubular cysts, suppurative inflammation and epithelial hyperplasia of the renal pelvis were observed. Epithelial hyperplasia and inflammation of the urinary bladder and suppurative inflammation of the prostate were seen in dosed male mice; and suppurative inflammation of the ovary, uterus and adrenal cortex was observed at increased incidence in high-dose female mice (National Toxicology Program, 1989).

Subcutaneous doses of furosemide at 5 or 15 mg/kg bw per day were given to Sprague-Dawley pups from day 4 to day 28 after birth. Increased urinary calcium and magnesium excretion was observed, and the total concentration of calcium and magnesium in bone was lower. The growth of the pups was inhibited in a dose-dependent manner, and bone mineral content was appropriate for the smaller bone mass (Koo *et al.*, 1986).

Furosemide at 0.5 mM reduced the viability of isolated mouse hepatocytes and induced ultrastructural changes related to toxicity (Massey *et al.*, 1987).

Haemodynamic effects include an increase in renal blood flow (Hook *et al.*, 1965) and decreases in mesenteric (Gaffney *et al.*, 1978), hepatic (Gaffney *et al.*, 1979) and splenic (Gaffney & Williamson, 1979) blood flow.

(iii) *Effects on reproduction and prenatal toxicity*

When CRCD rats were administered furosemide at 37.5, 75, 150 or 300 mg/kg bw twice daily on days 6-17 of gestation [route of administration unspecified], the two highest dose levels, which caused maternal deaths, resulted in increased resorption rates and decreased fetal weights. Dose-related increases in the frequency of wavy ribs occurred in all treatment groups. In addition, five of 176 fetuses in the group receiving 150 mg/kg bw had malformations of the scapula (Robertson *et al.*, 1981).

(iv) *Genetic and related effects*

Furosemide was not mutagenic to *Salmonella typhimurium* in plate incorporation tests in the presence or absence of an exogenous metabolic system (National Toxicology Program, 1989).

The urine of rats treated *in vivo* with furosemide at 45 mg/kg bw did not induce gene conversion in growing cells of *Saccharomyces cerevisiae* D4-RDII (Marquardt & Siebert, 1971).

Furosemide was reported to induce mutations to trifluorothymidine resistance in L5178Y mouse lymphoma cells in the presence of an exogenous metabolic system only at the highest concentration tested (1500 μg/ml). It was also reported to induce sister chromatid exchange and chromosomal aberrations in Chinese hamster CHO cells at 3750 and 5000 μg/ml in the presence and absence of an exogenous metabolic system (National Toxicology Program, 1989). [The Working Group noted the exceptionally high concentrations used in these studies, surpassing the solubility limits of the test substance, which preclude an assessment of the observed effects.] No sister chromatid exchange was induced in a diploid human fibroblast cell line (HE2144) by concentrations of up to 0.33 mg/ml (Sasaki *et al.*, 1980). Furosemide induced chromosomal damage in Chinese hamster lung fibroblasts *in vitro*, but only in the absence of an exogenous metabolic system (Matsuoka *et al.*, 1979; Ishidate, 1988). A concentration-dependent increase in the frequency of chromosomal aberrations was observed in human lymphocytes exposed *in vitro* to furosemide for 24 and 72 h (Jameela *et al.*, 1979). No such effect was detected in the human fibroblast cell line HE2144 (Sasaki *et al.*, 1980).

In male C3H/HE mice treated intraperitoneally with furosemide at 0.3-50 mg/kg bw, a non-dose-dependent increase in the percentage of meiotic cells with chromosomal aberrations was observed during the whole spermatogenic cycle, i.e., in weeks 1-5 after treatment (Subramanyam & Jameela, 1977). [The Working Group noted that only one mouse per dose per week was apparently used.]

(*b*) *Humans*

(i) *Pharmacokinetics*

In healthy subjects, the bioavailability of furosemide ranges from 60 to 69% (Kelly *et al.*, 1973; Rupp, 1974; Tilstone & Fine, 1978); but in end-stage renal failure its availability is reduced to 43-46% (Rane *et al.*, 1978; Tilstone & Fine, 1978). According to early reports, food does not alter bioavailability, although the rate of absorption is decreased (Kelly *et al.*, 1973). In a recent study, however, a reduction of approximately 30% in bioavailability, accompanied by a reduced diuretic effect, was observed when furosemide was given at 40 mg to ten healthy volunteers with breakfast as compared to when it was given in the fasting state (Beermann & Midskov, 1986).

About 99% of furosemide is bound to plasma proteins (Smith *et al.*, 1980), almost exclusively to albumin (Andreasen & Jacobsen, 1974; Prandota & Pruitt, 1975; Branch, 1983).

Two-compartment models are most often used to describe the kinetics of furosemide (Rupp, 1974; Beermann *et al.*, 1975). The half-time of the α-phase averages 10-15 min and that of the β-phase, 47-90 min (Beermann *et al.*, 1977; Mikkelsen & Andreasen, 1977; Rane *et al.*, 1978; Andreasen *et al.*, 1982). The apparent volume of distribution at steady state is approximately 190 ml/kg (Mikkelsen & Andreasen, 1977; Andreasen *et al.*, 1978). The plasma clearance of furosemide is 2.2-3.0 ml/min per kg (Mikkelsen & Andreasen, 1977; Andreasen *et al.*, 1978). A higher non-renal clearance ratio is seen after oral dosing (15.7 ± 4.8%) than after intravenous administration (11.2 ± 4.0%) (Zhu & Koizumi, 1987). Glucuronide conjugate is the only well documented metabolite of furosemide in man (Beermann *et al.*, 1975; Andreasen & Mikkelsen, 1977; Verbeeck *et al.*, 1982).

About 20% of furosemide is eliminated by renal glucuronidation (Smith *et al.*, 1980); it has been suggested that the remaining 25-30% may be secreted into the gut in unchanged and/or conjugated form (Branch, 1983). However, gastrointestinal elimination amounted to only 2% of renal clearance, and active secretion into the intestinal lumen did not occur in six healthy volunteers given furosemide as a 40-mg bolus followed by a continuous infusion of 0.55 mg/kg per h. Plasma clearance was 223 ± 15, renal clearance, 93.1 ± 21.2 and total clearance by the gastrointestinal tract, 2.1 ± 0.2 ml/min. There was no change in the intestinal clearance of furosemide after administration of probenecid, but plasma and renal clearance decreased by 48 and 70%, respectively. It was also shown that incubation of urine samples with β-glucuronidase increased furosemide levels (Valentine *et al.*, 1986).

The disposition of furosemide during renal insufficiency, nephrotic syndrome, cirrhosis and congestive heart failure has been reviewed (Brater, 1986). The mean plasma half-time of furosemide in patients with nephrosis does not differ from that in normal subjects but is prolonged about three fold in patients with uraemia (Rane *et al.*, 1978). A positive relationship between the renal clearance of creatinine and of furosemide has been shown (Beermann *et al.*, 1977). Liver disease may prolong plasma half-time by up to 4.3 h, depending on the degree of liver failure (Allgulander *et al.*, 1980; Fuller et al., 1981; Verbeeck *et al.*, 1982).

(ii) *Adverse effects*

The most common adverse effects of furosemide are fluid and electrolyte imbalance, including hyponatraemia, hypokalaemia and hypochloraemic alkalosis. Hyperuricaemia is relatively common, and a variety of uncommon adverse reactions have been reported (see Reynolds, 1989).

Signs of volume depletion and hypokalaemia have been reported in several studies (Greenblatt *et al.*, 1977; Naranjo *et al.*, 1978; Spino *et al.*, 1978; Lowe *et al.*, 1979). Rare adverse effects reported in patients receiving furosemide include skin rash, thrombocytopenia (Lowe *et al.*, 1979), gynaecomastia (Tuzel, 1981), temporary hearing impairment (Naranjo *et al.*, 1978; Spino *et al.*, 1978) and hepatic coma in cirrhotic patients (Naranjo *et al.*, 1978). Elevated serum concentrations of parathyroid hormone and alkaline phosphatase, together with decreased calcium concentration, were shown in 36 patients with congestive heart failure (Elmgreen *et al.*, 1980).

Renal calcification was documented in ten premature infants who had received furosemide in a dose of at least 2 mg/kg bw per day for at least 12 days (Hufnagle *et al.*, 1982).

(iii) *Effects on reproduction and prenatal toxicity*

No report of pregnancy outcomes following first-trimester use of furosemide has been found. Furosemide has been used extensively for treatment of oedema, hypertension and heart failure in the later stages of pregnancy, with no apparent adverse effect on the fetus or newborn (see review by Briggs *et al.*, 1986).

(iv) *Genetic and related effects*

No data were available to the Working Group.

3.3 Case reports and epidemiological studies of carcinogenicity to humans

In a hypothesis-generating cohort study designed to screen a large number of drugs for possible carcinogenicity [described in detail in the monograph on ampicillin], 2302 persons to whom at least one prescription for furosemide had been dispensed during 1969-73 were followed up for up to 15 years (Selby *et al.*, 1989). Increased risks were noted for cancer of the lung (50 observed, 25.4 expected; $p < 0.002$) and for cancers at all sites combined (233 observed, 164.5 expected; $p < 0.002$). [The Working Group noted that heart failure and cirrhosis of the liver, both of which are associated directly or indirectly with cigarette smoking, are frequent indications for prescribing furosemide, and confounding by cigarette smoking (which was not analysed in the study) may explain the observed associations.] In an earlier report with up to nine years of follow-up (Friedman & Ury, 1983), there was also an association with cancer of the liver (5 observed, 1.6 expected cases; $p < 0.05$). The medical records indicated that this association was due to underlying liver disease for which furosemide was prescribed. [The Working Group noted, as did the authors, that, since some 12 000 comparisons were made in this study, the associations should be verified independently. Data on duration of use were not provided.]

4. Summary of Data Reported and Evaluation

4.1 Exposure data

Furosemide is a diuretic. It has been used extensively since 1964 in the treatment of oedema and hypertension.

4.2 Experimental carcinogenicity data

Furosemide was tested for carcinogenicity by oral administration in one strain of mice and one strain of rats. A small increase in the incidence of mammary gland carcinomas was observed in female mice. No increase in the incidence of tumours was seen in rats.

4.3 Human carcinogenicity data

In one hypothesis-generating study in which many drugs were screened for possible carcinogenicity, associations with furosemide use were observed for cancers of the lung and of all sites combined, which could have been accounted for by smoking and/or chance.

4.4 Other relevant data

The data are inadequate to assess the effects of furosemide on human reproduction. In rats, the drug induces skeletal anomalies.

Furosemide is metabolized by mouse and human liver microsomes and binds covalently to proteins. Renal tubular hyperplasia and hepatic centrilobular necrosis have been observed after administration of large doses of furosemide to mice.

Studies on the induction by furosemide of chromosomal aberrations in mice were inconclusive. Reports of studies on chromosomal aberrations in human cells *in vitro* gave conflicting results; it induced chromosomal damage in hamster cells. Furosemide did not induce sister chromatid exchange in human cells *in vitro*; one study gave questionably positive results for sister chromatid exchange in Chinese hamster cells and for gene mutation in mouse lymphoma cells. The urine of rats treated with this drug did not induce gene conversion in *Saccharomyces cerevisiae*. It was not mutagenic to *Salmonella typhimurium*. (See Appendix 1.)

4.5 Evaluation[1]

There is *inadequate evidence* for the carcinogenicity of furosemide in humans.

There is *inadequate evidence* for the carcinogenicity of furosemide in experimental animals.

Overall evaluation

Furosemide *is not classifiable as to its carcinogenicity to humans (Group 3)*.

5. References

Allgulander, C., Beermann, G. & Sjögren, S. (1980) Frusemide pharmacokinetics in patients with liver disease. *Clin. Pharmacokinet.*, 5, 570-575

Andreasen, F. & Jakobsen, P. (1974) Determination of furosemide in blood plasma and its binding to proteins in normal plasma and in plasma from patients with acute renal failure. *Acta pharmacol. toxicol.*, 35, 49-57

Andreasen, F. & Mikkelsen, E. (1977) Distribution, elimination and effect of furosemide in normal subjects and in patients with heart failure. *Eur. J. clin. Pharmacol.*, 12, 15-22

Andreasen, F., Hansen, H.E. & Mikkelsen, E. (1978) Pharmacokinetics of furosemide in anephric patients and in normal subjects. *Eur. J. clin. Pharmacol.*, 13, 41-48

Andreasen, F., Kjeldahl Christensen, C., Kjær Jakobsen, F. & Mogensen, C.E. (1981) The use of HPLC to elucidate the metabolism and urinary excretion of furosemide and its metabolic products. *Acta pharmacol. toxicol.*, 49, 223-229

Andreasen, F., Kjeldahl-Christensen, C. Kjær-Jacobsen, F., Jansen, J., Mogensen, C.E. & Lederballe-Pedersen, O. (1982) The individual variation in pharmacokinetics and pharmacodynamics of furosemide in young normal male subjects. *Eur J. clin. Invest.*, 12, 247-255

Anon. (1979) *Pharmaceutical Codex*, 11th ed., London, The Pharmaceutical Press, pp. 374-376

Apoteksbolaget (1988) *Svensk Läkemedelsstatistic* [Swedish Drugs Statistics], Stockholm, Pharmaceutical Association of Sweden

Apoteksbolaget (1989) *Outprint of the Drug Data Base (17 October 1989)*, Stockholm, Pharmaceutical Association of Sweden

Barnhart, E. (1989) *Physicians' Desk Reference*, 43rd ed., Oradell, NJ, Medical Economics, p. 312

Beermann, B. & Midskov, C. (1986) Reduced bioavailability and effect of furosemide given with food. *Eur. J. clin. Pharmacol.*, 29, 725-727

---

[1]For description of the italicized terms, see Preamble, pp. 26–29.

Beermann, B., Dalen, E., Lindström, B. & Rosen, A. (1975) On the fate of furosemide in man. *Eur. J. clin. Pharmacol.*, *9*, 57-61

Beermann, B., Dalen, E. & Lindström, B. (1977) Elimination of furosemide in healthy subjects and in those with renal failure. *Clin. Pharmacol. Ther.*, *22*, 70-78

Branch, R.A. (1983) Role of binding in distribution of furosemide: where is nonrenal clearance? *Fed. Proc.*, *42*, 1699-1702

Brater, D.C. (1986) Disposition and response to bumetanide and furosemide. *Am. J. Cardiol.*, *57*, 20A-25A

Briggs, G.G., Freeman, R.K. & Yaffe, S.J. (1986) *Drugs in Pregnancy and Lactation*, 2nd ed., London, Williams & Wilkins, pp. 195-196

Chemical Information Services (1989-90) *Directory of World Chemical Producers*, Oceanside, NY

Dybing, E. (1977) Activation of α-methyldopa, paracetamol and furosemide by human liver microsomes. *Acta pharmacol. toxicol.*, *41*, 89-93

Elmgreen, J., Tougaard, L., Leth, A. & Christensen, M.S. (1980) Elevated serum parathyroid hormone concentration during treatment with high ceiling diuretics. *Eur. J. clin. Pharmacol.*, *18*, 363-364

Finnish Committee on Drug Information and Statistics (1987) *Finnish Statistics on Medicine*, Helsinki, National Board of Health

Friedman, G.D. & Ury, H.K. (1983) Screening for possible drug carcinogenicity: second report of findings. *J. natl Cancer Inst.*, *71*, 1165-1175

Fuller, R., Hoppel, C. & Ingalls, S.T. (1981) Furosemide kinetics in patients with hepatic cirrhosis with ascites. *Clin. Pharmacol. Ther.*, *30*, 461-467

Gaffney, G.R. & Wiliamson, H.E. (1979) Effect of furosemide on canine splenic arterial blood flow. *Res. Commun. chem. pathol. Pharmacol.*, *23*, 627-630

Gaffney, G.R., Day, D.K. & Williamson, H.E. (1978) Effect of furosemide on mesenteric blood flow in the dog. *Res. Commun. chem. Pathol. Pharmacol.*, *22*, 605-608

Gaffney, G.R., Betzer, L.K., Mow, M.T. & Williamson, H.E. (1979) Decrease in hepatic blood flow during furosemide-induced diuresis. *Arch. int. Pharmacodyn.*, *239*, 155-160

Goldenthal, E.I. (1971) A compilation of LD50 values in newborn and adult animals. *Toxicol. appl. Pharmacol.*, *18*, 185-207

Greenblatt, D.J., Duhme, D.W., Allen, M.D. & Koch-Weser, J. (1977) Clinical toxicity of furosemide in hospitalized patients. *Am. Heart J.*, *94*, 6-13

Hammarlund, M.M. & Paalzow, L.K. (1982) Dose-dependent pharmacokinetics of furosemide in the rat. *Biopharmacol. Drug Dispos*, *3*, 345-359

Hook, J.B. & Williamson, H.E. (1965) Influence of probenecid and alterations in acid-base balance of the saluretic activity of furosemide. *J. Pharmacol. exp. Ther.*, *149*, 404-408

Horioka, M., Saito, T., Takagi, K. & Takasugi, M. (1982) *Drugs in Japan (Ethical Drugs)*, Tokyo, Japan Pharmaceutical Information Center

Hufnagle, K.G., Khan, S.N., Penn, D., Caccearelli, A. & Williams, P. (1982) Renal calcifications: a comparison of long-term furosemide therapy in premature infants. *Pediatrics*, *70*, 360-363

IARC (1987) *IARC Monographs on the Evaluation of Carcinogenic Risks to Humans*, Suppl. 7, *Overall Evaluations of Carcinogenicity: An Updating of* IARC Monographs *Volumes 1 to 42*, Lyon, pp. 349-350

Ishidate, M., Jr (1988) Furosemide. In: *Data Book of Chromosomal Aberration Test* In Vitro, rev. ed., Amsterdam, Elsevier

Jameela, X., Subramanyam, S. & Sadasivan, G. (1979) Clastogenic effects of frusemide on human leukocytes in culture. *Mutat. Res.*, *66*, 69-74

Kelly, M.R., Cutler, R.E., Forrey, A.W. & Kimpel, B.M. (1973) Pharmacokinetics of orally administered furosemide. *Clin. Pharmacol. Ther.*, *15*, 178-186

Kitani, M., Ozaki, Y., Katayama, K., Kakemi, M. & Koizumi, T. (1988) A kinetic study on drug distribution: furosemide in rats. *Chem. pharm. Bull.*, *36*, 1053-1062

Koo, W.W.K., Guan, A.-P., Tsang, R.C., Laskarzewski, P. & Neumann, V. (1986) Growth failure and decreased bone mineral of newborn rats with chronic furosemide therapy. *Pediatr. Res.*, *20*, 74-78

La Piana Simonsen, L. (1989) Top 200 drugs of 1988. Branded new Rxs rise 4.0% and total Rxs move up 1.2%. *Pharm. Times*, *55*, 40-48

Lee, M.G. & Chiou, L.W. (1983) Evaluation of potential causes for the incomplete bioavailability of furosemide: gastric first-pass metabolism. *J. Pharmacokinet. Biopharmacol.*, *11*, 623-640

Lowe, J., Gray, J., Henry, D.A. & Lawson, D.H. (1979) Adverse reactions to frusemide in hospital inpatients. *Br. med. J.*, *ii*, 360-362

Marquardt, H. & Siebert, D. (1971) Ein neuer host mediated assay (Urinversuch) zum Nachweis mutagener Stoffe mit *Saccharomyces cerevisiae*. [A new host-mediated assay (urine test) for the detection of mutagenic material with *Saccharomyces cerevisiae* (Ger.).] *Naturwissenschaften*, *58*, 568

Massey, T.E., Walker, R.M., McElligott, T.F. & Racz, W.J. (1987) Furosemide toxicity in isolated mouse hepatocyte suspensions. *Toxicology*, *43*, 149-160

Matsuoka, A., Hayashi, M. & Ishidate, M., Jr (1979) Chromosomal aberration tests on 29 chemicals combined with S9 mix in vitro. *Mutat. Res.*, *66*, 277-290

Mikkelsen, E. & Andreasen, F. (1977) Simultaneous determination of furosemide and two of its possible metabolites in biological fluids. *Acta pharmacol. toxicol.*, *41*, 254-262

Mishra, P., Karolia, D. & Agrawal, R. (1989) Simple colorimetric estimation of furosemide in dosage forms: Part I. *Curr. Sci.*, *58*, 503-505

Mitchell, J.R., Potter, W.Z., Hinsen, J.A. & Jollow, D.J. (1974) Hepatic necrosis caused by furosemide. *Nature*, *251*, 508-511

Naranjo, C.A., Busto, U. & Cassis, L. (1978) Furosemide-induced adverse reactions during hospitalization. *Am. J. Hosp. Pharm.*, *35*, 294-298

National Toxicology Program (1989) *Toxicology and Carcinogenesis Studies of Furosemide (CAS No. 54-31-9) in F344/N Rats and B6C3F1 Mice (Feed Studies)* (Technical Report No. 356), Research Triangle Park, NC, US Department of Health and Human Services, pp. 1-90

Prandota, J. & Pruitt, A.W. (1975) Furosemide binding to human albumin and plasma of nephrotic children. *Clin. Pharmacol. Ther.*, *17*, 159-166

Rane, A., Villeneube, J.P., Stone, W.J., Nies, A.S., Wilkinson, G.R. & Branch, R.A. (1978) Plasma binding and disposition of furosemide in the nephrotic syndrome and in uremia. *Clin. pharmacol. Ther.*, 24, 199-207

Reynolds, J.E.F., ed. (1989) *Martindale. The Extra Pharmacopeia*, 29th ed., London, The Pharmaceutical Press, pp. 987-991

Robertson, R.T., Minsker, D.H., Bokelmann, D.L., Durand G. & Conquet, P. (1981) Potassium loss as a causative factor for skeletal malformations in rats produced by indacrinone: a new investigational loop diuretic. *Toxicol. appl. Pharmacol.*, 60, 142-150

Romanova, T.V. & Rudzit, E.A. (1985) Comparative study of the diuretic action of bumetanide and other antidiuretic agents in mice. *Pharm. Chem. J.*, 19, 706-708

Rupp, W. (1974) Pharmacokinetics and pharmacodynamics of Lasix. *Scott. med. J.*, 19, 5-13

Sasaki, M., Sugimura, K., Yoshida, M.A. & Abe, S. (1980) Cytogenetic effects of 60 chemicals on cultured human and Chinese hamster cells. *Kromosomo*, II-20, 574-584

Selby, J.V., Friedman, G.D. & Fireman, B.H. (1989) Screening prescription drugs for possible carcinogenicity: 11 to 15 years of follow-up. *Cancer Res.*, 49, 5736-5747

Shibata, M.A., Hagiwara, A., Tamano, S., Ono, S. & Fukushima, S. (1989) Lack of a modifying effect by the diuretic drug furosemide on the development of neoplastic lesions in rat two-stage urinary bladder carcinogenesis. *J. Toxicol. environ. Health*, 26, 255-265

Smith, D.E., Lin, E.T. & Benet, L.Z. (1980) Absorption and disposition of furosemide in healthy volunteers, measured with a metabolite-specific assay. *Drug Metab. Dispos.*, 8, 337-342

Sood, S.P., Green, V.I. & Norton, Z.M. (1987) Routine methods in toxicology and therapeutic drug monitoring by high performance liquid chromatography: III. A rapid microscale method for determination of furosemide in plasma and urine. *Ther. Drug Monit.*, 9, 484-488

Spino, M., Sellers, E.M., Kaplan, H.L., Stapleton, C. & MacLeod, S.M. (1978) Adverse biochemical and clinical consequences of furosemide administration. *Can. med. Assoc. J.*, 118, 1513-1518

Spitznagle, L.A., Wirth, P.J., Boobis, S.W., Thorgeirsson, S.S. & Nelson, W.L. (1977) The role of biliary excretion in the hepatotoxicity of furosemide in the mouse. *Toxicol. appl. Pharmacol.*, 39, 283-294

Sturm, K., Siedel, W. & Weyer, R. (1962) Sulphamoylanthranilic acids, FRG patent 1,122,541 (CA 56:14032-33, 1962)

Subramanyam, S. & Jameela (1977) Studies on cytological effects of frusemide on meiotic cells of male mice. *Indian J. med. Res.*, 66, 104-113

Tilstone, W.J. & Fine, A. (1978) Furosemide kinetics in renal failure. *Clin. Pharmacol. Ther.*, 23, 644-650

Tuzel, I.H. (1981) Comparison of adverse reactions to bumetanide and furosemide. *J. clin. Pharmacol.*, 21, 615-619

Uchino, K., Isozaki, S., Saitoh, Y., Nakagawa, F. & Tamura, Z. (1984) Quantitative determination of furosemide in plasma, plasma water, urine and ascites fluid by high performance liquid chromatography. *J. Chromatogr.*, 308, 241-249

US Pharmacopeial Convention, Inc. (1989) *US Pharmacopeia*, 22nd rev., Easton, PA, pp. 597-598

Valentine, J.F., Braterm, D.C. & Kreis, G.J. (1986) Clearance of furosemide by the gastrointestinal tract. *J. Pharmacol. exp. Ther.*, 236, 177-180

Verbeeck, R.K., Gerkens, J.F., Wilkinson, F.R. & Branch, R.A. (1981) Disposition of furosemide in functionally hepatectomized dogs. *J. Pharmacol. exp. Ther.*, 216, 479-483

Verbeeck, R.K., Patwardhan, R.V., Villeneuve, J-P., Wilkinson, F.R. & Branch, R.A. (1982) Furosemide disposition in cirrhosis. *Clin. Pharmacol. Ther.*, 31, 719-925

Weiner, I.M. & Mudge, G.H. (1985) Diuretics and other agents employed in the mobilization of edema fluid. In: Gilman, A.G., Goodman, L.S., Rall, T.W. & Murad, F., eds, *Goodman and Gilman's The Pharmacological Basis of Therapeutics*, 7th ed., New York, MacMillan, pp. 896-900

Windholz, M., ed. (1983) *The Merck Index*, 10th ed., Rahway, NJ, Merck & Co., p. 615

Wirth, P.J., Bettis, C.J. & Nelson, W.L. (1976) Microsomal metabolism of furosemide. Evidence for the nature of the reactive intermediate involved in covalent binding. *Mol. Pharmacol.*, 12, 759-768

Yakatan, G.J., Maness, D.D., Scholler, J., Johnston, J.T., Novick, W.J. & Doluisio, J.T. (1979) Plasma tissue levels of furosemide in dogs and monkeys following single and multiple oral doses. *Res. Commun. chem. pathol. Pharmacol.*, 24, 465-482

Zeiger, E., Anderson, B., Haworth, S., Lawlor, T., Mortelmans, K. & Speck, W. (1987) *Salmonella* mutagenicity tests: III. Results from the testing of 255 chemicals. *Environ. Mutagenesis*, 9 (Suppl. 9), 1-110

Zhu, J. & Koizumi, T. (1987) A study on furosemide disposition in man. *J. Pharmacobio-Dyn.*, 10, 370-376

HYDROCHLOROTHIAZIDE

1. Chemical and Physical Data

1.1 Synonyms

Chem. Abstr. Services Reg. No.: 58-93-5
Chem. Abstr. Name: 2*H*-1,2,4-Benzothiadiazine-7-sulfonamide, 6-chloro-3,4-dihydro-1,1-dioxide
Synonyms: 6-Chloro-3,4-dihydro-7-sulfamoyl-2*H*-1,2,4-benzothiadiazine 1,1-dioxide; 6-chloro-7-sulfamyl-3,4-dihydro-1,2,4-benzothiadiazine 1,1-dioxide-3,4-dihydrochlorothiazide; chlorosulfonamidodihydrobenzothiadiazine dioxide; chlorosulthiadil

1.2 Structural and molecular formula and molecular weight

$C_7H_8ClN_3O_4S$ Mol. wt: 297.72

1.3 Chemical and physical properties of the pure substance

From Deppeler (1981), unless otherwise specified
(a) *Description*: White, fluffy, microcrystalline powder
(b) *Melting-point*: 273-275 °C (Windholz, 1983)
(c) *Solubility*: Practically insoluble in water; soluble in dilute ammonia and sodium hydroxide; soluble in methanol, ethanol, acetone and acetonitrile
(d) *Spectroscopy data*: Infrared, ultraviolet, nuclear magnetic resonance and mass spectra have been reported.
(e) *Stability data*: Stable in bulk for five years at room temperature; at extremes of pH in aqueous solution, hydrolysed to formaldehyde and 6-chloro-2,4-disulfamoylaniline

(f) *Dissociation constant*: pK_a 7.2, 9.2 (Windholz, 1983)

1.4 Technical products and impurities

Trade names: Apo-Hydro; Aquarius; Atenadon; Bremil; Caturida; Chlorthia; Chlorzide; Cidrex; Cloredema; Delco-Retic; Dichlorosal; Dichlortride; Dichlotride; Diclotride; Didral; Diidrotiazide; Direma; Disalunil; Diu 25; Diucen-H; Diurex; Diursana-H; Dixidrasi; Edemex; Esidrex; Esidrix; Fluvin; Hidrenox; Hidroronol; Hidrosaluretil; Hydril; Hydro-Aquil; Hydro-Diuril; Hydro-MURIL; Hydrosaluric; Hydrothide; Hydro-Z; Hydrozide; Hypothiazide; Idrodiuvis; Idrofluin; Idrolisin; Ivaugan; Jen-diral; Lexor; Loqua; Maschitt; Mietrin; Natrimax; Nefrix; Neo-Codema; Neoflumen; Neo-Flumen; Neo Minzil; Newtolide; Novohydrazide; Oretic; Pantemon; Panurin; Ridaq; Ro-Hydrazide; Salupres; Serapres; SK-Hydrochlorothiazide; Tandiur; Thiaretic; Thiuretic; Urirex; Urodiazin; Urozide; Vetidrex

Hydrochlorothiazide is also contained in numerous multi-ingredient preparations.

Hydrochlorothiazide is available as tablets for oral use (25, 50 or 100 mg) containing calcium phosphate, D & C Yellow #6, gelatin, lactose, magnesium stearate, starch and talc (see IARC, 1987) (Barnhart, 1989).

2. Production, Occurrence, Use and Analysis

2.1 Production and occurrence

Hydrochlorothiazide in synthesized by either the reaction of *para*-formaldehyde with 5-chloro-2,4-disulfamoylaniline in nonaqueous media, or the reaction of formaldehyde with 6-chloro-7-sulfamoyl-2*H*-1,2,4-benzothiadiazine-1,1-dioxide in aqueous alkaline solution (Deppeler, 1981). It is synthesized in China, Hungary, India, Italy, Japan, Romania, Switzerland, the UK, the USA and Yugoslavia (Chemical Information Services, 1989-90).

Hydrochlorothiazide has been used as a diuretic and antihypertensive agent since 1957 (Reynolds, 1989). More prescriptions were written for hydrochlorthiazide/triamterene combination than for any other prescription drug product in the USA in 1984 and 1985 (Chappell, 1985), and hydrochlorothiazide was the sixth most frequently prescribed generic drug in 1987 and 1988 in the USA (La Piana Simonsen, 1989). In 1988, this drug was sold in Sweden at a level of 0.14 defined daily doses per 1000 inhabitants (Apoteksbolaget, 1988, 1989). In 1987, it was sold in Finland at a level of 2.06 defined daily doses per 1000 inhabitants (Finnish Committee on Drug Information and Statistics, 1987).

Hydrochlorothiazide is not known to occur as a natural product.

2.2 Use

Hydrochlorothiazide is a thiazide diuretic (Reynolds, 1989). It is used to reduce oedema associated with heart failure, as an antihypertensive agent, and for special indications such as Ménière's disease (Roydhouse, 1974) and reduction of the formation of renal calculi in patients with hypercalciuria (Yendt et al., 1970; Baggio et al., 1986). The daily dose of hydrochlorothiazide in treating oedema is 25-50 mg after an initial dose of twice this amount. The daily dose for children is 2.5 mg/kg bw and that for infants under six months, 3.5 mg/kg bw. The antihypertensive doses of hydrochlorothiazide vary between 25 and 200 mg daily (Reynolds, 1989).

2.3 Analysis

Hydrochlorothiazide can be analysed in urine and plasma by colorimetry, thin-layer chromatography and high-performance liquid chromatography (Sheppard et al., 1960; Redalieu et al., 1978; Suria, 1978; Koopmans et al., 1984; Alton et al., 1986; Fullinfaw et al., 1987; van der Meer & Brown, 1987). Analysis of hydrochlorothiazide in pharmaceutical preparations has also been reported (Cieri, 1988; US Pharmacopieal Convention, Inc., 1989).

3. Biological Data Relevant to the Evaluation of Carcinogenic Risk to Humans

3.1 Carcinogenicity studies in animals

(a) Oral administration

Mouse: Groups of 50 male and 50 female B6C3F1 mice, seven to eight weeks of age, were fed hydrochlorothiazide (> 98% pure) at 0, 2500 or 5000 mg/kg of diet for 103-104 weeks (average daily intake, 280 or 575 mg/kg bw), and all survivors were killed at weeks 113-114. Mean body weights were similar in control and treated mice. Survival in males was: control, 43/50; low-dose, 42/50 and high-dose, 43/50; that in females was: control, 38/50; low-dose, 40/50 and high-dose, 35/50. All animals were necropsied, and samples taken from all major organs, tissues and gross lesions were examined histologically. A significant increase in the incidence of hepatocellular adenomas and of combined adenomas and carcinomas (control, 7/48; low-dose, 10/49; high-dose, 21/50 ($p = 0.009$, incidental tumour test)) but not of carcinoma alone was observed in males. No increase in the incidence of any other neoplasm was observed (National Toxicology Program, 1989).

Rat: A group of 24 male and 24 female Fischer 344 rats, six to eight weeks of age, were fed hydrochlorothiazide [purity unspecified] at 1000 mg/kg of diet for 104 weeks (total intake: males, 21 g; females, 14 g). A control group of 24 male and 24 female rats remained untreated. Over 70% of the rats survived more than two years, with similar survival rates in all groups. All survivors were killed after 130 weeks; complete necropsies were performed on all animals, and major organs were examined histologically. No difference in overall tumour incidence or in the incidence of tumours at any site was observed between treated and control rats (Lijinsky & Reuber, 1987).

Four groups each of 50 male and 50 female Fischer 344/N rats, seven to eight weeks of age, were fed hydrochlorothiazide (>98% pure) at 0, 250, 500 or 2000 mg/kg of diet for 105-106 weeks (average daily intake, 11, 23 or 89 mg/kg bw), and all survivors were killed at weeks 113-114. Survival was—males: control, 18/50; low-dose, 16/50; mid-dose, 9/50; high-dose, 11/50; females: control, 31/50; low-dose, 25/50; mid-dose, 30/50; high-dose, 27/50. All animals were necropsied, and samples from all major organs, tissues and gross lesions were examined histologically. No increase in either overall tumour incidence or in the incidence of tumours at any site was observed (National Toxicology Program, 1989).

(b) *Administration in combination with other compounds*

Rat: In the experiment by Lijinsky and Reuber (1987), described above, three groups each of 24 male and 24 female Fischer 344 rats, six to eight weeks of age, were fed diets containing hydrochlorothiazide [purity unspecified] at 1000 mg/kg, sodium nitrite at 2000 mg/kg or hydrochlorothiazide at 1000 mg/kg plus sodium nitrite at 2000 mg/kg for 104 weeks. Over 70% of the rats survived more than two years, with similar survival rates in all groups. All survivors were killed after 130 weeks; complete necropsies were performed on all animals, and major organs were examined histologically. No difference in overall tumour incidence or in the incidence of tumours at any site was observed between treated and control rats.

3.2 Other relevant data

(a) *Experimental systems*

(i) *Absorption, distribution, excretion and metabolism*

No data were available to the Working Group.

(ii) *Toxic effects*

The oral LD_{50} for hydrochlorothiazide in mice was 3080 mg/kg bw (Barnes & Eltherington, 1965).

All 20 dogs receiving hydrochlorothiazide at daily doses of 50-200 mg for up to nine months had enlarged, hyperactive parathyroid glands (Pickleman *et al.*, 1969).

In male (but not female) Syrian golden hamsters receiving hydrochlorothiazide at 1 or 2 mg/kg bw by gavage for six months, increased total cholesterol and high-density lipoprotein cholesterol levels were observed. When a dose of 4 mg/kg bw was administered, a similar increase was seen in animals of each sex (Sarva *et al.*, 1985).

All male and female rats fed diets containing 3.125-50 g/kg (five dose levels) hydrochlorothiazide survived for 15 days. Thymic haemorrhage of slight to moderate severity was observed in animals receiving the highest doses, but no other toxic effect was observed (National Toxicology Program, 1989).

In groups of 24 male and 24 female rats fed hydrochlorotriazide at 1000 mg/kg of diet for two years, the incidence and severity of chronic progressive nephropathy and of lesions secondary to chronic renal disease, polyarteritis and mural thrombosis were increased (Lijinsky & Reuber, 1987).

In a two-year study (see section 3.1), there was a uniform reduction in the body weight of treated rats (male and female) at all doses. Chronic renal disease (cysts of the parenchyma and epithelial hyperplasia of the renal pelvis) was present in all groups of male and female rats, but it was more severe in dosed groups. Secondary signs of chronic renal disease, including parathyroid hyperplasia, mineralization in multiple organs and fibrous osteodystrophy, also occurred at increased frequency in dosed groups. No other lesion in rats appeared to be related to exposure to hydrochlorothiazide. In mice, a two-year exposure had only negligible effects on body weight. No increase in the frequency of non-neoplastic lesions in the kidney, urinary bladder or any other organ was attributed to hydrochlorothiazide administration (National Toxicology Program, 1989).

(iii) *Effects on reproduction and prenatal toxicity*

Hydrochlorothiazide was administered by gavage to pregnant CD rats at 100, 300 or 1000 mg/kg bw per day and to CD-1 mice at 300, 1000 or 3000 mg/kg bw per day on gestational days 6-15. No dose-related fetal toxicity or significant increase in the incidence of malformations was observed (National Toxicology Program, 1989).

(iv) *Genetic and related effects*

Hydrochlorothiozide did not induce reversion in an *arg⁻* strain of *Escherichia coli* (Hs30R) (Fujita, 1985). It was not mutagenic to *Salmonella typhimurium* in the presence or absence of an exogenous metabolic system (Waskell, 1978; Andrews *et al.*, 1984). [The Working Group noted that only one concentration was used in both studies.] In strain TA98, but not in TA1535, TA1537 or TA100, a small, reproducible, concentration-dependent increase in the mean number of revertants was observed in the absence, but not in the presence, of an exogenous metabolic system (Mortelmans *et al.*, 1986).

In a spot test, hydrochlorothiazide induced nondisjunction and mitotic crossing-over in *Aspergillus nidulans* (Bignami *et al.*, 1974).

Hydrochlorothiazide did not induce sex-linked recessive lethal mutations in *Drosophila melanogaster* either fed or injected with solutions of 10 mg/ml (Valencia *et al.*, 1985).

At concentrations above 500 µg/ml, hydrochlorothiazide produced cytotoxic effects and induced mutations to trifluorothymidine resistance in L5178Y mouse lymphoma cells in the absence of an exogenous metabolic system (National Toxicology Program, 1989). Significant, but not concentration-dependent, increases in the frequency of sister chromatid exchange were observed in Chinese hamster CHO cells in the presence and absence of an exogenous metabolic system (Galloway *et al.*, 1987). Chromosomal aberrations were not found in Chinese hamster lung CHL cells, but polyploidy was observed after 48 h treatment (Ishidate, 1988). Chromosomal aberrations were also not detected in Chinese hamster CHO cells in the presence or absence of an exogenous metabolic system at concentrations of up to 2600 µg/ml (Galloway *et al.*, 1987).

(*b*) *Humans*

(i) *Pharmacokinetics*

The pharmacokinetics of hydrochlorothiazide have been reviewed (Welling, 1986).

Hydrochlorothiazide is incompletely absorbed from the duodenum and upper jejunum (Beermann *et al.*, 1976), and plasma concentrations, peaking at about 2-3 h after intake, are proportional to the dose within the range 25-100 mg (Patel *et al.*, 1984). Administration with food either enhances (Beermann & Groschinsky-Grind, 1978) or reduces (Barbhaiya *et al.*, 1982) the absorption of hydrochlorothiazide, as compared with fasting conditions. The discrepancy is partly attributable to differences in fasting states in these experiments. Food might delay passage through the small intestine; patients with intestinal shunt surgery and accelerated intestinal passage have shown reduced absorption of hydrochlorothiazide (Backman *et al.*, 1979).

Hydrochlorothiazide is concentrated in red blood cells (Beermann *et al.*, 1976; Redalieu *et al.*, 1985). It is excreted almost entirely unchanged in urine; its renal clearance rate (about 300 ml/min) indicates combined glomerular filtration and tubular secretion (Barbhaiya *et al.*, 1982). Its plasma elimination half-time is about 6 h initially but up to 15 h terminally (Patel *et al.*, 1984). In patients with decreased renal function, the plasma half-time of hydrochlorothiazide is prolonged to 20 h (Niemeyer *et al.*, 1983).

Concentrations of hydrochlorothiazide in maternal plasma and umbilical cord plasma were similar (Beermann *et al.*, 1980) and were lower than those in amniotic fluid (Mulley *et al.*, 1978). The drug was detected in the milk of nursing mothers treated with it, but no measurable concentration was found in nursing infants (detection limit, 20 ng/ml) (Miller *et al.*, 1982).

(ii) *Adverse effects*

Administration of large doses of hydrochlorothiazide often leads to electrolyte imbalance, including hypochloraemic alkalosis, hyponatraemia, hypokalaemia and hypercalcaemia (Porter *et al.*, 1978; Zalin *et al.*, 1984; Bayer *et al.*, 1986; Reynolds, 1989).

Like other thiazide diuretics, hydrochlorotriazide is known to produce metabolic effects, such as hyperglycaemia and glycosuria, in diabetic and other susceptible patients (Flamenbaum, 1983; Freis, 1986). It produces asymptomatic hyperuricaemia in many patients, although actual attacks of gout are not common (Anon., 1987).

Hyperparathyroidism associated with prolonged intake of thiazides, including hydrochlorothiazide, has been reported (Paloyan & Pickleman, 1969; Christensson *et al.*, 1977; Klimiuk *et al.*, 1981).

A number of skin diseases of an allergic and idiosyncratic nature have been reported among patients treated with thiazide diuretics (Ebstein & Wintroub, 1985; Reed *et al.*, 1985; Hardwick & Saxe, 1986).

Interstitial nephritis (Linton *et al.*, 1980; Scully *et al.*, 1983), idiosyncratic pneumonitis (Piper *et al.*, 1983; Parfrey & Herlong, 1984), thrombocytopenia (Eisner & Crowell, 1971), intravascular haemolysis (Beck *et al.*, 1984) and pancreatitis (Cornish *et al.*, 1961) have been reported in patients treated with thiazide diuretics.

(iii) *Effects on reproduction and prenatal toxicity*

In the Collaborative Perinatal Project, in which drug intake and pregnancy outcome were studied in a series of 50 282 women in 1959-65, 107 women had been exposed to hydrochlorothiazide during the first trimester of pregnancy. There were nine malformed children in the exposed group, giving a nonsignificant standardized relative risk of 1.2 (Heinonen *et al.*, 1977).

(iv) *Genetic and related effects*

No data were available to the Working Group.

3.3 Case reports and epidemiological studies of carcinogenicity to humans

In a hypothesis-generating cohort study designed to screen a large number of drugs for possible carcinogenicity (described in detail in the monograph on ampicillin), 12 799 persons to whom at least one prescription for a thiazide diuretic had been dispensed during 1969-73 were followed up for up to 15 years (Selby *et al.*, 1989). Hydrochlorothiazide was the predominant drug used in this group.

Increased risks were noted for cancer of the prostate (53 cases observed, 38.2 expected; $p < 0.05$) during follow-up of up to seven years (Friedman & Ury, 1980) and for cancers at all sites combined (1209 observed, 1132.9 expected; $p < 0.05$) during follow-up of up to 15 years (Selby *et al.*, 1989). The association with prostatic cancer diminished in later follow-up. [The Working Group noted that prostatic cancer may be diagnosed more readily in patients under more intensive medical care. In addition, as also noted by the authors, since some 12 000 comparisons were made in this hypothesis-generating study, the associations should be verified independently. Data on duration of use were not provided.]

4. Summary of Data Reported and Evaluation

4.1 Exposure data

Hydrochlorothiazide has been used extensively since 1957 as a diuretic and antihypertensive agent.

4.2 Experimental carcinogenicity data

Hydrochlorothiazide was tested for carcinogenicity by oral administration in one strain of mice and one strain of rats. An increase in the incidence of hepatocellular adenomas was observed in male mice. No increase in the incidence of tumours at any site was observed in two studies in rats.

4.3 Human carcinogenicity data

In one hypothesis-generating study in which many drugs were screened for possible carcinogenicity, associations with hydrochlorothiazide use were observed for cancers of the prostate and of all sites combined, which could be accounted for by chance.

4.4 Other relevant data

One study provided no evidence that use of hydrochlorothiazide in the first trimester of pregnancy is associated with the induction of birth defects. In rats, no teratogenic, embryotoxic or fetotoxic effect was observed.

Hydrochlorothiazide induced gene mutations in mouse lymphoma cells and sister chromatid exchange in Chinese hamster cells. It did not induce chromosomal aberrations in Chinese hamster cells *in vitro* or sex-linked recessive lethal mutations in *Drosophila*. Hydrochlorothiazide induced mitotic recombination and nondisjunction in *Aspergillus nidulans*. It was not mutagenic to *Salmonella typhimurium* or *Escherichia coli*. (See Appendix 1.)

4.5 Evaluation[1]

There is *inadequate evidence* for the carcinogenicity of hydrochlorothiazide in humans.

There is *inadequate evidence* for the carcinogenicity of hydrochlorothiazide in experimental animals.

Overall evaluation

Hydrochlorothiazide *is not classifiable as to its carcinogenicity to humans (Group 3)*.

5. References

Alton, K.B., Desrivieres, D. & Patrick, J.E. (1986) High-performance liquid chromatographic assay for hydrochlorothiazide in human urine. *J. Chromatogr.*, 374, 103-110

Andrews, A.W., Lijinsky, W. & Snyder, S.W. (1984) Mutagenicity of amine drugs and their products of nitrosation. *Mutat. Res.*, 135, 105-108

Anon. (1987) Uric acid in hypertension. *Lancet*, i, 1124-1125

Apoteksbolaget (1988) *Svensk Läkemedelsstatistic* [Swedish Drugs Statistics], Stockholm, Pharmaceutical Association of Sweden

Apoteksbolaget (1989) *Outprint of the Drug Data Base (17 October 1989)*, Stockholm, Pharmaceutical Association of Sweden

Backman, L., Beermann, B., Groschinsky-Grind, M. & Hallberg, D. (1979) Malabsorption of hydrochlorothiazide following intestinal shunt surgery. *Clin. Pharmacokinet.*, 4, 63-68

Baggio, B., Gambaro, G., Marchini, F., Cicerello, E., Tenconi, R., Clementi, M. & Borsatti, A. (1986) An inheritable anomaly of red-cell oxalate transport in 'primary' calcium nephrolithiasis correctable with diuretics. *New Engl. J. Med.*, 314, 599-604

Barbhaiya, R.H., Graig, W.A., Corrick-West, H.P. & Welling, P.G. (1982) Pharmacokinetics of hydrochlorothiazide in fasted and nonfasted subjects: a comparison of plasma level and urinary excretion methods. *J. pharm. Sci.*, 71, 245-248

Barnes, C.D. & Eltherington, L.G. (1965) *Drug Dosages in Laboratory Animals, A Handbook*, Berkeley, CA, University of California Press, p. 73

---

[1]For description of the italicized terms, see Preamble, pp. 26–29.

Barnhart, E. (1989) *Physicians' Desk Reference*, 43rd ed., Oradell, NJ, Medical Economics, p. 314

Bayer, A.J., Garag, R., Browne, S. & Pathy, M.S.J. (1986) Plasma electrolytes in elderly patients taking fixed combination diuretics. *Postgrad. med. J.*, 62, 159-162

Beck, M.L., Cline, J.F., Hardman, J.T., Racela, L.S. & Davis, J.W. (1984) Fatal intravascular immune hemolysis induced by hydrochlorothiazide. *Am. J. clin. Pathol.*, 81, 791-794

Beermann, B. & Groschinsky-Grind, M. (1978) Gastrointestinal absorption of hydrochlorothiazide enhanced by concomitant intake of food. *Eur. J. clin. Pharmacol.*, 13, 125-128

Beermann, B., Groschinsky-Grind, M. & Rosen, A. (1976) Absorption, metabolism and excretion of hydrochlorothiazide. *Clin. pharmacol. Ther.*, 19, 531-537

Beermann, B., Fåhraeus, L., Groschinsky-Grind, M. & Lindström, B. (1980) Placental transfer of hydrochlorothiazide. *Gynaecol. obstet. Invest.*, 11, 45-48

Bignami, M., Morpurgo, G., Pagliani, R., Carere, A., Conti, G. & Di Giuseppe, G. (1974) Non-disjunction and crossing-over induced by pharmaceutical drugs in *Aspergillus nidulans*. *Mutat. Res.*, 26, 159-170

Chappell, S.C. (1985) 1st 6 months of 1985: RPhs are decision-makers in 20% of new Rxs compared with only 17% one year ago. *Pharm. Times*, 51, 122-130

Chemical Information Services (1989-90) *Directory of World Chemical Producers*, Oceanside, NY

Christensson, T., Hällström, K. & Wengle, B. (1977) Hypercalcemia and primary hyperparathyroidism. Prevalence in patients receiving thiazides as detected in a health screen. *Arch. intern. Med.*, 137, 1138-1142

Cieri, U.R. (1988) Determination of reserpine and hydrochlorothiazide in commercial tablets by liquid chromatography with fluorescence and UV absorption detectors in series. *J. Assoc. off. anal. Chem.*, 71, 515-518

Cornish, A.L., McClellan, J.T. & Johnston, D.H. (1961) Effects of chlorothiazide on the pancreas. *New Engl. J. Med.*, 265, 673-675

Deppeler, H.P. (1981) Hydrochlorothiazide. *Anal. Profiles Drug Subst.*, 10, 405-441

Ebstein, J.E. & Wintroub, B.U. (1985) Photosensitivity due to drugs. *Drugs*, 30, 42-57

Eisner, E.V. & Crowell, E.B. (1971) Hydrochlorothiazide-dependent thrombocytopenia due to IgM antibody. *J Am. med. Assoc.*, 215, 480-482

Finnish Committee on Drug Information and Statistics (1987) *Finnish Statistics on Medicine*, Helsinki, National Board of Health

Flamenbaum, W. (1983) Metabolic consequences of antihypertensive therapy. *Ann. intern. Med.*, 98, 239-244

Freis, E.D. (1986) The cardiovascular risk of thiazide diuretics. *Clin. pharmacol. Ther.*, 39, 239-244

Friedman, G.D. & Ury, H.K. (1980) Initial screening for carcinogenicity of commonly used drugs. *J. natl Cancer Inst.*, 65, 723-733

Fujita, H. (1985) Arginine reversion and lambda induction in *E. coli* with benzothiadiazine diuretics irradiated with near-ultraviolet light. *Mutat. Res.*, 158, 135-139

Fullinfaw, R.O., Bury, R.W. & Moulds, R.F.W. (1987) Liquid chromatographic screening of diuretics in urine. *J. Chromatogr.*, *415*, 347-356

Galloway, S.M., Armstrong, M.J., Reuben, C., Colman, S., Brown, B., Cannon, C., Bloom, A.D., Nakamura, F., Ahmed, M., Duk, S., Rimpo, J., Margolin, B.H., Resnick, M.A., Anderson, B. & Zeiger, E. (1987) Chromosome aberrations and sister chromatid exchanges in Chinese hamster ovary cells: evaluations of 108 chemicals. *Environ. mol. Mutagenesis*, *10 (Suppl. 10)*, 1-175

Hardwick, N. & Saxe, N. (1986) Patterns of dermatology referrals in a general hospital. *Br. J. Dermatol.*, *115*, 167-176

Heinonen, O.P., Slone, D. & Shapiro, S. (1977) *Birth Defects and Drugs in Pregnancy*, Littleton, MA, Publishing Sciences Group, pp. 371-376

IARC (1987) *IARC Monographs on the Evaluation of Carcinogenic Risks to Humans*, Suppl. 7, *Overall Evaluations of Carcinogenicity: An Updating of IARC Monographs Volumes 1 to 42*, Lyon, pp. 349-350

Ishidate, M., Jr (1988) *Data Book of Chromosomal Aberration Test* In Vitro, rev. ed., Amsterdam, Elsevier

Klimiuk, P.S., Davies, M. & Adams, P.H. (1981) Primary parathyroidism and thiazide diuretics. *Postgrad. med. J.*, *57*, 80-83

Koopmans, P.P., Tan, Y. & van Ginneken, C.A.M. (1984) High-performance liquid chromatographic determination of hydrochlorothiazide in plasma and urine. *J. Chromatogr.*, *307*, 445-450

La Piana Simonsen, L. (1989) Top 200 drugs of 1988. Branded new Rxs rise 4.0% and total Rxs move up 1.2%. *Pharm. Times*, *55*, 40-48

Lijinsky, W. & Reuber, M.D. (1987) Pathologic effects of chronic administration of hydrochlorothiazide, with and without sodium nitrite, to F344 rats. *Toxicol. ind. Health*, *3*, 413-422

Linton, A.L., Clark, W.F., Driedger, A.A., Turnbull, D.I. & Lindsay, R.M. (1980) Acute interstitial nephritis due to drugs. *Ann. intern. Med.*, *93*, 735-741

van der Meer, M.J. & Brown, L.W. (1987) Simultaneous determination of amiloride and hydrochlorothiazide in plasma by reversed-phase high-performance liquid chromatography. *J. Chromatogr.*, *423*, 351-357

Miller, M.E., Cohn, R.D. & Burghart, P.H. (1982) Hydrochlorothiazide disposition in a mother and her breast-fed infant. *J. Pediatr.*, *101*, 789-791

Mortelmans, K., Haworth, S., Lawlor, T., Speck, W., Tainer, B. & Zeiger, E. (1986) *Salmonella* mutagenicity tests: II. Results from the testing of 270 chemicals. *Environ. Mutagenesis*, *8 (Suppl. 7)*, 1-119

Mulley, B.A., Parr, G.D., Pau, W.K., Rye, R.M., Mould, J.J. & Siddle, N.C. (1978) Placental transfer of chlorthalidone and its elimination in maternal milk. *Eur. J. clin. Pharmacol.*, *13*, 129-131

National Toxicology Program (1989) *Toxicology and Carcinogenesis Studies of Hydrochlorothiazide (CAS No. 58-93-5) in F344/N Rats and B6C3F$_1$ Mice (Feed Studies)* (Technical Report Series No. 357), Springfield, VA, National Technical Information Service

Niemeyer, C., Hasenfuss, G., Wais, U., Knauf, H., Schäfer-Korting, M. & Mutschler, E. (1983) Pharmacokinetics of hydrochlorothiazide in relation to renal function. *Eur. J. clin. Pharmacol.*, 24, 661-665

Paloyan, E. & Pickleman, J. (1969) Hyperparathyroidism coexisting with hypertension and prolonged thiazide administration. *J. Am. med. Assoc.*, 210, 1243-1245

Parfrey, N.A. & Herlong, H.F. (1984) Pulmonary oedema after hydrochlorothiazide. *Br. med. J.*, 288, 1880

Patel, R.B., Patel, U.R., Rogge, M.C., Shah, V.P., Prasad, V.K., Selen, A. & Welling, P.G. (1984) Bioavailability of hydrochlorothiazide from tablets and suspensions. *J. pharm. Sci.*, 73, 359-361

Pickleman, J.R., Straus, F.H., II, Forland, M. & Paloyan, E. (1969) Thiazide-induced parathyroid stimulation. *Metabolism*, 18, 867-873

Piper, C., Wallem, D., Wesche, D., Brattig, N., Diao, G.-J. & Berg, P.A. (1983) Lungenödem nach Einnahme von Hydrochlorothiazid. Eine seltene, vital bedrohende Nebenwirkung. [Pulmonary oedema after intake of hydrochlorothiazide. A rare life-threatening side-effect (Ger.).] *Dtsch. med. Wochenschr.*, 108, 1480-1483

Porter, R.H., Cox, B.G., Heaney, D., Hostetter, T.H., Stinebauch, B.J. & Suki, W.N. (1978) Treatment of hypoparathyroid patients with chlorthalidone. *New Engl. J. Med.*, 298, 577-581

Redalieu, E., Tipnis, V.V. & Wagner, W.E., Jr (1978) Determination of plasma hydrochlorothiazide levels in humans. *J. pharm. Sci.*, 67, 726-728

Redalieu, E., Chan, K.K.H., Tipnis, V., Zak, S.B., Gilleran, T.G., Wagner, W.E., Jr & LeSher, A.R. (1985) Kinetics of hydrochlorothiazide absorption in humans. *J. pharm. Sci.*, 74, 765-767

Reed, B.R., Huff, J.C., Jones, S.K., Orton, P.W., Lee, L.A. & Norris, D.A. (1985) Subacute cutaneous lupus erythematosus associated with hydrochlorothiazide therapy. *Ann. intern. Med.*, 103, 49-51

Reynolds, J.E.F., ed. (1989) *Martindale. The Extra Pharmacopoeia*, 29th ed., London, The Pharmaceutical Press, pp. 991-993

Roydhouse, N. (1974) Vertigo and its treatment. *Drugs*, 7, 297-309

Sarva, R.P., Gavaler, J.S. & Van Thiel, D.H. (1985) Thiazide-induced hypercholesterolemia: sex differences. *Life Sci.*, 37, 1817-1822

Scully, R.E., Mark, E.J. & McNeely, B.U. (1983) Case records of the Massachusetts General Hospital. Case 42-1983. *New Engl. J. Med.*, 309, 970-978

Selby, J.V., Friedman, G.D. & Fireman, B.H. (1989) Screening prescription drugs for possible carcinogenicity: 11 to 15 years of follow-up. *Cancer Res.*, 49, 5736-5747

Sheppard, H., Mowles, T.F. & Plummer, A.J. (1960) Determination of hydrochlorothiazide in urine. *J. Am. pharm. Assoc. Sci. Ed.*, 49, 722-723

Suria, D. (1978) Quantitative determination of thiazides in urine by a sensitive colorimetric method. *Clin. Biochem.*, 11, 222

US Pharmacopeial Convention, Inc. (1989) *US Pharmacopeia*, 22nd rev., Easton, PA, pp. 647-648

Valencia, R., Mason, J.M., Woodruff, R.C. & Zimmering, S. (1985) Chemical mutagenesis testing in *Drosophila*. III. Results of 48 coded compounds tested for the National Toxicology Program. *Environ. Mutagenesis*, 7, 325-348

Waskell, L. (1978) A study of the mutagenicity of anesthetics and their metabolites. *Mutat. Res.*, 57, 141-153

Welling, P.G. (1986) Pharmacokinetics of the thiazide diuretics. *Biopharm. Drug Dispos.*, 7, 501-535

Windholz, M., ed. (1983) *The Merck Index*, 10th ed., Rahway, NJ, Merck & Co., pp. 692-693

Yendt, E., Guay, G.R. & Garcia, D.A. (1970) The use of thiazides in the prevention of renal calculi. *Can. med. Assoc. J.*, 102, 614-620

Zalin, A.M., Hutchinson, C.E., Jong, M. & Matthews, K. (1984) Hyponatraemia during treatment with chlorpropamide and Moduretic (amiloride plus hydrochlorothiazide). *Br. med. J.*, 289, 659

PARACETAMOL (ACETAMINOPHEN)

1. Chemical and Physical Data

1.1 Synonyms and trade names

Chem. Abstr. Services Reg. No.: 103-90-2

Chem. Abstr. Name: Acetamide, *N*-(4-hydroxyphenyl)-

Synonyms: 4'-Hydroxy-acetanilide; *para*-acetaminophenol; acetophenum; *para*-acetylamidophenol; *N*-acetyl-*para*-aminophenol; *para*-acetylaminophenol; *para*-hydroxyacetanilide; *N-para*-hydroxyphenylacetamide

A large number of fixed combinations containing paracetamol are available.

1.2 Structural and molecular formula and molecular weight

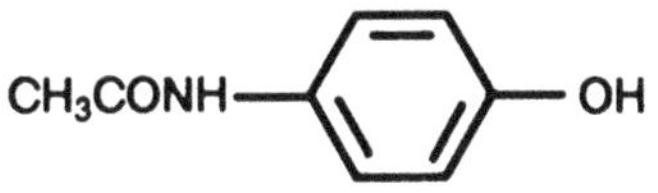

CH_3CONH—⟨ ⟩—OH

$C_8H_9NO_2$ Mol. wt: 151.16

1.3 Chemical and physical properties of the pure substance

From Fairbrother (1974) and El-Obeid and Al-Badr (1985)

(a) *Description*: White odourless crystalline powder; large monoclinic prisms from water

(b) *Melting-point*: 169-170.5°C

(c) *Solubility*: Soluble in water (1:70, 1:20 at 100°C), ethanol (1:7), acetone (1:13), chloroform (1:50), glycerol (1:40), methanol (1:10), propylene glycol (1:9) and solutions of alkali hydroxides; insoluble in diethyl ether. A saturated aqueous solution has a pH of ~6.

(d) *Spectroscopy data*: Infrared, ultraviolet, nuclear magnetic resonance, fluorescence and mass spectra have been reported.

(e) *Stability:* Dry, pure paracetamol is stable to 45°C. Contamination with traces of *para*-aminophenol, and humid conditions that cause hydrolysis to *para*-aminophenol, result in further degradation and discoloration. Slightly light-sensitive in solution, and degradation is catalysed by acids or bases.

(f) *Dissociation constant*: pK_a = 9.0-9.5

(g) *Partition coefficient*: P_c = 6.237 (octanol: pH 7.2 buffer)

1.4 Technical products and impurities

Paracetamol is available in pure form as numerous trade-name preparations for oral use. It is also found combined in over 200 preparations with other drugs.

Trade names: Abensanil; Acamol; Acephen; Acetalgin; Acetamol; Aferadol; Alba-Temp; Alpiny; Alvedon; Amadil; Anacin-3; Anaflon; Anhiba; Anuphen; Apamide; APAP; Atasol; Ben-u-ron; Bickie-mol; Bramcetamol; Calip; Calpol; Calpon; Campain; Capital; Captin; Ceetamol; Cetadol; Cetamol; Cetapon; Claradol; Claratal; Custodial; Dafalgan; Datril; Dial-a-gesix; Dirox; Disprol Paediatric; Dolamin; Dolanex; Doliprane; Doloral; Dolorol; Dolprone; Dorcol Children's Fever and Pain Reducer; Doregrippin; Dymadon; Efferalgan; Enelfa; Eneril; Ennagesic; Eu-Med; Exdol; Fanalgic; Febrigesic; Febrilix; Fendon; Fevamol; Finimal; Fonafor; Gelocatil; Glenpar; Gynospasmine; Hedex; Homoolan; Kinderfinimal; Kinder-Finiweh; Korum; Liquiprin; Lyteca; Malgis; Melabon; Momentum; Napamol; Naprinol; Nebs; Neuridal; Nevral; Nina 120; Nobedon; Ophinal; Oraphen; Pacemo; Pacemol; Painamol; Painaway; Paldesic; Pamol; Panado; Panadol; Panaleve; Panamax; Panasorb; Panets; Panex; Panodil; Panofen; Pantalgin; Paracet; Paracetamolum; Paraclear; Paralgin; Parapain; Paraprom; Parasin; Paraspen; Paratol; Parmol; Pasolind; Phendex; Pinex; Placemol; Praecimed; Proval; Puernol; Pyragesic; Pyralen; Reliv; Repamol; Resolve; Robigesic; Rounox; Salzone; Schmerzex; Sedapyren; Servigesic; Setamol; SK-APAP; Summadol; Tabalgin; Tachipirina; Tapar; Temlo; Tempra; Tenasfen; Ticelgesic; Tralgon; Treupel; Treuphadol; Tricocetamol; Tylenol; Tymol; Valadol; Zolben

Paracetamol is available as 325-mg or 500-mg tablets, which may include calcium stearate or magnesium stearate, cellulose, docusate sodium and sodium benzoate or sodium lauryl sulfate, starch, hydroxypropyl methylcellulose, propylene glycol, sodium starch glycolate, polyethylene glycol and Red #40.

It is also available as 500-mg gelatin capsules and as a mint-flavoured liquid containing 500 mg/15 ml solution, which can include 7% ethanol, citric acid, glycerine, polyethylene glycol, sodium benzoate, sorbitol, sucrose, Yellow #6, #10 and Blue #1. For children, drops (80 mg/0.8 ml), chewable tablets (80 mg), elixir (160 mg/5 ml) and coated capsules (160 mg/capsule) are available (Barnhart, 1989).

Characteristic impurities may include *para*-nitrophenol, *para*-aminophenol, *para*-chloroaniline, *ortho*-acetyl paracetamol, azobenzene (see IARC, 1975), azoxybenzene, quinone (see IARC, 1977), quinonimine, inorganic chloride, inorganic sulfate, inorganic sulfide and water (Fairbrother, 1974).

2. Production, Occurrence, Use and Analysis

2.1 Production and occurrence

Paracetamol may be made by acetylation of *para*-aminophenol (obtained by reduction of *para*-nitrophenol) with acetic acid or acetic anhydride. A number of other synthetic routes have been described (Fairbrother, 1974).

Paracetamol is synthesized in Argentina, Brazil, China, Colombia, France, the Federal Republic of Germany, India, Japan, Mexico, Poland, Republic of Korea, Romania, Taiwan, Turkey, the UK and the USA (Chemical Information Services Ltd, 1989-90).

In Sweden, paracetamol sales in 1988 were 20.02 defined daily doses per 1000 inhabitants (Apoteksbolaget, 1988, 1989).

Paracetamol is not known to occur naturally, but it is the major metabolite of phenacetin (see IARC, 1980, 1987).

2.2 Use

Paracetamol is used as an analgesic and antipyretic drug. It is the preferred alternative analgesic-antipyretic to aspirin (acetylsalicylic acid), particularly in patients with coagulation disorders, individuals with a history of peptic ulcer or who cannot tolerate aspirin, as well as in children (American Medical Association, 1986). Paracetamol was first used in clinical medicine in 1893. Following initial use as a prescription product in the USA in 1951, it subsequently became available without prescription in 1955 (Ameer & Greenblatt, 1977). In many countries, it is widely available without prescription.

The conventional oral dose for adults is 500-1000 mg. Dosing may be repeated every 4 h as necessary, but the total daily dose should not exceed 4000 mg. For children, the recommended dose is 10-15 mg/kg bw; no more than five doses should be administered over 24 h. Prolonged use (for more than ten days) and use for young children is not recommended (Flower *et al.*, 1985).

The usual dose for rectal administration is equal to that for oral administration (American Medical Association, 1986).

2.3 Analysis

Methods for the analysis of paracetamol have been reviewed (El-Obeid and Al-Badr, 1985).

Paracetamol and its metabolites can be analysed in biological fluids by high-performance liquid chromatography (HPLC; Manno *et al.*, 1981; Kinney & Kelly, 1987; Aguilar *et al.*, 1988; Meatherall & Ford, 1988), HPLC-mass spectrometry (Betowski *et al.*, 1987) and fluorescence polarization immunoassay (Koizumi *et al.*, 1988). It can be analysed in pharmaceutical preparations by HPLC (Biemer, 1987) and spectrophotometric (US Pharmacopeial Convention, Inc., 1989) methods.

3. Biological Data Relevant to the Evaluation of Carcinogenic Risk to Humans

3.1 Carcinogenicity studies in animals

Since paracetamol is a metabolite of phenacetin (Reynolds, 1989), carcinogenicity studies of phenacetin result in exposure of animals to paracetamol. For the results of studies on phenacetin, see IARC (1987).

(a) Oral administration

Mouse: Groups of 60 male and 60 female young adult IF strain mice were fed paracetamol (>98% pure; dissolved in acetone then evaporated) at 5000 or 10 000 mg/kg of diet for 18 months (approximate daily intake, 250 or 500 mg/kg bw, respectively). A group of 52 males and 52 females fed basal diet served as controls. Shortly after the beginning of treatment, 33 males and seven females in the higher-dose group died from liver necrosis. Subsequent survival in all groups was high. All survivors were killed at 18 months after the beginning of the experiment, and complete necropsy was carried out with histological examination of the liver, lungs, pancreas, kidneys, spleen, bladder and adrenal glands. The effective numbers of animals were 50 male and 48 female controls, 54 males and 57 females in the lower-dose group and 23 males and 47 females in the higher-dose group. The incidences of large, often multiple liver neoplasms (adenomas and carcinomas combined) were 20/23 (87%: 15 adenomas, 5 carcinomas) in higher-dose males, 9/47 (7 adenomas, 2 carcinomas) in higher-dose females, 1/54 (adenoma) in lower-dose males, 0/57 in lower-dose females, 1/50 (adenoma) in control males and 0/48 in control females (Flaks & Flaks, 1983). [The Working Group noted that the high dose produced early lethal hepatotoxicity in half the males.]

Groups of 50 and 55 male or female (C57Bl/6 × C3H/He)F1 (B6C3F1) mice, eight to nine weeks of age, were fed paracetamol (>98% pure) at 3000 and 6000 mg/kg of diet, respectively. The total intake of paracetamol in the high-dose groups was 863 g/kg bw for males and 675 g/kg bw for females. Two groups of 50 males and females were maintained on basal diet. All survivors were killed at 134 weeks. Survival among males was 43/50 (controls), 39/50 (low-dose) and 45/55 (high-dose), and that among females was 49/50 (controls), 46/50 (low-dose) and 50/55 (high-dose). The numbers of mice scored for tumours were 27/43 control males, 32/49 control females, 21/39 low-dose males, 33/46 low-dose females, 23/45 high-dose males and 33/50 high-dose females. No difference was found in the incidence of tumours at any site between treated and control mice (Amo & Matsuyama, 1985).

Groups of 60 and 120 male B6C3F1 mice, six weeks of age, received paracetamol at 5000 or 10 000 mg/kg of diet, respectively, for up to 70 weeks, at which time the remaining animals were killed. A group of 30 mice served as controls. Survival in the high-dose group was less than 50% at 24 weeks and 16% at 72 weeks; in the low-dose group, the survival was greater than 90%. Severe hepatotoxicity was a common finding in mice that died. No increased incidence of neoplasms was observed (Hagiwara & Ward, 1986). [The Working Group noted the poor survival in the high-dose group.]

Rat: Groups of 30 male SPF Sprague-Dawley rats, six weeks of age, were fed paracetamol (99.5-99.7% pure) at 0 or 5350 mg/kg of diet for 117 weeks (total paracetamol intake, 86.5 g per rat). All animals were necropsied, and kidneys, urinary bladder, adrenal glands, liver, stomach, spleen, lungs, heart and any grossly abnormal organs or tissues were examined histologically. No significant difference in survival rates was observed. In the treated group, 4/30 rats developed bladder papillomatosis or tumours *versus* 2/30 controls (Johansson, 1981). [The Working Group noted the relatively small number of animals used in the study.]

Groups of 50 male and 50 female Fischer 344/DuCrj rats, five weeks of age were fed pharmacopoeial-grade paracetamol at 0, 4500 or 9000 mg/kg (males) and 0, 6500 or 13 000 mg/kg (females) of diet for 104 weeks and were then observed for a further 26 weeks (average daily intakes: lower-dose males, 195 mg/kg bw; lower-dose females, 336 mg/kg bw; higher-dose males, 402 mg/kg bw; higher-dose females, 688 mg/kg bw), at which time all survivors were killed. Survival rates at 104 weeks varied between 86 and 90% in males and 80 and 82% in females, with no significant difference between treated and control rats. All rats were necropsied, and major organs, tissues and gross abnormalities were examined histologically. No difference was seen in tumour incidence between the groups (Hiraga & Fujii, 1985).

Groups of 50 male and 50 female young adult Leeds inbred rats were fed paracetamol (>98% pure) at 5000 or 10 000 mg/kg of diet for up to 18 months (mean daily intake, 300 and 600 mg/kg bw, respectively), at which time all survivors were killed. A group of 40 males and 40 females fed basal diet alone served as controls. Survival was high: male controls, 40/40; female controls, 40/40; lower-dose males, 48/50; lower-dose females, 49/50; higher-dose males, 45/50; and higher-dose females, 49/50. All animals were necropsied, and samples from each liver lobe, lungs, kidneys, pancreas, mammary glands, spleen, adrenal glands and from grossly visible lesions were examined histologically. No tumour was observed among controls. In treated animals, no hepatocellular carcinoma was observed, but hepatocellular neoplastic nodules occurred in 0/40, 1/48 and 9/45 control, lower-dose and higher-dose males and 0/40, 0/49 and 10/49 control, lower-dose and higher-dose females; and 20-25% of rats in each treated group developed hyperplasia of the bladder epithelium. Bladder calculi were present in about 30% of all treated male animals and in 6% of females; no clear association was seen between hyperplasia and the presence of bladder calculi. Bladder papillomas were observed in 5/49 higher-dose males and bladder carcinomas in 1/49 higher-dose males; the total bladder tumour incidence was significantly higher [$p = 0.02$, Fisher's exact test] among high-dose males. In the low-dose group, 4/49 females developed bladder papillomas and 1/49 females developed bladder carcinoma. Total bladder tumour incidence was significantly higher in low-dose female rats [$p = 0.045$, Fisher's exact test] (Flaks et al., 1985). [The Working Group noted that there were increased incidences of calculi, hyperplasia and tumours of the bladder in treated animals but there was no relationship between the presence of calculi and the presence of either hyperplasia or tumours.]

(b) *Administration with known carcinogens*

Mouse: Groups of 30 and 60 male B6C3F1 mice, six weeks of age, received paracetamol at 5000 or 10 000 mg/kg of diet, respectively, continuously for up to 70 weeks following a single intraperitoneal injection of 40 mg/kg bw N-nitrosodiethylamine at four weeks of age. A group of 30 mice that received N-nitrosodiethylamine alone served as controls. Mice were sacrificed at either 24 or 72 weeks after injection of the nitrosamine. Survival in the higher-dose group was very poor; severe hepatotoxicity was a common finding in mice that died. No increased incidence of neoplasms was found (Hagiwara & Ward, 1986).

Rat: Two groups of 25 or 30 male Fisher 344 rats weighing 150 g were administered N-nitrosoethyl-N-hydroxyethylamine (NEHEA) at 0 or 0.1% (v/v) in drinking-water for two weeks and one week later were fed diets containing paracetamol [purity unspecified] at 1.3% for 29 weeks. One group of 25 rats received NEHEA in the drinking-water followed by no further treatment. All animals were killed at the end of week 32, and samples from liver, kidneys and other organs with gross abnormalities were examined histologically.

γ-Glutamyltranspeptidase foci, hyperplastic nodules, hepatocellular carcinomas, renal-cell carcinomas, as well as 'atypical cell foci' and adenomas were measured. Paracetamol inhibited the formation of NEHEA-induced γ-glutamyltranspeptidase foci, hyperplastic nodules and carcinomas in comparison with animals treated with NEHEA only. No liver lesion was found in any animal treated with paracetamol only. In contrast, the incidence and multiplicity of preneoplastic renal lesions and renal-cell adenomas were significantly increased in NEHEA-initiated animals treated with paracetamol in comparison with animals treated with NEHEA only. No such renal lesion was observed in groups treated with paracetamol alone (Tsuda et al., 1984). [The Working Group noted that the progression of the lesions described as preneoplastic to neoplasms was not documented.]

Groups of 25 male Fischer 344 rats, seven weeks old, were administered N-nitrosobutyl-N-(4-hydroxybutyl)amine at 0 or 0.05% (v/v) in the drinking-water for four weeks to initiate bladder carcinogenesis and were then fed paracetamol [purity unspecified] at 13 000 mg/kg of diet for a further 32 weeks, at which time all rats were killed. One group received treatment with the nitrosamine only. Urinary bladders, livers and kidneys were examined histologically. No significant difference in the incidence of bladder tumours was observed between the groups (Kurata et al., 1986).

Groups of male Fischer 344 rats [numbers unspecified], six weeks of age, were subjected to a two-thirds partial hepatectomy and 24 h later received either intragastric intubations of paracetamol (purity, >99%) at 0 or 1000 mg/kg bw in 0.2% tragacanth gum twice a week for five weeks, or a single intragastric instillation of paracetamol at 500 mg/kg bw. Two weeks after the end of paracetamol treatment, the animals were administered phenobarbital (pharmacopoeial grade) at 0 or 1 mg/ml drinking-water for 12 weeks. The experiment was terminated at the end of phenobarbital treatment (weeks 13 and 18). Livers, kidneys, thyroid glands and any gross lesions were examined histologically. The tumour-initiating activity of paracetamol was evaluated by the formation of placental-type glutathione S-transferase-positive foci in liver cells; treatment with paracetamol did not result in the induction of such foci (Hasegawa et al., 1988). [The Working Group noted that the rate of absorption of paracetamol from the tragacanth suspension was not measured, and the limited reporting of the experiment.]

To examine possible interference with the activation of 2-acetylaminofluorene, groups of 20 female SPF CD rats were given diets containing acetylaminofluorene at 250 mg/kg alone or with paracetamol at 11 000 mg/kg for 20 weeks and were observed for an additional ten weeks. Mammary tumours were seen in 14/20 females given acetylaminofluorene and in 7/20 ($p = 0.028$, Fisher's exact test) animals given acetylaminofluorene and paracetamol (Weisburger et al., 1973).

Hamster: Groups of 30 male and 30 female Syrian golden hamsters, six weeks old, were given *N*-hydroxyacetylaminofluorene at 430 mg/kg alone or with paracetamol at 11 000 mg/kg of diet for 39 weeks. The experiment was terminated at 47 weeks. The incidences of liver cholangiomas in animals treated with *N*-hydroxyacetylaminofluorene were 13/26 in males and 22/25 in females; in the group treated with *N*-hydroxyacetylaminofluorene and paracetamol, no liver tumour was seen in 24 males but two occurred in 24 females. Similar results were found in groups given acetylaminofluorene at 400 mg/kg alone or with paracetamol at 11 000 mg/kg: with acetylaminofluorene, the incidence of liver cholangiomas was 6/30 males and 28/30 females; in the group treated with acetylaminofluorene and paracetamol, the incidence was 0/29 males ($p = 0.013$, Fisher's exact test) and 4/28 females ($p < 0.001$, Fisher's exact test) (Weisburger *et al.*, 1973).

3.2 Other relevant data

(a) *Experimental systems*

(i) *Absorption, distribution, excretion and metabolism*

Dogs receiving a single oral administration of a wide range of doses of paracetamol excreted about 85% of the administered dose within the first 24 h (Savides *et al.*, 1984).

A summary of the proposed metabolic pathways of paracetamol is shown in Figure 1. The major urinary metabolites (the glucuronide, sulfate and 3-mercapto derivatives) are observed in most species, although there is much species variation regarding the percentages of these conjugates excreted in the urine (Davis *et al.*, 1976). Each of the other metabolites shown in Figure 1 has been identified in one species (see Gemborys & Mudge, 1981, for details). In rats, biliary excretion of the various metabolites of paracetamol increased from 20 to 49% as doses were increased from 37.5 to 600 mg/kg bw. The glucuronide conjugate was the major metabolite recovered in the bile at all doses (Hjelle & Klaassen, 1984). The putative reactive intermediates are not known but are thought to include benzoquinone (Hinson *et al.*, 1977).

A minor but important metabolic pathway involves the conversion of paracetamol to a reactive metabolite by the hepatic cytochrome P450-dependent mixed-function oxidase system (Mitchell *et al.*, 1973; Potter *et al.*, 1973). The reactive metabolite is thought to be either *N*-acetyl-*para*-benzoquinoneimine (Corcoran *et al.*, 1980) or the corresponding semiquinone free radical (De Vries, 1981; Nelson *et al.*, 1981). With low doses of paracetamol, a conjugate of reduced glutathione with the reactive metabolite is further transformed to cysteine and mercapturic acid conjugates, which are excreted. As the dose of paracetamol increases, hepatic glutathione stores are diminished and the glucuronidation and sulfation pathways

Fig. 1. Summary of metabolism of paracetamol based on data for different species[a]

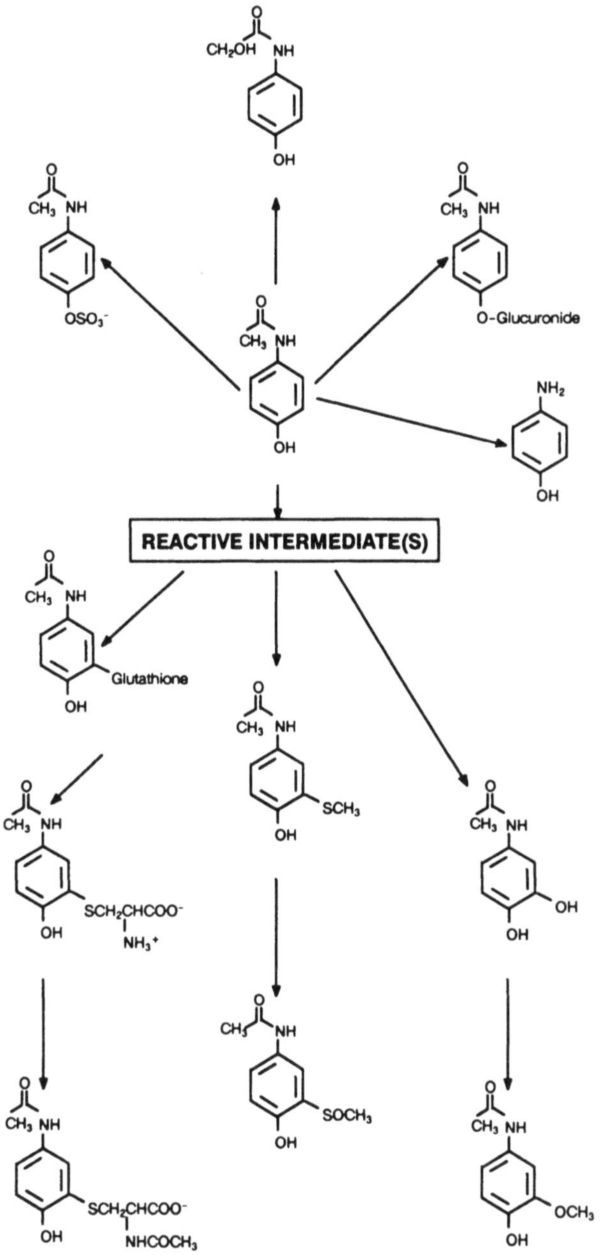

[a]From Jollow et al. (1974), Wong et al. (1976) and Gemborys & Mudge (1981)

become saturated (Galinsky & Levy, 1981). A correlation has been demonstrated between species sensitivity to the hepatotoxicity of paracetamol and the balance between two pathways: (i) formation of glutathione conjugates and the corresponding hydrolysis products (indicative of the 'toxic' pathway) and (ii) metabolism *via* formation of glucuronide and sulfate esters (the 'detoxification pathway') (Gregus *et al.*, 1988). Paracetamol-induced liver toxicity and depletion of glutathione may be partially prevented by provision of dietary methionine (Reicks *et al.*, 1988; McLean *et al.*, 1989). At sufficiently high doses of paracetamol, glutathione is depleted and the reactive metabolite binds covalently to cell macromolecules. It has also been noted that paracetamol and *N*-acetyl-*para*-benzoquinoneimine may exert their cytotoxic effects *via* disruption of Ca^{2+} homeostasis secondary to the depletion of soluble and protein-bound thiols (Moore *et al.*, 1985). These data indicate that oxidative or free-radical reactions initiated by paracetamol have a role in the hepatotoxicity of this drug (Birge *et al.*, 1988).

Radiolabel was bound covalently to hepatocellular proteins following incubation of mouse, rat, hamster, rabbit or guinea-pig liver microsomes with ^3H-paracetamol; the degree of binding was correlated with the susceptibility of the species to hepatotoxicity *in vivo* (Davis *et al.*, 1974). Similar covalent binding of radiolabel to liver proteins of rats 48 h after administration of [*ring*-^{14}C]-paracetamol was proportional to the extent of liver damage (Davis *et al.*, 1976). Covalent binding of radiolabel to liver plasma membranes and microsomes was demonstrated 2.5 h after oral administration of ^3H-paracetamol at 2.5 g/kg bw to rats (Tsokos-Kuhn *et al.*, 1988).

Paracetamol is activated in the kidney by an NADPH-dependent cytochrome P450 mechanism to an arylating agent which can bind covalently to cellular macromolecules (McMurty *et al.*, 1978). Studies in several species have suggested that formation of *para*-aminophenol may be of importance with respect to paracetamol nephrotoxicity. *para*-Aminophenol was identified as a urinary metabolite in hamsters (Gemborys & Mudge, 1981); the deacetylation of paracetamol to *para*-aminophenol has also been demonstrated in mouse renal cortical slices (Carpenter & Mudge, 1981). In comparison to acetyl-labelled paracetamol, ring-labelled paracetamol was preferentially bound to renal macromolecules in Fischer rats, which are sensitive to paracetamol nephrotoxicity, whereas binding of ring- and acetyl-labelled paracetamol to renal macromolecules was similar in non-susceptible Sprague-Dawley rats (Newton *et al.*, 1985). This suggests that *para*-aminophenol may be responsible for paracetamol-induced renal necrosis in Fischer 344 rats (Newton *et al.*, 1982).

(ii) *Toxic effects*

The single-dose oral LD_{50} of paracetamol in male rats was 3.7 g/kg bw (Boyd & Bereczky, 1966); the 100-day LD_{50} in rats was 400 mg per day (Boyd & Hogan, 1968).

Hepatic necrosis following administration of paracetamol was first reported in rats (Boyd & Bereczky, 1966). The main signs are hydropic vacuolation, centrilobular necrosis, macrophage infiltration and regenerative activity (Dixon *et al.*, 1971). Paracetamol-induced hepatotoxicity varies considerably among species: hamsters and mice are most sensitive, whereas rats, rabbits and guinea-pigs are resistant to paracetamol-induced liver injury (Davis *et al.*, 1974; Siegers *et al.*, 1978). Toxic effects in dogs and cats given a single oral dose of paracetamol (maximal doses, 500 and 120 mg/kg bw, respectively) included hepatic centrilobular pathology in dogs, while cats, which do not glucuronidate exogenous compounds, had more diffuse liver pathological changes (Savides *et al.*, 1984).

The hepatotoxic effects of paracetamol administered in the diet to mice have been examined histologically. After continuous exposure at 10 000 mg/kg diet for 72 weeks (Hagiwara & Ward, 1986), severe chronic hepatotoxicity was observed, with centrilobular hepatocytomegaly, cirrhosis, lipofuscin deposition and hepatocyte necrosis varying from focal to massive. With the same dose, Ham and Calder (1984) observed macroscopically and microscopically deformed livers with extensive lobular collapse, foci of hepatic necrosis and lymphoid aggregation in portal tracts after 32 weeks. At a lower dose (5000 mg/kg bw) and a shorter exposure time (24 weeks), histological changes were mild. Ultrastructural changes in the livers of rats administered paracetamol at 10 000 mg/kg diet for up to 18 months have been described (Flaks *et al.*, 1985).

Histopathological review of liver sections from B6C3F1 mice of each sex fed paracetamol at 3000, 6000 or 12 500 mg/kg diet for 41 weeks and from NIH general-purpose mice of each sex fed paracetamol at 11 000 mg/kg diet for 48 weeks indicated severe liver injury, characterized by centrilobular necrosis in animals receiving more than 10 000 mg/kg diet (Maruyama & Williams, 1988).

A single subcutaneous dose of paracetamol at 750 mg/kg bw to male Fischer 344 rats produced renal tubular necrosis restricted to the upper part of the proximal tubule (McMurty *et al.*, 1978). Chronic cortical and medullary damage has been produced in uninephrectomized homozygous Gunn rats by single doses of various analgesic preparations containing paracetamol (Henry & Tange, 1984).

In fasted adult male mice given paracetamol at 600 mg/kg bw orally and killed within 48 h after treatment, degenerative and necrotic changes were detected in the bronchial epithelium and in testicular and lymphoid tissue, in addition to renal and hepatic effects (Placke *et al.*, 1987).

When male rats were given paracetamol at 500 mg/kg bw per day orally for 70 days, a significant decrease in testicular weight was observed (Jacqueson et al., 1984).

(iii) *Effects on reproduction and prenatal toxicity*

In Sprague-Dawley rats administered paracetamol at 250 mg/kg bw orally on days 8 through 19 of gestation, embryo- and fetotoxic effects were not seen (Lubawy & Burriss Garret, 1977).

(iv) *Genetic and related effects*

Paracetamol was not mutagenic to *Salmonella typhimurium* at concentrations of up to 50 mg/plate in the presence or absence of an exogenous metabolic system (King et al., 1979; Wirth et al., 1980; Imamura et al., 1983; Dybing et al., 1984; Oldham et al., 1986; Jasiewicz & Richardson, 1987). It did not induce mutations in a liquid pre-incubation test with *Escherichia coli* in the presence or absence of an exogenous metabolic system (King et al., 1979). As reported in an abstract, paracetamol exhibited mutagenic activity towards *S. typhimurium* TA100 in the presence of an exogenous metabolic system (Tamura et al., 1980).

Feeding of male *Drosophila melanogaster* with a 40-mM solution of paracetamol did not induce sex-linked recessive mutations (King et al., 1979).

Treatment of Chinese hamster V79 cells with low concentrations (0.1-3.0 mM) of paracetamol inhibited DNA synthesis (Holme et al., 1988; Hongslo et al., 1988). Paracetamol at 10 mM had no effect on Reuber H4-II-E rat hepatoma cell DNA, as assayed by alkaline elution, but the toxic metabolite of paracetamol, *N*-acetyl-*para*-benzoquinoneimine, induced DNA strand breaks (Dybing et al., 1984). Treatment of Chinese hamster V79 cells induced DNA strand breaks at 3 and 10 mM but not at 1 mM (Hongslo et al., 1988). Analogous results were obtained with Chinese hamster ovary cells (Sasaki, 1986). Species specificity was observed in assays for unscheduled DNA synthesis *in vitro*. No unscheduled DNA synthesis was detected in Chinese hamster V79 cells (Hongslo et al., 1988), in Syrian hamster or guinea-pig primary hepatocytes (Holme & Soderlund, 1986) or in rat hepatocytes (Milam & Byard, 1985; Sasaki, 1986; Williams et al., 1989); however, a small but significant increase in unscheduled DNA synthesis was seen in rat primary hepatocytes and a marked increase in unscheduled DNA synthesis was observed in mouse hepatocytes (Holme & Soderlund, 1986).

Paracetamol did not induce mutations to ouabain-resistance in C3H/10T½ clone 8 mouse embryo cells (Patierno et al., 1989). It was reported in an abstract that paracetamol did not induce mutations at the *hprt* locus in Chinese hamster V79 cells (Sawada et al., 1985). It induced sister chromatid exchange in Chinese hamster V79 (Holme et al., 1988; Hongslo et al., 1988) and CHO cells (Sasaki, 1986). Micronuclei were induced by paracetamol in a rat kidney cell line (NRK-49F) at concentrations above 10 mM (Dunn *et al.*, 1987). Paracetamol induced chromosomal aberrations in three different Chinese hamster cell lines (Sasaki *et al.*, 1980; Sasaki, 1986; Ishidate, 1988) and in human lymphocytes (Watanabe, 1982). It weakly transformed C3H/10T½ clone 8 mouse embryo cells (Patierno *et al.*, 1989).

Paracetamol given twice at a dose of 3 mM (450 mg/kg bw) either intraperitoneally or orally to NMRI mice did not induce micronuclei (King *et al.*, 1979). Oral treatment of female Sprague-Dawley rats with paracetamol at 500 and 1000 mg/kg bw induced aneuploidy in 12-day embryos (Tsuruzaki *et al.*, 1982). Oral treatment of Swiss mice with single or three consecutive daily doses of aqueous solutions of up to 2.5 mg/0.5 ml did not lead to chromatid breaks in bone-marrow cells (Reddy, 1984) or meiotic cells of male Swiss mice (Reddy & Subramanyam, 1985). [The Working Group noted that the description of the doses used in the two last studies was unclear.]

(b) Humans

(i) *Pharmacokinetics*

Following an oral dose, paracetamol is absorbed rapidly from the small intestine. The rate of absorption depends on the rate of gastric emptying (Clements *et al.*, 1978). First-pass metabolism of paracetamol is dose-dependent: systemic availability ranges from 90% (with 1-2 g) to 68% (with 0.5 g). Plasma concentrations of paracetamol in fasting healthy subjects peaked within 1 h after treatment with 0.5 or 1.0 g but continued to rise up to 2 h after treatment with 2.0 g (Rawlings *et al.*, 1977).

Paracetamol is rapidly and relatively uniformly distributed throughout the body fluids (Gwilt *et al.*, 1963). Binding to plasma proteins is considered insignificant (Gazzard *et al.*, 1973). The apparent volume of distribution of paracetamol in man is about 0.9 l/kg bw (Forrest *et al.*, 1982). The decrease in paracetamol concentrations in plasma is multiphasic both after intravenous injections and after oral dosing with 500 and 1000 mg. When the data from six healthy volunteers were interpreted according to a two-compartment open model, the half-time of the first exponential ranged from 0.15 to 0.53 h and that of the second exponential from 2.24 to 3.30 h. The latter value was in agreement with that found after oral dosing. Mean clearance ($\pm$ SEM) after intravenous administration of 1000 mg was 352 ($\pm$ 40) ml/min (Rawlings *et al.*, 1977). Renal excretion of paracetamol involves glomerular filtration and passive reabsorption, and the sulfate conjugate is subject to active renal tubular secretion (Morris & Levy, 1984). Both these metabolites have been shown to accumulate in plasma in patients with renal failure who are taking paracetamol (Lowenthal *et al.*, 1976).

Paracetamol crosses the placenta in unconjugated form, and excretion in the urine of an exposed neonate was similar to that of a two- to three-day-old infant (Collins, 1981).

Paracetamol passes rapidly into milk, and the milk:plasma concentration ratio ranges from 0.7 to 1.1 (Berlin *et al.*, 1980; Notarianni *et al.*, 1987).

Paracetamol is metabolized predominantly to the glucuronide and sulfate conjugates in the human liver. A minor fraction is converted by cytochrome P450-dependent hepatic mixed-function oxidase to a highly reactive arylating metabolite, which is postulated to be *N*-acetyl-*para*-benzoquinoneimine (Miner & Kissenger, 1979). This metabolite is rapidly inactivated by conjugation with reduced glutathione and eventually excreted in the urine as acetyl cysteine and mercapturic acid conjugates. Large doses of paracetamol can deplete glutathione stores, and the excess of highly reactive intermediate binds covalently with vital cell elements, which may result in acute hepatic necrosis (Mitchell *et al.*, 1973, 1974). Only 2-5% of a therapeutic dose was excreted unchanged in the urine. In young healthy subjects, about 55, 30, 4 and 4% of a therapeutic dose was excreted after hepatic conjugation with glucuronic acid, sulfuric acid, cysteine and mercapturic acid, respectively (Forrest *et al.*, 1982).

The fractional recovery of mercapturic acid and cysteine conjugates after ingestion of paracetamol at 1500 mg was 9.3% in Caucasians compared with only 4.4-5.2% in Africans (Critchley *et al.*, 1986). This may reflect different susceptibility to paracetamol hepatotoxicity.

(ii) *Adverse effects*

The toxic effects of paracetamol have been reviewed (Flower *et al.*, 1985).

Reports on the acute toxicity, and in particular hepatotoxicity, of paracetamol have continued to appear since the reporting of the first two cases in 1966 (Davidson & Eastham, 1966). Initial symptoms of overdose are nausea, vomiting, diarrhoea and abdominal pain. Clinical indications of hepatic damage become manifest within two to four days after ingestion of toxic doses; in adults, a single dose of 10-15 g (200-250 mg/kg bw) is toxic. Serum transaminases, lactic dehydrogenase and bilirubin concentrations are elevated, and prothrombin time is prolonged (Koch-Weser, 1976). The severity of hepatic injury increases with the ingested dose and with previous consumption of other drugs that induce liver cytochrome P450 enzymes (Wright & Prescott, 1973). Biopsy of the liver reveals centrilobular necrosis with sparing of the periportal area (James *et al.*, 1975). In nonfatal cases, the hepatic lesions are reversible over a period of months, without development of cirrhosis (Hamlyn *et al.*, 1977).

Heavy alcohol consumption has been stated in several case reports to be related to more severe paracetamol hepatotoxicity than in non- or moderate drinkers (for review, see Black, 1984). Five cases of combined hepatocellular injury and renal tubular necrosis have been reported among patients with a history of chronic alcohol use who were receiving therapeutic doses of paracetamol (Kaysen et al., 1985).

(iii) *Effects on reproduction and prenatal toxicity*

No association of paracetamol use with congenital abnormalities or stillbirths was observed in a study on drug use in approximately 10 000 pregnancies in the UK (Crombie et al., 1970). In a case-control study of 458 mothers of malformed babies and 911 controls, there was no association of abnormalities with use of paracetamol during the first trimester (Nelson & Forfar, 1971). In the Collaborative Perinatal Project, in which drug intake and pregnancy outcome were studied in a series of 50 282 women in 1959-65, 226 women had been exposed to paracetamol during the first trimester of pregnancy. There were 17 malformed children in the exposed group, giving a nonsignificant standardized relative risk (RR) of 1.05 (Heinonen et al., 1977).

In a study of 280 000 women belonging to a prepaid health plan in Seattle, WA (USA), all drug prescriptions and all pregnancy outcomes were monitored between July 1977 and December 1979. Among the liveborn babies of 6837 women, 80 (1.2%) had major congenital malformations. Three of the infants born to 493 women for whom paracetamol had been prescribed in the first trimester had major malformations (types not specified), giving a prevalence of 6 per 1000, which was not significantly different from the overall prevalence in the total population studied (12 per 1000). A second group of 328 women were exposed to paracetamol with codeine in the first trimester. Five of these had malformed babies, giving a prevalence of 15 per 1000, which was not significantly different from that in controls (Jick et al., 1981).

In a second study of the same population, covering the period January 1980 to June 1982, 6509 women had pregnancies ending in livebirths; 105 (1.5%) of the infants had major congenital malformations. Two of the infants born to 350 women for whom paracetamol had been prescribed in the first trimester had major malformations (types not specified), giving a prevalence of 6 per 1000 compared with an overall prevalence in the entire group of 16 per 1000. Three of 347 women exposed to paracetamol with codeine had malformed babies, giving a prevalence of 9 per 1000 (not significant) (Aselton et al., 1985).

(iv) *Genetic and related effects*

Eleven healthy volunteers were given paracetamol at 1000 mg three times over a period of 8 h. The frequency of chromatid breaks in peripheral blood lymphocytes was significantly increased after one day but returned to normal one week later (Kocisova et al., 1988).

3.3 Case reports and epidemiological studies of carcinogenicity to humans

The Working Group considered only studies in which paracetamol was taken directly, either alone or in mixtures. Paracetamol may be taken by analgesic users who previously took phenacetin. Analgesic mixtures containing phenacetin are carcinogenic to humans; and phenacetin is probably carcinogenic to humans (IARC, 1980, 1987).

A population-based case-control study was conducted in Minnesota, USA, involving 495 cases of cancer of the renal parenchyma and 74 cases of cancer of the renal pelvis, diagnosed in 1974-79, and 697 controls (McLauglin *et al.*, 1983, 1984, 1985). An association between cancer of the renal pelvis and intensity and duration of use of paracetamol-containing drugs was seen in women (p for trend, < 0.05; RR in the highest exposure category, based on three exposed cases and eight exposed controls, 5.8; 95% confidence interval (CI), 0.8-40). [The Working Group noted that the trend test included unexposed cases and controls; if the unexposed are excluded, the trend is not statistically significant.] No other significant association was observed. Four of the five cases in the highest exposure category (two men, three women) who developed renal pelvic cancer had also taken phenacetin-containing analgesics; in the entire study, only two cases of cancer of the renal pelvis and seven controls had taken paracetamol alone.

Another population-based case control study was conducted among women aged 20-49 years in the state of New York (USA) involving 173 cases of bladder cancer diagnosed in 1975-79 and an equal number of controls matched for age and telephone area code (Piper *et al.*, 1985). A history of regular use of analgesics containing paracetamol (and not phenacetin) at least one year before diagnosis yielded a smoking-adjusted RR of 1.5 (95% CI, 0.4-7.2). In contrast, the risk for regular users of phenacetin-containing analgesics was significantly elevated whether they also regularly took paracetamol (RR, 3.8; 95% CI, 1.4-13.0) or not (RR, 6.5; 95% CI, 1.5-59.2).

A series of population-based case-control studies of urinary-tract cancer were conducted in New South Wales, Australia, involving cases identified in 1977-82 (McCredie *et al.*, 1983a,b, 1988; McCredie & Stewart, 1988). Ultimately, there were 360 cases of renal parenchymal cancer, 73 cases of renal pelvic cancer, 55 cases of ureteral cancer and 162 cases (women only) of bladder cancer. Controls (985 for renal parenchymal cancer and 689 for the other sites) were derived from electoral rolls. The only significant increase in risk for regular use of paracetamol (cumulative consumption of at least 0.1 kg) was with ureteral cancer (RR, 2.5; 95% CI, 1.1-5.9); this association was not further elevated in the subgroup with higher exposure (at least 1 kg; RR, 2.0; 95% CI, 0.8-4.5). The RR for cancer of the renal pelvis was 1.2 (95% CI, 0.6-2.3). These analyses were adjusted for cigarette smoking and the presence of urological disease.

A further population-based case-control study was conducted in Los Angeles County, USA, based on 187 cases of cancer of the renal pelvis or ureter diagnosed in 1978-82 and an equal number of neighbourhood controls (Ross et al., 1989). An association was found with use of nonprescription analgesics in general. The risks for use of analgesics containing paracetamol were nonsignificantly elevated, at 1.3 for use more than 30 days/year ($p = 0.34$) and 2.0 for use more than 30 consecutive days/year ($p = 0.08$). The analyses were controlled for cigarette smoking and history of urinary-tract stones. The authors noted that it was difficult to distinguish the effects of individual compounds in this study.

In a hypothesis-generating cohort study designed to screen a large number of drugs for possible carcinogenicity (described in detail in the monograph on ampicillin), 3238 persons to whom at least one prescription for paracetamol alone and 2612 to whom at least one prescription for paracetamol with codeine had been dispensed during 1969-73 were followed up for up to 15 years (Selby et al., 1989). No significant association with cancer at any site was seen for use of paracetamol with codeine. For paracetamol alone, a positive association was noted for melanoma (seven cases observed, 1.7 expected; RR, 4.1; 95% CI, 1.7-8.5), and negative associations for cancer of the colon (four observed, 12.1 expected; RR, 0.33; 95% CI, 0.1-0.85) and cancer of the uterine corpus (one observed, 6.5 expected; RR, 0.15; 95% CI, 0-0.86); but no association was seen for any cancer of the urinary tract or for all cancers combined (Friedman & Ury, 1980, 1983; Selby et al., 1989). [The Working Group noted that there was no information on non-prescription dispensing of paracetamol, which is the most common way that it is obtained. Since, as also noted by the authors, some 12 000 comparisons were made in this study, the associations should be verified independently. Data on duration of use were not provided.]

4. Summary of Data Reported and Evaluation

4.1 Exposure data

Paracetamol has been used extensively as an analgesic and antipyretic since 1946.

4.2 Experimental carcinogenicity data

Paracetamol was tested for carcinogenicity by oral administration in mice and rats. In one strain of mice, a significant increase in the incidence of multiple liver carcinomas and adenomas was observed in animals of each sex at a markedly toxic dose; in two studies on another strain, no increase in the incidence of any tumour was observed at a well-tolerated dose that was approximately half that in the preceding study. Administration of paracetamol to two different strains of rats did not increase tumour incidence. In a further strain of rats, the incidence of neoplastic liver nodules was increased in animals of each sex given the higher dose; the combined incidence of bladder papillomas and carcinomas (mostly papillomas) was significantly greater in high-dose male and in low-dose female rats. Although treatment increased the incidence of bladder calculi in treated rats, there was no relationship between the presence of calculi and of either hyperplasia or tumours in the bladder.

Oral administration of paracetamol to rats enhanced the incidence of renal adenomas induced by *N*-nitrosoethyl-*N*-hydroxyethylamine.

4.3 Human carcinogenicity data

A positive association between use of paracetamol and cancer of the ureter (but not of other sites in the urinary tract) was observed in an Australian case-control study. None of three other population-based case-control studies showed an association between paracetamol use and cancer in the urinary tract.

4.4 Other relevant data

One study provided no evidence that use of paracetamol in the first trimester of pregnancy is associated with an increase in the incidence of malformations. Paracetamol induced testicular atrophy in rats.

Hepatotoxicity has been reported repeatedly in people taking high doses of paracetamol; chronic alcohol users are particularly sensitive. Paracetamol is metabolized in humans and animals to reactive intermediates that bind to proteins. It is hepatotoxic to experimental animals and causes renal tubular necrosis in rats.

Paracetamol induced chromatid breaks in peripheral human lymphocytes *in vivo*. It induced aneuploidy in rat embryos treated transplacentally. It gave negative results in the micronucleus test in mice *in vivo*. It did not induce chromosomal aberrations in bone-marrow cells or spermatocytes of mice.

Paracetamol induced sister chromatid exchange and chromosomal aberrations in Chinese hamster cells, micronuclei in rat kidney cells and chromosomal aberrations in human lymphocytes *in vitro*. It did not induce point mutations in mouse or Chinese hamster cells. Paracetamol gave positive results in a transformation test in mouse cells *in vitro*. It induced unscheduled DNA synthesis in mouse and rat cells but not in Chinese or Syrian hamster or guinea-pig cells. Paracetamol did not induce sex-linked recessive lethal mutations in *Drosophila* and was not mutagenic to *Salmonella typhimurium* or *Escherichia coli*. (See Appendix 1.)

4.5 Evaluation[1]

There is *inadequate evidence* for the carcinogenicity of paracetamol in humans.

There is *limited evidence* for the carcinogenicity of paracetamol in experimental animals.

Overall evaluation

Paracetamol *is not classifiable as to its carcinogenicity to humans (Group 3)*.

5. References

Aguilar, M.I., Hart, S.J. & Calder, I.C. (1988) Complete separation of urinary metabolites of paracetamol and substituted paracetamols by reversed-phase ion-pair high-performance liquid chromatography. *J. Chromatogr.*, 426, 315-333

Ameer, B. & Greenblatt, D.J. (1977) Acetaminophen. *Ann. intern. Med.*, 87, 202-209

American Medical Association (1986) *AMA Drug Evaluations*, 6th ed., Philadelphia, W.B. Saunders, pp. 73-74

Amo, H. & Matsuyama, M. (1985) Subchronic and chronic effects of feeding of large amounts of acetaminophen in B6C3F1 mice. *Jpn. J. Hyg.*, 40, 567-574

Apoteksbolaget (1988) *Svensk Lälemedelsstatistik* [Swedish Drugs Statistics], Stockholm, Pharmaceutical Association of Sweden

Apoteksbolaget (1989) *Outprint of the Drug Data Base (17 October 1989)*, Stockholm, The Pharmaceutical Association of Sweden

Aselton, P., Jick, H., Milunsky, A., Hunter, J.R. & Stergachis, A. (1985) First trimester drug use and congenital disorders. *Obstet. Gynecol.*, 65, 451-455

Barnhart, E. (1989) *Physicians' Desk Reference*, 43rd ed., Oradell, NJ, Medical Economics, p. 301

Berlin, C.M., Jr, Yaffe, S.J. & Ragni, M. (1980) Disposition of acetaminophen in milk, saliva, and plasma of lactating women. *Pediatr. Pharmacol.*, 1, 135-141

Betowski, L.D., Korfmacher, W.A., Lay, J.O., Jr, Potter, D.W. & Hinson, J.A. (1987) Direct analysis of rat bile for acetaminophen and two of its conjugated metabolites via thermospray liquid chromatography/mass spectrometry. *Biomed. environ. mass Spectrom.*, 14, 705-709

Biemer, T.A. (1987) Simultaneous analysis of acetaminophen, pseudoephedrine hydrochloride and chlorpheniramine maleate in a cold tablet using an isocratic, mixed micellar high-performance liquid chromatographic mobile phase. *J. Chromatogr.*, 410, 206-210

---

[1]For description of the italicized terms, see Preamble, pp. 26-29.

Birge, R.B., Bartolone, J.B., Nishanian, E.V., Bruno, M.K., Mangold, J.B., Cohen, S.D. & Khairallah, E.A. (1988) Dissociation of covalent binding from the oxidative effects of acetaminophen. *Biochem. Pharmacol.*, 37, 3383-3393

Black, M. (1984) Acetaminophen hepatotoxicity. *Ann. Rev. Med.*, 35, 577-593

Boyd, E.M. & Bereczky, G.M. (1966) Liver necrosis from paracetamol. *Br. J. Pharmacol. Chemother.*, 26, 606-614

Boyd, E.M. & Hogan, S.E. (1968) The chronic oral toxicity of paracetamol at the range of the LD_{50} (100 days) in albino rats. *Can. J. Physiol. Pharmacol.*, 46, 239-245

Carpenter, H.M. & Mudge, G.H. (1981) Acetaminophen nephrotoxicity: studies on renal acetylation and deacetylation. *J. Pharmacol. exp. Ther.*, 218, 161-167

Chemical Information Services Ltd (1989-90) *Directory of World Chemical Producers*, Oceanside, NY

Clements, J.A., Heading, R.C., Nimmo, W.S. & Prescott, L.F. (1978) Kinetics of acetaminophen absorption and gastric emptying in man. *Clin. Pharmacol. Ther.*, 24, 420-431

Collins, E. (1981) Maternal and fetal effects of acetaminophen and salicylates in pregnancy. *Obstet. Gynaecol.*, 58 (Suppl. 5), 57s-62s

Corcoran, G.B., Mitchell, J.R., Vaishnav, Y.N. & Horning, E.C. (1980) Evidence that acetaminophen and *N*-hydroxyacetaminophen form a common arylating intermediate, *N*-acetyl-*para*-benzoquinoneimine. *Mol. Pharmacol.*, 18, 536-542

Critchley, J.A.J.H., Nimmo, G.R., Gregson, C.A., Woolhouse, N.M. & Prescott, L.F. (1986) Inter-subject and ethnic differences in paracetamol metabolism. *Br. J. clin. Pharmacol.*, 22, 649-657

Crombie, D.L., Pinsent, R.J.F.H., Slater, B.C., Fleming, D. & Cross, K.W. (1970) Teratogenic drugs. RCGP survey. *Br. med. J.*, iv, 178-179

Davidson, D.G.D. & Eastham, W.N. (1966) Acute liver necrosis following overdose of paracetamol. *Br. med. J.*, ii, 497-499

Davis, D.C., Potter, W.Z., Jollow, D.J. & Mitchell, J.R. (1974) Species differences in hepatic glutathione depletion, covalent binding and hepatic necrosis after acetaminophen. *Life Sci.*, 14, 2099-2109

Davis, M., Harrison, N.G., Ideo, G., Portman, B., Labadarios, D. & Williams, R. (1976) Paracetamol metabolism in the rat: relationship to covalent binding and hepatic damage. *Xenobiotica*, 6, 249-255

De Vries, J. (1981) Hepatotoxic metabolic activation of paracetamol and its derivatives phenacetin and benorilate: oxygenation or electron transfer? *Biochem. Pharmacol.*, 30, 399-402

Dixon, M.F., Nimmo, J. & Prescott, L.F. (1971) Experimental paracetamol-induced hepatic necrosis: a histopathological study. *J. Pathol.*, 103, 225-229

Dunn, T.L., Gardiner, R.A., Seymour, G.J. & Lavin, M.F. (1987) Genotoxicity of analgesic compounds assessed by an *in vitro* micronucleus assay. *Mutat. Res.*, 189, 299-306

Dybing, E., Holme, J.A., Gordon, W.P., Soderlund, E.J., Dahlin, D.C. & Nelson, S.D. (1984) Genotoxicity studies with paracetamol. *Mutat. Res.*, 138, 21-32

El-Obeid, H.A. & Al-Badr, A.A. (1985) Acetaminophen. *Anal. Profiles Drug Subst.*, *14*, 552-596

Fairbrother, J.E. (1974) Acetaminophen. *Anal. Profiles Drug Subst.*, *3*, 2-109

Flaks, A. & Flaks, B. (1983) Induction of liver cell tumours in IF mice by paracetamol. *Carcinogenesis*, *4*, 363-368

Flaks, B., Flaks, A. & Shaw, A.P.W. (1985) Induction by paracetamol of bladder and liver tumours in the rat. *Acta pathol. microbiol. immunol. scand. Sect. A*, *93*, 367-377

Flower, R.J., Moncada, S. & Vane, J.R. (1985) Analgesic-antipyretics and anti-inflammatory agents; drugs employed in the treatment of gout. In: Gilman, A.G., Goodman, L.S., Rall, T.W. & Murad, F., eds, *Goodman and Gilman's The Pharmacological Basis of Therapeutics*, 7th ed., New York, MacMillan, pp. 674-715

Forrest, J.A.H., Clements, J.A. & Prescott, L.F. (1982) Clinical pharmacokinetics of paracetamol. *Clin. Pharmacokinet.*, *7*, 93-107

Friedman, G.D. & Ury, H.K. (1980) Initial screening for carcinogenicity of commonly used drugs. *J. natl Cancer Inst.*, *65*, 723-733

Friedman, G.D. & Ury, H.K. (1983) Screening for possible drug carcinogenicity: second report of findings. *J. natl Cancer Inst.*, *71*, 1165-1175

Galinsky, R.E. & Levy, G. (1981) Dose and time-dependent elimination of acetaminophen in rats: pharmacokinetic implications of cosubstrate depletion. *J. Pharmacol. exp. Ther.*, *219*, 14-20

Gazzard, B.G., Ford-Hutchinson, A.W., Smith, M.J.H. & Williams, R. (1973) The binding of paracetamol to plasma proteins of man and pig. *J. Pharm. Pharmacol.*, *25*, 964-967

Gemborys, M.W. & Mudge, G.H. (1981) Formation and disposition of the minor metabolites of acetaminophen in the hamster. *Drug Metab. Dispos.*, *9*, 340-351

Gregus, Z., Madhu, C. & Klaassen, C.D. (1988) Species variation in toxication and detoxication of acetaminophen in vivo: a comparative study of biliary and urinary excretion of acetaminophen metabolites. *J. Pharmacol. exp. Ther.*, *244*, 91-99

Gwilt, J.R., Robertson, A. & McChaney, E.W. (1963) Determination of blood and other tissue concentrations of paracetamol in dog and man. *J. Pharm. Pharmacol.*, *15*, 440-444

Hagiwara, A. & Ward, J.M. (1986) The chronic hepatotoxic, tumor-promoting, and carcinogenic effects of acetaminophen in male B6C3F mice. *Fundam. appl. Toxicol.*, *7*, 376-386

Ham, K.N. & Calder, I.C. (1984) Tumor formation induced by phenacetin and its metabolites. *Adv. Inflammation Res.*, *6*, 139-148

Hamlyn, A.N., Douglas, A.P, James, O.F.W., Lesna, M. & Watson, A.J. (1977) Liver function and structure in survivors of acetaminophen poisoning: a follow-up of serum bile acids and liver histology. *Am. J. dig. Dis.*, *22*, 605-610

Hasegawa, R., Furukawa, F., Toyoda, K., Jang, J.J., Yamashita, K., Sato, S., Takahashi, M. & Hayashi, Y. (1988) Study for tumor-initiating effect of acetaminophen in two-stage liver carcinogenesis of male F344 rats. *Carcinogenesis*, *9*, 755-759

Heinonen, O.P., Slone, D. & Shapiro, S. (1977) *Birth Defects and Drugs in Pregnancy*, Littleton, MA, Publishing Sciences Group, pp. 286-295

Henry, M.A. & Tange, J.D. (1984) Chronic renal lesions in the uninephrectomized Gunn rat after analgesic mixtures. *Pathology*, 16, 278-284

Hinson, J.A., Nelson, S.D. & Mitchell, J.R. (1977) Studies on the microsomal formation of arylating metabolites of acetaminophen and phenacetin. *Mol. Pharmacol.*, 13, 625-633

Hiraga, K. & Fujii, T. (1985) Carcinogenicity testing of acetaminophen in F344 rats. *Jpn. J. Cancer Res. (Gann)*, 76, 79-85

Hjelle, J.J. & Klaassen, C.D. (1984) Glucuronidation and biliary excretion of acetaminophen in rats. *J. Pharmacol. exp. Ther.*, 228, 407-413

Holme, J.A. & Soderlund, E. (1986) Species differences in cytotoxic and genotoxic effects of phenacetin and paracetamol in primary monolayer cultures of hepatocytes. *Mutat. Res.*, 164, 167-175

Holme, J.A., Hongslo, J.K., Bjornstad, C., Harvison, P.J. & Nelson, S.D. (1988) Toxic effects of paracetamol and related structures in V79 Chinese hamster cells. *Mutagenesis*, 3, 51-56

Hongslo, J.K., Christensen, T., Brunborg, G., Bjornstad, C. & Holme, J.A. (1988) Genotoxic effects of paracetamol in V79 Chinese hamster cells. *Mutat. Res.*, 204, 333-341

IARC (1975) *IARC Monographs on the Evaluation of Carcinogenic Risk of Chemicals to Man*, Vol. 8, *Some Aromatic Azo Compounds*, Lyon, pp. 75-81

IARC (1977) *IARC Monographs on the Evaluation of the Carcinogenic Risk of Chemicals to Man*, Vol. 15, *Some Fumigants, the Herbicides 2,4-D and 2,4,5-T, Chlorinated Dibenzodioxins and Miscellaneous Industrial Chemicals*, Lyon, pp. 255-264

IARC (1980) *IARC Monographs on the Evaluation of the Carcinogenic Risk of Chemicals to Humans*, Vol. 24, *Some Pharmaceutical Drugs*, Lyon, pp. 135-161

IARC (1987) *IARC Monographs on the Evaluation of Carcinogenic Risks to Humans*, Suppl. 7, *Overall Evaluations of Carcinogenicity: An Updating of* IARC Monographs *Volumes 1 to 42*, pp. 310-312

Imamura, A., Kurumi, T., Danzuka, T., Kodama, M., Kawachi, T. & Nagao, M. (1983) Classification of compounds by cluster analysis of Ames test data. *Gann*, 74, 196-204

Ishidate, M., Jr (1988) *Data Book of Chromosomal Aberration Test In Vitro*, rev. ed., Amsterdam, Elsevier

Ishidate, M., Jr, Hayashi, M., Sawada, M., Matsuoka, A., Yoshikawa, K., Ono, M. & Nakadate, M. (1978) Cytotoxicity test on medical drugs—chromosome aberration tests with Chinese hamster cells *in vitro*. *Bull. natl Inst. Hyg. Sci. (Tokyo)*, 96, 55-61

Jacqueson, A., Semont H., Thevenin, M., Warnet, J.M., Prost, R. & Claude, J.R. (1984) Effects of daily high doses of paracetamol given orally during spermatogenesis in the rat testes. *Arch. Toxicol., Suppl. 7*, 164-166

James, O., Lesna, M., Roberts, S.H., Pulman, L., Douglas, A.P., Smith, P.A. & Watson, A.J. (1975) Liver damage after paracetamol overdose: comparison of liver function tests, fasting serum bile acids, and liver histology. *Lancet*, ii, 579-581

Jasiewicz, M.L. & Richardson, J.C. (1987) Absence of mutagenic activity of benorylate, paracetamol and aspirin in the *Salmonella*/mammalian microsome test. *Mutat. Res.*, 190, 95-100

Jick, H., Holmes, L.B., Hunter, J.R., Madsen, S. & Stergachis, A. (1981) First trimester drug use and congenital disorders. *J. Am. med. Assoc.*, *246*, 343-346

Johansson, S.L. (1981) Carcinogenicity of analgesics: long-term treatment of Sprague-Dawley rats with phenacetin, phenazone, caffeine and paracetamol (acetamidophen). *Int. J. Cancer*, *27*, 521-529

Jollow, D.J., Thorgeirsson, S.S., Potter, W.Z., Hashimoto, M. & Mitchell, J.R. (1974) Acetaminophen-induced hepatic necrosis. VI. Metabolic disposition of toxic and nontoxic doses of acetaminophen. *Pharmacology*, *12*, 251-271

Kaysen, G.A., Pond, S.M., Roper, M.H., Menki, D.J. & Marrama, M.A. (1985) Combined hepatic and renal injury in alcoholics during therapeutic use of acetaminophen. *Arch. intern. Med.*, *145*, 2019-2023

King, M.-T., Beikirch, H., Eckhardt, K., Gocke, E. & Wild, D. (1979) Mutagenicity studies with X-ray-contrast media, analgesics, antipyretics, antirheumatics and some other pharmaceutical drugs in bacterial, *Drosophila* and mammalian test systems. *Mutat. Res.*, *66*, 33-43

Kinney, C.D. & Kelly, J.G. (1987) Liquid chromatographic determination of paracetamol and dextropropoxyphene in plasma. *J. Chromatogr.*, *419*, 433-437

Koch-Weser, J. (1976) Drug therapy: acetaminophen. *New Engl. J. Med.*, *295*, 1297-1300

Kocisova, J., Rossner, P., Binkova, B., Bavorova, H. & Sram, R.J. (1988) Mutagenicity studies on paracetamol in human volunteers. I. Cytogenetic analysis of peripheral lymphocytes and lipid peroxidation in plasma. *Mutat. Res.*, *209*, 161-165

Koizumi, F., Kawamura, T., Ishimori, A., Ebina, H. & Satoh, M. (1988) Plasma paracetamol concentrations measured by fluorescence polarization immunoassay and gastric emptying time. *Tohoku J. exp. Med.*, *155*, 159-164

Kurata, Y., Asamoto, M., Hagiwara, A., Masui, T. & Fukushima S. (1986) Promoting effects of various agents in rat urinary bladder carcinogenesis initiated by N-butyl-N-(4-hydroxybutyl)nitrosamine. *Cancer Lett.*, *32*, 125-135

Lowenthal, D.T., Oie, S., Van Stone, J.C., Briggs, W.A. & Levy, G. (1976) Pharmacokinetics of acetaminophen elimination by anephric patients. *J. Pharmacol. exp. Ther.*, *196*, 570-578

Lubawy, W.C. & Burriss Garrett, R.J. (1977) Effects of aspirin and acetaminophen on fetal and placental growth in rats. *J. pharm. Sci.*, *66*, 111-113

Manno, B.R., Manno, J.E., Dempsey, C.A. & Wood, M.A. (1981) A high-pressure liquid chromatographic method for the determination of N-acetyl-p-aminophenol (acetaminophen) in serum or plasma using a direct injection technique. *J. anal. Toxicol.*, *5*, 24-28

Maruyama, H. & Williams, G.M. (1988) Hepatotoxicity of chronic high dose administration of acetaminophen to mice. A critical review and implications for hazard assessment. *Arch. Toxicol.*, *62*, 465-469

McCredie, M. & Stewart, J.H. (1988) Does paracetamol cause urothelial cancer or renal papillary necrosis? *Nephron*, *49*, 296-300

McCredie, M., Stewart, J., Ford, J. & MacLennan, R. (1983a) Phenacetin-containing analgesics and cancer of the bladder or renal pelvis in women. *Br. J. Urol.*, *55*, 220-224

McCredie, M., Stewart, J. & Ford, J. (1983b) Analgesics and tobacco as risk factors for cancer of the ureter and renal pelvis. *J. Urol.*, *130*, 28-30

McCredie, M., Ford, J.M. & Stewart, J.H. (1988) Risk factors for cancer of the renal parenchyma. *Int. J. Cancer*, *42*, 13-16

McLaughlin, J.K., Blot, W.J., Mandel, J.S., Schuman, L.M., Mehl, E.S. & Fraumeni, J.F., Jr (1983) Etiology of cancer of the renal pelvis. *J. natl Cancer Inst.*, *71*, 287-291

McLaughlin, J.K., Mandel, J.S., Blot, W.J., Schuman, L.M., Mehl, E.S. & Fraumeni, J.F., Jr (1984) A population-based case-control study of renal cell carcinoma. *J. natl Cancer Inst.*, *72*, 275-284

McLaughlin, J.K., Blot, W.J., Mehl, E.S., Mandel, J.S., Schuman, L.M. & Fraumeni, J.F., Jr (1985) Relation of analgesic use to renal cancer: population-based findings. *Natl Cancer Inst. Monogr.*, *69*, 217-222

McLean, A.E.M., Armstrong, A.R. & Beales, D. (1989) Effect of D- or L-methionine and cysteine on the growth inhibitory effects of feeding 1% paracetamol to rats. *Biochem. Pharmacol.*, *38*, 347-352

McMurty, R.J., Snodgrass, W.R. & Mitchell, J.R. (1978) Renal necrosis, glutathione depletion and covalent binding after acetaminophen. *Toxicol. appl. Pharmacol.*, *46*, 87-100

Meatherall, R. & Ford, D. (1988) Isocratic liquid chromatographic determination of theophylline, acetaminophen, chloramphenicol, caffeine, anticonvulsants, and barbiturates in serum. *Ther. Drug Monit.*, *10*, 101-115

Milam, K.M. & Byard, J.L. (1985) Acetaminophen metabolism, cytotoxicity, and genotoxicity in rat primary hepatocyte cultures. *Toxicol. appl. Pharmacol.*, *79*, 342-347

Miner, D.J. & Kissenger, P.T. (1979) Evidence for the involvement of N-acetyl-p-quinoneimine in paracetamol metabolism. *Biochem. Pharmacol.*, *28*, 3285-3290.

Mitchell, J.R., Jollow, D.J., Potter, W.Z., Davis, D.C., Gillette, J.R. & Brodie, B.B. (1973) Acetaminophen-induced hepatic necrosis. I. Role of drug metabolism. *J. Pharmacol. exp. Ther.*, *187*, 185-194

Mitchell, J.R., Thorgeirsson, S.S., Potter, W.Z., Jollow, D.J. & Keiser, H. (1974) Acetaminophen-induced hepatic injury: protective role of glutathione in man and rationale for therapy. *Clin. Pharmacol. Ther.*, *16*, 676-684

Moore, M., Thor, H., Moore, G., Nelson, S., Moldeus, P. & Orrenius, S. (1985) The toxicity of acetaminophen and *N*-acetyl-*p*-benzoquinoneimine in isolated hepatocytes is associated with thiol depletion and increased cytosolic Ca^{2+}. *J. biol. Chem.*, *260*, 13035-13039

Morris, M.E. & Levy, G. (1984) Renal clearance and serum protein binding of acetaminophen and its major conjugates in humans. *J. pharm. Sci.*, *73*, 1038-1041

Nelson, M.M. & Forfar, J.O. (1971) Association between drugs administered during pregnancy and congenital abnormalities of the fetus. *Br. med. J.*, *i*, 523-527

Nelson, S.D., Dahlin, D.C., Rauckman, E.J. & Rosen, G.M. (1981) Peroxidase-mediated formation of reactive metabolites of acetaminophen. *Mol. Pharmacol.*, *20*, 195-199

Newton, J.F., Kuo, C.-H., Gemborys, M.W., Mudge, G.H. & Hook, J.B. (1982) Nephrotoxicity of *p*-aminophenol, a metabolite of acetaminophen, in the Fischer 344 rat. *Toxicol. appl. Pharmacol.*, 65, 336-344

Newton, J.F., Pasino, D.A. & Hook, J.B. (1985) Acetaminophen nephrotoxicity in the rat: quantitation of renal metabolic activation *in vivo*. *Toxicol. appl. Pharmacol.*, 78, 39-46

Notarianni, L.J., Oldham, H.G. & Bennet, P.N. (1987) Passage of paracetamol into breast milk and its subsequent metabolism be the neonate. *Br. J. clin. Pharmacol.*, 24, 63-67.

Oldham, J.W., Preston, R.F. & Paulson, J.D (1986) Mutagenicity testing of selected analgesics in Ames *Salmonella* strains. *J. appl. Toxicol.*, 6, 237-243

Patierno, S.R., Lehman, N.L., Henderson, B.E. & Landolph, J.R. (1989) Study of the ability of phenacetin, acetaminophen, and aspirin to induce cytotoxicity, mutation, and morphological transformation in C3H/10T½ clone 8 mouse embryo cells. *Cancer Res.*, 49, 1038-1044

Piper, J.M., Tonascia, J. & Matanoski, G.M. (1985) Heavy phenacetin use and bladder cancer in women aged 20 to 49 years. *New Engl. J. Med.*, 313, 292-295

Placke, M.E., Wyand, D.S. & Cohen, S.D. (1987) Extrahepatic lesions induced by acetaminophen in the mouse. *Toxicol. Pathol.*, 15, 381-383

Potter, W.Z., Davis, D.C., Mitchell, H.R., Jollow, D.G., Gillette, J.R. & Brodie, B.B. (1973) Acetaminophen-induced hepatic necrosis. III. Cytochrome P-450-mediated covalent binding in vitro. *J. Pharmacol. exp. Ther.*, 187, 203-209

Rawlings, M.D., Henderson, D.B. & Hijab, A.R. (1977) Pharmacokinetics of paracetamol (acetaminophen) after intravenous and oral administration. *Eur. J. clin. Pharmacol.*, 11, 283-286

Reddy, G.A. (1984), Effects of paracetamol on chromosomes of bone marrow. *Caryologia*, 37, 127-132

Reddy, G.A. & Subramanyam, S. (1981) Response of mitotic cells of *Allium cepa* to paracetamol. In: Manna, G.K. & Sinha, U., eds, *Perspectives in Cytology and Genetics*, Vol. 3, Delhi, Hindasi Publishers, pp. 571-576

Reddy, G.A. & Subramanyam, S. (1985) Cytogenetic response of meiocytes of Swiss albino mice to paracetamol. *Caryologia*, 38, 347-355

Reicks, M., Calvert, R.J. & Hathcock, J.N. (1988) Effects of prolonged acetaminophen ingestion and dietary methionine on mouse liver glutathione. *Drug-Nutr. Interact.*, 5, 351-363

Reynolds, J.E.F., ed. (1989) *Martindale. The Extra Pharmacopoeia*, 29th ed., London, The Pharmaceutical Press, pp. 32-34

Ross, R.K., Paganini-Hill, A., Landolph, J., Gerkins, V. & Henderson, B.E. (1989) Analgesics, cigarette smoking and other risk factors for cancer of the renal pelvis and ureter. *Cancer Res.*, 49, 1045-1048

Sasaki, M. (1986) Enhancing effect of acetaminophen on mutagenesis. *Prog. clin. biol. Res.*, 209A, 365-372

Sasaki, M., Sugimura, K., Yoshida, M.A. & Abe, S. (1980) Cytogenetic effects of 60 chemicals on cultured human and Chinese hamster cells. *Kromosomo*, II-20, 574-584

Savides, M.C., Oehme, F.W., Nash, S.L. & Leipold, H.W. (1984) The toxicity and biotransformation of single doses of acetaminophen in dogs and cats. *Toxicol. appl. Pharmacol.*, 74, 26-34

Sawada, M., Matsuoka, A., Nohmi, T., Sofuni, T. & Ishidate, M., Jr (1985) Mutagenicity tests on phenacetin-related compounds in cultured mammalian cells (Abstract). *Mutat. Res.*, 147, 273

Selby, J.V., Friedman, G.D. & Fireman, B.H. (1989) Screening prescription drugs for possible carcinogenicity: 11 to 15 years of follow-up. *Cancer Res.*, 49, 5736-5747

Siegers, C.-P., Strublet, O. & Schutt, A. (1978) Relations between hepatotoxicity and pharmacokinetics of paracetamol in rats and mice. *Pharmacology*, 16, 273-278

Tamura, T., Fijii, A. & Kuboyama, N. (1980) Pharmacological studies on the mutagenicity: I. Analgesics and antiinflammatory drugs and their derivatives. *Jpn. J. Pharmacol.*, 30 (*Suppl.*), 238P

Tsokos-Kuhn, J.O., Hughes, H., Smith, C.V. & Mitchell, J.R. (1988) Alkylation of the liver plasma membrane and inhibition of the Ca^{2+} ATPase by acetaminophen. *Biochem. Pharmacol.*, 37, 2125-2131

Tsuda, H., Sakata, T., Masui, T., Imaida, K. & Ito, N. (1984) Modifying effects of butylated hydroxyanisole, ethoxyquin and acetaminophen on induction of neoplastic lesions in rat liver and kidney initiated by N-ethyl-N-hydroxyethylnitrosamine. *Carcinogenesis*, 5, 525-531

Tsuruzaki, T., Yamamoto, M. & Watanabe, G. (1982) Maternal consumption of antipyretic analgesics produces chromosome anomalies in F_1 rat embryos. *Teratology*, 26, 42A

US Pharmacopeial Convention, Inc. (1989) *US Pharmacopeia*, 22nd rev., Easton, PA, pp. 12-15

Watanabe, M. (1982) The cytogenetic effects of aspirin and acetaminophen on *in vitro* human lymphocytes. *Jpn. J. Hyg.*, 37, 673-685

Weisburger, J.H., Weisburger, E.K., Madison, R.M., Wenk, M.L. & Klein, D.S. (1973) Effect of acetanilide and p-hydroxy-acetanilide on the carcinogenicity of N-2-fluoronylacetamide and N-hydroxy-N-2-fluorenylacetamide in mice, hamsters and female rats. *J. natl Cancer Inst.*, 51, 235-240

Williams, G.M., Mori, H. & McQueen, C.A. (1989) Structure-activity relationship in the rat hepatocyte DNA repair test for 300 chemicals. *Mutat. Res.*, 221, 263-286

Wirth, P.J., Dybing, E., von Bahr, C. & Thorgeirsson, S.S. (1980) Mechanism of N-hydroxyacetylarylamine mutagenicity in the *Salmonella* test system: metabolic activation of N-hydroxyphenacetin by liver and kidney fractions from rat, mouse, hamster, and man. *Mol. Pharmacol.*, 18, 117-127

Wong, L.T., Solomonraj, G. & Thomas, B.H. (1976) Metabolism of [^{14}C]paracetamol and its interactions with aspirin in hamsters. *Xenobiotica*, 6, 575-584

Wright, N. & Prescott, L.F. (1973) Potentiation by previous drug therapy of hepatotoxicity following paracetamol overdosage. *Scott. med. J.*, 18, 56-58

SUMMARY OF FINAL EVALUATIONS

Agent	Evidence for carcinogenicity		Overall evaluation
	Humans	Animals	
Ampicillin	Inadequate	Limited	Not classifiable (3)
Azacitidine	No data	Sufficient	Probably carcinogenic (2A)
Chloramphenicol	Limited	Inadequate	Probably carcinogenic (2A)
Chlorozotocin	No data	Sufficient	Probably carcinogenic (2A)
Ciclosporin	Sufficient	Limited	Carcinogenic (1)
Cimetidine	Inadequate	Inadequate	Not classifiable (3)
Dantron (Chrysazin; 1,8–Dihydroxy-anthraquinone)	No data	Sufficient	Possibly carcinogenic (2B)
Furosemide (Frusemide)	Inadequate	Inadequate	Not classifiable (3)
Hydrochlorothiazide	Inadequate	Inadequate	Not classifiable (3)
Nitrofural (Nitrofurazone)	Inadequate	Limited	Not classifiable (3)
Nitrofurantoin	Inadequate	Limited	Not classifiable (3)
Paracetamol (Acetaminophen)	Inadequate	Limited	Not classifiable (3)
Prednimustine	No data	Inadequate	Not classifiable (3)
Thiotepa	Sufficient	Sufficient	Carcinogenic (1)
Trichlormethine (Trimustine hydrochloride)	No data	Sufficient	Possibly carcinogenic (2B)

Appendix 1. Summary table of genetic and related effects

	Nonmammalian systems												Mammalian systems																							
	Prokaryotes			Lower eukaryotes			Plants			Insects			In vitro																In vivo						
													Animal cells										Human cells							Animals					Humans				
	D	G	R	G	A	D	D	G	C	C	R	G	C	A	D	G	S	M	C	A	T	I	D	G	S	M	C	A	T	D	G	S	M	C	DL	D	S	M	C	A
Antineoplastic and immunosuppressive agents																																								
Azacitidine	+			+¹	+¹	−¹				+¹	+¹	+¹			+¹	+	+		+¹	+	+		+¹	+¹	?		?								−¹					
Chlorozotocin	+			+¹					+¹			+¹			+¹	+¹	+¹		+¹					+¹						+¹										
Ciclosporin	−¹														−¹	−¹								+																?
Thiotepa	+	+¹								+					+	+	+		+	+¹			+¹	+¹	+		+			+¹	+¹	+¹	+	+						+¹
Trichlormethine															+¹																				+¹					
Antimicrobial agents																																								
Ampicillin	−	−							+¹						−	−¹	−¹	−¹						−¹	−¹	?														
Chloramphenicol	−	?					−¹		+	−					−	+	+¹	−¹		−			?	?	?	?	−							?	?					
Nitrofural	+	+¹		?					+			−¹			?	?	+¹	+	+¹				?	?	−¹	−¹	−¹							−	−					
Nitrofurantoin	+	+		?					?						?	+¹	+¹	+¹					?	−¹	−¹		−¹			+	−¹	+¹	−	−¹	−					

Appendix 1 (contd)

	Nonmammalian systems																	Mammalian systems																						
	Prokaryotes		Lower eukaryotes				Plants				Insects				In vitro																			In vivo						
															Animal cells								Human cells								Animals							Humans				
	D	G	D	R	G	A	D	G	C	R	G	C	A	D	G	S	M	C	A	T	I	D	G	S	M	C	A	T	I	D	G	S	M	C	DL	A	D	S	M	C	A
Other drugs																																									
Cimetidine	−													−ª																											
N-Nitrosocimetidine	+	+												+¹	+¹	+		+		+¹		+		+¹																	
Dantron	+	+¹												?						+¹	?								+¹							−¹					
Furosemide	−¹															?	?	+						−¹				?													
Hydrochlorothiazide	+¹	+¹									−¹				+¹	+¹	−										+¹														
Paracetamol	−	−									−¹			?	−¹	+	+¹	+		+¹								+¹		−	−					+¹				+¹	

A, aneuploidy; C, chromosomal aberrations; D, DNA damage; DL, dominant lethal mutation; G, gene mutation; I, inhibition of intercellular communication; M, micronuclei; R, mitotic recombination and gene conversion; S, sister chromatid exchange; T, cell transformation

In completing the tables, the following symbols indicate the consensus of the Working Group with regard to the results for each endpoint:

+ considered to be positive for the specific endpoint and level of biological complexity
+¹ considered to be positive, but only one valid study was available to the Working Group
− considered to be negative
−¹ considered to be negative, but only one valid study was available to the Working Group
? considered to be equivocal or inconclusive (e.g., there were contradictory results from different laboratories; there were confounding exposures; the results were equivocal)

ªCimetidine hydrochloride gave a positive result.

APPENDIX 2

ACTIVITY PROFILES
FOR GENETIC AND RELATED EFFECTS

Methods

The x-axis of the activity profile (Waters *et al.*, 1987, 1988) represents the bioassays in phylogenetic sequence by endpoint, and the values on the y-axis represent the logarithmically transformed lowest effective doses (LED) and highest ineffective doses (HID) tested. The term 'dose', as used in this report, does not take into consideration length of treatment or exposure and may therefore be considered synonymous with concentration. In practice, the concentrations used in all the in-vitro tests were converted to µg/ml, and those for in-vivo tests were expressed as mg/kg bw. Because dose units are plotted on a log scale, differences in molecular weights of compounds do not, in most cases, greatly influence comparisons of their activity profiles. Conventions for dose conversions are given below.

Profile-line height (the magnitude of each bar) is a function of the LED or HID, which is associated with the characteristics of each individual test system – such as population size, cell-cycle kinetics and metabolic competence. Thus, the detection limit of each test system is different, and, across a given activity profile, responses will vary substantially. No attempt is made to adjust or relate responses in one test system to those of another.

Line heights are derived as follows: for negative test results, the highest dose tested without appreciable toxicity is defined as the HID. If there was evidence of extreme toxicity, the next highest dose is used. A single dose tested with a negative result is considered to be equivalent to the HID. Similarly, for positive results, the LED is recorded. If the original data were analysed statistically by the author, the dose recorded is that at which the response was significant ($p < 0.05$). If the available data were not analysed statistically, the dose required to produce an effect is estimated as follows: when a dose-related positive response is observed with two or more doses, the lower of the doses is taken as the LED; a single dose resulting in a positive response is considered to be equivalent to the LED.

In order to accommodate both the wide range of doses encountered and positive and negative responses on a continuous scale, doses are transformed logarithmically, so that effective (LED) and ineffective (HID) doses are represented by positive and negative numbers, respectively. The response, or logarithmic dose unit (LDU_{ij}), for a given test system i and chemical j is represented by the expressions

$LDU_{ij} = -\log_{10}$ (dose), for HID values; LDU ≤ 0
and (1)
$LDU_{ij} = -\log_{10}$ (dose x 10^{-5}), for LED values; LDU ≥ 0.

These simple relationships define a dose range of 0 to -5 logarithmic units for ineffective doses (1–100 000 µg/ml or mg/kg bw) and 0 to $+8$ logarithmic units for effective doses (100 000–0.001 µg/ml or mg/kg bw). A scale illustrating the LDU values is shown in Figure 1. Negative responses at doses less than 1 µg/ml (mg/kg bw) are set equal to 1. Effectively, an LED value $\geq 100\,000$ or an HID value ≤ 1 produces an LDU = 0; no quantitative information is gained from such extreme values. The dotted lines at the levels of log dose units 1 and -1 define a 'zone of uncertainty' in which positive results are reported at such high doses (between 10 000 and 100 000 µg/ml or mg/kg bw) or negative results are reported at such low dose levels (1 to 10 µg/ml or mg/kg bw) as to call into question the adequacy of the test.

Fig. 1. Scale of log dose units used on the y-axis of activity profiles

Positive (µg/ml or mg/kg bw)		Log dose units	
0.001		8	—
0.01		7	—
0.1		6	—
1.0		5	—
10		4	—
100		3	—
1000		2	—
10 000		1	—
100 000	1	0	—
	10	−1	—
	100	−2	—
	1000	−3	—
	10 000	−4	—
	100 000	−5	—

Negative
(µg/ml or mg/kg bw)

LED and HID are expressed as µg/ml or mg/kg bw.

In practice, an activity profile is computer generated. A data entry programme is used to store abstracted data from published reports. A sequential file (in ASCII) is created for each compound, and a record within that file consists of the name and Chemical Abstracts Service number of the compound, a three-letter code for the test system (see below), the qualitative test result (with and without an exogenous metabolic system), dose (LED or HID), citation number and additional source information. An abbreviated citation for each publication is stored in a segment of a record accessing both the test data file and the citation file. During processing of the data file, an average of the logarithmic values of the data subset is calculated, and the length of the profile line represents this average value. All dose values are plotted for each profile line, regardless of whether results are positive or negative. Results obtained in the absence of an exogenous metabolic system are indicated by a bar (-), and results obtained in the presence of an exogenous metabolic system are indicated by an upward-directed arrow (↑). When all results for a given assay are either positive or negative, the mean of the LDU values is plotted as a solid line; when conflicting data are reported for the same assay (i.e., both positive and negative results), the majority data are shown by a solid line and the minority data by a dashed line (drawn to the extreme conflicting response). In the few cases in which the numbers of positive and negative results are equal, the solid line is drawn in the positive direction and the maximal negative response is indicated with a dashed line.

Profile lines are identified by three-letter code words representing the commonly used tests. Code words for most of the test systems in current use in genetic toxicology were defined for the US Environmental Protection Agency's GENE-TOX Program (Waters, 1979; Waters & Auletta, 1981). For IARC Monographs Supplement 6, Volume 44 and subsequent volumes, including this publication, codes were redefined in a manner that should facilitate inclusion of additional tests. If a test system is not defined precisely, a general code is used that best defines the category of the test. Naming conventions are described below.

Data listings are presented with each activity profile and include endpoint and test codes, a short test code definition, results [either with (M) or without (NM) an exogenous activation system], the associated LED or HID value and a short citation. Test codes are organized phylogenetically and by endpoint from left to right across each activity profile and from top to bottom of the corresponding data listing. Endpoints are defined as follows: A, aneuploidy; C, chromosomal aberrations; D, DNA damage; F, assays of body fluids; G, gene mutation; H, host-mediated assays; I, inhibition of intercellular communication; M, micronuclei; P, sperm morphology; R, mitotic recombination or gene conversion; S, sister chromatid exchange; and T, cell transformation.

Dose conversions for activity profiles

Doses are converted to µg/ml for in-vitro tests and to mg/kg bw per day for in-vivo experiments.

1. In-vitro test systems

    (a) Weight/volume converts directly to µg/ml.

    (b) Molar (M) concentration × molecular weight = mg/ml = 10^3 µg/ml; mM concentration × molecular weight = µg/ml.

    (c) Soluble solids expressed as % concentration are assumed to be in units of mass per volume (i.e., 1% = 0.01 g/ml = 10 000 µg/ml; also, 1 ppm = 1 µg/ml).

    (d) Liquids and gases expressed as % concentration are assumed to be given in units of volume per volume. Liquids are converted to weight per volume using the density (D) of the solution (D = g/ml). Gases are converted from volume to mass using the ideal gas law, $PV = nRT$. For exposure at 20–37°C at standard atmospheric pressure, 1% (v/v) = 0.4 µg/ml × molecular weight of the gas. Also, 1 ppm (v/v) = 4×10^{-5} µg/ml × molecular weight.

    (e) In microbial plate tests, it is usual for the doses to be reported as weight/plate, whereas concentrations are required to enter data on the activity profile chart. While remaining cognisant of the errors involved in the process, it is assumed that a 2-ml volume of top agar is delivered to each plate and that the test substance remains in solution within it; concentrations are derived from the reported weight/plate values by dividing by this arbitrary volume. For spot tests, a 1-ml volume is used in the calculation.

    (f) Conversion of particulate concentrations given in µg/cm^2 are based on the area (A) of the dish and the volume of medium per dish; i.e., for a 100-mm dish: $A = \pi R^2 = \pi \times (5 \text{ cm})^2 = 78.5 \text{ cm}^2$. If the volume of medium is 10 ml, then 78.5 cm^2 = 10 ml and 1 cm^2 = 0.13 ml.

2. In-vitro systems using in-vivo activation

    For the body fluid-urine (BF-) test, the concentration used is the dose (in mg/kg bw) of the compound administered to test animals or patients.

3. In-vivo test systems

    (a) Doses are converted to mg/kg bw per day of exposure, assuming 100% absorption. Standard values are used for each sex and species of rodent, including body weight and average intake per day, as reported by Gold *et al.* (1984). For example, in a test using male mice fed 50 ppm of the agent in the diet, the standard food intake per day is 12% of body weight, and the conversion is dose = 50 ppm × 12% = 6 mg/kg bw per day.

Standard values used for humans are: weight – males, 70 kg; females, 55 kg; surface area, 1.7 m^2; inhalation rate, 20 l/min for light work, 30 l/min for mild exercise.

(b) When reported, the dose at the target site is used. For example, doses given in studies of lymphocytes of humans exposed *in vivo* are the measured blood concentrations in µg/ml.

Codes for test systems

For specific nonmammalian test systems, the first two letters of the three-symbol code word define the test organism (e.g., SA- for *Salmonella typhimurium*, EC- for *Escherichia coli*). If the species is not known, the convention used is -S-. The third symbol may be used to define the tester strain (e.g., SA8 for *S. typhimurium* TA1538, ECW for *E. coli* WP2uvrA). When strain designation is not indicated, the third letter is used to define the specific genetic endpoint under investigation (e.g., —D for differential toxicity, —F for forward mutation, —G for gene conversion or genetic crossing-over, —N for aneuploidy, —R for reverse mutation, —U for unscheduled DNA synthesis). The third letter may also be used to define the general endpoint under investigation when a more complete definition is not possible or relevant (e.g., —M for mutation, —C for chromosomal aberration).

For mammalian test systems, the first letter of the three-letter code word defines the genetic endpoint under investigation: A— for aneuploidy, B— for binding, C— for chromosomal aberration, D— for DNA strand breaks, G— for gene mutation, I— for inhibition of intercellular communication, M— for micronucleus formation, R— for DNA repair, S— for sister chromatid exchange, T— for cell transformation and U— for unscheduled DNA synthesis.

For animal (i.e., non-human) test systems *in vitro*, when the cell type is not specified, the code letters -IA are used. For such assays *in vivo*, when the animal species is not specified, the code letters -VA are used. Commonly used animal species are identified by the third letter (e.g., —C for Chinese hamster, —M for mouse, —R for rat, —S for Syrian hamster).

For test systems using human cells *in vitro*, when the cell type is not specified, the code letters -IH are used. For assays on humans *in vivo*, when the cell type is not specified, the code letters -VH are used. Otherwise, the second letter specifies the cell type under investigation (e.g., -BH for bone marrow, -LH for lymphocytes).

Some other specific coding conventions used for mammalian systems are as follows: BF- for body fluids, HM- for host-mediated, —L for leucocytes or lymphocytes *in vitro* (-AL, animals; -HL, humans), -L- for leucocytes *in vivo* (-LA, animals; -LH, humans), —T for transformed cells.

Note that these are examples of major conventions used to define the assay code words. The alphabetized listing of codes must be examined to confirm a specific code word. As might be expected from the limitation to three symbols, some codes do not fit the naming conventions precisely. In a few cases, test systems are defined by first-letter code words, for example: MST, mouse spot test; SLP, mouse specific locus test, postspermatogonia; SLO, mouse specific locus test, other stages; DLM, dominant lethal test in mice; DLR, dominant lethal test in rats; MHT, mouse heritable translocation test.

The genetic activity profiles and listings that follow were prepared in collaboration with Environmental Health Research and Testing Inc. (EHRT) under contract to the US Environmental Protection Agency; EHRT also determined the doses used. The references cited in each genetic activity profile listing can be found in the list of references in the appropriate monograph.

References

Garrett, N.E., Stack, H.F., Gross, M.R. & Waters, M.D. (1984) An analysis of the spectra of genetic activity produced by known or suspected human carcinogens. *Mutat. Res.*, 134, 89-111

Gold, L.S., Sawyer, C.B., Magaw, R., Backman, G.M., de Veciana, M., Levinson, R., Hooper, N.K., Havender, W.R., Bernstein, L., Peto, R., Pike, M.C. &Ames, B.N. (1984) A carcinogenic potency database of the standardized results of animal bioassays. *Environ. Health Perspect.*, 58, 9-319

Waters, M.D. (1979) *The GENE-TOX program*. In: Hsie, A.W., O'Neill, J.P. & McElheny, V.K., eds, *Mammalian Cell Mutagenesis: The Maturation of Test Systems (Banbury Report 2)*, Cold Spring Harbor, NY, CHS Press, pp. 449-467

Waters, M.D. & Auletta, A. (1981) The GENE-TOX program: genetic activity evaluation. *J. chem. Inf. comput. Sci.*, 21, 35-38

Waters, M.D., Stack, H.F., Brady, A.L., Lohman, P.H.M., Haroun, L. & Vainio, H. (1987) Appendix 1: Activity profiles for genetic and related tests. In: *IARC Monographs on the Evaluation of the Carcinogenic Risk of Chemicals to Humans*, Suppl. 6, *Genetic and Related Effects: An Update of Selected* IARC Monographs *from Volumes 1 to 42*, Lyon, IARC, pp. 687-696

Waters, M.D., Stack, H.F., Brady, A.L., Lohman, P.H.M., Haroun, L. & Vainio, H. (1988) Use of computerized data listings and activity profiles of genetic and related effects in the review of 195 compounds. *Mutat. Res.*, 205, 295-312

APPENDIX 2

AZACITIDINE

Test system	Result without exogenous metabolic system	Result with exogenous metabolic system	Dose LED/HID	Reference
RVA, virus, mutation	+	0	5 μg/ml	Halle (1968)
PRB, Prophage induction	+	0	20 μg/ml	Barbe et al. (1986)
ECB, Escherichia coli, DNA damage (dcm+/recA56)	+	0	2.0 μg/ml	Bhagwat & Roberts (1987)
SAF, Salmonella typhimurium TM677, forward mutation	+	0	0.24 μg/ml	Call et al. (1986)
SA0, Salmonella typhimurium TA100, reverse mutation	–	0	10 μg/ml	Marquardt & Marquardt (1977)
SA0, Salmonella typhimurium TA100, reverse mutation	–	0	5 μg/ml	Podger (1983)
SA0, Salmonella typhimurium TA100, reverse mutation	+	0	6 μg/ml	Schmuck et al. (1986)
SA2, Salmonella typhimurium TA102, reverse mutation	+	0	2.4 μg/ml	Schmuck et al. (1986)
SA4, Salmonella typhimurium TA104, reverse mutation	+	0	2.4 μg/ml	Schmuck et al. (1986)
SA5, Salmonella typhimurium TA1535, reverse mutation	–	0	24 μg/ml	Schmuck et al. (1986)
SA8, Salmonella typhimurium TA1538, reverse mutation	–	0	25 μg/ml	Schmuck et al. (1986)
SA9, Salmonella typhimurium TA98, reverse mutation	–	0	5 μg/ml	Podger (1983)
SA9, Salmonella typhimurium TA98, reverse mutation	–	0	25 μg/ml	Schmuck et al. (1986)
SA9, Salmonella typhimurium TA98, reverse mutation	–	0	12.5 μg/ml	Levin & Ames (1986)
SAS, Salmonella typhimurium miscellaneous strains, reverse mutation	+	0	0.5 μg/ml	Podger (1983)
SAS, Salmonella typhimurium TA2638, reverse mutation	+	0	2.4 μg/ml	Schmuck et al. (1986)
SAS, Salmonella typhimurium TA92, reverse mutation	–	0	12 μg/ml	Schmuck et al. (1986)
SAS, Salmonella typhimurium TA2640, reverse mutation	–	0	25 μg/ml	Schmuck et al. (1986)
SAS, Salmonella typhimurium TA96, TA97, hisG428, hisG46, hisG1775, reverse mutation	–	0	12.5 μg/ml	Levin & Ames (1986)
SAS, Salmonella typhimurium TA2661, reverse mutation	+	0	12.5 μg/ml	Levin & Ames (1986)
SAS, Salmonella typhimurium TA4006, reverse mutation	+	0	12.5 μg/ml	Levin & Ames (1986)
EC2, Escherichia coli WP2, reverse mutation	–	0	4 μg/ml	Fucik et al. (1965)
ECF, Escherichia coli exclusive of strain K12, forward mutation	+	0	0.1 μg/ml	Lal et al. (1988)
ECR, Escherichia coli other miscellaneous strains, reverse mutation	+	0	0.4 μg/ml	Fucik et al. (1965)
SCH, Saccharomyces cerevisiae, mitotic recombination	+	0	2500 μg/ml	Zimmermann & Scheel (1984)
SCG, Saccharomyces cerevisiae, mitotic gene conversion	+	0	1000 μg/ml	Zimmermann & Scheel (1984)
SCR, Saccharomyces cerevisiae, reverse mutation	+	0	1000 μg/ml	Zimmermann & Scheel (1984)
SCN, Saccharomyces cerevisiae, aneuploidy	–	0	5000 μg/ml	Zimmermann & Scheel (1984)
VFC, Vicia faba, chromosomal aberrations	–	0	24 μg/ml	Fucik et al. (1970)
DMM, Drosophila melanogaster, wing-spot assay (somatic mutation and recombination)	+	0	244 μg/ml	Katz (1985)
G9H, Gene mutation, Chinese hamster lung V79 cells, hprt locus	–	0	0.7 μg/ml	Landolph & Jones (1982)

AZACITIDINE (contd)

Test system	Result		Dose LED/HID	Reference
	Without exogenous metabolic system	With exogenous metabolic system		
G9O, Gene mutation, Chinese hamster lung V79 cells, ouabain resistance	+	0	1 μg/ml	Marquart & Marquart (1977)
G9O, Gene mutation, Chinese hamster lung V79 cells, ouabain resistance	–	0	0.7 μg/ml	Landolph & Jones (1982)
G5T, Gene mutation, mouse lymphoma L5178Y cells in vitro, tk locus	+	–	0.02 μg/ml	Amacher & Turner (1987)
G5T, Gene mutation, mouse lymphoma L5178Y cells in vitro, tk locus	+	0	0.01 μg/ml	McGregor et al. (1989)
GIA, Gene mutation, mouse C3H/10 T1/2 cells, ouabain resistance	–	0	2.4 μg/ml	Landolph & Jones (1982)
GIA, Gene mutation, BHK cells, hprt locus	–	0	2.4 μg/ml	Bouck et al. (1984)
GIA, Gene mutation, BHK cells, ouabain resistance	–	0	2.4 μg/ml	Bouck et al. (1984)
GIA, Gene mutation, primary rat tracheal epithelial cells, ouabain resistance/hprt locus	–	0	1 μg/ml	Walker & Nettesheim (1986)
GIA, Gene mutation, mouse lymphoma L5178Y cells in vitro, hprt locus	–	0	0.33 μg/ml	McGregor et al. (1989)
SIT, Sister chromatid exchange, hamster cells in vitro	+	0	1.00 μg/ml	Banerjee & Benedict (1979)
SIC, Sister chromatid exchange, hamster cells in vitro	+	0	0.24 μg/ml	Hori (1983)
CIC, Chromosomal aberrations, Chinese hamster Don cells in vitro	+	0	10 μg/ml	Karon & Benedict (1972)
CIC, Chromosomal aberrations, Chinese hamster embryo fibroblasts (CHEF/18) in vitro	+	0	0.73 μg/ml	Harrison et al. (1983)
CIT, Chromosomal aberrations, hamster cells in vitro	(+)	0	2.5 μg/ml	Benedict et al. (1977)
TBM, Cell transformation, BALB/c 3T3 mouse cells	+	0	1.2 μg/ml	Yasutake et al. (1987)
TCM, Cell transformation, C3H 10T1/2 mouse cells	+	0	0.25 μg/ml	Benedict et al. (1977)
TCL, Cell transformation, Chinese hamster embryo fibroblasts (CHEF/18)	+	0	0.73 μg/ml	Harrison et al. (1983)
TCL, Cell transformation, primary rat tracheal epithelial cells	+	0	0.24 μg/ml	Walker & Nettesheim (1986)
DIH, DNA strand breaks, HeLa cells	+	0	48 μg/ml	Snyder & Lachmann (1989)
GIH, Gene mutation, human cells in vitro, hprt locus	+	0	0.12 μg/ml	Call et al. (1986)
GIH, Gene mutation, human cells in vitro, tk locus	+	0	0.024 μg/ml	Call et al. (1986)
SHL, Sister chromatid exchange, human lymphocytes in vitro	+	0	1.95 μg/ml	Lavia et al. (1985)
CHL, Chromosomal aberrations, human lymphocytes in vitro	+	0	1.95 μg/ml	Lavia et al. (1985)
CFT, Chromosomal aberrations, transformed human cells in vitro	–	0	2.4 μg/ml	Call et al. (1986)
DLM, Dominant lethal test, mice	–	0	10 mg/kg × 1, i.p.	Epstein et al. (1972)

APPENDIX 2

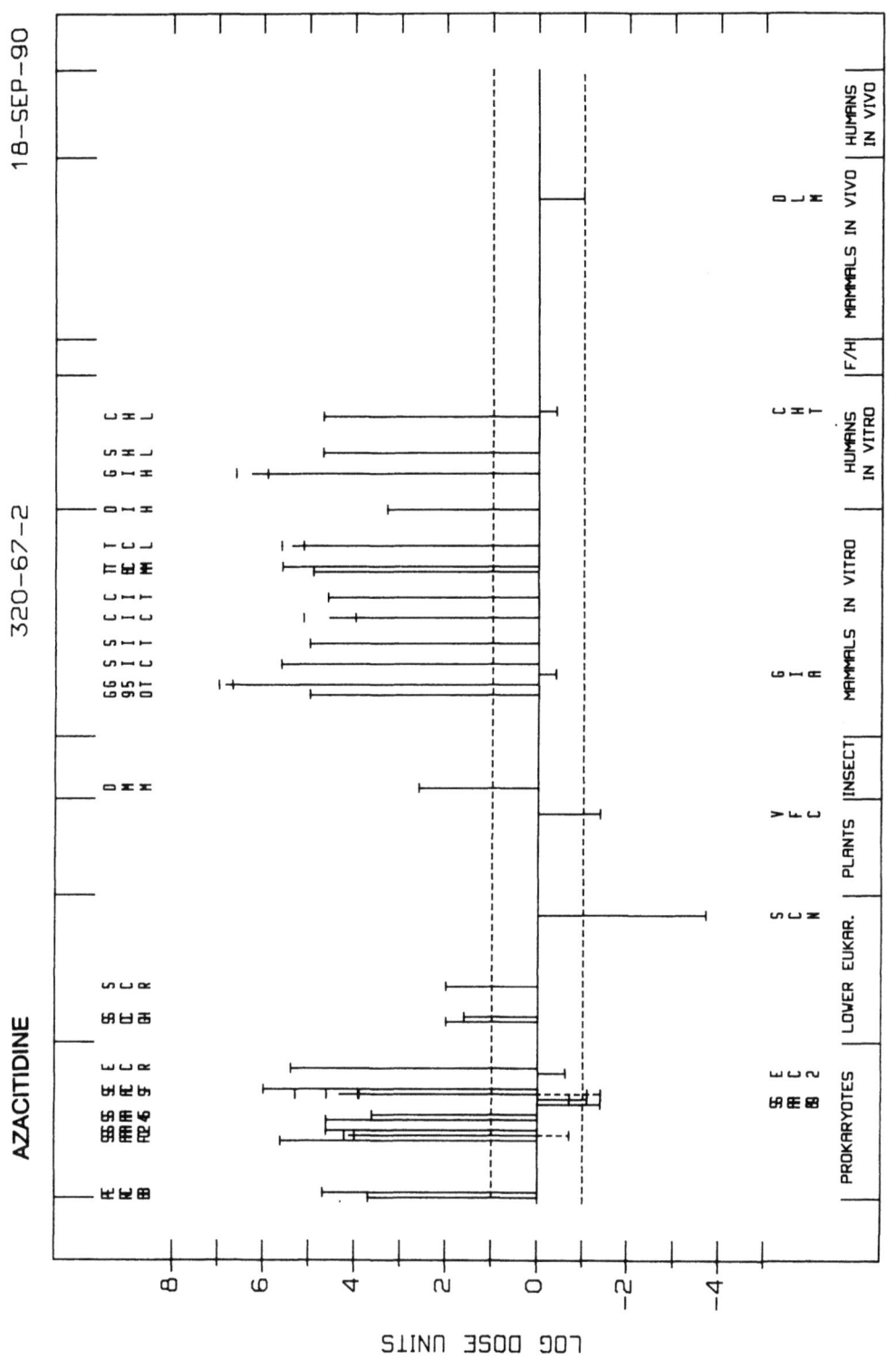

CHLOROZOTOCIN

Test system	Result		Dose LED/HID	Reference
	Without exogenous metabolic system	With exogenous metabolic system		
PRB, strand breaks in PM2-CCC DNA	+	0	1570 µg/ml	Lown & McLaughlin (1979)
PRB, Plasmid pBR 322 DNA strand breaks	+	0	2857 µg/ml	Vadi & Reed (1983)
Plasmid pBR 322 DNA alkylation	+	0	2857 µg/ml	Vadi & Reed (1983)
PRB, Plasmid pBR 322 DNA interstrand cross-links	+	0	2857 µg/ml	Vadi & Reed (1983)
DNA cross-links, calf thymus	+	0	1570 µg/ml	Alexander et al. (1986)
SA0, Salmonella typhimurium TA100, reverse mutation	+	+	31 µg/ml	Franza et al. (1980)
SA5, Salmonella typhimurium TA1535, reverse mutation	+	+	0	Franza et al. (1980)
SA5, Salmonella typhimurium TA1535, reverse mutation	+	+	50 µg/ml	Suling et al. (1983)
SA8, Salmonella typhimurium TA1538, reverse mutation	–	–	62 µg/ml	Franza et al. (1980)
SA9, Salmonella typhimurium TA98, reverse mutation	–	–	62 µg/ml	Franza et al. (1980)
SAS, Salmonella typhimurium hisG46, reverse mutation	+	0	100 µg/ml	Zimmer & Bhuyan (1976)
SCG, Saccharomyces cerevisiae, gene conversion	+	0	314 µg/ml	Siebert & Eisenbrand (1977)
DMX, Drosophila melanogaster, sex-linked recessive lethal mutation	+	0	31.4 µg/ml	Kortselius (1978)
DIA, DNA cross-links and strand breaks, mouse leukaemia L1210 cells	+	0	7.85 µg/ml	Ewig & Kohn (1977)
DIA, DNA strand breaks, Chinese hamster V79 cells	+	0	4 µg/ml	Erickson et al. (1978)
DIA, DNA strand breaks, mouse leukaemia L1210 cells	+	0	15.7 µg/ml	Alexander et al. (1986)
G9H, Gene mutation, Chinese hamster lung V79 cells, hprt locus	+	0	6.28 µg/ml	Bradley et al. (1980)
SIM, Sister chromatid exchange, mouse leukaemia L1210 cells	+	0	0.1 µg/ml	Siddiqui et al. (1988)
SIT, Sister chromatid exchange, 9L rat brain tumour cells	+	0	0.3 µg/ml	Tofilon et al. (1983)
DIH, DNA cross-links, human cells in vitro	+	0	15.7 µg/ml	Erickson et al. (1980)
DVA, DNA interstrand cross-links, strand breaks, rat bone-marrow cells in vivo	+	0	31.4 mg/kg x 1, i.p.	Bedford & Eisenbrand (1984)
BVD, DNA binding in vitro	+	0	24 µg/ml	Panasci et al. (1979)
BVD, DNA binding in vitro	+	0	24 µg/ml	Ahlgren et al. (1982)

APPENDIX 2

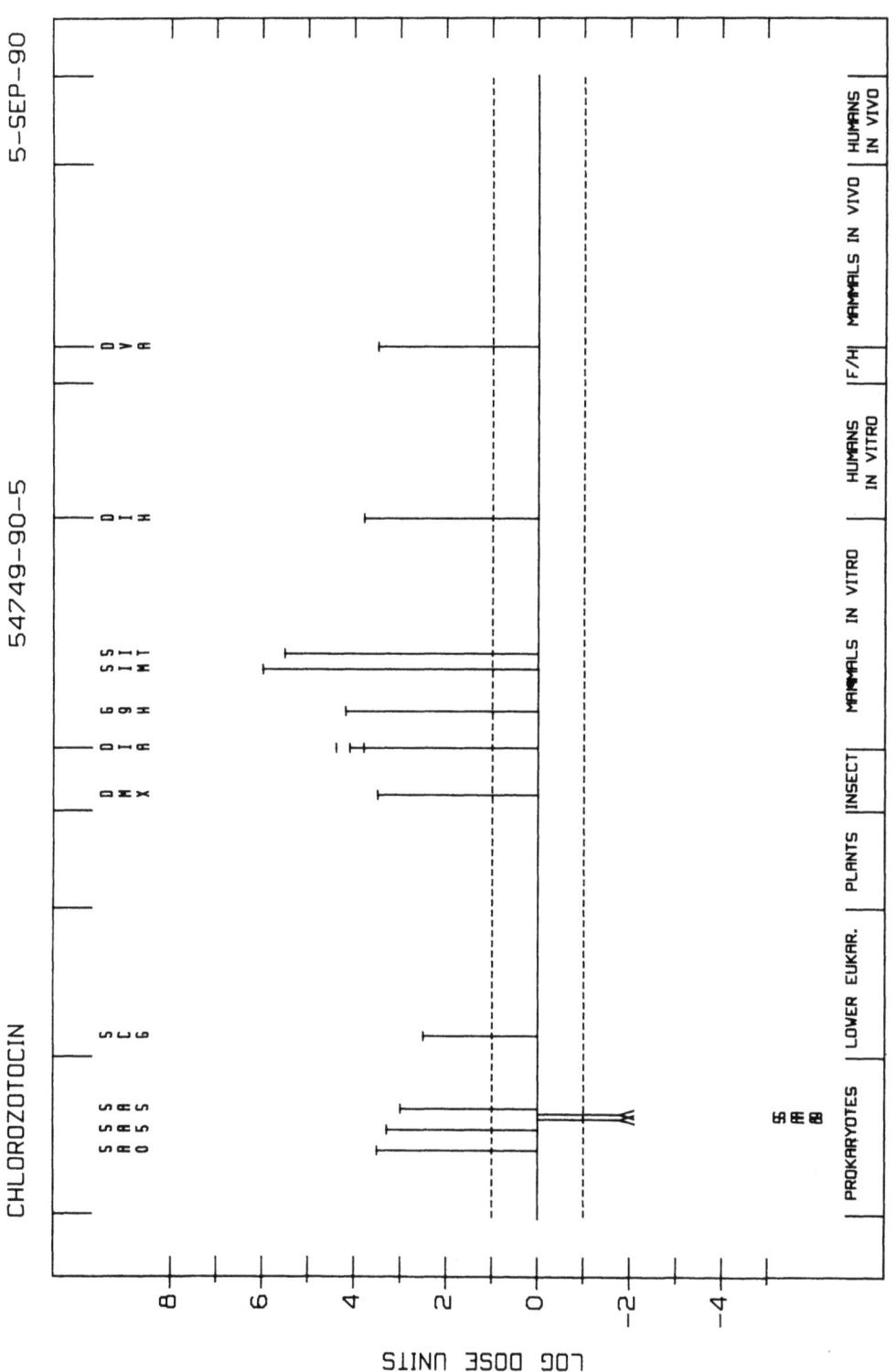

CICLOSPORIN

Test system	Result		Dose LED/HID	Reference
	Without exogenous metabolic system	With exogenous metabolic system		
SA0, Salmonella typhimurium TA100, reverse mutation	–	–	15000 µg/ml	Matter et al. (1982)
SA5, Salmonella typhimurium TA1535, reverse mutation	–	–	15000 µg/ml	Matter et al. (1982)
SA7, Salmonella typhimurium TA1537, reverse mutation	–	–	15000 µg/ml	Matter et al. (1982)
SA8, Salmonella typhimurium TA1538, reverse mutation	–	–	15000 µg/ml	Matter et al. (1982)
SAS, Salmonella typhimurium miscellaneous strains, reverse mutation	–	–	15000 µg/ml	Matter et al. (1982)
G9H, Gene mutation, Chinese hamster lung V79 cells, hprt locus	–	–	250 µg/ml	Zwanenburg et al. (1988)
SHL, Sister chromatid exchange, human lymphocytes in vitro	(+)	0	1 µg/ml	Yuzawa et al. (1986)
SHL, Sister chromatid exchange, human lymphocytes in vitro	(+)	0	1 µg/ml	Yuzawa et al. (1987)
UVR, Unscheduled DNA synthesis, mouse cells in vivo	–	0	0	Matter et al. (1982)
MVM, Micronucleus test, mice in vivo	–	0	1500 mg/kg x 1, p.o.	Matter et al. (1982)
MVC, Micronucleus test, hamsters in vivo	–	0	1500 mg/kg x 1, p.o.	Matter et al. (1982)
CBA, Chromosomal aberrations, animal bone-marrow cells in vivo	–	0	1500 mg/kg x 1, p.o.	Matter et al. (1982)
DLM, Dominant lethal test, mice	–	0	1000 mg/kg x 1, p.o.	Matter et al. (1982)
UVH, Unscheduled DNA synthesis, human lymphocytes in vivo	+	0	0	Petitjean et al. (1986)
CLH, Chromosomal aberrations, human lymphocytes in vivo	(+)	0	9.5 mg/kg[a]	Fukuda et al. (1987)
CLH, Chromosomal aberrations, human lymphocytes in vivo	(+)	0	9 mg/kg[b]	Fukuda et al. (1988)

[a] Tapering to 5–6 mg/kg per day; prednisolone was also given at 10 mg/person per day.
[b] Tapering to 4 mg/kg per day after one year; prednisolone was also given at 50 mg/person/day and tapering to 10 mg/person per day.

APPENDIX 2

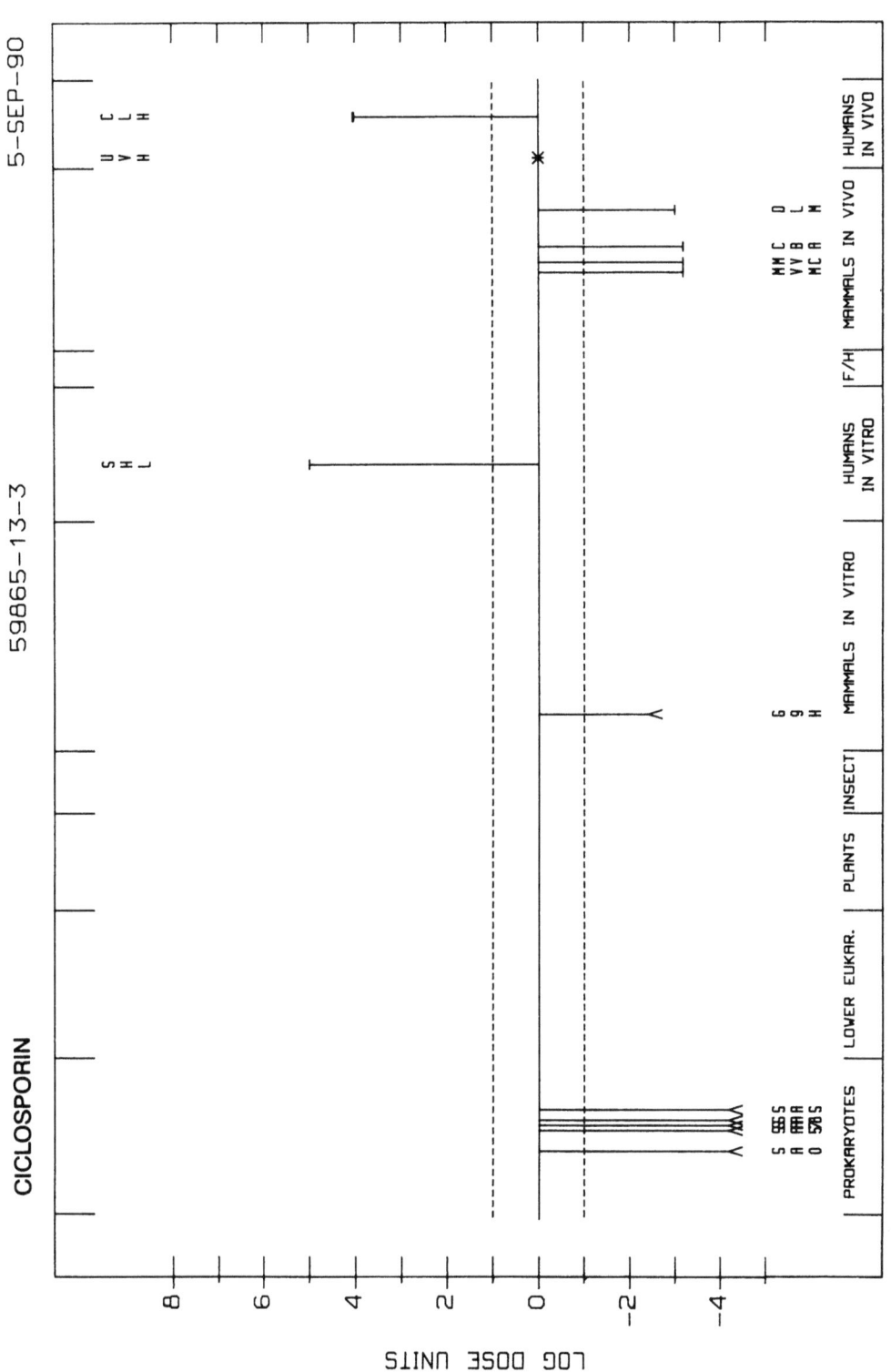

THIOTEPA

Test system	Result		Dose LED/HID	Reference
	Without exogenous metabolic system	With exogenous metabolic system		
SA0, Salmonella typhimurium TA100, reverse mutation	+	0	250 μg/ml	Pak et al. (1979)
SA5, Salmonella typhimurium TA1535, reverse mutation	+	0	50 μg/ml	Benedict et al. (1977a)
SA9, Salmonella typhimurium TA98, reverse mutation	+	0	250 μg/ml	Bruce & Heddle (1979)
SA9, Salmonella typhimurium TA98, reverse mutation	–	0	500 μg/ml	Pak et al. (1979)
ANF, Aspergillus nidulans, forward mutation	+	0	12.5 μg/ml	Bignami et al. (1982)
VFS, Vicia faba, sister chromatid exchange	+	0	37.8 μg/ml	Kihlman (1975)
VFC, Vicia faba, chromosomal aberrations	+	0	37.8 μg/ml	Kihlman (1975)
VFC, Vicia faba, chromosomal aberrations	+	0	95 μg/ml	Sturelid & Kihlman (1975)
VFC, Vicia faba, chromosomal aberrations	+	0	19 μg/ml	Popa et al. (1976)
DMX, Drosophila melanogaster, sex-linked recessive lethal mutations	+	0	0.23 μg/ml	Lüers & Röhrborn (1965)
DMX, Drosophila melanogaster, sex-linked recessive lethal mutations	+	0	1.9 μg/ml	Fahmy & Fahmy (1970)
G9H, Gene mutation, Chinese hamster V79 lung cells, hprt locus	+	0	2 μg/ml	Paschin & Kozachenko (1982)
SIC, Sister chromatid exchange, Chinese hamster cells in vitro	+	0	2.5 μg/ml	Chebotarev & Selezneva (1979)
SIC, Sister chromatid exchange, Chinese hamster cells in vitro	+	0	0.05 μg/ml	Chebotarev et al. (1980)
SIC, Sister chromatid exchange, Chinese hamster cells in vitro	+	0	0.06 μg/ml	Selezneva et al. (1982)
SIT, Sister chromatid exchange, mouse cells in vitro	+	0	0.2 μg/ml	Andersen (1983)
SIT, Sister chromatid exchange, cloned hamster cells in vitro	+	0	0.01 μg/ml	Banerjee & Benedict (1979)
SIA, Sister chromatid exchange, rhesus monkey cells in vitro	+	0	2.5 μg/ml	Kuzin et al. (1987)
CIC, Chromosomal aberrations, Chinese hamster cells in vitro	+	0	2 μg/ml	Sturelid (1976)
CIC, Chromosomal aberrations, Chinese hamster cells in vitro	+	0	10 μg/ml	Maier & Schmid (1976)
CIC, Chromosomal aberrations, Chinese hamster cells in vitro	+	0	3.78 μg/ml	Sturelid & Kihlman (1975)
CIT, Chromosomal aberrations, cloned hamster cells in vitro	+	0	0.5 μg/ml	Benedict et al. (1977b)
CIA, Chromosomal aberrations, rabbit cells in vitro	+	0	5 μg/ml	Bochkov et al. (1982)
CIA, Chromosomal aberrations, rhesus monkey cells in vitro	+	0	2.5 μg/ml	Kuzin et al. (1987)
TCM, Cell transformation, C3H 10T1/2 mouse cells	+	0	0.1 μg/ml	Benedict et al. (1977a)
UHL, Unscheduled DNA synthesis, human lymphocytes in vitro	+	0	1 μg/ml	Titenko (1983)
SHL, Sister chromatid exchange, human lymphocytes in vitro	+	0	2.5 μg/ml	Littlefield et al. (1979)
SHL, Sister chromatid exchange, human lymphocytes in vitro	+	0	0.03 μg/ml	Mourelatos (1979)
SHL, Sister chromatid exchange, human lymphocytes in vitro	+	0	5 μg/ml	Chebotarev & Listopad (1980)
SHL, Sister chromatid exchange, human lymphocytes in vitro	+	0	1 μg/ml	Listopad & Chebotarev (1982)
SHL, Sister chromatid exchange, human lymphocytes in vitro	+	0	2.8 μg/ml	Shcheglova & Chebotarev (1983a)
CHL, Chromosomal aberrations, human lymphocytes in vitro	+	0	3 μg/ml	Hampel et al. (1966)
CHL, Chromosomal aberrations, human lymphocytes in vitro	+	0	1 μg/ml	Bochkov & Kuleshov (1972)
CHL, Chromosomal aberrations, human lymphocytes in vitro	+	0	10 μg/ml	Bochkov et al. (1972)

APPENDIX 2

THIOTEPA (contd)

Test system	Result		Dose LED/HID	Reference
	Without exogenous metabolic system	With exogenous metabolic system		
CHL, Chromosomal aberrations, human lymphocytes in vitro	+	0	8 μg/ml	Chebotarev (1974)
CHL, Chromosomal aberrations, human lymphocytes in vitro	+	0	20 μg/ml	Kirichenko (1974)
CHL, Chromosomal aberrations, human lymphocytes in vitro	+	0	10 μg/ml	Kirichenko & Chebotarev (1976)
CHL, Chromosomal aberrations, human lymphocytes in vitro	+	0	6 μg/ml	Yakovenko & Nazarenko (1977)
CHL, Chromosomal aberrations, human lymphocytes in vitro	+	0	6 μg/ml	Bochkov et al. (1979)
CHL, Chromosomal aberrations, human lymphocytes in vitro	+	0	200 μg/ml	Wolff & Arutyunyan (1979)
CHL, Chromosomal aberrations, human lymphocytes in vitro	+	0	10 μg/ml	Yakovenko & Kagramanyan (1982)
CHL, Chromosomal aberrations, human lymphocytes in vitro	+	0	6.6 μg/ml	Shcheglova & Chebotarev (1983a)
HMA, Host-mediated assay, mouse leukaemia L5178Y cells in mice	+	0	7.5 mg/kg x 1, s.c.	Lee (1973)
HMM, Host-mediated assay, Salmonella typhimurium in mice	+	0	12.4 mg/kg x 3, i.p.	Arni et al. (1977)
HMM, Host-mediated assay, Salmonella typhimurium in mice	+	0	2.5 mg/kg x 2, p.o.	Devi & Reddy (1980)
SVA, Sister chromatid exchange, mouse bone-marrow cells in vivo	+	0	2 mg/kg x 1, i.v.	Shcheglova & Chebotarev (1983b)
SVA, Sister chromatid exchange, rhesus monkey lymphocytes in vivo	+	0	3 mg/kg x 1, i.v.	Kuzin et al. (1987)
MVM, Micronucleus test, mice in vivo	+	0	1 mg/kg x 2, i.p.	Maier & Schmid (1976)
MVM, Micronucleus test, mice in vivo	+	0	20 mg/kg x 1, i.p.	Ioan et al. (1977)
MVM, Micronucleus test, mice in vivo	+	0	2.5 mg/kg x 5, i.p.	Bruce & Heddle (1979)
MVM, Micronucleus test, mice in vivo	+	0	2.5 mg/kg x 1, i.p.	Leonard et al. (1979)
MVR, Micronucleus test, rat in vivo	+	0	4 mg/kg x 1, i.p.	Setnikar et al. (1976)
CBA, Chromosomal aberrations, mouse bone-marrow cells in vivo	+	0	0.32 mg/kg x 1, i.p.	Malashenko & Surkova (1974b)
CBA, Chromosomal aberrations, mouse bone-marrow cells in vivo	+	0	2 mg/kg x 1, i.p.	Malashenko & Surkova (1975)
CBA, Chromosomal aberrations, mouse bone-marrow cells in vivo	+	0	1.25 mg/kg x 1, i.p.	Leonard et al. (1979)
CBA, Chromosomal aberrations, mouse bone-marrow cells in vivo	+	0	1 mg/kg x 1, i.p.	Shcheglova & Chebotarev (1983b)
CCC, Chromosomal aberrations, mouse spermatocytes in vivo	+	0	1.66 mg/kg x 2, p.o.	Devi & Reddy (1980)
CCC, Chromosomal aberrations, mouse spermatocytes in vivo	+	0	20 mg/kg x 1, i.p.	Meistrich et al. (1982)
CGG, Chromosomal aberrations, mouse spermatogonia in vivo	+	0	1 mg/kg x 1, i.p.	Malashenko & Beskova (1988)
CVA, Chromosomal aberrations, mouse liver cells in vivo	+	0	8 mg/kg x 1, i.p.	Korogodina & Lil'p (1978)
COE, Chromosomal aberrations, preimplantation mouse embryos in vivo	+	0	1.25 mg/kg x 1, i.p.	Malashenko et al. (1978)
CVF, Chromosomal aberrations, embryonal mouse liver in vivo	+	0	2.5 mg/kg x 1, i.p.	Korogodina et al. (1979)
COE, Chromosomal aberrations, preimplantation mouse embryos in vivo	+	0	1.25 mg/kg x 1, i.p.	Semenov & Malashenko (1979)
COE, Chromosomal aberrations, embryonal mouse liver in vivo	+	0	2.5 mg/kg x 1, i.p.	Korogodina & S'yakste (1981)
CLA, Chromosomal aberrations, rabbit lymphocytes in vivo	+	0	3 mg/kg x 1, i.v.	Bochkov et al. (1982)
CVA, Chromosomal aberrations, rhesus monkey lymphocytes in vivo	+	0	5 mg/kg x 1, i.v.	Kuzin et al. (1987)
DLM, Dominant lethal test, mice	+	0	5 mg/kg x 1, i.p.	Machemer & Hess (1971)
DLM, Dominant lethal test, mice	+	0	5 mg/kg x 1, i.p.	Epstein et al. (1972)

THIOTEPA (contd)

Test system	Result		Dose LED/HID	Reference
	Without exogenous metabolic system	With exogenous metabolic system		
DLM, Dominant lethal test, mice	+	0	0.2 mg/kg x 10, i.p.	Sram (1976)
DLM, Dominant lethal test, mice	+	0	1.25 µg/kg x 1, i.p.	Malashenko et al. (1978)
DLM, Dominant lethal test, mice	+	0	2.5 mg/kg x 1, i.p.	Semenov & Malashenko (1981)
MHT, Mouse heritable translocation test	+	0	5 mg/kg x 1, i.p.	Malashenko & Surkova (1974a)
MHT, Mouse heritable translocation test	+	0	1.25 mg/kg x 1, i.p.	Semenov & Malashenko (1977)
MHT, Mouse heritable translocation test	+	0	1.25 mg/kg x 1, i.p.	Malashenko et al. (1978)
CLH, Chromosomal aberrations, human lymphocytes in vivo	+	0	1.25 mg/kg x 1, i.p.	Malashenko & Goetz (1981)
			0.14 mg/kg x 4 - x 10, i.m.	Selezneva & Korman (1973)
SPM, Sperm morphology, mice in vivo	+	0	2.5 mg/kg x 5, i.v.	Bruce & Heddle (1979)

APPENDIX 2

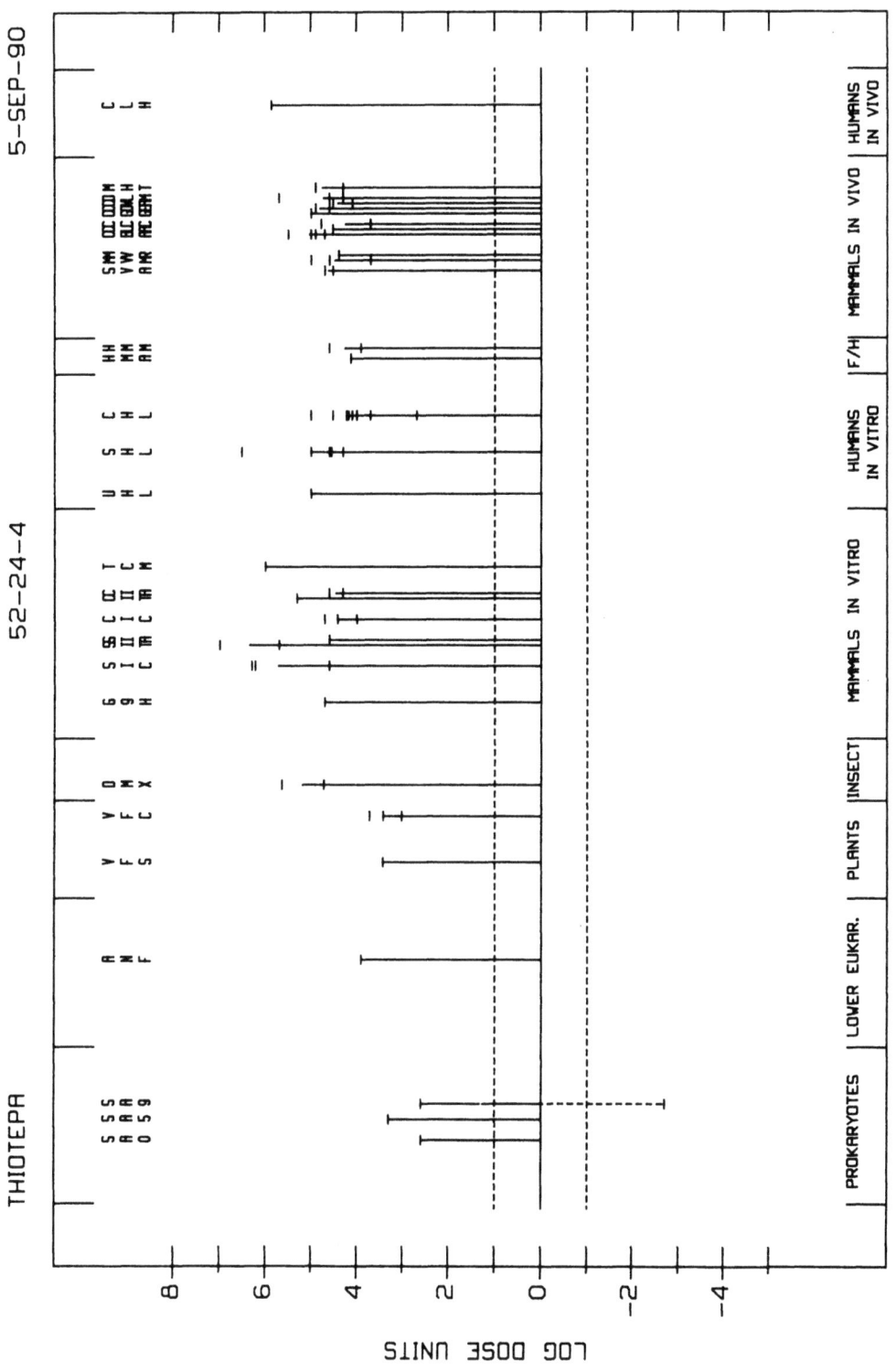

TRICHLORMETHINE

Test system	Result		Dose LED/HID	Reference
	Without exogenous metabolic system	With exogenous metabolic system		
CSH, Gene mutation, Chinese hamster lung V79 cells, hprt locus	+	0	3 µg/ml	Slamenova et al. (1983)
CIT, Chromosomal aberrations, Walker 256 cells	+	0	1 mg/kg x 4 - x 10, i.p.	Boyland et al. (1948)
CIT, Chromosomal aberrations, Walker 256 cells	+	0	0	Koller (1969)
DLM, Dominant lethal test, mice	+	0	5 mg/kg x 1, i.p.	Sykora & Gandalovicova (1978)

APPENDIX 2

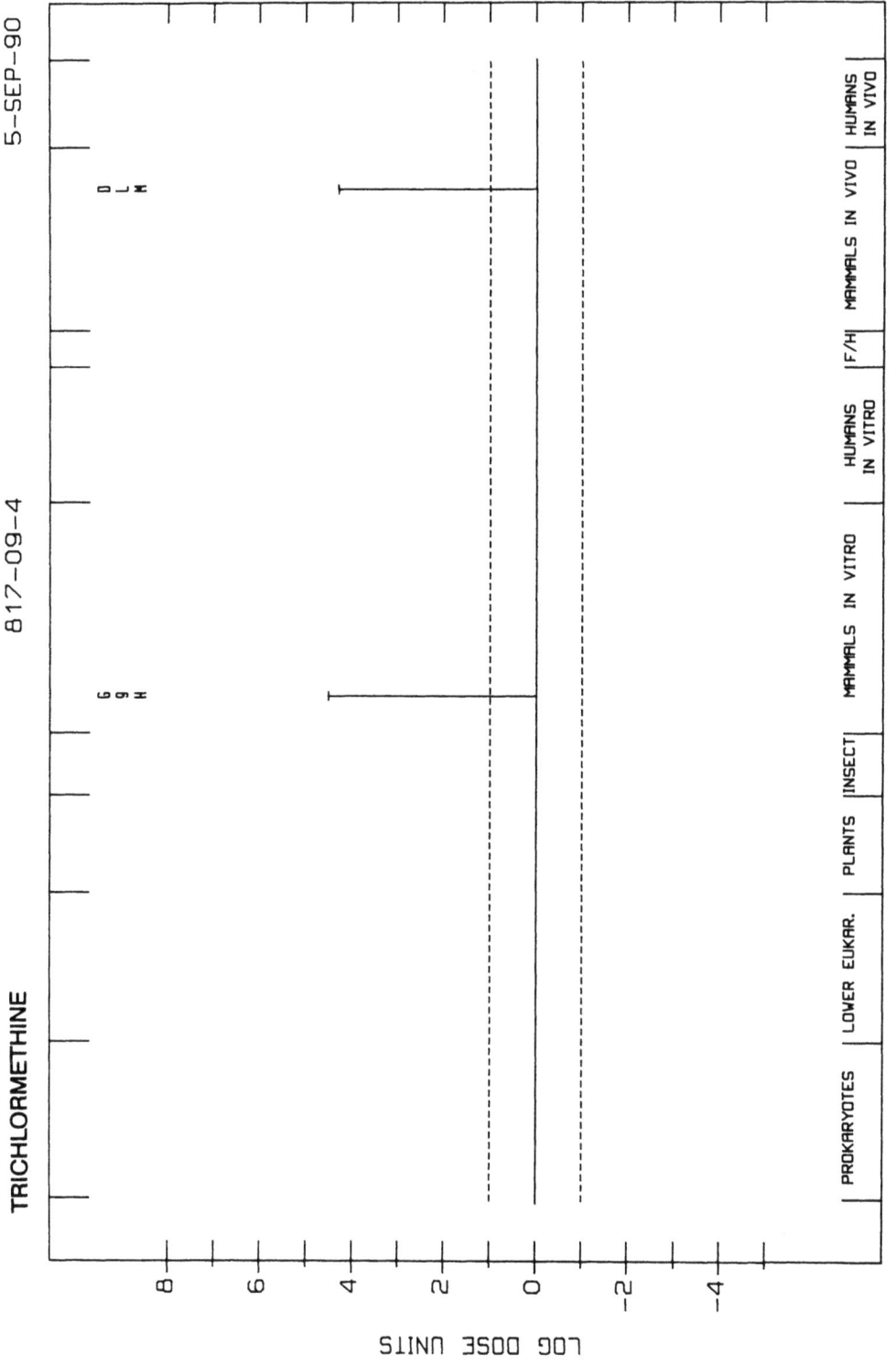

AMPICILLIN

Test system	Result		Dose LED/HID	Reference
	Without exogenous metabolic system	With exogenous metabolic system		
PRB, Staphylococcus aureus, prophage induction	+	0	5 μg/ml	Manthey et al. (1975)
PRB, Escherichia coli PQ37, SOS induction	–	0	417 μg/ml	Venier et al. (1989)
ERD, Escherichia coli, DNA repair	–	–	100 μg/ml	Green & Tweats (1981)
ECB, Escherichia coli, DNA repair	0	–	100 μg/ml	Tweats et al. (1981)
ECB, Escherichia coli, DNA repair	–	–	2 μg/ml	De Flora et al. (1984)
SA0, Salmonella typhimurium TA100, reverse mutation	–	0	0.00	De Flora et al. (1984)
SA0, Salmonella typhimurium TA100, reverse mutation	–	–	167 μg/ml	Mortelmans et al. (1986)
SA5, Salmonella typhimurium TA1535, reverse mutation	–	0	0.00	De Flora et al. (1984)
SA5, Salmonella typhimurium TA1535, reverse mutation	–	–	1 μg/ml	Mortelmans et al. (1986)
SA7, Salmonella typhimurium TA1537, reverse mutation	–	0	0.00	De Flora et al. (1984)
SA7, Salmonella typhimurium TA1537, reverse mutation	–	–	1 μg/ml	Mortelmans et al. (1986)
SA8, Salmonella typhimurium TA1538, reverse mutation	–	0	0.00	De Flora et al. (1984)
SA9, Salmonella typhimurium TA98, reverse mutation	–	0	0.00	De Flora et al. (1984)
SA9, Salmonella typhimurium TA98, reverse mutation	–	–	167 μg/ml	Mortelmans et al. (1986)
SAS, Salmonella typhimurium TA97, reverse mutation	–	0	0.00	De Flora et al. (1984)
VFC, Vicia faba, aberrant cell division	+	–	5000 μg/ml	Prasad (1977)
G5T, Gene mutation, mouse lymphoma L5178Y cells, TK locus	–	–	5000 μg/ml	National Toxicology Program (1987)
SIC, Sister chromatid exchange, Chinese hamster cells in vitro	–	–	1500 μg/ml	National Toxicology Program (1987)
CIC, Chromosomal aberrations, Chinese hamster cells in vitro	–	–	1500 μg/ml	National Toxicology Program (1987)
SHL, Sister chromatid exchange, human lymphocytes in vitro	–	0	28 μg/ml	Jaju et al. (1984)
CHF, Chromosomal aberrations, human fibroblasts in vitro	+	0	4000 μg/ml	Byarugaba et al. (1975)
CHL, Chromosomal aberrations, human lymphocytes in vitro	+	0	28 μg/ml	Jaju et al. (1984)

APPENDIX 2

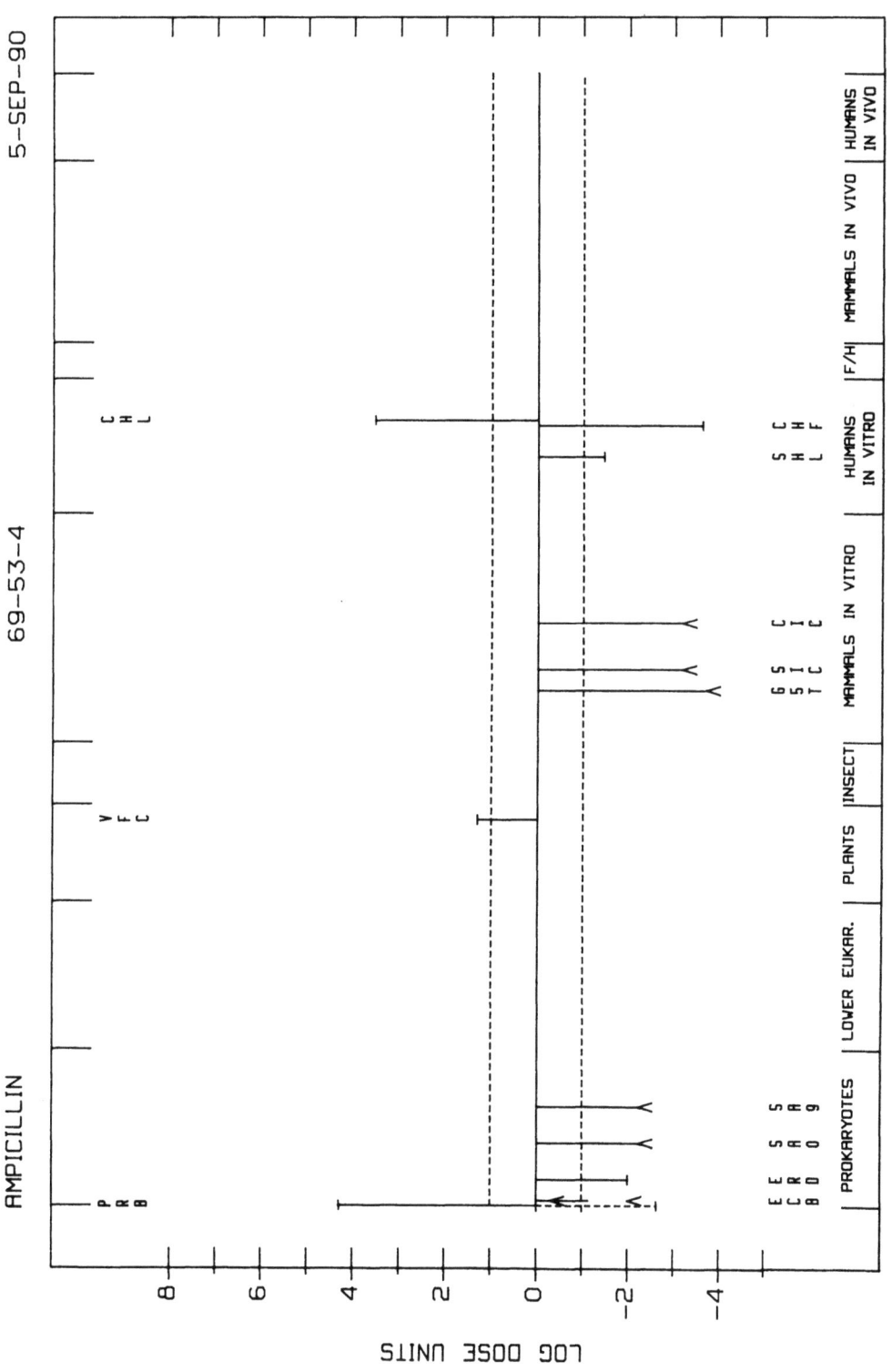

CHLORAMPHENICOL

Test system	Result		Dose LED/HID	Reference
	Without exogenous metabolic system	With exogenous metabolic system		
PRB, Prophage induction, SOS repair test, DNA strand breaks	–	0	10 μg/ml	Manthey et al. (1975)
PRB, Escherichia coli, DNA damage	–	0	30 μg/ml	Mamber et al. (1986)
Salmonella typhimurium, DNA breaks	±	0	0	Jackson et al. (1977)
ECB, Escherichia coli, DNA breaks	+	0	1615 μg/ml	Jackson et al. (1977)
SAD, Salmonella typhimurium, differential toxicity	–	0	15 μg/ml	Russell et al. (1980)
SAD, Salmonella typhimurium, differential toxicity	–	0	5 μg/ml	Nader et al. (1981)
ECD, Escherichia coli pol A, differential toxicity (spot test)	–	0	30 μg/ml	Longnecker et al. (1974)
ECD, Escherichia coli pol A, differential toxicity (spot test)	–	0	30 μg/ml	Nestmann et al. (1979)
ECD, Escherichia coli pol A, differential toxicity (spot test)	–	0	30 μg/ml	Boyle & Simpson (1980)
ECD, Escherichia coli pol A, differential toxicity (spot test)	–	0	30 μg/ml	Leifer et al. (1981)
ECL, Escherichia coli pol A, differential toxicity (liquid)	–	0	20 μg/ml	Leifer et al. (1981)
ECD, Escherichia coli, differential toxicity	–	0	30 μg/ml	Slater et al. (1971)
ECD, Escherichia coli, differential toxicity	–	0	0	Venturini & Monti-Bragadin (1978)
ERD, Escherichia coli rec, differential toxicity	+	0	0.6 μg/ml	Suter & Jaeger (1982)
BSD, Bacillus subtilis, differential toxicity	–	0	1000 μg/ml	Shimizu & Rosenberg (1973)
BSD, Bacillus subtilis, differential toxicity	–	0	2.5 μg/ml	Sekizawa & Shibamoto (1982)
BSD, Bacillus subtilis, differential toxicity	–	0	2.5 μg/ml	Suter & Jaeger (1982)
BRD, Bacteria (other), differential toxicity	–	0	500 μg/ml	Adler et al. (1976)
BRD, Bacteria (other), differential toxicity	–	0	20 μg/ml	Leifer et al. (1981)
SA0, Salmonella typhimurium TA100, reverse mutation	0	–	0	Jackson et al. (1977)
SA0, Salmonella typhimurium TA100, reverse mutation	0	–	2.5 μg/ml	McCann et al. (1975)
SA0, Salmonella typhimurium TA100, reverse mutation	–	–	333 μg/ml	Mortelmans et al. (1986)
SA3, Salmonella typhimurium TA1530, reverse mutation	–	0	30 μg/ml	Brem et al. (1974)
SA2, Salmonella typhimurium TA102, reverse mutation	–	–	5 μg/ml	Albertini & Gocke (1988)
SA5, Salmonella typhimurium TA1535, reverse mutation	–	0	30 μg/ml	Brem et al. (1974)
SA5, Salmonella typhimurium TA1535, reverse mutation	0	–	2.5 μg/ml	McCann et al. (1975)
SA5, Salmonella typhimurium TA1535, reverse mutation	–	0	0	Jackson et al. (1977)
SA5, Salmonella typhimurium TA1535, reverse mutation	–	–	333 μg/ml	Mortelmans et al. (1986)
SA7, Salmonella typhimurium TA1537, reverse mutation	0	–	2.5 μg/ml	McCann et al. (1975)
SA7, Salmonella typhimurium TA1537, reverse mutation	–	–	333 μg/ml	Mortelmans et al. (1986)
SA8, Salmonella typhimurium TA1538, reverse mutation	–	0	30 μg/ml	Brem et al. (1974)
SA9, Salmonella typhimurium TA98, reverse mutation	0	0	2.5 μg/ml	McCann et al. (1975)
SA9, Salmonella typhimurium TA98, reverse mutation	(+)	(+)	9 μg/ml	Mitchell et al. (1980)

APPENDIX 2

CHLORAMPHENICOL (contd)

Test system	Result without exogenous metabolic system	Result with exogenous metabolic system	Dose LED/HID	Reference
SA9, Salmonella typhimurium TA98, reverse mutation	–	–	333 µg/ml	Mortelmans et al. (1986)
SA9, Salmonella typhimurium TA98, reverse mutation	+	0	0	Jackson et al. (1977)
ECF, Escherichia coli, forward mutation	+	0	10 µg/ml	Mitchell et al. (1980)
ECF, Escherichia coli WP2, forward mutation	+	0	27 µg/ml	Mitchell & Gilbert (1985)
ECF, Escherichia coli CM891, forward mutation	(+)	0	27 µg/ml	Mitchell & Gilbert (1985)
EC2, Escherichia coli WP2, reverse mutation	–	0	200 µg/ml	Hemmerly & Demerec (1955)
EC2, Escherichia coli WP2, reverse mutation	–	0	27 µg/ml	Mitchell & Gilbert (1985)
ECR, Escherichia coli CM891, reverse mutation	–	0	200 µg/ml	Hemmerly & Demerec (1955)
ECR, Escherichia coli CM891, reverse mutation	+	0	27 µg/ml	Mitchell & Gilbert (1985)
SCF, Saccharomyces cerevisiae D1121, petite mutations	(+)	0	4000 µg/ml	Weislogel & Butow (1970)
SCF, Saccharomyces cerevisiae D35 and 44, petite mutations	(–)	0	3000 µg/ml	Carnevali et al. (1971)
SCF, Saccharomyces cerevisiae, petite mutations	(+)	0	3000 µg/ml	Williamson et al. (1971)
ASM, Arabidopsis species, mutation	–	0	1620 µg/ml	Müller (1965)
TSI, Tradescantia paludosa, micronuclei	–	0	1615 µg/ml	Ma et al. (1984)
HSC, Hordeum species, chromosomal aberrations	+	0	300 µg/ml	Yoshida et al. (1972)
VFC, Vicia faba, chromosomal aberrations	+	0	5000 µg/ml	Prasad (1977)
DMX, Drosophila melanogaster, sex-linked recessive lethal mutation	–	0	2500 µg/ml	Clark (1963)
DMX, Drosophila melanogaster, sex-linked recessive lethal mutation	–	0	100000 µg/ml	Nasrat (1977)
DML, Drosophila melanogaster, dominant lethal test	–	0	100000 µg/ml	Nasrat (1977)
UIA, Unscheduled DNA synthesis, Syrian hamster cells in vitro	–	–	1000 µg/ml	Suzuki (1987)
G5T, Gene mutation, mouse lymphoma L5178Y cells, TK locus	+	+	3000 µg/ml	Mitchell et al. (1988)
G5T, Gene mutation, mouse lymphoma L5178Y cells, TK locus	+	+	2000 µg/ml	Myhr & Caspary (1988)
SIS, Sister chromatid exchange, Syrian hamster cells in vitro	+	0	30 µg/ml	Suzuki (1987)
CIA, Chromosomal aberrations, other animal cells in vitro	+	0	500 µg/ml	Quéinnec et al. (1975)
TCS, Cell transformation, Syrian hamster embryo cells	(–)	0	1000 µg/ml	Suzuki (1987)
T7S, Cell transformation, SA7/Syrian hamster embryo cells	(+)	0	3490 µg/ml	Hatch et al. (1986)
DIH, DNA strand breaks, human lymphocytes in vitro	–	0	646 µg/ml	Yunis et al. (1987)
DIH, DNA strand breaks, human lymphocytes in vitro	–	0	258 µg/ml	Isildar et al. (1988)
DIH, DNA strand breaks, human lymphoblastoid cells in vitro	–	0	258 µg/ml	Isildar et al. (1988)
DIH, DNA strand breaks, human bone-marrow cells in vitro	–	0	258 µg/ml	Isildar et al. (1988)
SHL, Sister chromatid exchange, human lymphocytes in vitro	–	0	200 µg/ml	Pant et al. (1976)
CHF, Chromosomal aberrations, human fibroblasts in vitro	–	0	625 µg/ml	Byarugaba et al. (1975)
CHL, Chromosomal aberrations, human lymphocytes in vitro	+	0	10 µg/ml	Mitus & Coleman (1970)
CHL, Chromosomal aberrations, human lymphocytes in vitro	–	0	500 µg/ml	Jensen (1972)

CHLORAMPHENICOL (contd)

Test system	Result		Dose LED/HID	Reference
	Without exogenous metabolic system	With exogenous metabolic system		
CHL, Chromosomal aberrations, human lymphocytes in vitro	+	0	100 µg/ml	Sasaki & Tonomura (1973)
CHL, Chromosomal aberrations, human lymphocytes in vitro	+	0	80 µg/ml	Goh (1979)
CHL, Chromosomal aberrations, human lymphocytes in vitro	+	0	200 µg/ml	Pant et al. (1976)
CBA, Chromosomal aberrations, animal bone-marrow cells in vivo	–	0	1000 mg/kg x 3, i.m.	Jensen (1972)
CBA, Chromosomal aberrations, animal bone-marrow cells in vivo	(+)	0	50 mg/kg x 1, i.m.	Manna & Bardhan (1973)
CBA, Chromosomal aberrations, animal bone-marrow cells in vivo	(+)	0	50 mg/kg x 1, i.m.	Manna & Bardhan (1977)
CGG, Chromosomal aberrations, Swiss mouse meiotic cells in vivo	(+)	0	50 mg/kg x 1, i.m.	Roy & Manna (1981)
CCC, Chromosomal aberrations, Swiss mouse meiotic cells in vivo	(+)	0	50 mg/kg x 1, i.m.	Roy & Manna (1981)
DLM, Dominant lethal test, mice	–	0	333 mg/kg x 1, i.p.	Epstein & Shafner (1968)
DLM, Dominant lethal test (101xC3H)F1 mice	–	0	1500 mg/kg x 1, i.p.	Ehling (1971)
DLM, Dominant lethal test, mice	–	0	666 mg/kg x 1, i.p.	Epstein et al. (1972)
DLM, Dominant lethal test, mice	+	0	500 mg/kg x 1, i.p.	Sram (1972)

APPENDIX 2

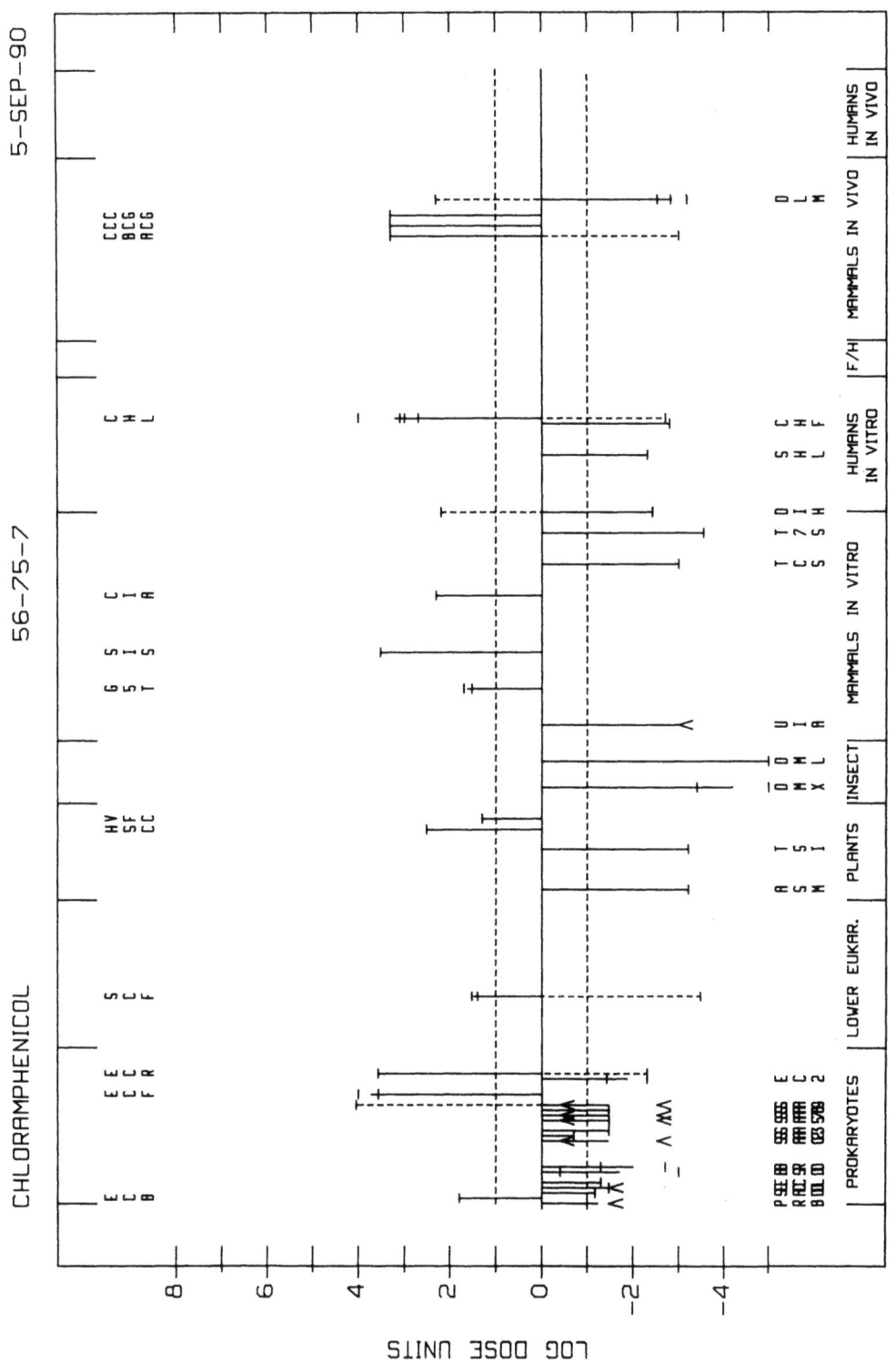

NITROFURAL (NITROFURAZONE)

Test system		Result		Dose LED/HID	Reference
		Without exogenous metabolic system	With exogenous metabolic system		
PRB,	Escherichia coli T44(1), prophage induction	+	0	1.0 μg/ml	McCalla & Voutsinos (1974)
ECB,	Escherichia coli B/R, DNA strand breaks	+	0	25 μg/ml	McCalla et al. (1971)
ECB,	Escherichia coli c1256, DNA strand breaks	+	0	75 μg/ml	Tu & McCalla (1975)
ECB,	Escherichia coli WP2A, DNA strand breaks	+	0	15 μg/ml	Wentzell & McCalla (1980)
ECB,	Escherichia coli nfr-207, DNA strand breaks	–	0	50 μg/ml	McCalla et al. (1971)
SAD,	Salmonella typhimurium TA1975, DNA strand breaks	+	0	50 μg/ml	McCalla et al. (1975)
SAD,	Salmonella typhimurium TA1975, differential toxicity	–	0	100 μg/ml	Yahagi et al. (1974)
ERD,	Escherichia coli WP100, differential toxicity	+	0	10 μg/ml	Haveland-Smith et al. (1979)
ERD,	Escherichia coli WP67, differential toxicity	?	0	10 μg/ml	Haveland-Smith et al. (1979)
ERD,	Escherichia coli, differential toxicity	+	0	100 μg/ml	Yahagi et al. (1974)
ERD,	Escherichia coli, differential toxicity	+	0	1 μg/ml	Ebringer & Bencova (1980)
BSD,	Bacillus subtilis HLl3g vs HJ-15, differential toxicity	+	0	500 μg/ml	Tanooka (1977)
BSM,	Bacillus subtilis TKJ5211, mutation	+	0	500 μg/ml	Tanooka (1977)
SA0,	Salmonella typhimurium TA100, fluctuation test	+	0	0.0001 μg/ml	Green et al. (1977)
SA0,	Salmonella typhimurium TA100, reverse mutation	+	+	0.15 μg/ml	National Toxicology Program (1988)
SA0,	Salmonella typhimurium TA100, reverse mutation	+	0	0.25 μg/ml	Goodman et al. (1977)
SA0,	Salmonella typhimurium TA100, reverse mutation (spot test)	+	0	1 μg/ml	Yahagi et al. (1976)
SA0,	Salmonella typhimurium TA100, reverse mutation	+	0	0.198 μg/ml	Chin et al. (1978)
SA0,	Salmonella typhimurium TA100, reverse mutation	+	0	1.98 μg/ml	Rosin & Stich (1978)
SA0,	Salmonella typhimurium TA100, reverse mutation	+	0	2 μg/ml	Bruce & Heddle (1979)
SA0,	Salmonella typhimurium TA100, reverse mutation	+	0	10 μg/ml	Ebringer & Bencova (1980)
SA5,	Salmonella typhimurium TA1535, fluctuation test	(+)	+	0.1 μg/ml	Green et al. (1977)
SA5,	Salmonella typhimurium TA1535, reverse mutation	(+)	+	16 μg/ml	National Toxicology Program (1988)
SA5,	Salmonella typhimurium TA1535, reverse mutation	–	0	2.5 μg/ml	McCalla et al. (1975)
SA5,	Salmonella typhimurium TA1535, reverse mutation	+	0	59.4 μg/ml	Yahagi et al. (1974)
SA5,	Salmonella typhimurium TA1535, reverse mutation	(+)	0	1 μg/ml	Yahagi et al. (1976)
SA7,	Salmonella typhimurium TA1537, reverse mutation	–	0	33 μg/ml	National Toxicology Program (1988)
SA7,	Salmonella typhimurium TA1537, reverse mutation	–	0	59.4 μg/ml	Yahagi et al. (1974)
SA8,	Salmonella typhimurium TA1538, reverse mutation	–	0	2.5 μg/ml	McCalla et al. (1975)
SA8,	Salmonella typhimurium TA1538, reverse mutation	–	0	59.4 μg/ml	Yahagi et al. (1974)
SA9,	Salmonella typhimurium TA98, reverse mutation	+	+	2.5 μg/ml	Ni et al. (1987)
SA9,	Salmonella typhimurium TA98, reverse mutation	+	+	1.5 μg/ml	National Toxicology Program (1988)
SA9,	Salmonella typhimurium TA98, reverse mutation	+	0	0.5 μg/ml	Goodman et al. (1977)
SA9,	Salmonella typhimurium TA98, reverse mutation	+	0	2 μg/ml	Bruce & Heddle (1979)

APPENDIX 2

NITROFURAL (NITROFURAZONE) (contd)

Test system	Result without exogenous metabolic system	Result with exogenous metabolic system	Dose LED/HID	Reference
SAS, Salmonella typhimurium TA98NR, reverse mutation	+	+	1 µg/ml	Ni et al. (1987)
SAS, Salmonella typhimurium TA98/1,8-DNP6, reverse mutation	+	+	1 µg/ml	Ni et al. (1987)
SAS, Salmonella typhimurium TA1536, reverse mutation	–	0	59.4 µg/ml	Yahagi et al. (1974)
SAS, Salmonella typhimurium TA97, reverse mutation (fluct. test)	+	0	0.32 µg/ml	Obaseiki-Ebor & Akerele (1986)
ECF, Escherichia coli 343/113/R-9, forward mutation	–	+	40 µg/ml	Baars et al. (1980)
ECW, Escherichia coli WP2uvrA, reverse mutation (spot test)	+	0	50 µg/ml	McCalla & Voutsinos (1974)
ECW, Escherichia coli WP2uvrA, reverse mutation	–	0	8 µg/ml	McCalla & Voutsinos (1974)
ECW, Escherichia coli WP2uvrA, reverse mutation (fluctuation test)	+	0	0.01 µg/ml	Green et al. (1977)
ECW, Escherichia coli WP2uvrA, reverse mutation	+	0	0.25 µg/ml	Haveland-Smith et al. (1979)
ECW, Escherichia coli WP2uvrA, reverse mutation	+	0	2.5 µg/ml	McCalla et al. (1975)
ECW, Escherichia coli WP2uvrA, reverse mutation	–	0	59.4 µg/ml	Yahagi et al. (1974)
ECW, Escherichia coli WP2uvrA, reverse mutation	+	0	10 µg/ml	Lu et al. (1979)
EC2, Escherichia coli WP2, reverse mutation (spot test)	(+)	0	100 µg/ml	McCalla & Voutsinos (1974)
EC2, Escherichia coli WP2, reverse mutation	–	0	16 µg/ml	McCalla & Voutsinos (1974)
EC2, Escherichia coli WP2, reverse mutation (fluctuation test)	(+)	0	0.04 µg/ml	Obaseiki-Ebor & Akerele (1986)
ECR, Escherichia coli nfr 343, reverse mutation	–	0	10 µg/ml	McCalla & Voutsinos (1974)
ECR, Escherichia coli nfr 343, reverse mutation	–	0	2.5 µg/ml	McCalla et al. (1975)
ECR, Escherichia coli nfr 345, reverse mutation	–	0	10 µg/ml	McCalla & Voutsinos (1974)
ECR, Escherichia coli CM561, reverse mutation	–	0	100 µg/ml	McCalla & Voutsinos (1974)
ECR, Escherichia coli CM571, reverse mutation	–	0	100 µg/ml	McCalla & Voutsinos (1974)
ECR, Escherichia coli CM611, reverse mutation	–	0	50 µg/ml	McCalla & Voutsinos (1974)
ECR, Escherichia coli S, Lac, reverse mutation	+	0	50 µg/ml	Zampieri & Greenberg (1964)
ECR, Escherichia coli CM611, reverse mutation (fluctuation test)	+	0	0.01 µg/ml	Green et al. (1977)
ECR, Escherichia coli EE97, reverse mutation (fluctuation test)	+	0	0.02 µg/ml	Obaseiki-Ebor & Akerele (1986)
ECR, Escherichia coli 343/113/R-9, reverse mutation	–	+	40 µg/ml	Baars et al. (1980)
ANF, Aspergillus nidulans, forward mutation	+	0	1000 µg/ml	Bignami et al. (1982)
NCR, Neurospora crassa, reverse mutation	+	0	198 µg/ml	Ong (1977)
DMX, Drosophila melanogaster, sex-linked recessive lethal mutation	–	0	990 µg/ml	Kramers (1982)
DIA, DNA single strand breaks, mouse L929 cells in vitro	+	0	49.5 µg/ml	Olive & McCalla (1975)
DIA, DNA single strand breaks, hamster BHK-21 cells in vitro	+	0	49.5 µg/ml	Olive & McCalla (1975)
DIA, DNA single strand breaks, mouse L929 cells in vitro	–	+	39.6 µg/ml	Olive (1978)
URP, Unscheduled DNA synthesis, rat primary hepatocytes	+	0	0.011 µg/ml	Mori et al. (1987)
UIA, Unscheduled DNA synthesis, mouse hepatocytes in vitro	+	0	0.011 µg/ml	Mori et al. (1987)
GCO, Gene mutation, Chinese hamster ovary cells in vitro	–	–	200 µg/ml	Anderson & Phillips (1985)
GIA, Gene mutation, Chinese hamster V79 cells, 6-thioguanine res.	+	0	150 µg/ml	Olive (1981)

NITROFURAL (NITROFURAZONE) (contd)

Test system	Result		Dose LED/HID	Reference
	Without exogenous metabolic system	With exogenous metabolic system		
GST, Gene mutation, mouse lymphoma L5178Y cells, TK locus	+	0	50 µg/ml	National Toxicology Program (1988)
SIC, Sister chromatid exchange, Chinese hamster CHO cells in vitro	+	0	0.83 µg/ml	National Toxicology Program (1988)
SIC, Sister chromatid exchange, Chinese hamster CHO cells in vitro	0	+	83.3 µg/ml	National Toxicology Program (1988)
CIC, Chromosomal aberrations, Chinese hamster lung cells in vitro	+	+	150 µg/ml	Ishidate (1988)
CIC, Chromosomal aberrations, Chinese hamster ovary cells in vitro	+	+	100 µg/ml	Anderson & Phillips (1985)
CIC, Chromosomal aberrations, Chinese hamster ovary cells in vitro	+	0	25 µg/ml	National Toxicology Program (1988)
CIC, Chromosomal aberrations, Chinese hamster ovary cells in vitro	0	–	600 µg/ml	National Toxicology Program (1988)
CIC, Chromosomal aberrations, Chinese hamster CHL cells in vitro	–	+	100 µg/ml	Matsuoka et al. (1979)
DIH, DNA single strand breaks, human KB cells in vitro	+	0	49.5 µg/ml	Olive & McCalla (1975)
UHF, Unscheduled DNA synthesis, normal human fibroblasts in vitro	–	0	23.8 µg/ml	Tonomura & Sasaki (1973)
UHF, Unscheduled DNA synthesis, human XP fibroblasts in vitro	–	0	23.8 µg/ml	Tonomura & Sasaki (1973)
CHL, Chromosomal aberrations, human lymphocytes in vitro	–	0	23.8 µg/ml	Tonomura & Sasaki (1973)
DVA, DNA strand breaks, mouse tissue in vivo	+	0	120 mg/kg x 25, p.o.	Olive (1978)
MVM, Micronucleus test, mice in vivo	–	0	150 mg/kg x 5, i.p.	Bruce & Heddle (1978)
MVR, Micronucleus test, Sprague-Dawley rats in vivo	–	0	60 mg/kg x 1, i.p.	Goodman et al. (1977)
MVR, Micronucleus test, Long-Evans rats in vivo	–	0	60 mg/kg x 1, i.p.	Goodman et al. (1977)
CBA, Chromosomal aberrations, rat bone-marrow cells in vivo	–	0	60 mg/kg x 1, i.p.	Goodman et al. (1977)
CBA, Chromosomal aberrations, rat bone-marrow cells in vivo	–	0	400 mg/kg x 1, p.o.	Anderson & Phillips (1985)
CBA, Chromosomal aberrations, rat bone-marrow cells in vivo	–	0	150 mg/kg x 5, p.o.	Anderson & Phillips (1985)
SPF, Sperm morphology, F1 mice in vivo	–	0	150 mg/kg x 5, i.p.	Bruce & Heddle (1978)

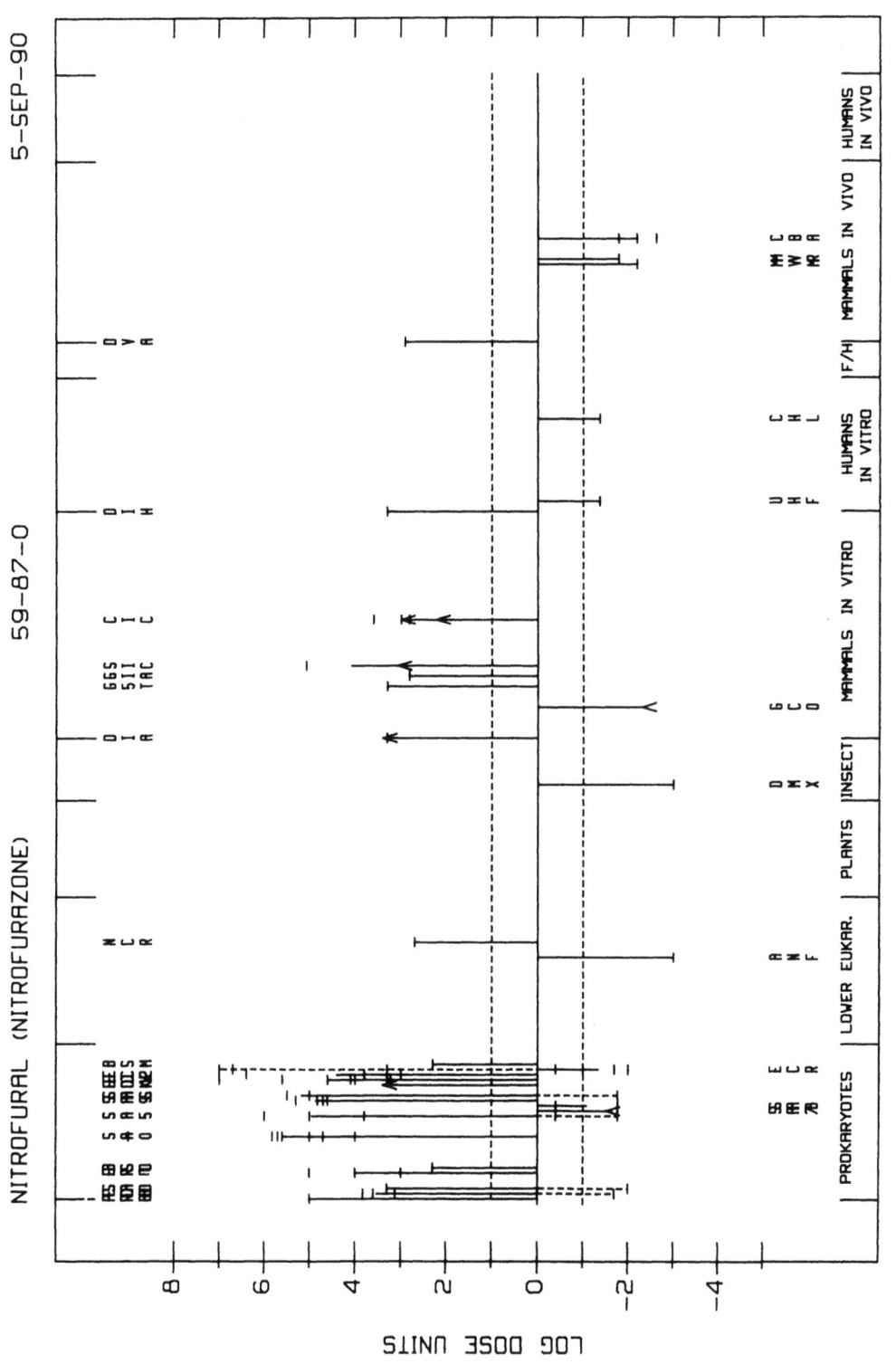

NITROFURANTOIN

Test system		Result		Dose LED/HID	Reference
		Without exogenous metabolic system	With exogenous metabolic system		
SA0,	Salmonella typhimurium, differential toxicity	+	0	119 µg/ml	Yahagi et al. (1974)
ECB,	Escherichia coli DNA strand breaks	(+)	0	50 µg/ml	McCalla et al. (1971)
ECD,	Escherichia coli W3110 vs p3478 differential toxicity	+	0	10 µg/ml	McCarroll et al. (1981a)
ERD,	Escherichia coli WP2 vs WPuvrA, differential toxicity	+	0	10 µg/ml	Ebringer & Bencova (1980)
ERD,	Escherichia coli WP2 vs WPuvrA, differential toxicity	+	0	3 µg/ml	McCarroll et al. (1981a)
ERD,	Escherichia coli WP2 vs WP67, differential toxicity	–	0	30 µg/ml	McCarroll et al. (1981a)
ERD,	Escherichia coli WP2 vs CM611 differential toxicity	–	0	3 µg/ml	McCarroll et al. (1981a)
ERD,	Escherichia coli WP2 vs WP100, differential toxicity	+	0	0.1 µg/ml	McCarroll et al. (1981a)
ERD,	Escherichia coli WP2 vs WP67, differential toxicity	+	+	6.25 µg/ml	De Flora et al. (1984)
ERD,	Escherichia coli WP2 vs CM871, differential toxicity	+	+	0.4 µg/ml	De Flora et al. (1984)
ERD,	Escherichia coli, differential toxicity	+	0	119 µg/ml	Yahagi et al. (1974)
ERD,	Escherichia coli, differential toxicity	+	0	0	McCarroll et al. (1981b)
BSD,	Bacillus subtilis, H-17 vs M-45, differential toxicity	+	0	20 µg/ml	Suter & Jaeger (1982)
BSD,	Bacillus subtilis, rec strains, differential toxicity	+	0	0	Suter & Jaeger (1982)
SA0,	Salmonella typhimurium TA100, reverse mutation	+	0	0.15 µg/ml	Wang & Lee (1976)
SA0,	Salmonella typhimurium TA100, reverse mutation	+	+	0.025 µg/ml	De Flora (1979)
SA0,	Salmonella typhimurium TA100, reverse mutation	+	+	0.15 µg/ml	Haworth et al. (1983)
SA0,	Salmonella typhimurium TA100, reverse mutation	+	0	0.125 µg/ml	Goodman et al. (1977)
SA0,	Salmonella typhimurium TA100, reverse mutation	+	+	1 µg/ml	Rosenkranz & Speck (1976)
SA0,	Salmonella typhimurium TA100, reverse mutation	+	0	0.119 µg/ml	Shirai & Wang (1980)
SA0,	Salmonella typhimurium TA100, reverse mutation	+	0	1 µg/ml	Yahagi et al. (1974)
SA0,	Salmonella typhimurium TA100, reverse mutation	+	–	1 µg/ml	Ebringer & Bencova (1980)
SA5,	Salmonella typhimurium TA1535, reverse mutation	–	–	16 µg/ml	Haworth et al. (1983)
SA5,	Salmonella typhimurium TA1535, reverse mutation	–	0	71 µg/ml	Yahagi et al. (1974)
SA7,	Salmonella typhimurium TA1537, reverse mutation	–	–	8 µg/pl	Haworth et al. (1983)
SA7,	Salmonella typhimurium TA1537, reverse mutation	–	0	71 µg/ml	Yahagi et al. (1974)
SA8,	Salmonella typhimurium TA1538, reverse mutation	–	0	71 µg/ml	Yahagi et al. (1974)
SA9,	Salmonella typhimurium TA98, reverse mutation	+	+	0.15 µg/ml	Haworth et al. (1983)
SA9,	Salmonella typhimurium TA98, reverse mutation	+	+	1 µg/ml	Ni et al. (1987)
SA9,	Salmonella typhimurium TA98, reverse mutation	+	0	0.5 µg/ml	Goodman et al. (1977)
SAS,	Salmonella typhimurium TA100FR1, reverse mutation	+	+	1.5 µg/ml	Wang & Lee (1976)
SAS,	Salmonella typhimurium TA98NR, reverse mutation	+	+	50 µg/ml	Ni et al. (1987)
SAS,	Salmonella typhimurium TA98/1,8-DNP6, reverse mutation	+	+	1 µg/ml	Ni et al. (1987)

APPENDIX 2

NITROFURANTOIN (contd)

Test system		Result		Dose LED/HID	Reference
		Without exogenous metabolic system	With exogenous metabolic system		
SAS,	Salmonella typhimurium TA1536, reverse mutation	–	0	71 μg/ml	Yahagi et al. (1974)
SAS,	Salmonella typhimurium TA97, reverse mutation (fluct. test)	+	0	0.32 μg/ml	Obaseiki-Ebor & Akerele (1986)
SAS,	Salmonella typhimurium TA100FR1, reverse mutation	+	+	5 μg/ml	Rosenkranz & Speck (1976)
ECW,	Escherichia coli WP2 uvrA, reverse mutation	+	0	71 μg/ml	Yahagi et al. (1974)
ECW,	Escherichia coli WP2 uvrA, reverse mutation	+	0	10 μg/ml	McCalla & Vouteinos (1974)
ECW,	Escherichia coli WP2 uvrA, reverse mutation	+	0	7.14 μg/ml	Lu et al. (1979)
EC2,	Escherichia coli WP2, reverse mutation (fluctuation test)	–	0	0.4 μg/ml	Obaseiki-Ebor & Akerele (1986)
EC2,	Escherichia coli WP2, reverse mutation	(+)	0	19 μg/ml	McCalla & Vouteinos (1974)
ECR,	Escherichia coli EE97, reverse mutation (fluctuation test)	+	0	0.1 μg/ml	Obaseiki-Ebor & Akerele (1986)
SCG,	Saccharomyces cerevisiae D4-RDII, mitotic gene conversion	–	0	23.8 μg/ml	Siebert et al. (1979)
SCG,	Saccharomyces cerevisiae D4-RDII, mitotic gene conversion	0	+	238 μg/ml	Siebert et al. (1979)
SCG,	Saccharomyces cerevisiae D7, mitotic gene conversion	+	0	476 μg/ml	Callen (1981)
ANG,	Aspergillus nidulans, crossing over	–	0	0	Bignami et al. (1974)
SCG,	Saccharomyces cerevisiae D4, reverse mutation/gene conversion	–	0	238 μg/ml	Setnikar et al. (1976)
DMX,	Drosophila melanogaster, sex-linked recessive lethal mutation	(+)	0	214 μg/ml	Kramers (1982)
DMX,	Drosophila melanogaster, sex-linked recessive lethal mutation	–	0	2000 μg/ml (food)	Zimmering et al. (1985)
DMX,	Drosophila melanogaster, sex-linked recessive lethal mutation	–	0	10000 μg/ml (injection)	Zimmering et al. (1985)
DMM,	Drosophila melanogaster, somatic mutation	+	0	1190 μg/ml	Graf et al. (1989)
DIA,	DNA single strand breaks, mouse L cells in vitro	+	0	102 μg/ml	Olive & McCalla (1977)
URP,	Unscheduled DNA synthesis, rat primary hepatocytes	–	0	23.8 μg/ml	Williams et al (1989)
SIC,	Sister chromatid exchange, Chinese hamster CHO cells in vitro	+	0	9.5 μg/ml	Shirai & Wang (1980)
CIC,	Chromosomal aberrations, Chinese hamster lung cells in vitro	+	0	60 μg/ml	Ishidate (1988)
UHF,	Unscheduled DNA synthesis, human fibroblasts in vitro	–	0	20 μg/ml	Tonomura & Sasaki (1973)
UHF,	Unscheduled DNA synthesis, human XP fibroblasts in vitro	–	0	20 μg/ml	Tonomura & Sasaki (1973)
SIH,	Sister chromatid exchange, human HE2144 cells in vitro	+	0	2.38 μg/ml	Sasaki et al. (1980)
CHL,	Chromosomal aberrations, human lymphocytes in vitro	–	0	20 μg/ml	Wang et al. (1977)
CIH,	Chromosomal aberrations, human HE2144 cells in vitro	–	0	2.38 μg/ml	Sasaki et al. (1980)
BFA,	Salmonella typhimurium TA100, reverse mutation (rat urine)	(+)	0	600 mg/kg x 4, p.o.	Wang & Lee (1976)
BFA,	Salmonella typhimurium TA100FR1, reverse mutation (rat urine)	+	0	600 mg/kg x 4, p.o.	Wang & Lee (1976)
BFA,	Saccharomyces cerevisiae D4-RDII, mitotic gene conversion	+	0	500 mg/kg x 1, p.o.	Siebert et al. (1979)
BFH,	Salmonella typhimurium TA100, reverse mutation (human urine)	+	0	1.6 mg/kg x 1, p.o.	Wang et al. (1977)
BFH,	Salmonella typhimurium TA100FR1, reverse mutation (human urine)	(+)	0	1.6 mg/kg x 1, p.o.	Wang et al. (1977)
HPM,	Saccharomyces cerevisiae D4, reverse mutation/gene conversion	–	0	71 mg/kg x 1, p.o.	Setnikar et al. (1976)
HPM,	Saccharomyces cerevisiae D4-RDII, mitotic gene conversion	–	0	500 mg/kg x 1, p.o. 6 h	Siebert et al. (1979)

NITROFURANTOIN (contd)

Test system	Result without exogenous metabolic system	Result with exogenous metabolic system	Dose LED/HID	Reference
HMM, Saccharomyces cerevisiae D4-RDII, mitotic gene conversion	+	0	500 mg/kg x 1, p.o. 8h	Siebert et al. (1979)
DVA, DNA damage, Sprague-Dawley rats in vivo	+	0	56 mg/kg x 1, i.p.	Russo et al. (1982)
DVA, DNA damage, Sprague-Dawley rats in vivo	+	0	14 mg/kg x 1, i.p.	Parodi et al. (1983)
DVA, DNA damage, mouse bone-marrow cells in vivo	+	0	64 mg/kg x 1, i.p.	Parodi et al. (1983)
MST, Mouse spot test	–	0	80 mg/kg x 1, i.p.	Gocke et al. (1983)
SVA, Sister chromatid exchange, mouse bone-marrow cells in vivo	+	0	32 mg/kg x 1, i.p.	Parodi et al. (1983)
MVR, Micronucleus test, Sprague-Dawley rats in vivo	–	0	400 mg/kg x 1, p.o.	Setnikar et al. (1976)
MVR, Micronucleus test, Sprague-Dawley rats in vivo	–	0	200 mg/kg x 1, i.p.	Goodman et al. (1977)
CCC, Chromosomal aberrations, male NMRI mice meiotic cells	?	0	40 mg/kg x 2, i.p.	Fonatsch (1977)
DLM, Dominant lethal test, ICR/Ha Swiss mice	–	0	80 mg/kg x 1, i.p.	Epstein et al. (1972)
DLM, Dominant lethal test, NMRI mice	–	0	17.5 mg/kg x 1, p.o.	Setnikar et al. (1976)

APPENDIX 2

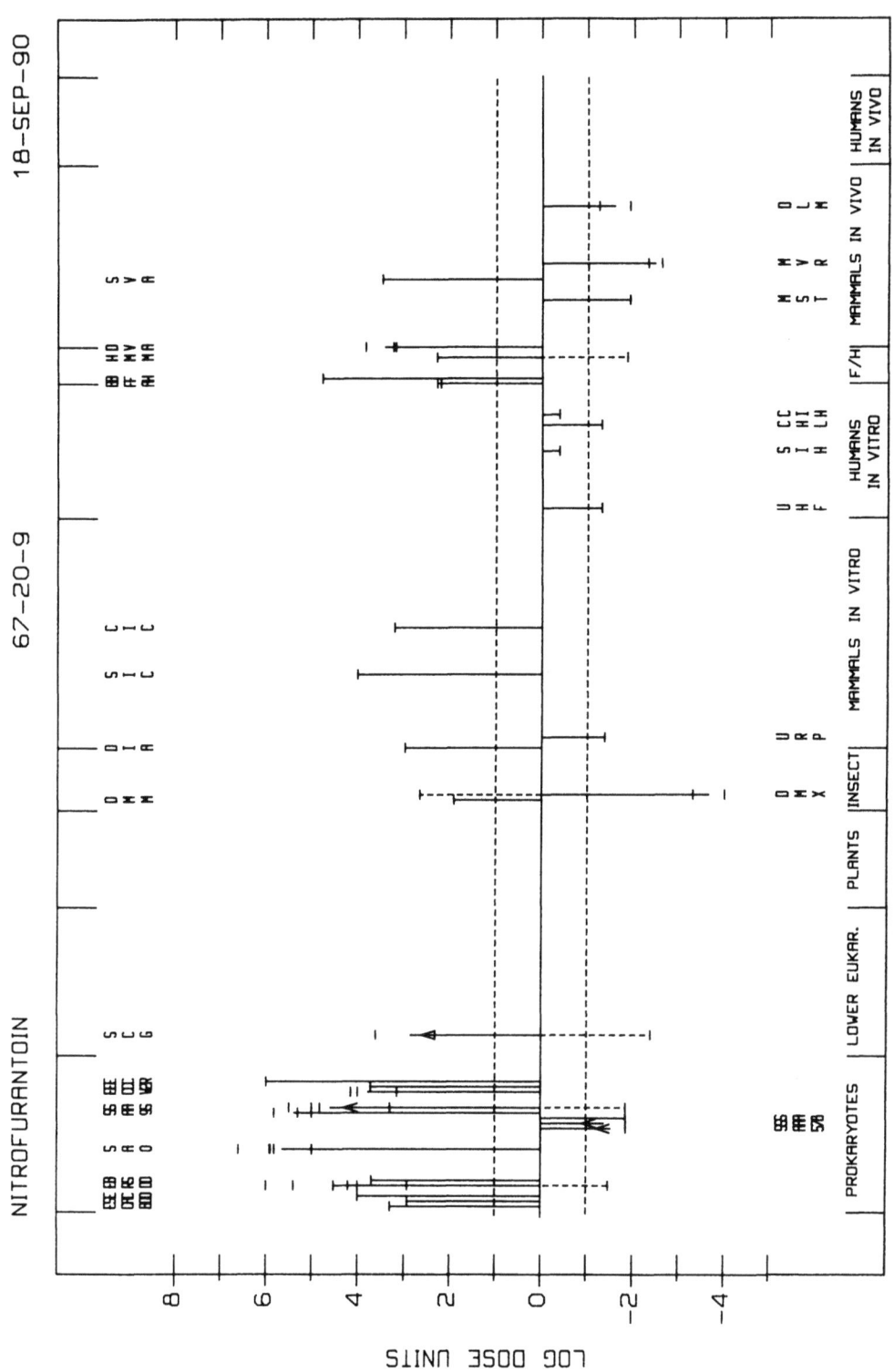

CIMETIDINE

Test system	Result		Dose LED/HID	Reference
	Without exogenous metabolic system	With exogenous metabolic system		
ERD, Escherichia coli, differential toxicity	–	0	60 μg/ml	Pool et al. (1979)
ERD, Escherichia coli, differential toxicity	–	0	1250 μg/ml	De Flora (1981)
SA0, Salmonella typhimurium TA100, reverse mutation	–	–	10000 μg/ml	De Flora & Picciotto (1980)
SA5, Salmonella typhimurium TA1535, reverse mutation	–	–	10000 μg/ml	De Flora & Picciotto (1980)
SA7, Salmonella typhimurium TA1537, reverse mutation	–	–	10000 μg/ml	De Flora & Picciotto (1980)
SA8, Salmonella typhimurium TA1538, reverse mutation	–	–	10000 μg/ml	De Flora & Picciotto (1980)
SA9, Salmonella typhimurium TA98, reverse mutation	–	–	10000 μg/ml	De Flora & Picciotto (1980)
DIA, DNA strand breaks, transformed mouse epithelial cells in vitro	–	0	1260 μg/ml	Schwarz et al. (1980)
DIA, DNA damage, rat hepatocytes in vitro	+	0	756 μg/ml[a]	Martelli et al. (1983)
URP, Unscheduled DNA synthesis, rat primary hepatocytes	+	0	83 μg/ml[a]	Martelli et al. (1983)
URP, Unscheduled DNA synthesis, rat primary hepatocytes	–	0	2520 μg/ml[a]	Lefevre & Ashby (1985)
URP, Unscheduled DNA synthesis, rat primary hepatocytes	+	0	25.2 μg/ml[a]	Lefevre & Ashby (1985)
DIH, DNA damage, human hepatocytes in vitro	–	0	2268 μg/ml[a]	Martelli et al. (1986)
UIH, Unscheduled DNA synthesis, human hepatocytes in vitro	–	0	2268 μg/ml	Martelli et al. (1986)
SHL, Sister chromatid exchange, human lymphocytes in vitro	–	0	252 μg/ml	Inoue et al. (1985)
DVA, DNA damage, rat liver cells in vivo	–	0	250 mg/kg x1 – x20 p.o.[b]	Brambilla et al. (1982)
DVA, DNA damage, rat gastric mucosa in vivo	–	0	250 mg/kg x 1 p.o.[b]	Pino & Robbiano (1983)

[a] Cimetidine hydrochloride
[b] With NaNO$_2$, 80 mg/kg

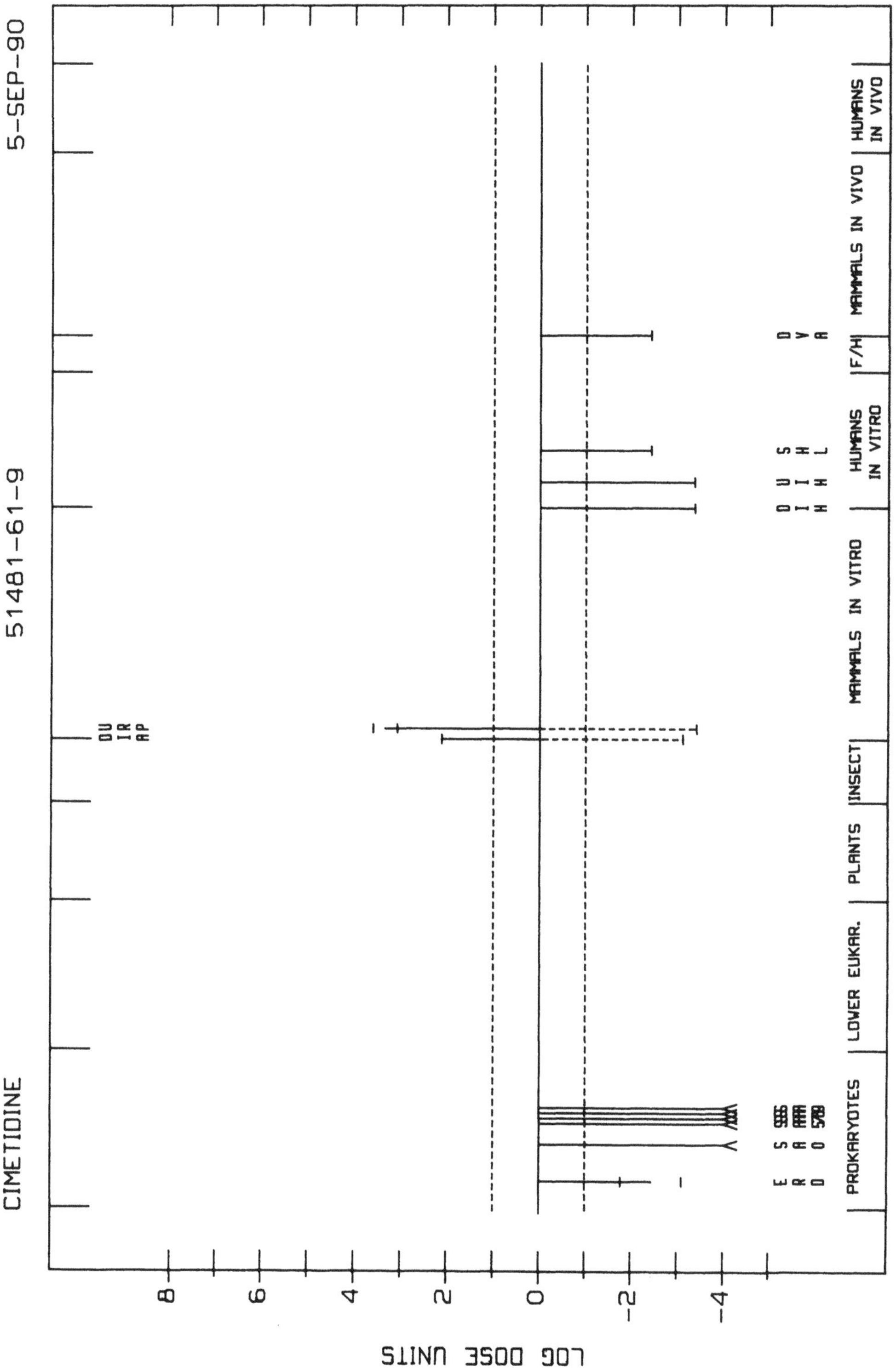
CIMETIDINE
51481-61-9
5-SEP-90
PROKARYOTES
LOWER EUKAR.
PLANTS
INSECT
MAMMALS IN VITRO
HUMANS IN VITRO
F/H
MAMMALS IN VIVO
HUMANS IN VIVO
8
6
4
2
0
-2
-4
LOG DOSE UNITS

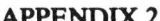

N-NITROSOCIMETIDINE/CIMETIDINE PLUS NITRITE

Test system	Result without exogenous metabolic system	Result with exogenous metabolic system	Dose LED/HID	Reference
ERD, Escherichia coli, differential toxicity	+	0	6 μg/ml	Pool et al. (1979)
ERD, Escherichia coli, differential toxicity	+	0	1250 μg/ml[a]	De Flora (1981)
ERD, Escherichia coli, differential toxicity	+	0	60000 μg/ml[b]	Ichinotsubo et al. (1981)
ERD, Escherichia coli, differential toxicity	+	0	200 μg/ml[c]	Ichinotsubo et al. (1981)
ERD, Escherichia coli (WP2 trp-) strains, differential toxicity	+	0	30000 μg/ml[b]	Ichinotsubo et al. (1981)
ERD, Escherichia coli (WP2 trp-) strains, differential toxicity	+	0	300 μg/ml[c]	Ichinotsubo et al. (1981)
ECF, Escherichia coli, forward mutation	+	0	112 μg/ml	Alldrick et al. (1984)
SA0, Salmonella typhimurium TA100, reverse mutation	+	0	155 μg/ml[d]	De Flora & Picciotto (1980)
SA0, Salmonella typhimurium TA100, reverse mutation	+	+	10000 μg/ml[b]	De Flora & Picciotto (1980)
SA0, Salmonella typhimurium TA100, reverse mutation	+	0	50 μg/ml	De Flora (1981)
SA0, Salmonella typhimurium TA100, reverse mutation	+	0	17500 μg/ml[b]	Ichinotsubo et al. (1981)
SA0, Salmonella typhimurium TA100, reverse mutation	+	0	1000 μg/ml[c]	Ichinotsubo et al. (1981)
SA5, Salmonella typhimurium TA1535, reverse mutation	+	0	15 μg/ml	Pool et al. (1979)
SA5, Salmonella typhimurium TA1535, reverse mutation	+	+	10000 μg/ml[d]	De Flora & Picciotto (1980)
SA5, Salmonella typhimurium TA1535, reverse mutation	+	0	15000 μg/ml[b]	Ichinotsubo et al. (1981)
SA5, Salmonella typhimurium TA1535, reverse mutation	+	0	300 μg/ml[c]	Ichinotsubo et al. (1981)
SA7, Salmonella typhimurium TA1537, reverse mutation	+	+	10000 μg/ml[d]	De Flora & Picciotto (1980)
SA8, Salmonella typhimurium TA1538, reverse mutation	+	+	10000 μg/ml[d]	De Flora & Picciotto (1980)
SA9, Salmonella typhimurium TA98, reverse mutation	+	+	10000 μg/ml[d]	De Flora & Picciotto (1980)
DIA, DNA damage, transformed mouse epithelial cells	+	0	252 μg/ml	Schwarz et al. (1980)
GIA, Gene mutation, BHK-21/C113 hamster cells in vitro	+	0	5 μg/ml	Barrows et al. (1982)
SIC, Sister chromatid exchange, Chinese hamster CHO cells in vitro	+	0	0.03 μg/ml[b]	Athanasiou & Kyrtopoulos (1981)
SIC, Sister chromatid exchange, Chinese hamster CHO cells in vitro	+	0	0.23 μg/ml[b]	Ichinotsubo et al. (1981)
SIC, Sister chromatid exchange, Chinese hamster CHO cells in vitro	+	0	0.017 μg/ml[c]	Ichinotsubo et al. (1981)
CIC, Chromosomal aberrations, Chinese hamster CHO cells in vitro	+	0	0.03 μg/ml	Athanasiou & Kyrtopoulos (1981)
CIC, Chromosomal aberrations, Chinese hamster CHO cells in vitro	+	0	23.18 μg/ml[b]	Ichinotsubo et al. (1981)
CIC, Chromosomal aberrations, Chinese hamster CHO cells in vitro	+	0	0.65 μg/ml[c]	Ichinotsubo et al. (1981)
TCL, Cell transformation, BHK-21/C113 hamster cells	+	0	5 μg/ml	Barrows et al. (1982)
DIH, DNA damage, human lymphoblastoid cell line in vitro	+	0	88 μg/ml	Henderson et al. (1981)
UIH, Unscheduled DNA synthesis, human leukocytes in vitro	+	0	45 μg/ml	Henderson et al. (1981)
UIH, Unscheduled DNA synthesis, human lymphoblasts in vitro	+	0	45 μg/ml	Henderson et al. (1981)
SHL, Sister chromatid exchange, human lymphocytes in vitro	+	0	3.28 μg/ml	Inoue et al. (1985)
SHL, Sister chromatid exchange, human lymphocytes in vitro	+	0	2.37 μg/ml[e]	Inoue et al. (1985)
HMM, Host-mediated assay, Salmonella typhimurium in mice	–	0	350 mg/kg	Baumeister (1982)

N-NITROSOCIMETIDINE/CIMETIDINE PLUS NITRITE (contd)

Test system	Result		Dose LED/HID	Reference
	Without exogenous metabolic system	With exogenous metabolic system		
DVA, DNA damage, rat liver cells in vivo	–	0	250 mg/kg[f] x1 – x20 p.o.	Brambilla et al. (1982)
DVA, DNA damage, rat gastric mucosa in vivo	–	0	250 mg/kg[f] x 1 p.o.	Pino & Robbiano (1983)

[a] With 2.5 mg $NaNO_2$, pH 3, 1 h
[b] Mononitrosocimetidine
[c] Dinitrosocimetidine
[d] With 5 mg $NaNO_2$, human gastric juice, pH 1.37, 1 h, 37°C
[e] With 60/120 mg/kg $NaNO_2$
[f] With 80 mg/kg $NaNO_2$

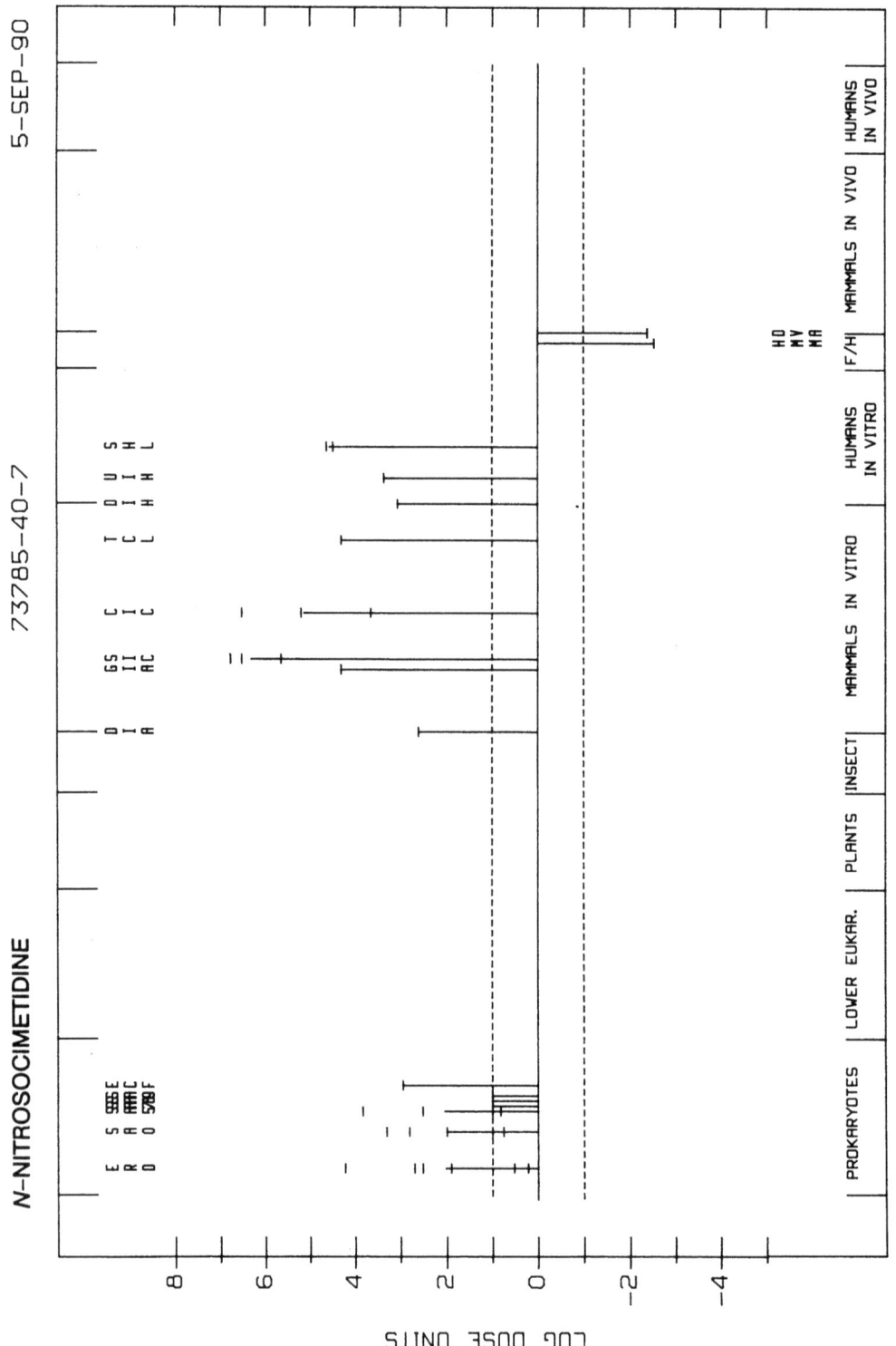

DANTRON (1,8-DIHYDROXYANTHRAQUINONE)

Test system	Result without exogenous metabolic system	Result with exogenous metabolic system	Dose LED/HID	Reference
SA0, Mutation, Salmonella typhimurium TA100	–	–	1000 µg/ml	Brown & Brown (1976)
SA0, Mutation, Salmonella typhimurium TA100	–	–	10 µg/ml	Liberman et al. (1982)
SA0, Mutation, Salmonella typhimurium TA100	–	–	50 µg/ml	Tikkanen et al. (1983)
SA2, Mutation, Salmonella typhimurium TA102	–	+	15 µg/ml	Levin et al. (1984)
SA5, Mutation, Salmonella typhimurium TA1535	–	–	500 µg/ml	Brown & Brown (1976)
SA5, Mutation, Salmonella typhimurium TA1535	–	–	10 µg/ml	Liberman et al. (1982)
SA7, Mutation, Salmonella typhimurium TA1537	+	+	50 µg/ml	Brown & Brown (1976)
SA7, Mutation, Salmonella typhimurium TA1537	+	+	1 µg/ml	Liberman et al. (1982)
SA8, Mutation, Salmonella typhimurium TA1538	–	–	1000 µg/ml	Brown & Brown (1976)
SA8, Mutation, Salmonella typhimurium TA1538	–	–	50 µg/ml	Liberman et al. (1982)
SA9, Mutation, Salmonella typhimurium TA98	–	–	1000 µg/ml	Brown & Brown (1976)
SA9, Mutation, Salmonella typhimurium TA98	–	–	10 µg/ml	Liberman et al. (1982)
SA9, Mutation, Salmonella typhimurium TA98	–	–	50 µg/ml	Tikkanen et al. (1983)
SAS, Mutation, Salmonella typhimurium TA104	0	+	4.8 µg/ml	Chesis et al. (1984)
SAS, Mutation, Salmonella typhimurium TA2637	–	+	1 µg/ml	Tikkanen et al. (1983)
SCR, Saccharomyces cerevisiae, forward mutation	+	0	0	Zetterberg & Swanbeck (1971)
URP, Unscheduled DNA synthesis, rat primary hepatocytes	–	0	120 µg/ml	Probst et al. (1981)
URP, Unscheduled DNA synthesis, rat primary hepatocytes	+	0	4.8 µg/ml	Mori et al. (1984)
URP, Unscheduled DNA synthesis, rat primary hepatocytes	+	0	12 µg/ml	Kawai et al. (1986)
UIA, Unscheduled DNA synthesis, mouse hepatocytes	+	0	4.8 µg/ml	Mori et al. (1984)
CHL, Chromosomal aberrations, human lymphocytes in vitro	+	0	10 µg/ml	Carballo et al. (1981)
ICR, Inhibition of intercellular communication, animal cells in vitro	–	0	3 µg/ml	Zeilmaker & Yamasaki (1986)
ICR, Inhibition of intercellular communication, animal cells in vitro	–	0	2.4 µg/ml	Si et al. (1988)

376

IARC MONOGRAPHS VOLUME 50

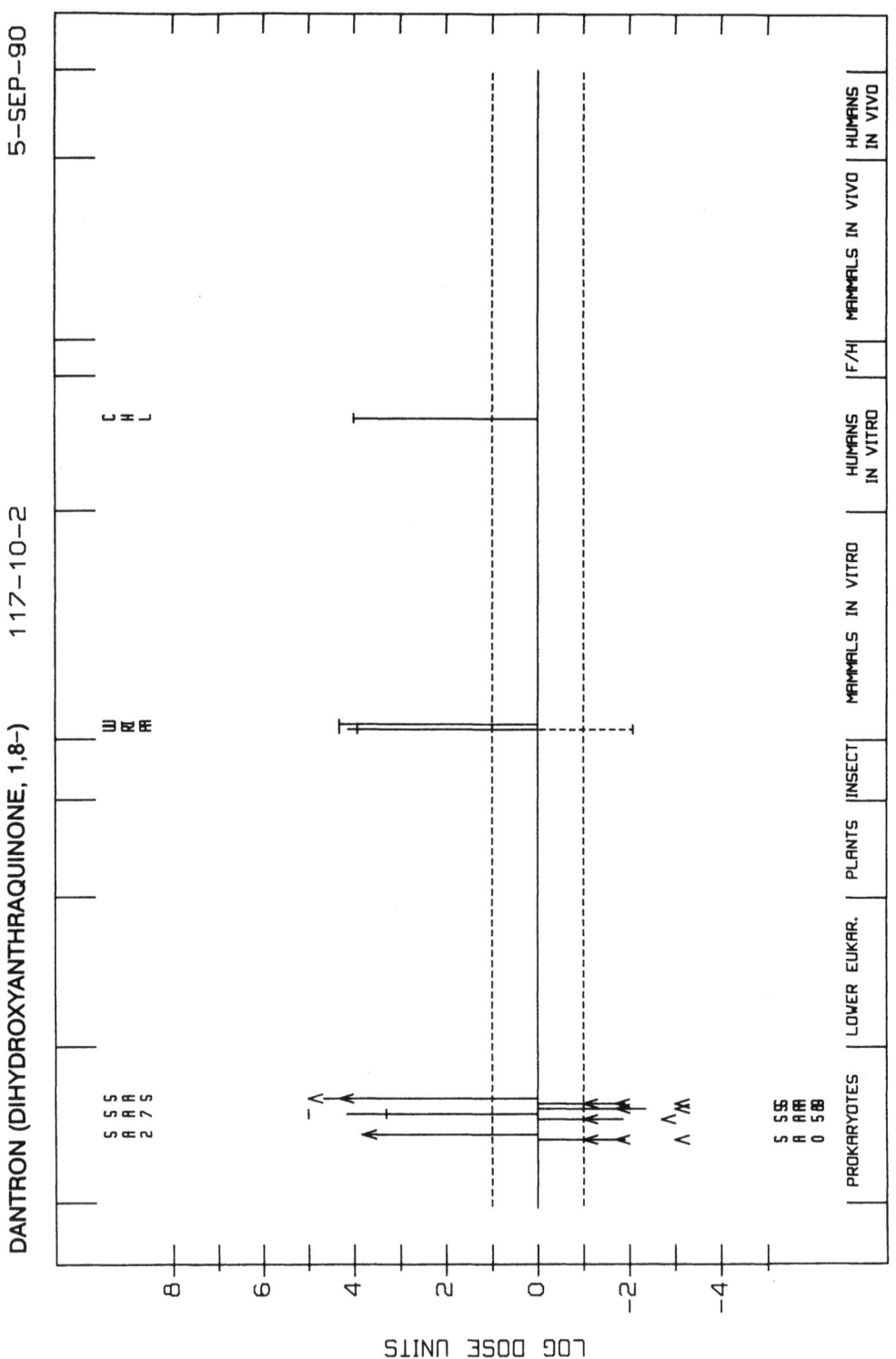

FUROSEMIDE

Test system	Result without exogenous metabolic system	Result with exogenous metabolic system	Dose LED/HID	Reference
SA0, Salmonella typhimurium TA100, reverse mutation	–	–	5000 µg/ml	National Toxicology Program (1989)
SA5, Salmonella typhimurium TA1535, reverse mutation	–	–	5000 µg/ml	National Toxicology Program (1989)
SA7, Salmonella typhimurium TA1537, reverse mutation	–	–	5000 µg/ml	National Toxicology Program (1989)
SA9, Salmonella typhimurium TA98, reverse mutation	–	–	5000 µg/ml	National Toxicology Program (1989)
G51, Gene mutation mouse lymphoma L5178Y cells	–	(+)	1500 µg/ml	National Toxicology Program (1989)
SIC, Sister chromatid exchange, Chinese hamster ovary cells	(+)	(+)	750 µg/ml	National Toxicology Program (1989)
CIC, Chromosomal aberrations, Chinese hamster lung cells in vitro	(+)	0	2000 µg/ml	Ishidate (1988)
CIC, Chromosomal aberrations, Chinese hamster lung cells in vitro	(+)	–	500 µg/ml	Matsuoka et al. (1979)
SHF, Sister chromatid exchange, Chinese hamster ovary cells	–	(+)	3750 µg/ml	National Toxicology Program (1989)
CHF, Chromosomal aberrations, human fibroblasts in vitro	–	0	1654 µg/ml	Sasaki et al. (1980)
CIH, Chromosomal aberrations, human fibroblasts in vitro	–	0	1654 µg/ml	Sasaki et al. (1980)
CIH, Chromosomal aberrations, human leukocytes in vitro	+	0	200 µg/ml	Jameela et al. (1979)
CCC, Chromosomal aberrations, C3H/He mouse germ cells in vivo	+	0	50 mg/kg x 1, i.p.	Subramanyam & Jameela (1977)
BFA, Saccharomyces cerevisiae D4-RDII, gene conversion mouse urine	–	0	45 mg/kg x 1, i.p.	Marquardt & Siebert (1971)

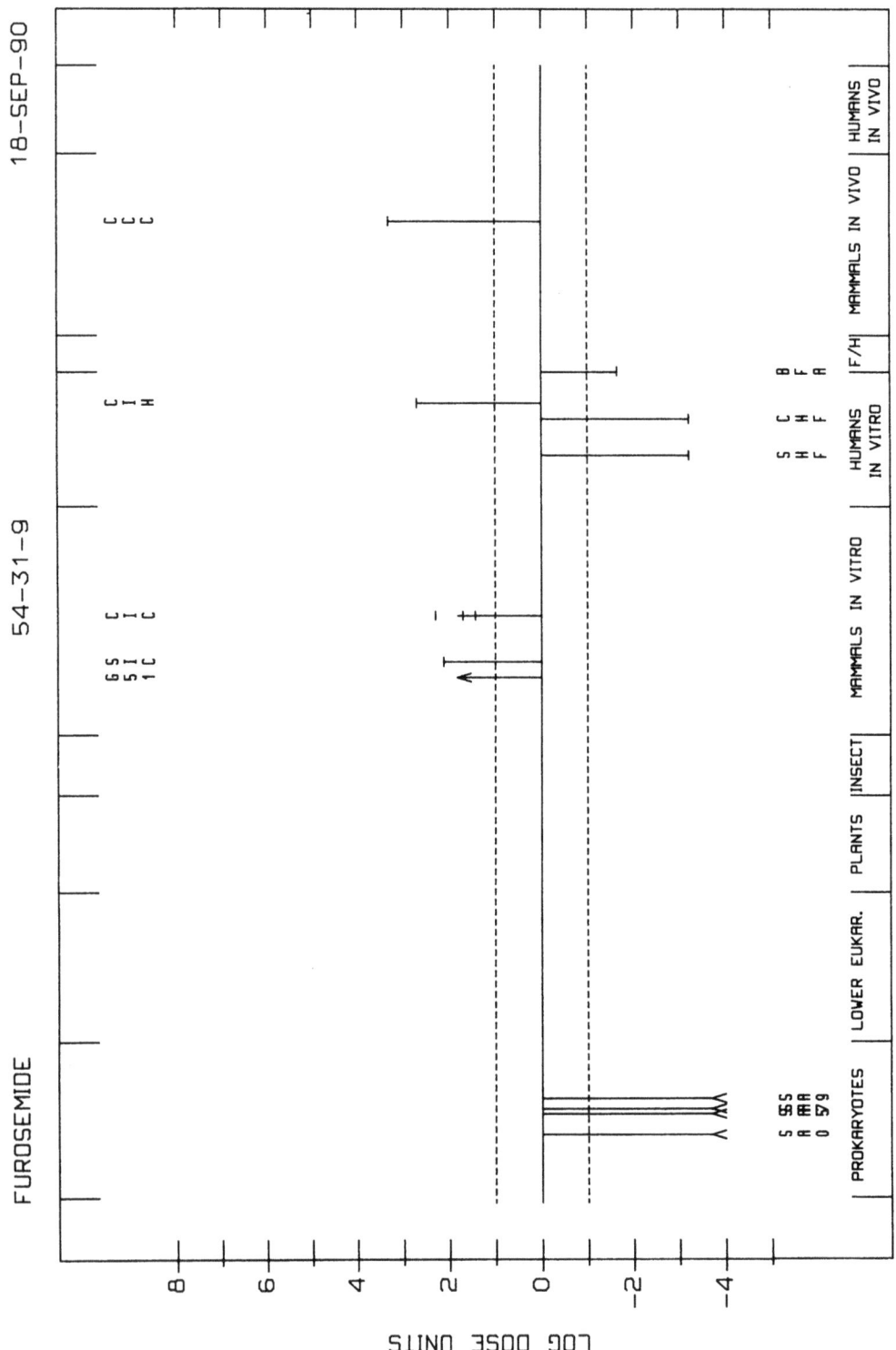

APPENDIX 2

HYDROCHLOROTHIAZIDE

Test system	Result		Dose LED/HID	Reference
	Without exogenous metabolic system	With exogenous metabolic system		
ECR, Escherichia coli Hs30R, reverse mutation	–	0	77.5 μg/ml	Fujita (1985)
SA0, Salmonella typhimurium TA100, reverse mutation	–	–	5000 μg/ml	Mortelmans et al. (1986)
SA0, Salmonella typhimurium TA100, reverse mutation	–	–	2500 μg/ml	Waskell (1978)
SA0, Salmonella typhimurium TA100, reverse mutation	–	–	500 μg/ml	Andrews et al. (1984)
SA5, Salmonella typhimurium TA1535, reverse mutation	–	–	5000 μg/ml	Mortelmans et al. (1986)
SA5, Salmonella typhimurium TA1535, reverse mutation	–	–	500 μg/ml	Andrews et al. (1984)
SA7, Salmonella typhimurium TA1537, reverse mutation	–	–	5000 μg/ml	Mortelmans et al. (1986)
SA8, Salmonella typhimurium TA1538, reverse mutation	–	–	500 μg/ml	Andrews et al. (1984)
SA9, Salmonella typhimurium TA98, reverse mutation	?	–	5000 μg/ml	Mortelmans et al. (1986)
SA9, Salmonella typhimurium TA98, reverse mutation	–	–	2500 μg/ml	Waskell (1978)
SA9, Salmonella typhimurium TA98, reverse mutation	–	–	500 μg/ml	Andrews et al. (1984)
ANG, Aspergillus nidulans, non-disjunction and mitotic crossing-over	+	0	0.00	Bignami et al. (1974)
DMX, Drosophila melanogaster, sex-linked recessive lethal mutation	–	0	10000 μg/ml	Valencia et al. (1985)
G51, Gene mutation, mouse lymphoma L5178Y cells	+	0	500 μg/ml	National Toxicology Program (1989)
SIC, Sister chromatid exchange, Chinese hamster ovary cells in vitro	+	+	500 μg/ml	Galloway et al. (1987)
CIC, Chromosomal aberrations, Chinese hamster ovary cells in vitro	–	0	2600 μg/ml	National Toxicology Program (1989)
CIC, Chromosomal aberrations, Chinese hamster lung cell	–	0	500 μg/ml	Ishidate (1988)

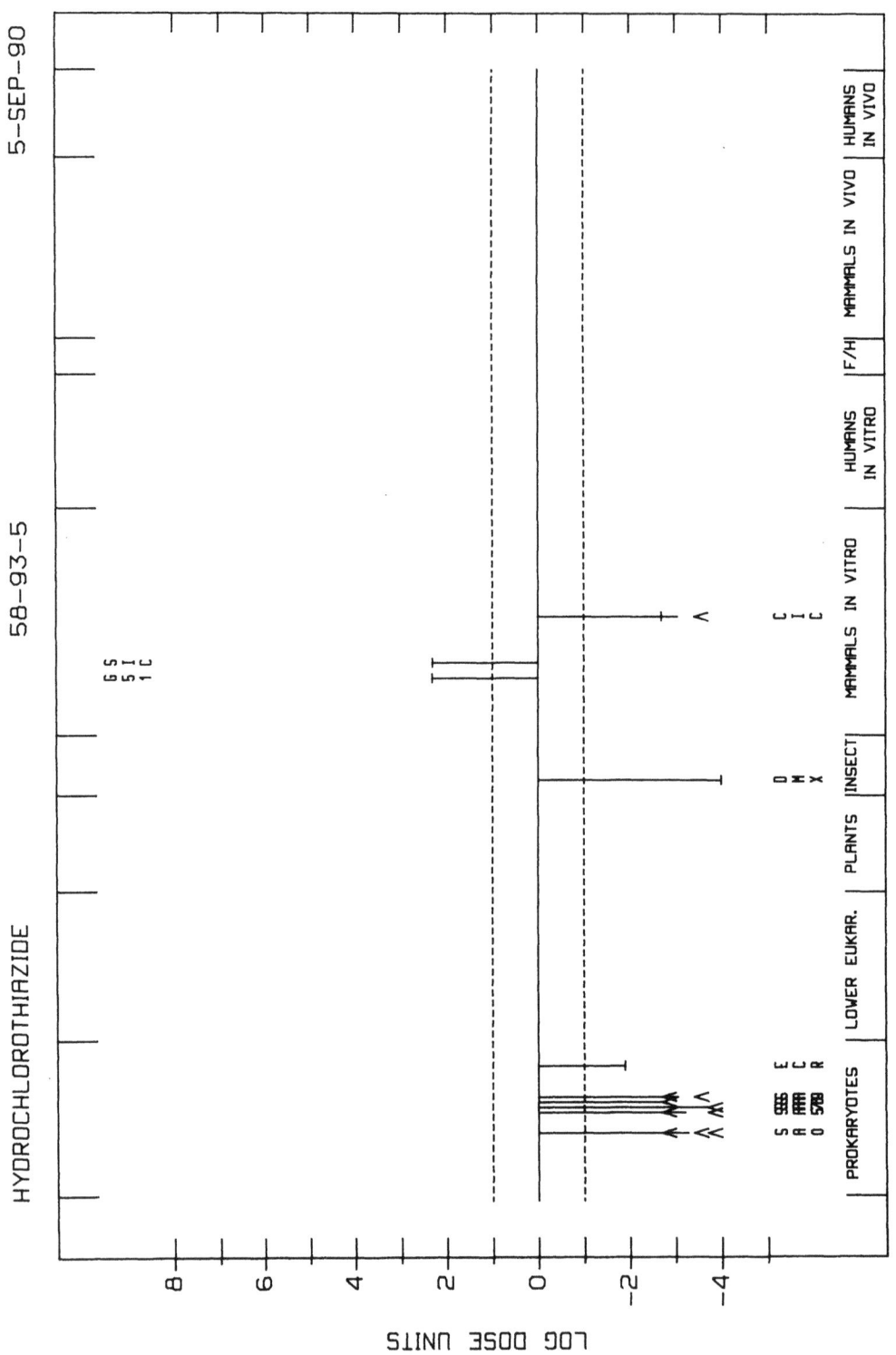

APPENDIX 2

PARACETAMOL

Test system	Result without exogenous metabolic system	Result with exogenous metabolic system	Dose LED/HID	Reference
SA0, Salmonella typhimurium TA100, reverse mutation	–	–	3576 μg/ml	King et al. (1979)
SA0, Salmonella typhimurium TA100, reverse mutation	–	–	0	Wirth et al. (1980)
SA0, Salmonella typhimurium TA100, reverse mutation	0	–	3020	Dybing et al. (1984)
SA0, Salmonella typhimurium TA100, reverse mutation	–	–	2500 μg/ml	Oldham et al. (1986)
SA0, Salmonella typhimurium TA100, reverse mutation	–	–	5000 μg/ml	Jasiewicz & Richardson (1987)
SA2, Salmonella typhimurium TA102, reverse mutation	0	–	3020 μg/ml	Dybing et al. (1984)
SA5, Salmonella typhimurium TA1535, reverse mutation	–	–	3576 μg/ml	King et al. (1979)
SA5, Salmonella typhimurium TA1535, reverse mutation	–	–	2500 μg/ml	Oldham et al. (1986)
SA5, Salmonella typhimurium TA1535, reverse mutation	–	–	500 μg/ml	Jasiewicz & Richardson (1987)
SA7, Salmonella typhimurium TA1537, reverse mutation	–	–	3576 μg/ml	King et al. (1979)
SA7, Salmonella typhimurium TA1537, reverse mutation	–	–	2500 μg/ml	Oldham et al. (1986)
SA7, Salmonella typhimurium TA1537, reverse mutation	–	–	2500 μg/ml	Jasiewicz & Richardson (1987)
SA8, Salmonella typhimurium TA1538, reverse mutation	–	–	3576 μg/ml	King et al. (1979)
SA8, Salmonella typhimurium TA1538, reverse mutation	–	–	2500 μg/ml	Oldham et al. (1986)
SA8, Salmonella typhimurium TA1538, reverse mutation	–	–	2500 μg/ml	Jasiewicz & Richardson (1987)
SA9, Salmonella typhimurium TA98, reverse mutation	–	–	3576 μg/ml	King et al. (1979)
SA9, Salmonella typhimurium TA98, reverse mutation	–	–	500 μg/ml	Wirth et al. (1980)
SA9, Salmonella typhimurium TA98, reverse mutation	0	–	3020 μg/ml	Dybing et al. (1984)
SA9, Salmonella typhimurium TA98, reverse mutation	–	–	2500 μg/ml	Oldham et al. (1986)
SA9, Salmonella typhimurium TA98, reverse mutation	–	–	5000 μg/ml	Jasiewicz & Richardson (1987)
SAS, Salmonella typhimurium TA97, reverse mutation	–	–	2500 μg/ml	Jasiewicz & Richardson (1987)
ECK, Escherichia coli K12/343/113, mutation	–	–	8940 μg/ml	King et al. (1979)
ACC, Allium cepa root cells, chromosomal aberrations	+	0	5000 μg/ml	Reddy & Subramanyam (1981)
DMX, Drosophila melanogaster, sex-linked recessive lethal mutation	–	0	11920 μg/ml	King et al. (1979)
DIA, DNA damage, Reuber hepatoma cells in vitro	–	0	1510 μg/ml	Dybing et al. (1984)
DIA, DNA damage, Chinese hamster V79 cells in vitro	(+)	0	1510 μg/ml	Hongslo et al. (1988)
URP, Unscheduled DNA synthesis, rat hepatocytes in vitro	(+)	0	1057 μg/ml	Milam & Byard (1985)
URP, Unscheduled DNA synthesis, rat hepatocytes in vitro	–	0	1510 μg/ml	Holme & Soderlund (1986)
UIA, Unscheduled DNA synthesis, mouse hepatocytes in vitro	+	0	755 μg/ml	Dybing et al. (1984)
UIA, Unscheduled DNA synthesis, mouse hepatocytes in vitro	+	0	755 μg/ml	Holme & Soderlund (1986)
UIA, Unscheduled DNA synthesis, hamster hepatocytes in vitro	–	0	1510 μg/ml	Holme & Soderlund (1986)
UIA, Unscheduled DNA synthesis, guinea-pig hepatocytes in vitro	–	0	1510 μg/ml	Holme & Soderlund (1986)
UIA, Unscheduled DNA synthesis, Chinese hamster V79 cells in vitro	–	0	1510 μg/ml	Hongslo et al. (1988)
GIA, Gene mutation, mouse C3H 10T1/2 clone 8 cells in vitro	–	0	1000 μg/ml	Patierno et al. (1989)

PARACETAMOL (contd)

Test system	Result		Dose LED/HID	Reference
	Without exogenous metabolic system	With exogenous metabolic system		
SIC, Sister chromatid exchange, Chinese hamster V79 cells in vitro	+	+	453 μg/ml	Hongslo et al. (1988)
SIC, Sister chromatid exchange, Chinese hamster V79 cells in vitro	+	0	151 μg/ml	Holme et al. (1988)
MIA, Micronucleus test, rat kidney cells in vitro	+	0	1510 μg/ml	Dunn et al. (1987)
CIC, Chromosomal aberrations, Chinese hamster lung cells in vitro	(+)	0	60 μg/ml	Ishidate et al. (1978)
CIC, Chromosomal aberrations, Chinese hamster Don-6 cells in vitro	+	0	75 μg/ml	Sasaki et al. (1980)
TCM, Cell transformation, C3H 10T1/2 clone 8 cells in vitro	(+)	+	1000 μg/ml	Patierno et al. (1989)
CHL, Chromosomal aberrations, human lymphocytes in vitro	+	0	200 μg/ml	Watanabe (1982)
MVM, Micronucleus test, NMRI mice in vivo	−		894 mg/kg x 2, i.p.	King et al. (1979)
CBA, Chromosomal aberrations, Swiss mice bone-marrow cells in vivo	(+)		100 mg/kg x 3, p.o.	Reddy (1984)
CCC, Chromosomal aberrations, male Swiss mice germ cells in vivo	?		100 mg/kg x 3, p.o.	Reddy & Subramanyam (1985)
AVA, Aneuploidy, rat embryos in vivo	+		500 mg/kg x 25, p.o.	Tsuruzaki et al. (1982)
CLH, Chromosomal aberrations, human lymphocytes in vivo	+		50 mg/kg x 1, p.o.	Kocisova et al. (1988)

APPENDIX 2

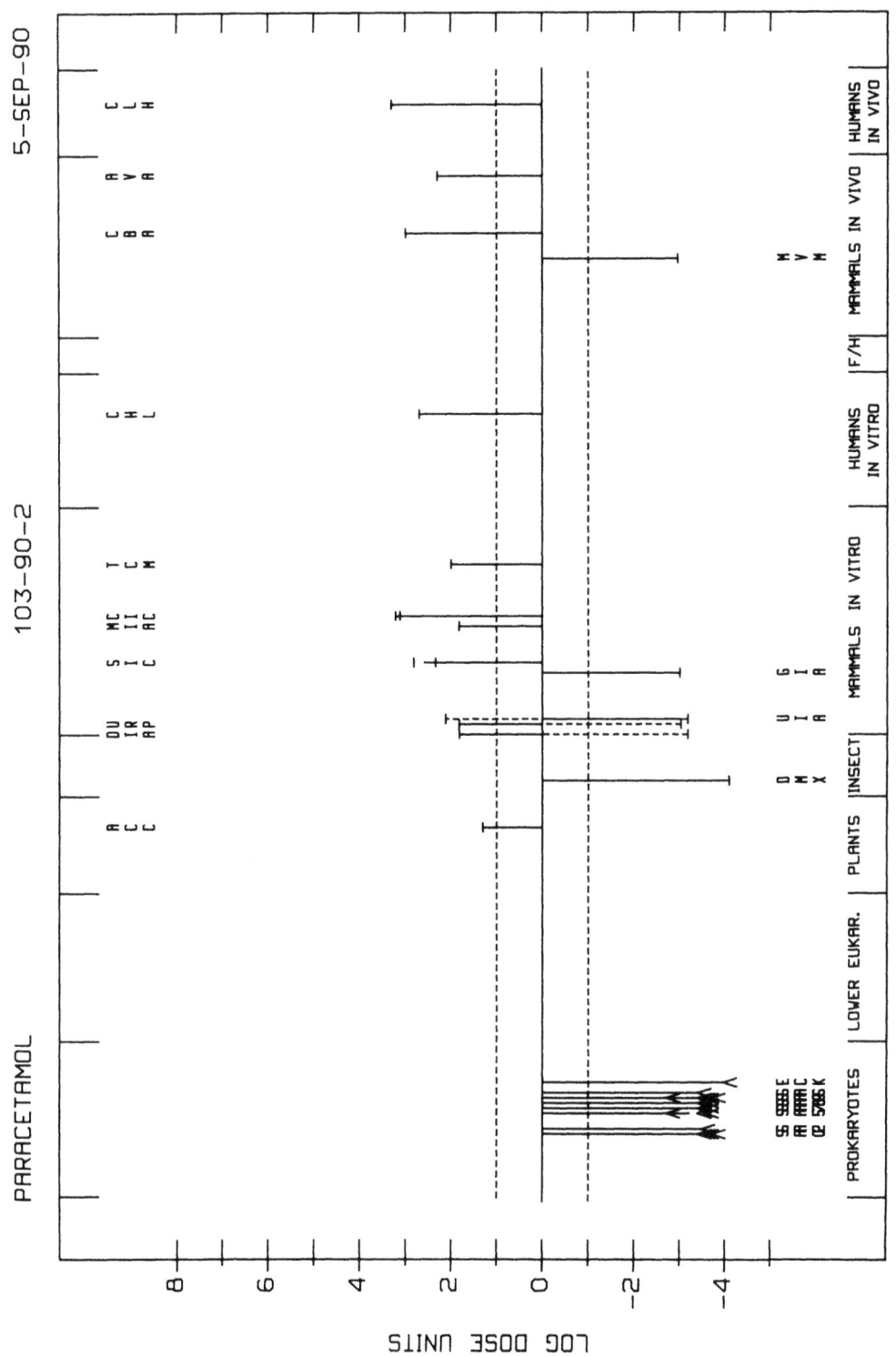

SUPPLEMENTARY CORRIGENDA TO VOLUMES 1–49

Corrigenda to Volumes 1–43 are listed in Volume 42, pp. 251–264; additional corrigenda are given in Volume 43, p. 261, in Volume 45, p. 283, in Volume 46, p. 419 and in Volume 47, p. 505.

Volume 47

p. 499	G9H	Paschin & Bahitova (1982)	*Replace* + 0 *by* 0 +
	SHL	Jansson *et al.* (1986)	*Replace* 2.0000 *by* 188.0000
	SHL	Erexson *et al.* (1985)	*Replace* 0.0050 *by* 0.5000
	SHL	Morimoto *et al.* (1983)	*Replace* 3.0000 *by* 282.0000

CUMULATIVE CROSS INDEX TO *IARC MONOGRAPHS ON THE EVALUATION OF CARCINOGENIC RISKS TO HUMANS*

The volume, page and year are given. References to corrigenda are given in parentheses.

A

A-α-C	*40*, 245 (1986); *Suppl. 7*, 56 (1987)
Acetaldehyde	*36*, 101 (1985) (*corr. 42*, 263); *Suppl. 7*, 77 (1987)
Acetaldehyde formylmethylhydrazone (*see* Gyromitrin)	
Acetamide	*7*, 197 (1974); *Suppl. 7*, 389 (1987)
Acetaminophen (*see* Paracetamol)	
Acridine orange	*16*, 145 (1978); *Suppl. 7*, 56 (1987)
Acriflavinium chloride	*13*, 31 (1977); *Suppl. 7*, 56 (1987)
Acrolein	*19*, 479 (1979); *36*, 133 (1985); *Suppl. 7*, 78 (1987);
Acrylamide	*39*, 41 (1986); *Suppl. 7*, 56 (1987)
Acrylic acid	*19*, 47 (1979); *Suppl. 7*, 56 (1987)
Acrylic fibres	*19*, 86 (1979); *Suppl. 7*, 56 (1987)
Acrylonitrile	*19*, 73 (1979); *Suppl. 7*, 79 (1987)
Acrylonitrile-butadiene-styrene copolymers	*19*, 91 (1979); *Suppl. 7*, 56 (1987)
Actinolite (*see* Asbestos)	
Actinomycins	*10*, 29 (1976) (*corr. 42*, 255); *Suppl. 7*, 80 (1987)
Adriamycin	*10*, 43 (1976); *Suppl. 7*, 82 (1987)
AF-2	*31*, 47 (1983); *Suppl. 7*, 56 (1987)
Aflatoxins	*1*, 145 (1972) (*corr. 42*, 251); *10*, 51 (1976); *Suppl. 7*, 83 (1987)
Aflatoxin B_1 (*see* Aflatoxins)	
Aflatoxin B_2 (*see* Aflatoxins)	
Aflatoxin G_1 (*see* Aflatoxins)	
Aflatoxin G_2 (*see* Aflatoxins)	
Aflatoxin M_1 (*see* Aflatoxins)	
Agaritine	*31*, 63 (1983); *Suppl. 7*, 56 (1987)

-387-

Alcohol drinking	*44*
Aldrin	5, 25 (1974); *Suppl. 7*, 88 (1987)
Allyl chloride	36, 39 (1985); *Suppl. 7*, 56 (1987)
Allyl isothiocyanate	36, 55 (1985); *Suppl. 7*, 56 (1987)
Allyl isovalerate	36, 69 (1985); *Suppl. 7*, 56 (1987)
Aluminium production	34, 37 (1984); *Suppl. 7*, 89 (1987)
Amaranth	8, 41 (1975); *Suppl. 7*, 56 (1987)
5-Aminoacenaphthene	16, 243 (1978); *Suppl. 7*, 56 (1987)
2-Aminoanthraquinone	27, 191 (1982); *Suppl. 7*, 56 (1987)
para-Aminoazobenzene	8, 53 (1975); *Suppl. 7*, 390 (1987)
ortho-Aminoazotoluene	8, 61 (1975) *(corr. 42, 254)*;. *Suppl.* 7, 56 (1987)
para-Aminobenzoic acid	16, 249 (1978); *Suppl. 7*, 56 (1987)
4-Aminobiphenyl	1, 74 (1972) *(corr. 42, 251)*; *Suppl.* 7, 91 (1987)
2-Amino-3,4-dimethylimidazo[4,5-*f*]quinoline (*see* MeIQ)	
2-Amino-3,8-dimethylimidazo[4,5-*f*]quinoxaline (*see* MeIQx)	
3-Amino-1,4-dimethyl-5*H*-pyrido[4,3-*b*]indole (*see* Trp-P-1)	
2-Aminodipyrido[1,2-*a*:3',2'-*d*]imidazole (*see* Glu-P-2)	
1-Amino-2-methylanthraquinone	27, 199 (1982); *Suppl. 7*, 57 (1987)
2-Amino-3-methylimidazo[4,5-*f*]quinoline (*see* IQ)	
2-Amino-6-methyldipyrido[1,2-*a*:3',2'-*d*]-imidazole (*see* Glu-P-1)	
2-Amino-3-methyl-9*H*-pyrido[2,3-*b*]indole (*see* MeA-α-C)	
3-Amino-1-methyl-5*H*-pyrido[4,3-*b*]indole (*see* Trp-P-2)	
2-Amino-5-(5-nitro-2-furyl)-1,3,4-thiadiazole	7, 143 (1974); *Suppl. 7*, 57 (1987)
4-Amino-2-nitrophenol	16, 43 (1978); *Suppl.7*, 57 (1987)
2-Amino-5-nitrothiazole	31, 71 (1983); *Suppl. 7*, 57 (1987)
2-Amino-9*H*-pyrido[2,3-*b*]indole [*see* A-α-C]	
11-Aminoundecanoic acid	39, 239 (1986); *Suppl. 7*, 57 (1987)
Amitrole	7, 31 (1974); 41, 293 (1986) *Suppl. 7*, 92 (1987)
Ammonium potassium selenide (*see* Selenium and selenium compounds)	
Amorphous silica (*see also* Silica)	*Suppl. 7*, 341 (1987)
Amosite (*see* Asbestos)	
Ampicillin	50, 153 (1990)
Anabolic steroids (*see* Androgenic (anabolic) steroids)	
Anaesthetics, volatile	11, 285 (1976); *Suppl. 7*, 93 (1987)
Analgesic mixtures containing phenacetin (*see also* Phenacetin)	*Suppl. 7*, 310 (1987)
Androgenic (anabolic) steroids	*Suppl. 7*, 96 (1987)
Angelicin and some synthetic derivatives (*see also* Angelicins)	40, 291 (1986)
Angelicin plus ultraviolet radiation (*see also* Angelicin and some synthetic derivatives)	*Suppl. 7*, 57 (1987)
Angelicins	*Suppl. 7*, 57 (1987)

Aniline	*4*, 27 (1974) (*corr.* 42, 252); 27, 39 (1982); *Suppl. 7*, 99 (1987)
ortho-Anisidine	27, 63 (1982); *Suppl. 7*, 57 (1987)
para-Anisidine	27, 65 (1982); *Suppl. 7*, 57 (1987)
Anthanthrene	*32*, 95 (1983); *Suppl. 7*, 57 (1987)
Anthophyllite (*see* Asbestos)	
Anthracene	*32*, 105 (1983); *Suppl. 7*, 57 (1987)
Anthranilic acid	*16*, 265 (1978); *Suppl. 7*, 57 (1987)
Antimony trioxide	*47*, 291 (1989)
Antimony trisulfide	*47*, 291 (1989)
ANTU (*see* 1-Naphthylthiourea)	
Apholate	*9*, 31 (1975); *Suppl. 7*, 57 (1987)
Aramite®	*5*, 39 (1974); *Suppl. 7*, 57 (1987)
Areca nut (*see* Betel quid)	
Arsanilic acid (*see* Arsenic and arsenic compounds)	
Arsenic and arsenic compounds	*1*, 41 (1972); *2*, 48 (1973); *23*, 39 (1980); *Suppl. 7*, 100 (1987)
Arsenic pentoxide (*see* Arsenic and arsenic compounds)	
Arsenic sulphide (*see* Arsenic and arsenic compounds)	
Arsenic trioxide (*see* Arsenic and arsenic compounds)	
Arsine (*see* Arsenic and arsenic compounds)	
Asbestos	*2*, 17 (1973) (*corr.* 42, 252); *14* (1977) (*corr.* 42, 256); Suppl. 7, 106 (1987) (*corr.* 45, 283)
Attapulgite	*42*, 159 (1987); *Suppl. 7*, 117 (1987)
Auramine (technical-grade)	*1*, 69 (1972) (*corr.* 42, 251); *Suppl. 7*, 118 (1987)
Auramine, manufacture of (*see also* Auramine, technical-grade)	*Suppl. 7*, 118 (1987)
Aurothioglucose	*13*, 39 (1977); *Suppl. 7*, 57 (1987)
Azacitidine	*26*, 37 (1981); *Suppl. 7*, 57 (1987); *50*, 47 (1990)
5-Azacytidine (*see* Azacitidine)	
Azaserine	*10*, 73 (1976) (*corr.* 42, 255); *Suppl. 7*, 57 (1987)
Azathioprine	*26*, 47 (1981); *Suppl. 7*, 119 (1987)
Aziridine	*9*, 37 (1975); *Suppl. 7*, 58 (1987)
2-(1-Aziridinyl)ethanol	*9*, 47 (1975); *Suppl. 7*, 58 (1987)
Aziridyl benzoquinone	*9*, 51 (1975); *Suppl. 7*, 58 (1987)
Azobenzene	*8*, 75 (1975); *Suppl. 7*, 58 (1987)

B

Barium chromate (*see* Chromium and chromium compounds)
Basic chromic sulphate (*see* Chromium and chromium compounds)

BCNU (see Bischloroethyl nitrosourea)
Benz[a]acridine   32, 123 (1983); Suppl. 7, 58 (1987)
Benz[c]acridine   3, 241 (1973); 32, 129 (1983);
                                                        Suppl. 7, 58 (1987)
Benzal chloride (see also α-Chlorinated toluenes)   29, 65 (1982); Suppl. 7, 148 (1987)
Benz[a]anthracene   3, 45 (1973); 32, 135 (1983);
                                                        Suppl. 7, 58 (1987)
Benzene   7, 203 (1974) (corr. 42, 254); 29, 93,
                                                        391 (1982); Suppl. 7, 120 (1987)
Benzidine   1, 80 (1972); 29, 149, 391 (1982);
                                                        Suppl. 7, 123 (1987)
Benzidine-based dyes   Suppl. 7, 125 (1987)
Benzo[b]fluoranthene   3, 69 (1973); 32, 147 (1983);
                                                        Suppl. 7, 58 (1987)
Benzo[j]fluoranthene   3, 82 (1973); 32, 155 (1983); Suppl.
                                                        7, 58 (1987)
Benzo[k]fluoranthene   32, 163 (1983); Suppl. 7, 58 (1987)
Benzo[ghi]fluoranthene   32, 171 (1983); Suppl. 7, 58 (1987)
Benzo[a]fluorene   32, 177 (1983); Suppl. 7, 58 (1987)
Benzo[b]fluorene   32, 183 (1983); Suppl. 7, 58 (1987)
Benzo[c]fluorene   32, 189 (1983); Suppl. 7, 58 (1987)
Benzo[ghi]perylene   32, 195 (1983); Suppl. 7, 58 (1987)
Benzo[c]phenanthrene   32, 205 (1983); Suppl. 7, 58 (1987)
Benzo[a]pyrene   3, 91 (1973); 32, 211 (1983);
                                                        Suppl. 7, 58 (1987)
Benzo[e]pyrene   3, 137 (1973); 32, 225 (1983);
                                                        Suppl. 7, 58 (1987)
para-Benzoquinone dioxime   29, 185 (1982); Suppl. 7, 58 (1987)
Benzotrichloride (see also α-Chlorinated toluenes)   29, 73 (1982); Suppl. 7, 148 (1987)
Benzoyl chloride   29, 83 (1982) (corr. 42, 261); Suppl.
                                                        7, 126 (1987)
Benzoyl peroxide   36, 267 (1985); Suppl. 7, 58 (1987)
Benzyl acetate   40, 109 (1986); Suppl. 7, 58 (1987)
Benzyl chloride (see also α-Chlorinated toluenes)   11, 217 (1976) (corr. 42, 256); 29,
                                                        49 (1982); Suppl. 7, 148 (1987)
Benzyl violet 4B   16, 153 (1978); Suppl. 7, 58 (1987)
Bertrandite (see Beryllium and beryllium compounds)
Beryllium and beryllium compounds   1, 17 (1972); 23, 143 (1980) (corr.
                                                        42, 260); Suppl. 7, 127 (1987)

Beryllium acetate (see Beryllium and beryllium compounds)
Beryllium acetate, basic (see Beryllium and beryllium compounds)
Beryllium–aluminium alloy (see Beryllium and beryllium
    compounds)
Beryllium carbonate (see Beryllium and beryllium compounds)
Beryllium chloride (see Beryllium and beryllium compounds)

Beryllium-copper alloy (*see* Beryllium and beryllium compounds)
Beryllium-copper-cobalt alloy (*see* Beryllium and beryllium compounds)
Beryllium fluoride (*see* Beryllium and beryllium compounds)
Beryllium hydroxide (*see* Beryllium and beryllium compounds)
Beryllium-nickel alloy (*see* Beryllium and beryllium compounds)
Beryllium oxide (*see* Beryllium and beryllium compounds)
Beryllium phosphate (*see* Beryllium and beryllium compounds)
Beryllium silicate (*see* Beryllium and beryllium compounds)
Beryllium sulphate (*see* Beryllium and beryllium compounds)
Beryl ore (*see* Beryllium and beryllium compounds)

Betel quid	*37*, 141 (1985); *Suppl. 7*, 128 (1987)
Betel-quid chewing (*see* Betel quid)	
BHA (*see* Butylated hydroxyanisole)	
BHT (*see* Butylated hydroxytoluene)	
Bis(1-aziridinyl)morpholinophosphine sulphide	*9*, 55 (1975); *Suppl. 7*, 58 (1987)
Bis(2-chloroethyl)ether	*9*, 117 (1975); *Suppl. 7*, 58 (1987)
N,N-Bis(2-chloroethyl)-2-naphthylamine	*4*, 119 (1974) (*corr. 42*, 253); *Suppl. 7*, 130 (1987)
Bischloroethyl nitrosourea (*see also* Chloroethyl nitrosoureas)	*26*, 79 (1981); *Suppl. 7*, 150 (1987)
1,2-Bis(chloromethoxy)ethane	*15*, 31 (1977); *Suppl. 7*, 58 (1987)
1,4-Bis(chloromethoxymethyl)benzene	*15*, 37 (1977); *Suppl. 7*, 58 (1987)
Bis(chloromethyl)ether	*4*, 231 (1974) (*corr. 42*, 253); *Suppl. 7*, 131 (1987)
Bis(2-chloro-1-methylethyl)ether	*41*, 149 (1986); *Suppl. 7*, 59 (1987)
Bis(2,3-epoxycyclopentyl)ether	*47*, 231 (1989)
Bitumens	*35*, 39 (1985); *Suppl. 7*, 133 (1987)
Bleomycins	*26*, 97 (1981); *Suppl. 7*, 134 (1987)
Blue VRS	*16*, 163 (1978); *Suppl. 7*, 59 (1987)
Boot and shoe manufacture and repair	*25*, 249 (1981); *Suppl. 7*, 232 (1987)
Bracken fern	*40*, 47 (1986); *Suppl. 7*, 135 (1987)
Brilliant Blue FCF	*16*, 171 (1978) (*corr. 42*, 257); *Suppl. 7*, 59 (1987)
1,3-Butadiene	*39*, 155 (1986) (*corr. 42*, 264); *Suppl. 7*, 136 (1987)
1,4-Butanediol dimethanesulphonate	*4*, 247 (1974); *Suppl. 7*, 137 (1987)
n-Butyl acrylate	*39*, 67 (1986); *Suppl. 7*, 59 (1987)
Butylated hydroxyanisole	*40*, 123 (1986); *Suppl. 7*, 59 (1987)
Butylated hydroxytoluene	*40*, 161 (1986); *Suppl. 7*, 59 (1987)
Butyl benzyl phthalate	*29*, 193 (1982) (*corr. 42*, 261); *Suppl. 7*, 59 (1987)
β-Butyrolactone	*11*, 225 (1976); *Suppl. 7*, 59 (1987)
γ-Butyrolactone	*11*, 231 (1976); *Suppl. 7*, 59 (1987)

C

Cabinet-making (*see* Furniture and cabinet-making)

Cadmium acetate (*see* Cadmium and cadmium compounds)
Cadmium and cadmium compounds   2, 74 (1973); *11*, 39 (1976)
                                                 (*corr. 42*, 255);
                                                 Suppl. 7, 139 (1987)

Cadmium chloride (*see* Cadmium and cadmium compounds)
Cadmium oxide (*see* Cadmium and cadmium compounds)
Cadmium sulphate (*see* Cadmium and cadmium compounds)
Cadmium sulphide (*see* Cadmium and cadmium compounds)
Calcium arsenate (*see* Arsenic and arsenic compounds)
Calcium chromate (*see* Chromium and chromium compounds)
Calcium cyclamate (*see* Cyclamates)
Calcium saccharin (*see* Saccharin)
Cantharidin   *10*, 79 (1976); *Suppl. 7*, 59 (1987)
Caprolactam   *19*, 115 (1979) (*corr. 42*, 258);
                                                 39, 247 (1986) (*corr. 42*, 264);
                                                 Suppl. 7, 390 (1987)

Captan   *30*, 295 (1983); *Suppl. 7*, 59 (1987)
Carbaryl   *12*, 37 (1976); *Suppl. 7*, 59 (1987)
Carbazole   *32*, 239 (1983); *Suppl. 7*, 59 (1987)
3-Carbethoxypsoralen   *40*, 317 (1986); *Suppl. 7*, 59 (1987)
Carbon blacks   *3*, 22 (1973); *33*, 35 (1984); *Suppl.
                                                 7*, 142 (1987)
Carbon tetrachloride   *1*, 53 (1972); *20*, 371 (1979);
                                                 Suppl. 7, 143 (1987)
Carmoisine   *8*, 83 (1975); *Suppl. 7*, 59 (1987)
Carpentry and joinery   *25*, 139 (1981); *Suppl. 7*, 378 (1987)
Carrageenan   *10*, 181 (1976) (*corr. 42*, 255); *31*,
                                                 79 (1983); *Suppl. 7*, 59 (1987)

Catechol   *15*, 155 (1977); *Suppl. 7*, 59 (1987)
CCNU (*see* 1-(2-Chloroethyl)-3-cyclohexyl-1-nitrosourea)
Ceramic fibres (*see* Man-made mineral fibres)
Chemotherapy, combined, including alkylating agents
    (*see* MOPP and other combined chemotherapy including
    alkylating agents)
Chlorambucil   *9*, 125 (1975); *26*, 115 (1981);
                                                 Suppl. 7, 144 (1987)
Chloramphenicol   *10*, 85 (1976); *Suppl. 7*, 145 (1987);
                                                 50, 169 (1990)
Chlorendic acid   *48*, 45 (1990)
Chlordane (*see also* Chlordane/Heptachlor)   *20*, 45 (1979) (*corr. 42*, 258)
Chlordane/Heptachlor   *Suppl. 7*, 146 (1987)
Chlordecone   *20*, 67 (1979); *Suppl. 7*, 59 (1987)
Chlordimeform   *30*, 61 (1983); *Suppl. 7*, 59 (1987)
Chlorinated dibenzodioxins (other than TCDD)   *15*, 41 (1977); *Suppl. 7*, 59 (1987)
Chlorinated paraffins   *48*, 55 (1990)

α-Chlorinated toluenes	*Suppl. 7*, 148 (1987)
Chlormadinone acetate (*see also* Progestins; Combined oral contraceptives)	*6*, 149 (1974); *21*, 365 (1979)
Chlornaphazine (*see N,N*-Bis(2-chloroethyl)-2-naphthylamine)	
Chlorobenzilate	*5*, 75 (1974); *30*, 73 (1983); *Suppl. 7*, 60 (1987)
Chlorodifluoromethane	*41*, 237 (1986); *Suppl. 7*, 149 (1987)
1-(2-Chloroethyl)-3-cyclohexyl-1-nitrosourea (*see also* Chloroethyl nitrosoureas)	*26*, 137 (1981) (*corr. 42*, 260); *Suppl. 7*, 150 (1987)
1-(2-Chloroethyl)-3-(4-methylcyclohexyl)-1-nitrosourea (*see also* Chloroethyl nitrosoureas)	*Suppl. 7*, 150 (1987)
Chloroethyl nitrosoureas	*Suppl. 7*, 150 (1987)
Chlorofluoromethane	*41*, 229 (1986); *Suppl. 7*, 60 (1987)
Chloroform	*1*, 61 (1972); *20*, 401 (1979); *Suppl. 7*, 152 (1987)
Chloromethyl methyl ether (technical-grade) (*see also* Bis(chloromethyl)ether)	*4*, 239 (1974)
(4-Chloro-2-methylphenoxy)acetic acid (*see* MCPA)	
Chlorophenols	*Suppl. 7*, 154 (1987)
Chlorophenols (occupational exposures to)	*41*, 319 (1986)
Chlorophenoxy herbicides	*Suppl. 7*, 156 (1987)
Chlorophenoxy herbicides (occupational exposures to)	*41*, 357 (1986)
4-Chloro-*ortho*-phenylenediamine	*27*, 81 (1982); *Suppl. 7*, 60 (1987)
4-Chloro-*meta*-phenylenediamine	*27*, 82 (1982); *Suppl. 7*, 60 (1987)
Chloroprene	*19*, 131 (1979); *Suppl. 7*, 160 (1987)
Chloropropham	*12*, 55 (1976); *Suppl. 7*, 60 (1987)
Chloroquine	*13*, 47 (1977); *Suppl. 7*, 60 (1987)
Chlorothalonil	*30*, 319 (1983); *Suppl. 7*, 60 (1987)
para-Chloro-*ortho*-toluidine and its strong acid salts (*see also* Chlordimeform)	*16*, 277 (1978); *30*, 65 (1983); *Suppl. 7*, 60 (1987); *48*, 123 (1990)
Chlorotrianisene (*see also* Nonsteroidal oestrogens)	*21*, 139 (1979)
2-Chloro-1,1,1-trifluoroethane	*41*, 253 (1986); *Suppl. 7*, 60 (1987)
Chlorozotocin	*50*, 65 (1990)
Cholesterol	*10*, 99 (1976); *31*, 95 (1983); *Suppl. 7*, 161 (1987)
Chromic acetate (*see* Chromium and chromium compounds)	
Chromic chloride (*see* Chromium and chromium compounds)	
Chromic oxide (*see* Chromium and chromium compounds)	
Chromic phosphate (*see* Chromium and chromium compounds)	
Chromite ore (*see* Chromium and chromium compounds)	
Chromium and chromium compounds	*2*, 100 (1973); *23*, 205 (1980); *Suppl. 7*, 165 (1987); *49*, 49 (1990)
Chromium carbonyl (*see* Chromium and chromium compounds)	
Chromium potassium sulphate (*see* Chromium and chromium compounds)	

Chromium sulphate (see Chromium and chromium compounds)	
Chromium trioxide (see Chromium and chromium compounds)	
Chrysazin (see Dantron)	
Chrysene	3, 159 (1973); 32, 247 (1983); Suppl. 7, 60 (1987)
Chrysoidine	8, 91 (1975); Suppl. 7, 169 (1987)
Chrysotile (see Asbestos)	
Ciclosporin	50, 77 (1990)
CI Disperse Yellow 3	8, 97 (1975); Suppl. 7, 60 (1987)
Cimetidine	50, 235 (1990)
Cinnamyl anthranilate	16, 287 (1978); 31, 133 (1983); Suppl. 7, 60 (1987)
Cisplatin	26, 151 (1981); Suppl. 7, 170 (1987)
Citrinin	40, 67 (1986); Suppl. 7, 60 (1987)
Citrus Red No. 2	8, 101 (1975) (corr. 42, 254); Suppl. 7, 60 (1987)
Clofibrate	24, 39 (1980); Suppl. 7, 171 (1987)
Clomiphene citrate	21, 551 (1979); Suppl. 7, 172 (1987)
Coal gasification	34, 65 (1984); Suppl. 7, 173 (1987)
Coal-tar pitches (see also Coal-tars)	Suppl. 7, 174 (1987)
Coal-tars	35, 83 (1985); Suppl. 7, 175 (1987)
Cobalt-chromium alloy (see Chromium and chromium compounds)	
Coke production	34, 101 (1984); Suppl. 7, 176 (1987)
Combined oral contraceptives (see also Oestrogens, progestins and combinations)	Suppl. 7, 297 (1987)
Conjugated oestrogens (see also Steroidal oestrogens)	21, 147 (1979)
Contraceptives, oral (see Combined oral contraceptives; Sequential oral contraceptives)	
Copper 8-hydroxyquinoline	15, 103 (1977); Suppl. 7, 61 (1987)
Coronene	32, 263 (1983); Suppl. 7, 61 (1987)
Coumarin	10, 113 (1976); Suppl. 7, 61 (1987)
Creosotes (see also Coal-tars)	Suppl. 7, 177 (1987)
meta-Cresidine	27, 91 (1982); Suppl. 7, 61 (1987)
para-Cresidine	27, 92 (1982); Suppl. 7, 61 (1987)
Crocidolite (see Asbestos)	
Crude oil	45, 119 (1989)
Crystalline silica (see also Silica)	Suppl. 7, 341 (1987)
Cycasin	1, 157 (1972) (corr. 42, 251); 10, 121 (1976); Suppl. 7, 61 (1987)
Cyclamates	22, 55 (1980); Suppl. 7, 178 (1987)
Cyclamic acid (see Cyclamates)	
Cyclochlorotine	10, 139 (1976); Suppl. 7, 61 (1987)
Cyclohexanone	47, 157 (1989)
Cyclohexylamine (see Cyclamates)	

Cyclopenta[*cd*]pyrene	*32*, 269 (1983); *Suppl. 7*, 61 (1987)
Cyclopropane (*see* Anaesthetics, volatile)	
Cyclophosphamide	*9*, 135 (1975); *26*, 165 (1981); *Suppl. 7*, 182 (1987)

D

2,4-D (*see also* Chlorophenoxy herbicides; Chlorophenoxy herbicides, occupational exposures to)	*15*, 111 (1977)
Dacarbazine	*26*, 203 (1981); *Suppl. 7*, 184 (1987)
Dantron	*50*, 265 (1990)
D & C Red No. 9	*8*, 107 (1975); *Suppl. 7*, 61 (1987)
Dapsone	*24*, 59 (1980); *Suppl. 7*, 185 (1987)
Daunomycin	*10*, 145 (1976); *Suppl. 7*, 61 (1987)
DDD (*see* DDT)	
DDE (*see* DDT)	
DDT	*5*, 83 (1974) (*corr. 42*, 253); *Suppl. 7*, 186 (1987)
Decabromodiphenyl oxide	*48*, 73 (1990)
Diacetylaminoazotoluene	*8*, 113 (1975); *Suppl. 7*, 61 (1987)
N,N'-Diacetylbenzidine	*16*, 293 (1978); *Suppl. 7*, 61 (1987)
Diallate	*12*, 69 (1976); *30*, 235 (1983); *Suppl. 7*, 61 (1987)
2,4-Diaminoanisole	*16*, 51 (1978); *27*, 103 (1982); *Suppl. 7*, 61 (1987)
4,4'-Diaminodiphenyl ether	*16*, 301 (1978); *29*, 203 (1982); *Suppl. 7*, 61 (1987)
1,2-Diamino-4-nitrobenzene	*16*, 63 (1978); *Suppl. 7*, 61 (1987)
1,4-Diamino-2-nitrobenzene	*16*, 73 (1978); *Suppl. 7*, 61 (1987)
2,6-Diamino-3-(phenylazo)pyridine (*see* Phenazopyridine hydrochloride)	
2,4-Diaminotoluene (*see also* Toluene diisocyanates)	*16*, 83 (1978); *Suppl. 7*, 61 (1987)
2,5-Diaminotoluene (*see also* Toluene diisocyanates)	*16*, 97 (1978); *Suppl. 7*, 61 (1987)
ortho-Dianisidine (*see* 3,3'-Dimethoxybenzidine)	
Diazepam	*13*, 57 (1977); *Suppl. 7*, 189 (1987)
Diazomethane	*7*, 223 (1974); *Suppl. 7*, 61 (1987)
Dibenz[*a,h*]acridine	*3*, 247 (1973); *32*, 277 (1983); *Suppl. 7*, 61 (1987)
Dibenz[*a,j*]acridine	*3*, 254 (1973); *32*, 283 (1983); *Suppl. 7*, 61 (1987)
Dibenz[*a,c*]anthracene	*32*, 289 (1983) (*corr. 42*, 262); *Suppl. 7*, 61 (1987)
Dibenz[*a,h*]anthracene	*3*, 178 (1973) (*corr. 43*, 261); *32*, 299 (1983); *Suppl. 7*, 61 (1987)

Dibenz[a,j]anthracene	32, 309 (1983); *Suppl. 7*, 61 (1987)
7H-Dibenzo[c,g]carbazole	3, 260 (1973); 32, 315 (1983); *Suppl. 7*, 61 (1987)
Dibenzodioxins, chlorinated (other than TCDD) (*see* Chlorinated dibenzodioxins (other than TCDD))	
Dibenzo[a,e]fluoranthene	32, 321 (1983); *Suppl. 7*, 61 (1987)
Dibenzo[h,rst]pentaphene	3, 197 (1973); *Suppl. 7*, 62 (1987)
Dibenzo[a,e]pyrene	3, 201 (1973); 32, 327 (1983); *Suppl. 7*, 62 (1987)
Dibenzo[a,h]pyrene	3, 207 (1973); 32, 331 (1983); *Suppl. 7*, 62 (1987)
Dibenzo[a,i]pyrene	3, 215 (1973); 32, 337 (1983); *Suppl. 7*, 62 (1987)
Dibenzo[a,l]pyrene	3, 224 (1973); 32, 343 (1983); *Suppl. 7*, 62 (1987)
1,2-Dibromo-3-chloropropane	15, 139 (1977); 20, 83 (1979); *Suppl. 7*, 191 (1987)
Dichloroacetylene	39, 369 (1986); *Suppl. 7*, 62 (1987)
ortho-Dichlorobenzene	7, 231 (1974); 29, 213 (1982); *Suppl. 7*, 192 (1987)
para-Dichlorobenzene	7, 231 (1974); 29, 215 (1982); *Suppl. 7*, 192 (1987)
3,3'-Dichlorobenzidine	4, 49 (1974); 29, 239 (1982); *Suppl. 7*, 193 (1987)
trans-1,4-Dichlorobutene	15, 149 (1977); *Suppl. 7*, 62 (1987)
3,3'-Dichloro-4,4'-diaminodiphenyl ether	16, 309 (1978); *Suppl. 7*, 62 (1987)
1,2-Dichloroethane	20, 429 (1979); *Suppl. 7*, 62 (1987)
Dichloromethane	20, 449 (1979); 41, 43 (1986); *Suppl. 7*, 194 (1987)
2,4-Dichlorophenol (*see* Chlorophenols; Chlorophenols, occupational exposures to)	
(2,4-Dichlorophenoxy)acetic acid (*see* 2,4-D)	
2,6-Dichloro-*para*-phenylenediamine	39, 325 (1986); *Suppl. 7*, 62 (1987)
1,2-Dichloropropane	41, 131 (1986); *Suppl. 7*, 62 (1987)
1,3-Dichloropropene (technical-grade)	41, 113 (1986); *Suppl. 7*, 195 (1987)
Dichlorvos	20, 97 (1979); *Suppl. 7*, 62 (1987)
Dicofol	30, 87 (1983); *Suppl. 7*, 62 (1987)
Dicyclohexylamine (*see* Cyclamates)	
Dieldrin	5, 125 (1974); *Suppl. 7*, 196 (1987)
Dienoestrol (*see also* Nonsteroidal oestrogens)	21, 161 (1979)
Diepoxybutane	11, 115 (1976) (*corr.* 42, 255); *Suppl. 7*, 62 (1987)
Diesel and gasoline engine exhausts	46, 41 (1989)
Diesel fuels	45, 219 (1989) (*corr.* 47, 505)
Diethyl ether (*see* Anaesthetics, volatile)	

Di(2-ethylhexyl)adipate	29, 257 (1982); *Suppl. 7*, 62 (1987)
Di(2-ethylhexyl)phthalate	29, 269 (1982) (*corr. 42*, 261); *Suppl. 7*, 62 (1987)
1,2-Diethylhydrazine	4, 153 (1974); *Suppl. 7*, 62 (1987)
Diethylstilboestrol	6, 55 (1974); 21, 173 (1979) (*corr. 42*, 259); *Suppl. 7*, 273 (1987)
Diethylstilboestrol dipropionate (*see* Diethylstilboestrol)	
Diethyl sulphate	4, 277 (1974); *Suppl. 7*, 198 (1987)
Diglycidyl resorcinol ether	11, 125 (1976); 36, 181 (1985); *Suppl. 7*, 62 (1987)
Dihydrosafrole	1, 170 (1972); 10, 233 (1976); *Suppl. 7*, 62 (1987)
1,8-Dihydroxyanthraquinone (*see* Dantron)	
Dihydroxybenzenes (*see* Catechol; Hydroquinone; Resorcinol)	
Dihydroxymethylfuratrizine	24, 77 (1980); *Suppl. 7*, 62 (1987)
Dimethisterone (*see also* Progestins; Sequential oral contraceptives)	6, 167 (1974); 21, 377 (1979)
Dimethoxane	15, 177 (1977); *Suppl. 7*, 62 (1987)
3,3'-Dimethoxybenzidine	4, 41 (1974); *Suppl. 7*, 198 (1987)
3,3'-Dimethoxybenzidine-4,4'-diisocyanate	39, 279 (1986); *Suppl. 7*, 62 (1987)
para-Dimethylaminoazobenzene	8, 125 (1975); *Suppl. 7*, 62 (1987)
para-Dimethylaminoazobenzenediazo sodium sulphonate	8, 147 (1975); *Suppl. 7*, 62 (1987)
trans-2-[(Dimethylamino)methylimino]-5-[2-(5-nitro-2-furyl)-vinyl]-1,3,4-oxadiazole	7, 147 (1974) (*corr. 42*, 253); *Suppl. 7*, 62 (1987)
4,4'-Dimethylangelicin plus ultraviolet radiation (*see also* Angelicin and some synthetic derivatives)	*Suppl. 7*, 57 (1987)
4,5'-Dimethylangelicin plus ultraviolet radiation (*see also* Angelicin and some synthetic derivatives)	*Suppl. 7*, 57 (1987)
Dimethylarsinic acid (*see* Arsenic and arsenic compounds)	
3,3'-Dimethylbenzidine	1, 87 (1972); *Suppl. 7*, 62 (1987)
Dimethylcarbamoyl chloride	12, 77 (1976); *Suppl. 7*, 199 (1987)
Dimethylformamide	47, 171 (1989)
1,1-Dimethylhydrazine	4, 137 (1974); *Suppl. 7*, 62 (1987)
1,2-Dimethylhydrazine	4, 145 (1974) (*corr. 42*, 253); *Suppl. 7*, 62 (1987)
Dimethyl hydrogen phosphite	48, 85 (1990)
1,4-Dimethylphenanthrene	32, 349 (1983); *Suppl. 7*, 62 (1987)
Dimethyl sulphate	4, 271 (1974); *Suppl. 7*, 200 (1987)
3,7-Dinitrofluoranthene	46, 189 (1989)
3,9-Dinitrofluoranthene	46, 195 (1989)
1,3-Dinitropyrene	46, 201 (1989)
1,6-Dinitropyrene	46, 215 (1989)
1,8-Dinitropyrene	33, 171 (1984); *Suppl. 7*, 63 (1987); 46, 231 (1989)
Dinitrosopentamethylenetetramine	11, 241 (1976); *Suppl. 7*, 63 (1987)

1,4-Dioxane	*11*, 247 (1976); *Suppl. 7*, 201 (1987)
2,4'-Diphenyldiamine	*16*, 313 (1978); *Suppl. 7*, 63 (1987)
Direct Black 38 (*see also* Benzidine-based dyes)	*29*, 295 (1982) (*corr. 42*, 261)
Direct Blue 6 (*see also* Benzidine-based dyes)	*29*, 311 (1982)
Direct Brown 95 (*see also* Benzidine-based dyes)	*29*, 321 (1982)
Disperse Blue 1	*48*, 139 (1990)
Disperse Yellow 3	*48*, 149 (1990)
Disulfiram	*12*, 85 (1976); *Suppl. 7*, 63 (1987)
Dithranol	*13*, 75 (1977); *Suppl. 7*, 63 (1987)
Divinyl ether (*see* Anaesthetics, volatile)	
Dulcin	*12*, 97 (1976); *Suppl. 7*, 63 (1987)

E

Endrin	*5*, 157 (1974); *Suppl. 7*, 63 (1987)
Enflurane (*see* Anaesthetics, volatile)	
Eosin	*15*, 183 (1977); *Suppl. 7*, 63 (1987)
Epichlorohydrin	*11*, 131 (1976) (*corr. 42*, 256); *Suppl. 7*, 202 (1987)
1,2-Epoxybutane	*47*, 217 (1989)
1-Epoxyethyl-3,4-epoxycyclohexane	*11*, 141 (1976); *Suppl. 7*, 63 (1987)
3,4-Epoxy-6-methylcyclohexylmethyl-3,4-epoxy-6-methyl-cyclohexane carboxylate	*11*, 147 (1976); *Suppl. 7*, 63 (1987)
cis-9,10-Epoxystearic acid	*11*, 153 (1976); *Suppl. 7*, 63 (1987)
Erionite	*42*, 225 (1987); *Suppl. 7*, 203 (1987)
Ethinyloestradiol (*see also* Steroidal oestrogens)	*6*, 77 (1974); *21*, 233 (1979)
Ethionamide	*13*, 83 (1977); *Suppl. 7*, 63 (1987)
Ethyl acrylate	*19*, 57 (1979); *39*, 81 (1986); *Suppl. 7*, 63 (1987)
Ethylene	*19*, 157 (1979); *Suppl. 7*, 63 (1987)
Ethylene dibromide	*15*, 195 (1977); *Suppl. 7*, 204 (1987)
Ethylene oxide	*11*, 157 (1976); *36*, 189 (1985) (*corr. 42*, 263); *Suppl. 7*, 205 (1987)
Ethylene sulphide	*11*, 257 (1976); *Suppl. 7*, 63 (1987)
Ethylene thiourea	*7*, 45 (1974); *Suppl. 7*, 207 (1987)
Ethyl methanesulphonate	*7*, 245 (1974); *Suppl. 7*, 63 (1987)
N-Ethyl-*N*-nitrosourea	*1*, 135 (1972); *17*, 191 (1978); *Suppl. 7*, 63 (1987)
Ethyl selenac (*see also* Selenium and selenium compounds)	*12*, 107 (1976); *Suppl. 7*, 63 (1987)
Ethyl tellurac	*12*, 115 (1976); *Suppl. 7*, 63 (1987)
Ethynodiol diacetate (*see also* Progestins; Combined oral contraceptives)	*6*, 173 (1974); *21*, 387 (1979)
Eugenol	*36*, 75 (1985); *Suppl. 7*, 63 (1987)
Evans blue	*8*, 151 (1975); *Suppl. 7*, 63 (1987)

F

Fast Green FCF	16, 187 (1978); *Suppl. 7*, 63 (1987)
Ferbam	12, 121 (1976) (*corr. 42*, 256); *Suppl. 7*, 63 (1987)
Ferric oxide	1, 29 (1972); *Suppl. 7*, 216 (1987)
Ferrochromium (*see* Chromium and chromium compounds)	
Fluometuron	30, 245 (1983); *Suppl. 7*, 63 (1987)
Fluoranthene	32, 355 (1983); *Suppl. 7*, 63 (1987)
Fluorene	32, 365 (1983); *Suppl. 7*, 63 (1987)
Fluorides (inorganic, used in drinking-water)	27, 237 (1982); *Suppl. 7*, 208 (1987)
5-Fluorouracil	26, 217 (1981); *Suppl. 7*, 210 (1987)
Fluorspar (*see* Fluorides)	
Fluosilicic acid (*see* Fluorides)	
Fluroxene (*see* Anaesthetics, volatile)	
Formaldehyde	29, 345 (1982); *Suppl. 7*, 211 (1987)
2-(2-Formylhydrazino)-4-(5-nitro-2-furyl)thiazole	7, 151 (1974) (*corr. 42*, 253); *Suppl. 7*, 63 (1987)
Frusemide (*see* Furosemide)	
Fuel oils (heating oils)	45, 239 (1989) (*corr. 47*, 505)
Furazolidone	31, 141 (1983); *Suppl. 7*, 63 (1987)
Furniture and cabinet-making	25, 99 (1981); *Suppl. 7*, 380 (1987)
Furosemide	50, 277 (1990)
2-(2-Furyl)-3-(5-nitro-2-furyl)acrylamide (*see* AF-2)	
Fusarenon-X	11, 169 (1976); 31, 153 (1983); *Suppl. 7*, 64 (1987)

G

Gasoline	45, 159 (1989) (*corr. 47*, 505)
Gasoline engine exhaust (*see* Diesel and gasoline engine exhausts)	
Glass fibres (*see* Man-made mineral fibres)	
Glasswool (*see* Man-made mineral fibres)	
Glass filaments (*see* Man-made mineral fibres)	
Glu-P-1	40, 223 (1986); *Suppl. 7*, 64 (1987)
Glu-P-2	40, 235 (1986); *Suppl. 7*, 64 (1987)
L-Glutamic acid, 5-[2-(4-hydroxymethyl)phenylhydrazide] (*see* Agaratine)	
Glycidaldehyde	11, 175 (1976); *Suppl. 7*, 64 (1987)
Some glycidyl ethers	47, 237 (1989)
Glycidyl oleate	11, 183 (1976); *Suppl. 7*, 64 (1987)
Glycidyl stearate	11, 187 (1976); *Suppl. 7*, 64 (1987)
Griseofulvin	10, 153 (1976); *Suppl. 7*, 391 (1987)
Guinea Green B	16, 199 (1978); *Suppl. 7*, 64 (1987)
Gyromitrin	31, 163 (1983); *Suppl. 7*, 391 (1987)

H

Haematite	*1*, 29 (1972); *Suppl. 7*, 216 (1987)
Haematite and ferric oxide	*Suppl. 7*, 216 (1987)
Haematite mining, underground, with exposure to radon	*1*, 29 (1972); *Suppl. 7*, 216 (1987)
Hair dyes, epidemiology of	*16*, 29 (1978); *27*, 307 (1982)
Halothane (*see* Anaesthetics, volatile)	
α-HCH (*see* Hexachlorocyclohexanes)	
β-HCH (*see* Hexachlorocyclohexanes)	
γ-HCH (*see* Hexachlorocyclohexanes)	
Heating oils (*see* Fuel oils)	
Heptachlor (*see also* Chlordane/Heptachlor)	*5*, 173 (1974); *20*, 129 (1979)
Hexachlorobenzene	*20*, 155 (1979); *Suppl. 7*, 219 (1987)
Hexachlorobutadiene	*20*, 179 (1979); *Suppl. 7*, 64 (1987)
Hexachlorocyclohexanes	*5*, 47 (1974); *20*, 195 (1979) (*corr. 42*, 258); *Suppl. 7*, 220 (1987)
Hexachlorocyclohexane, technical-grade (*see* Hexachlorocyclohexanes)	
Hexachloroethane	*20*, 467 (1979); *Suppl. 7*, 64 (1987)
Hexachlorophene	*20*, 241 (1979); *Suppl. 7*, 64 (1987)
Hexamethylphosphoramide	*15*, 211 (1977); *Suppl. 7*, 64 (1987)
Hexoestrol (*see* Nonsteroidal oestrogens)	
Hycanthone mesylate	*13*, 91 (1977); *Suppl. 7*, 64 (1987)
Hydralazine	*24*, 85 (1980); *Suppl. 7*, 222 (1987)
Hydrazine	*4*, 127 (1974); *Suppl. 7*, 223 (1987)
Hydrochlorothiazide	*50*, 293 (1990)
Hydrogen peroxide	*36*, 285 (1985); *Suppl. 7*, 64 (1987)
Hydroquinone	*15*, 155 (1977); *Suppl. 7*, 64 (1987)
4-Hydroxyazobenzene	*8*, 157 (1975); *Suppl. 7*, 64 (1987)
17α-Hydroxyprogesterone caproate (*see also* Progestins)	*21*, 399 (1979) (*corr. 42*, 259)
8-Hydroxyquinoline	*13*, 101 (1977); *Suppl. 7*, 64 (1987)
8-Hydroxysenkirkine	*10*, 265 (1976); *Suppl. 7*, 64 (1987)

I

Indeno[1,2,3-*cd*]pyrene	*3*, 229 (1973); *32*, 373 (1983); *Suppl. 7*, 64 (1987)
IQ	*40*, 261 (1986); *Suppl. 7*, 64 (1987)
Iron and steel founding	*34*, 133 (1984); *Suppl. 7*, 224 (1987)
Iron-dextran complex	*2*, 161 (1973); *Suppl. 7*, 226 (1987)
Iron-dextrin complex	*2*, 161 (1973) (*corr. 42*, 252); *Suppl. 7*, 64 (1987)
Iron oxide (*see* Ferric oxide)	
Iron oxide, saccharated (*see* Saccharated iron oxide)	
Iron sorbitol-citric acid complex	*2*, 161 (1973); *Suppl. 7*, 64 (1987)

Isatidine	*10*, 269 (1976); *Suppl. 7*, 65 (1987)
Isoflurane (*see* Anaesthetics, volatile)	
Isoniazid (*see* Isonicotinic acid hydrazide)	
Isonicotinic acid hydrazide	*4*, 159 (1974); *Suppl. 7*, 227 (1987)
Isophosphamide	*26*, 237 (1981); *Suppl. 7*, 65 (1987)
Isopropyl alcohol	*15*, 223 (1977); *Suppl. 7*, 229 (1987)
Isopropyl alcohol manufacture (strong-acid process) (*see also* Isopropyl alcohol)	*Suppl. 7*, 229 (1987)
Isopropyl oils	*15*, 223 (1977); *Suppl. 7*, 229 (1987)
Isosafrole	*1*, 169 (1972); *10*, 232 (1976); *Suppl. 7*, 65 (1987)

J

Jacobine	*10*, 275 (1976); *Suppl. 7*, 65 (1987)
Jet fuel	*45*, 203 (1989)
Joinery (*see* Carpentry and joinery)	

K

Kaempferol	31, 171 (1983); *Suppl. 7*, 65 (1987)
Kepone (*see* Chlordecone)	

L

Lasiocarpine	*10*, 281 (1976); *Suppl. 7*, 65 (1987)
Lauroyl peroxide	*36*, 315 (1985); Suppl. 7, 65 (1987)
Lead acetate (*see* Lead and lead compounds)	
Lead and lead compounds	*1*, 40 (1972) (*corr. 42*, 251); *2*, 52, 150 (1973); *12*, 131 (1976); *23*, 40, 208, 209, 325 (1980); *Suppl. 7*, 230 (1987)
Lead arsenate (*see* Arsenic and arsenic compounds)	
Lead carbonate (*see* Lead and lead compounds)	
Lead chloride (*see* Lead and lead compounds)	
Lead chromate (*see* Chromium and chromium compounds)	
Lead chromate oxide (*see* Chromium and chromium compounds)	
Lead naphthenate (*see* Lead and lead compounds)	
Lead nitrate (*see* Lead and lead compounds)	
Lead oxide (*see* Lead and lead compounds)	
Lead phosphate (*see* Lead and lead compounds)	
Lead subacetate (*see* Lead and lead compounds)	
Lead tetroxide (*see* Lead and lead compounds)	
Leather goods manufacture	*25*, 279 (1981); *Suppl. 7*, 235 (1987)

Leather industries	25, 199 (1981); *Suppl. 7*, 232 (1987)
Leather tanning and processing	25, 201 (1981); *Suppl. 7*, 236 (1987)
Ledate (*see also* Lead and lead compounds)	12, 131 (1976)
Light Green SF	16, 209 (1978); *Suppl. 7*, 65 (1987)
Lindane (*see* Hexachlorocyclohexanes)	
The lumber and sawmill industries (including logging)	25, 49 (1981); *Suppl. 7*, 383 (1987)
Luteoskyrin	10, 163 (1976); *Suppl. 7*, 65 (1987)
Lynoestrenol (*see also* Progestins; Combined oral contraceptives)	21, 407 (1979)

M

Magenta	4, 57 (1974) (*corr.* 42, 252); *Suppl. 7*, 238 (1987)
Magenta, manufacture of (*see also* Magenta)	*Suppl. 7*, 238 (1987)
Malathion	30, 103 (1983); *Suppl. 7*, 65 (1987)
Maleic hydrazide	4, 173 (1974) (*corr.* 42, 253); *Suppl. 7*, 65 (1987)
Malonaldehyde	36, 163 (1985); *Suppl. 7*, 65 (1987)
Maneb	12, 137 (1976); *Suppl. 7*, 65 (1987)
Man-made mineral fibres	43, 39 (1988)
Mannomustine	9, 157 (1975); *Suppl. 7*, 65 (1987)
MCPA (*see also* Chlorophenoxy herbicides; Chlorophenoxy herbicides, occupational exposures to)	30, 255 (1983)
MeA-α-C	40, 253 (1986); *Suppl. 7*, 65 (1987)
Medphalan	9, 168 (1975); *Suppl. 7*, 65 (1987)
Medroxyprogesterone acetate	6, 157 (1974); 21, 417 (1979) (*corr.* 42, 259); *Suppl. 7*, 289 (1987)
Megestrol acetate (*see* also Progestins; Combined oral contraceptives)	
MeIQ	40, 275 (1986); *Suppl. 7*, 65 (1987)
MeIQx	40, 283 (1986); *Suppl. 7*, 65 (1987)
Melamine	39, 333 (1986); *Suppl. 7*, 65 (1987)
Melphalan	9, 167 (1975); *Suppl. 7*, 239 (1987)
6-Mercaptopurine	26, 249 (1981); *Suppl. 7*, 240 (1987)
Merphalan	9, 169 (1975); *Suppl. 7*, 65 (1987)
Mestranol (*see also* Steroidal oestrogens)	6, 87 (1974); 21, 257 (1979) (*corr.* 42, 259)
Methanearsonic acid, disodium salt (*see* Arsenic and arsenic compounds)	
Methanearsonic acid, monosodium salt (*see* Arsenic and arsenic compounds	
Methotrexate	26, 267 (1981); *Suppl. 7*, 241 (1987)
Methoxsalen (*see* 8-Methoxypsoralen)	
Methoxychlor	5, 193 (1974); 20, 259 (1979); *Suppl. 7*, 66 (1987)

Methoxyflurane (*see* Anaesthetics, volatile)	
5-Methoxypsoralen	*40*, 327 (1986); *Suppl. 7*, 242 (1987)
8-Methoxypsoralen (*see also* 8-Methoxypsoralen plus ultraviolet radiation)	*24*, 101 (1980)
8-Methoxypsoralen plus ultraviolet radiation	*Suppl. 7*, 243 (1987)
Methyl acrylate	*19*, 52 (1979); *39*, 99 (1986); *Suppl. 7*, 66 (1987)
5-Methylangelicin plus ultraviolet radiation (*see also* Angelicin and some synthetic derivatives)	*Suppl. 7*, 57 (1987)
2-Methylaziridine	*9*, 61 (1975); *Suppl. 7*, 66 (1987)
Methylazoxymethanol acetate	*1*, 164 (1972); *10*, 131 (1976); *Suppl. 7*, 66 (1987)
Methyl bromide	*41*, 187 (1986) (*corr. 45*, 283); *Suppl. 7*, 245 (1987)
Methyl carbamate	*12*, 151 (1976); *Suppl. 7*, 66 (1987)
Methyl-CCNU [*see* 1-(2-Chloroethyl)-3-(4-methylcyclohexyl)-1-nitrosourea]	
Methyl chloride	*41*, 161 (1986); *Suppl. 7*, 246 (1987)
1-, 2-, 3-, 4-, 5- and 6-Methylchrysenes	*32*, 379 (1983); *Suppl. 7*, 66 (1987)
N-Methyl-*N*,4-dinitrosoaniline	*1*, 141 (1972); *Suppl. 7*, 66 (1987)
4,4'-Methylene bis(2-chloroaniline)	*4*, 65 (1974) (*corr. 42*, 252); *Suppl. 7*, 246 (1987)
4,4'-Methylene bis(*N*,*N*-dimethyl)benzenamine	*27*, 119 (1982); *Suppl. 7*, 66 (1987)
4,4'-Methylene bis(2-methylaniline)	*4*, 73 (1974); *Suppl. 7*, 248 (1987)
4,4'-Methylenedianiline	*4*, 79 (1974) (*corr. 42*, 252); *39*, 347 (1986); *Suppl. 7*, 66 (1987)
4,4'-Methylenediphenyl diisocyanate	*19*, 314 (1979); *Suppl. 7*, 66 (1987)
2-Methylfluoranthene	*32*, 399 (1983); *Suppl. 7*, 66 (1987)
3-Methylfluoranthene	*32*, 399 (1983); *Suppl. 7*, 66 (1987)
Methyl iodide	*15*, 245 (1977); *41*, 213 (1986); *Suppl. 7*, 66 (1987)
Methyl methacrylate	*19*, 187 (1979); *Suppl. 7*, 66 (1987)
Methyl methanesulphonate	*7*, 253 (1974); *Suppl. 7*, 66 (1987)
2-Methyl-1-nitroanthraquinone	*27*, 205 (1982); *Suppl. 7*, 66 (1987)
N-Methyl-*N*'-nitro-*N*-nitrosoguanidine	*4*, 183 (1974); *Suppl. 7*, 248 (1987)
3-Methylnitrosaminopropionaldehyde (*see* 3-(*N*-Nitrosomethylamino)propionaldehyde)	
3-Methylnitrosaminopropionitrile (*see* 3-(*N*-Nitrosomethylamino)propionitrile)	
4-(Methylnitrosamino)-4-(3-pyridyl)-1-butanal (*see* 4-(*N*-Nitrosomethylamino)-4-(3-pyridyl)-1-butanal)	
4-(Methylnitrosamino)-1-(3-pyridyl)-1-butanone (*see* 4-(*N*-Nitrosomethylamino)-1-(3-pyridyl)-1-butanone)	
N-Methyl-*N*-nitrosourea	*1*, 125 (1972); *17*, 227 (1978); *Suppl. 7*, 66 (1987)

N-Methyl-N-nitrosourethane	4, 211 (1974); Suppl. 7, 66 (1987)
Methyl parathion	30, 131 (1983); Suppl. 7, 392 (1987)
1-Methylphenanthrene	32, 405 (1983); Suppl. 7, 66 (1987)
7-Methylpyrido[3,4-c]psoralen	40, 349 (1986); Suppl. 7, 71 (1987)
Methyl red	8, 161 (1975); Suppl. 7, 66 (1987)
Methyl selenac (see also Selenium and selenium compounds)	12, 161 (1976); Suppl. 7, 66 (1987)
Methylthiouracil	7, 53 (1974); Suppl. 7, 66 (1987)
Metronidazole	13, 113 (1977); Suppl. 7, 250 (1987)
Mineral oils	3, 30 (1973); 33, 87 (1984) (corr. 42, 262); Suppl. 7, 252 (1987)
Mirex	5, 203 (1974); 20, 283 (1979) (corr. 42, 258); Suppl. 7, 66 (1987)
Mitomycin C	10, 171 (1976); Suppl. 7, 67 (1987)
MNNG (see N-Methyl-N'-nitro-N-nitrosoguanidine)	
MOCA (see 4,4'-Methylene bis(2-chloroaniline))	
Modacrylic fibres	19, 86 (1979); Suppl. 7, 67 (1987)
Monocrotaline	10, 291 (1976); Suppl. 7, 67 (1987)
Monuron	12, 167 (1976); Suppl. 7, 67 (1987)
MOPP and other combined chemotherapy including alkylating agents	Suppl. 7, 254 (1987)
Morpholine	47, 199 (1989)
5-(Morpholinomethyl)-3-[(5-nitrofurfurylidene)amino]-2-oxazolidinone	7, 161 (1974); Suppl. 7, 67 (1987)
Mustard gas	9, 181 (1975) (corr. 42, 254); Suppl. 7, 259 (1987)
Myleran (see 1,4-Butanediol dimethanesulphonate)	

N

Nafenopin	24, 125 (1980); Suppl. 7, 67 (1987)
1,5-Naphthalenediamine	27, 127 (1982); Suppl. 7, 67 (1987)
1,5-Naphthalene diisocyanate	19, 311 (1979); Suppl. 7, 67 (1987)
1-Naphthylamine	4, 87 (1974) (corr. 42, 253); Suppl. 7, 260 (1987)
2-Naphthylamine	4, 97 (1974); Suppl. 7, 261 (1987)
1-Naphthylthiourea	30, 347 (1983); Suppl. 7, 263 (1987)
Nickel acetate (see Nickel and nickel compounds)	
Nickel ammonium sulphate (see Nickel and nickel compounds)	
Nickel and nickel compounds	2, 126 (1973) (corr. 42, 252); 11, 75 (1976); Suppl. 7, 264 (1987) (corr. 45, 283); 49, 257 (1990)
Nickel carbonate (see Nickel and nickel compounds)	
Nickel carbonyl (see Nickel and nickel compounds)	
Nickel chloride (see Nickel and nickel compounds)	
Nickel-gallium alloy (see Nickel and nickel compounds)	

Nickel hydroxide (see Nickel and nickel compounds)
Nickelocene (see Nickel and nickel compounds)
Nickel oxide (see Nickel and nickel compounds)
Nickel subsulphide (see Nickel and nickel compounds)
Nickel sulphate (see Nickel and nickel compounds)

Niridazole	*13*, 123 (1977); *Suppl. 7*, 67 (1987)
Nithiazide	*31*, 179 (1983); *Suppl. 7*, 67 (1987)
Nitrilotriacetic acid and its salts	*48*, 181 (1990)
5-Nitroacenaphthene	*16*, 319 (1978); *Suppl. 7*, 67 (1987)
5-Nitro-*ortho*-anisidine	*27*, 133 (1982); *Suppl. 7*, 67 (1987)
9-Nitroanthracene	*33*, 179 (1984); *Suppl. 7*, 67 (1987)
7-Nitrobenz[*a*]anthracene	*46*, 247 (1989)
6-Nitrobenzo[*a*]pyrene	*33*, 187 (1984); *Suppl. 7*, 67 (1987); *46*, 255 (1989)
4-Nitrobiphenyl	*4*, 113 (1974); *Suppl. 7*, 67 (1987)
6-Nitrochrysene	*33*, 195 (1984); *Suppl. 7*, 67 (1987); *46*, 267 (1989)
Nitrofen (technical-grade)	*30*, 271 (1983); *Suppl. 7*, 67 (1987)
3-Nitrofluoranthene	*33*, 201 (1984); *Suppl. 7*, 67 (1987)
2-Nitrofluorene	*46*, 277 (1989)
Nitrofural	*7*, 171 (1974); *Suppl. 7*, 67 (1987); *50*, 195 (1990)
5-Nitro-2-furaldehyde semicarbazone (see Nitrofural)	
Nitrofurantoin	*50*, 211 (1990)
Nitrofurazone (see Nitrofural)	
1-[(5-Nitrofurfurylidene)amino]-2-imidazolidinone	*7*, 181 (1974); *Suppl. 7*, 67 (1987)
N-[4-(5-Nitro-2-furyl)-2-thiazolyl]acetamide	*1*, 181 (1972); *7*, 185 (1974); *Suppl. 7*, 67 (1987)
Nitrogen mustard	*9*, 193 (1975); *Suppl. 7*, 269 (1987)
Nitrogen mustard *N*-oxide	*9*, 209 (1975); *Suppl. 7*, 67 (1987)
1-Nitronaphthalene	*46*, 291 (1989)
2-Nitronaphthalene	*46*, 303 (1989)
3-Nitroperylene	*46*, 313 (1989)
2-Nitropropane	*29*, 331 (1982); *Suppl. 7*, 67 (1987)
1-Nitropyrene	*33*, 209 (1984); *Suppl. 7*, 67 (1987); *46*, 321 (1989)
2-Nitropyrene	*46*, 359 (1989)
4-Nitropyrene	*46*, 367 (1989)
N-Nitrosatable drugs	*24*, 297 (1980) *(corr. 42*, 260)
N-Nitrosatable pesticides	*30*, 359 (1983)
N'-Nitrosoanabasine	*37*, 225 (1985); *Suppl. 7*, 67 (1987)
N'-Nitrosoanatabine	*37*, 233 (1985); *Suppl. 7*, 67 (1987)
N-Nitrosodi-*n*-butylamine	*4*, 197 (1974); *17*, 51 (1978); *Suppl. 7*, 67 (1987)
N-Nitrosodiethanolamine	*17*, 77 (1978); *Suppl. 7*, 67 (1987)

N-Nitrosodiethylamine	1, 107 (1972) (corr. 42, 251); 17, 83 (1978) (corr. 42, 257); Suppl. 7, 67 (1987)
N-Nitrosodimethylamine	1, 95 (1972); 17, 125 (1978) (corr. 42, 257); Suppl. 7, 67 (1987)
N-Nitrosodiphenylamine	27, 213 (1982); Suppl. 7, 67 (1987)
para-Nitrosodiphenylamine	27, 227 (1982) (corr. 42, 261); Suppl. 7, 68 (1987)
N-Nitrosodi-n-propylamine	17, 177 (1978); Suppl. 7, 68 (1987)
N-Nitroso-N-ethylurea (see N-Ethyl-N-nitrosourea)	
N-Nitrosofolic acid	17, 217 (1978); Suppl. 7, 68 (1987)
N-Nitrosoguvacine	37, 263 (1985); Suppl. 7, 68 (1987)
N-Nitrosoguvacoline	37, 263 (1985); Suppl. 7, 68 (1987)
N-Nitrosohydroxyproline	17, 304 (1978); Suppl. 7, 68 (1987)
3-(N-Nitrosomethylamino)propionaldehyde	37, 263 (1985); Suppl. 7, 68 (1987)
3-(N-Nitrosomethylamino)propionitrile	37, 263 (1985); Suppl. 7, 68 (1987)
4-(N-Nitrosomethylamino)-4-(3-pyridyl)-1-butanal	37, 205 (1985); Suppl. 7, 68 (1987)
4-(N-Nitrosomethylamino)-1-(3-pyridyl)-1-butanone	37, 209 (1985); Suppl. 7, 68 (1987)
N-Nitrosomethylethylamine	17, 221 (1978); Suppl. 7, 68 (1987)
N-Nitroso-N-methylurea (see N-Methyl-N-nitrosourea)	
N-Nitroso-N-methylurethane (see N-Methyl-N-methylurethane)	
N-Nitrosomethylvinylamine	17, 257 (1978); Suppl. 7, 68 (1987)
N-Nitrosomorpholine	17, 263 (1978); Suppl. 7, 68 (1987)
N'-Nitrosonornicotine	17, 281 (1978); 37, 241 (1985); Suppl. 7, 68 (1987)
N-Nitrosopiperidine	17, 287 (1978); Suppl. 7, 68 (1987)
N-Nitrosoproline	17, 303 (1978); Suppl. 7, 68 (1987)
N-Nitrosopyrrolidine	17, 313 (1978); Suppl. 7, 68 (1987)
N-Nitrososarcosine	17, 327 (1978); Suppl. 7, 68 (1987)
Nitrosoureas, chloroethyl (see Chloroethyl nitrosoureas)	
5-Nitro-ortho-toluidine	48, 169 (1990)
Nitrous oxide (see Anaesthetics, volatile)	
Nitrovin	31, 185 (1983); Suppl. 7, 68 (1987)
NNA (see 4-(N-Nitrosomethylamino)-4-(3-pyridyl)-1-butanal)	
NNK (see 4-(N-Nitrosomethylamino)-1-(3-pyridyl)-1-butanone)	
Nonsteroidal oestrogens (see also Oestrogens, progestins and combinations)	Suppl. 7, 272 (1987)
Norethisterone (see also Progestins; Combined oral contraceptives)	6, 179 (1974); 21, 461 (1979)
Norethynodrel (see also Progestins; Combined oral contraceptives	6, 191 (1974); 21, 461 (1979) (corr. 42, 259)
Norgestrel (see also Progestins, Combined oral contraceptives)	6, 201 (1974); 21, 479 (1979)
Nylon 6	19, 120 (1979); Suppl. 7, 68 (1987)

O

Ochratoxin A	*10*, 191 (1976); *31*, 191 (1983) (*corr.* *42*, 262); *Suppl. 7*, 271 (1987)
Oestradiol-17β (*see also* Steroidal oestrogens)	*6*, 99 (1974); *21*, 279 (1979)
Oestradiol 3-benzoate (*see* Oestradiol-17β)	
Oestradiol dipropionate (*see* Oestradiol-17β)	
Oestradiol mustard	*9*, 217 (1975)
Oestradiol-17β-valerate (*see* Oestradiol-17β)	
Oestriol (*see also* Steroidal oestrogens)	*6*, 117 (1974); *21*, 327 (1979)
Oestrogen-progestin combinations (*see* Oestrogens, progestins and combinations)	
Oestrogen-progestin replacement therapy (*see also* Oestrogens, progestins and combinations)	*Suppl. 7*, 308 (1987)
Oestrogen replacement therapy (*see also* Oestrogens, progestins and combinations)	*Suppl. 7*, 280 (1987)
Oestrogens (*see* Oestrogens, progestins and combinations)	
Oestrogens, conjugated (*see* Conjugated oestrogens)	
Oestrogens, nonsteroidal (*see* Nonsteroidal oestrogens)	
Oestrogens, progestins and combinations	*6* (1974); *21* (1979); *Suppl. 7*, 272 (1987)
Oestrogens, steroidal (*see* Steroidal oestrogens)	
Oestrone (*see also* Steroidal oestrogens)	*6*, 123 (1974); *21*, 343 (1979) (*corr.* *42*, 259)
Oestrone benzoate (*see* Oestrone)	
Oil Orange SS	*8*, 165 (1975); *Suppl. 7*, 69 (1987)
Oral contraceptives, combined (*see* Combined oral contraceptives)	
Oral contraceptives, investigational (*see* Combined oral contraceptives)	
Oral contraceptives, sequential (*see* Sequential oral contraceptives)	
Orange I	*8*, 173 (1975); *Suppl. 7*, 69 (1987)
Orange G	*8*, 181 (1975); *Suppl. 7*, 69 (1987)
Organolead compounds (*see also* Lead and lead compounds)	*Suppl. 7*, 230 (1987)
Oxazepam	*13*, 58 (1977); *Suppl. 7*, 69 (1987)
Oxymetholone (*see also* Androgenic (anabolic) steroids)	*13*, 131 (1977)
Oxyphenbutazone	*13*, 185 (1977); *Suppl. 7*, 69 (1987)

P

Paint manufacture and painting (occupational exposures in)	*47*, 329 (1989)
Panfuran S (*see also* Dihydroxymethylfuratrizine)	*24*, 77 (1980); *Suppl. 7*, 69 (1987)
Paper manufacture (*see* Pulp and paper manufacture)	
Paracetamol	*50*, 307 (1990)
Parasorbic acid	*10*, 199 (1976) (*corr.* *42*, 255); *Suppl. 7*, 69 (1987)

Parathion	30, 153 (1983); Suppl. 7, 69 (1987)
Patulin	10, 205 (1976); 40, 83 (1986); Suppl. 7, 69 (1987)
Penicillic acid	10, 211 (1976); Suppl. 7, 69 (1987)
Pentachloroethane	41, 99 (1986); Suppl. 7, 69 (1987)
Pentachloronitrobenzene (see Quintozene)	
Pentachlorophenol (see also Chlorophenols; Chlorophenols, occupational exposures to)	20, 303 (1979)
Perylene	32, 411 (1983); Suppl. 7, 69 (1987)
Petasitenine	31, 207 (1983); Suppl. 7, 69 (1987)
Petasites japonicus (see Pyrrolizidine alkaloids)	
Petroleum refining (occupational exposures in)	45, 39 (1989)
Some petroleum solvents	47, 43 (1989)
Phenacetin	13, 141 (1977); 24, 135 (1980); Suppl. 7, 310 (1987)
Phenanthrene	32, 419 (1983); Suppl. 7, 69 (1987)
Phenazopyridine hydrochloride	8, 117 (1975); 24, 163 (1980) (corr. 42, 260); Suppl. 7, 312 (1987)
Phenelzine sulphate	24, 175 (1980); Suppl. 7, 312 (1987)
Phenicarbazide	12, 177 (1976); Suppl. 7, 70 (1987)
Phenobarbital	13, 157 (1977); Suppl. 7, 313 (1987)
Phenol	47, 263 (1989)
Phenoxyacetic acid herbicides (see Chlorophenoxy herbicides)	
Phenoxybenzamine hydrochloride	9, 223 (1975); 24, 185 (1980); Suppl. 7, 70 (1987)
Phenylbutazone	13, 183 (1977); Suppl. 7, 316 (1987)
meta-Phenylenediamine	16, 111 (1978); Suppl. 7, 70 (1987)
para-Phenylenediamine	16, 125 (1978); Suppl. 7, 70 (1987)
N-Phenyl-2-naphthylamine	16, 325 (1978) (corr. 42, 257); Suppl. 7, 318 (1987)
ortho-Phenylphenol	30, 329 (1983); Suppl. 7, 70 (1987)
Phenytoin	13, 201 (1977); Suppl. 7, 319 (1987)
Piperazine oestrone sulphate (see Conjugated oestrogens)	
Piperonyl butoxide	30, 183 (1983); Suppl. 7, 70 (1987)
Pitches, coal-tar (see Coal-tar pitches)	
Polyacrylic acid	19, 62 (1979); Suppl. 7, 70 (1987)
Polybrominated biphenyls	18, 107 (1978); 41, 261 (1986); Suppl. 7, 321 (1987)
Polychlorinated biphenyls	7, 261 (1974); 18, 43 (1978) (corr. 42, 258); Suppl. 7, 322 (1987)
Polychlorinated camphenes (see Toxaphene)	
Polychloroprene	19, 141 (1979); Suppl. 7, 70 (1987)
Polyethylene	19, 164 (1979); Suppl. 7, 70 (1987)

Polymethylene polyphenyl isocyanate	*19*, 314 (1979); *Suppl. 7*, 70 (1987)
Polymethyl methacrylate	*19*, 195 (1979); *Suppl. 7*, 70 (1987)
Polyoestradiol phosphate (*see* Oestradiol-17β)	
Polypropylene	*19*, 218 (1979); *Suppl. 7*, 70 (1987)
Polystyrene	*19*, 245 (1979); *Suppl. 7*, 70 (1987)
Polytetrafluoroethylene	*19*, 288 (1979); *Suppl. 7*, 70 (1987)
Polyurethane foams	*19*, 320 (1979); *Suppl. 7*, 70 (1987)
Polyvinyl acetate	*19*, 346 (1979); *Suppl. 7*, 70 (1987)
Polyvinyl alcohol	*19*, 351 (1979); *Suppl. 7*, 70 (1987)
Polyvinyl chloride	*7*, 306 (1974); *19*, 402 (1979); *Suppl. 7*, 70 (1987)
Polyvinyl pyrrolidone	*19*, 463 (1979); *Suppl. 7*, 70 (1987)
Ponceau MX	*8*, 189 (1975); *Suppl. 7*, 70 (1987)
Ponceau 3R	*8*, 199 (1975); *Suppl. 7*, 70 (1987)
Ponceau SX	*8*, 207 (1975); *Suppl. 7*, 70 (1987)
Potassium arsenate (*see* Arsenic and arsenic compounds)	
Potassium arsenite (*see* Arsenic and arsenic compounds)	
Potassium bis(2-hydroxyethyl)dithiocarbamate	*12*, 183 (1976); *Suppl. 7*, 70 (1987)
Potassium bromate	*40*, 207 (1986); *Suppl. 7*, 70 (1987)
Potassium chromate (*see* Chromium and chromium compounds)	
Potassium dichromate (*see* Chromium and chromium compounds)	
Prednimustine	*50*, 115 (1990)
Prednisone	*26*, 293 (1981); *Suppl. 7*, 326 (1987)
Procarbazine hydrochloride	*26*, 311 (1981); *Suppl. 7*, 327 (1987)
Proflavine salts	*24*, 195 (1980); *Suppl. 7*, 70 (1987)
Progesterone (*see also* Progestins; Combined oral contraceptives)	*6*, 135 (1974); *21*, 491 (1979) (*corr. 42*, 259)
Progestins (*see also* Oestrogens, progestins and combinations)	*Suppl. 7*, 289 (1987)
Pronetalol hydrochloride	*13*, 227 (1977) (*corr. 42*, 256); *Suppl. 7*, 70 (1987)
1,3-Propane sultone	*4*, 253 (1974) (*corr. 42*, 253); *Suppl. 7*, 70 (1987)
Propham	*12*, 189 (1976); *Suppl. 7*, 70 (1987)
β-Propiolactone	*4*, 259 (1974) (*corr. 42*, 253); *Suppl. 7*, 70 (1987)
n-Propyl carbamate	*12*, 201 (1976); *Suppl. 7*, 70 (1987)
Propylene	*19*, 213 (1979); *Suppl. 7*, 71 (1987)
Propylene oxide	*11*, 191 (1976); *36*, 227 (1985) (*corr. 42*, 263); *Suppl. 7*, 328 (1987)
Propylthiouracil	*7*, 67 (1974); *Suppl. 7*, 329 (1987)
Ptaquiloside (*see also* Bracken fern)	*40*, 55 (1986); *Suppl. 7*, 71 (1987)
Pulp and paper manufacture	*25*, 157 (1981); *Suppl. 7*, 385 (1987)
Pyrene	*32*, 431 (1983); *Suppl. 7*, 71 (1987)
Pyrido[3,4-c]psoralen	*40*, 349 (1986); *Suppl. 7*, 71 (1987)
Pyrimethamine	*13*, 233 (1977); *Suppl. 7*, 71 (1987)

Pyrrolizidine alkaloids (*see* Hydroxysenkirkine; Isatidine;
Jacobine; Lasiocarpine; Monocrotaline; Retrorsine; Riddelliine;
Seneciphylline; Senkirkine)

Q

Quercetin (*see also* Bracken fern)	*31*, 213 (1983); *Suppl. 7*, 71 (1987)
para-Quinone	*15*, 255 (1977); *Suppl. 7*, 71 (1987)
Quintozene	*5*, 211 (1974); *Suppl. 7*, 71 (1987)

R

Radon	*43*, 173 (1988) (*corr. 45*, 283)
Reserpine	*10*, 217 (1976); *24*, 211 (1980) (*corr. 42*, 260); *Suppl. 7*, 330 (1987)
Resorcinol	*15*, 155 (1977); *Suppl. 7*, 71 (1987)
Retrorsine	*10*, 303 (1976); *Suppl. 7*, 71 (1987)
Rhodamine B	*16*, 221 (1978); *Suppl. 7*, 71 (1987)
Rhodamine 6G	*16*, 233 (1978); *Suppl. 7*, 71 (1987)
Riddelliine	*10*, 313 (1976); *Suppl. 7*, 71 (1987)
Rifampicin	*24*, 243 (1980); *Suppl. 7*, 71 (1987)
Rockwool (*see* Man-made mineral fibres)	
The rubber industry	*28* (1982) (*corr. 42*, 261); *Suppl. 7*, 332 (1987)
Rugulosin	*40*, 99 (1986); *Suppl. 7*, 71 (1987)

S

Saccharated iron oxide	*2*, 161 (1973); *Suppl. 7*, 71 (1987)
Saccharin	*22*, 111 (1980) (*corr. 42*, 259); *Suppl. 7*, 334 (1987)
Safrole	*1*, 169 (1972); *10*, 231 (1976); *Suppl. 7*, 71 (1987)
The sawmill industry (including logging) (*see* The lumber and sawmill industry (including logging))	
Scarlet Red	*8*, 217 (1975); *Suppl. 7*, 71 (1987)
Selenium and selenium compounds	*9*, 245 (1975) (*corr. 42*, 255); *Suppl. 7*, 71 (1987)
Selenium dioxide (*see* Selenium and selenium compounds)	
Selenium oxide (*see* Selenium and selenium compounds)	
Semicarbazide hydrochloride	*12*, 209 (1976) (*corr. 42*, 256); *Suppl. 7*, 71 (1987)
Senecio jacobaea L. (*see* Pyrrolizidine alkaloids)	
Senecio longilobus (*see* Pyrrolizidine alkaloids)	

Seneciphylline	*10*, 319, 335 (1976); *Suppl. 7*, 71 (1987)
Senkirkine	*10*, 327 (1976); *31*, 231 (1983); *Suppl. 7*, 71 (1987)
Sepiolite	*42*, 175 (1987); *Suppl. 7*, 71 (1987)
Sequential oral contraceptives (*see also* Oestrogens, progestins and combinations)	*Suppl. 7*, 296 (1987)
Shale-oils	*35*, 161 (1985); *Suppl. 7*, 339 (1987)
Shikimic acid (*see also* Bracken fern)	*40*, 55 (1986); *Suppl. 7*, 71 (1987)
Shoe manufacture and repair (*see* Boot and shoe manufacture and repair)	
Silica (*see also* Amorphous silica; Crystalline silica)	*42*, 39 (1987)
Slagwool (*see* Man-made mineral fibres)	
Sodium arsenate (*see* Arsenic and arsenic compounds)	
Sodium arsenite (*see* Arsenic and arsenic compounds)	
Sodium cacodylate (*see* Arsenic and arsenic compounds)	
Sodium chromate (*see* Chromium and chromium compounds)	
Sodium cyclamate (*see* Cyclamates)	
Sodium dichromate (*see* Chromium and chromium compounds)	
Sodium diethyldithiocarbamate	*12*, 217 (1976); *Suppl. 7*, 71 (1987)
Sodium equilin sulphate (*see* Conjugated oestrogens)	
Sodium fluoride (*see* Fluorides)	
Sodium monofluorophosphate (*see* Fluorides)	
Sodium oestrone sulphate (*see* Conjugated oestrogens)	
Sodium *ortho*-phenylphenate (*see also ortho*-Phenylphenol)	*30*, 329 (1983); *Suppl. 7*, 392 (1987)
Sodium saccharin (*see* Saccharin)	
Sodium selenate (*see* Selenium and selenium compounds)	
Sodium selenite (*see* Selenium and selenium compounds)	
Sodium silicofluoride (*see* Fluorides)	
Soots	*3*, 22 (1973); *35*, 219 (1985); *Suppl. 7*, 343 (1987)
Spironolactone	*24*, 259 (1980); *Suppl. 7*, 344 (1987)
Stannous fluoride (*see* Fluorides)	
Steel founding (*see* Iron and steel founding)	
Sterigmatocystin	*1*, 175 (1972); *10*, 245 (1976); *Suppl. 7*, 72 (1987)
Steroidal oestrogens (*see also* Oestrogens, progestins and combinations)	*Suppl. 7*, 280 (1987)
Streptozotocin	*4*, 221 (1974); *17*, 337 (1978); *Suppl. 7*, 72 (1987)
Strobane® (*see* Terpene polychlorinates)	
Strontium chromate (*see* Chromium and chromium compounds)	
Styrene	*19*, 231 (1979) (*corr. 42*, 258); *Suppl. 7*, 345 (1987)
Styrene-acrylonitrile copolymers	*19*, 97 (1979); *Suppl. 7*, 72 (1987)

Styrene-butadiene copolymers	19, 252 (1979); *Suppl. 7*, 72 (1987)
Styrene oxide	11, 201 (1976); 19, 275 (1979); 36, 245 (1985); *Suppl. 7*, 72 (1987)
Succinic anhydride	15, 265 (1977); *Suppl. 7*, 72 (1987)
Sudan I	8, 225 (1975); *Suppl. 7*, 72 (1987)
Sudan II	8, 233 (1975); *Suppl. 7*, 72 (1987)
Sudan III	8, 241 (1975); *Suppl. 7*, 72 (1987)
Sudan Brown RR	8, 249 (1975); *Suppl. 7*, 72 (1987)
Sudan Red 7B	8, 253 (1975); *Suppl. 7*, 72 (1987)
Sulfafurazole	24, 275 (1980); *Suppl. 7*, 347 (1987)
Sulfallate	30, 283 (1983); *Suppl. 7*, 72 (1987)
Sulfamethoxazole	24, 285 (1980); *Suppl. 7*, 348 (1987)
Sulphisoxazole (*see* Sulfafurazole)	
Sulphur mustard (*see* Mustard gas)	
Sunset Yellow FCF	8, 257 (1975); *Suppl. 7*, 72 (1987)
Symphytine	31, 239 (1983); *Suppl. 7*, 72 (1987)

T

2,4,5-T (*see also* Chlorophenoxy herbicides; Chlorophenoxy herbicides, occupational exposures to)	15, 273 (1977)
Talc	42, 185 (1987); *Suppl. 7*, 349 (1987)
Tannic acid	10, 253 (1976) (*corr.* 42, 255); *Suppl. 7*, 72 (1987)
Tannins (*see also* Tannic acid)	10, 254 (1976); *Suppl. 7*, 72 (1987)
TCDD (*see* 2,3,7,8-Tetrachlorodibenzo-*para*-dioxin)	
TDE (*see* DDT)	
Terpene polychlorinates	5, 219 (1974); *Suppl. 7*, 72 (1987)
Testosterone (*see also* Androgenic (anabolic) steroids)	6, 209 (1974); 21, 519 (1979)
Testosterone oenanthate (*see* Testosterone)	
Testosterone propionate (*see* Testosterone)	
2,2',5,5'-Tetrachlorobenzidine	27, 141 (1982); *Suppl. 7*, 72 (1987)
2,3,7,8-Tetrachlorodibenzo-*para*-dioxin	15, 41 (1977); *Suppl. 7*, 350 (1987)
1,1,1,2-Tetrachloroethane	41, 87 (1986); *Suppl. 7*, 72 (1987)
1,1,2,2-Tetrachloroethane	20, 477 (1979); *Suppl. 7*, 354 (1987)
Tetrachloroethylene	20, 491 (1979); *Suppl. 7*, 355 (1987)
2,3,4,6-Tetrachlorophenol (*see* Chlorophenols; Chlorophenols, occupational exposures to)	
Tetrachlorvinphos	30, 197 (1983); *Suppl. 7*, 72 (1987)
Tetraethyllead (*see* Lead and lead compounds)	
Tetrafluoroethylene	19, 285 (1979); *Suppl. 7*, 72 (1987)
Tetrakis(hydroxymethyl) phosphonium salts	48, 95 (1990)
Tetramethyllead (*see* Lead and lead compounds)	
Textile manufacturing industry, exposures in	48, 215 (1990)
Thioacetamide	7, 77 (1974); *Suppl. 7*, 72 (1987)

4,4'-Thiodianiline	16, 343 (1978); 27, 147 (1982); Suppl. 7, 72 (1987)
Thiotepa	9, 85 (1975); Suppl. 7, 368 (1987); 50, 123 (1990)
Thiouracil	7, 85 (1974); Suppl. 7, 72 (1987)
Thiourea	7, 95 (1974); Suppl. 7, 72 (1987)
Thiram	12, 225 (1976); Suppl. 7, 72 (1987)
Titanium dioxide	47, 307 (1989)
Tobacco habits other than smoking (see Tobacco products, smokeless)	
Tobacco products, smokeless	37 (1985) (corr. 42, 263); Suppl. 7, 357 (1987)
Tobacco smoke	38 (1986) (corr. 42, 263); Suppl. 7, 357 (1987)
Tobacco smoking (see Tobacco smoke)	
ortho-Tolidine (see 3,3'-Dimethylbenzidine)	
2,4-Toluene diisocyanate (see also Toluene diisocyanates)	19, 303 (1979); 39, 287 (1986)
2,6-Toluene diisocyanate (see also Toluene diisocyanates)	19, 303 (1979); 39, 289 (1986)
Toluene	47, 79 (1989)
Toluene diisocyanates	39, 287 (1986) (corr. 42, 264); Suppl. 7, 72 (1987)
Toluenes, α-chlorinated (see α-Chlorinated toluenes)	
ortho-Toluenesulphonamide (see Saccharin)	
ortho-Toluidine	16, 349 (1978); 27, 155 (1982); Suppl. 7, 362 (1987)
Toxaphene	20, 327 (1979); Suppl. 7, 72 (1987)
Tremolite (see Asbestos)	
Treosulphan	26, 341 (1981); Suppl. 7, 363 (1987)
Triaziquone (see Tris(aziridinyl)-para-benzoquinone)	
Trichlorfon	30, 207 (1983); Suppl. 7, 73 (1987)
Trichlormethine	9, 229 (1975); Suppl. 7, 73 (1987); 50, 143 (1990)
1,1,1-Trichloroethane	20, 515 (1979); Suppl. 7, 73 (1987)
1,1,2-Trichloroethane	20, 533 (1979); Suppl. 7, 73 (1987)
Trichloroethylene	11, 263 (1976); 20, 545 (1979); Suppl. 7, 364 (1987)
2,4,5-Trichlorophenol (see also Chlorophenols; Chlorophenols occupational exposures to)	20, 349 (1979)
2,4,6-Trichlorophenol (see also Chlorophenols; Chlorophenols, occupational exposures to)	20, 349 (1979)
(2,4,5-Trichlorophenoxy)acetic acid (see 2,4,5-T)	
Trichlorotriethylamine hydrochloride (see Trichlormethine)	
T_2-Trichothecene	31, 265 (1983); Suppl. 7, 73 (1987)
Triethylene glycol diglycidyl ether	11, 209 (1976); Suppl. 7, 73 (1987)

4,4',6-Trimethylangelicin plus ultraviolet radiation (*see also* Angelicin and some synthetic derivatives)	*Suppl. 7*, 57 (1987)
2,4,5-Trimethylaniline	27, 177 (1982); *Suppl. 7*, 73 (1987)
2,4,6-Trimethylaniline	27, 178 (1982); *Suppl. 7*, 73 (1'987)
4,5',8-Trimethylpsoralen	40, 357 (1986); *Suppl. 7*, 366 (1987)
Trimustine hydrochloride (*see* Trichlormethine)	
Triphenylene	32, 447 (1983); *Suppl. 7*, 73 (1987)
Tris(aziridinyl)-*para*-benzoquinone	9, 67 (1975); *Suppl. 7*, 367 (1987)
Tris(1-aziridinyl)phosphine oxide	9, 75 (1975); *Suppl. 7*, 73 (1987)
Tris(1-aziridinyl)phosphine sulphide (*see* Thiotepa)	
2,4,6-Tris(1-aziridinyl)-*s*-triazine	9, 95 (1975); *Suppl. 7*, 73 (1987)
Tris(2-chloroethyl) phosphate	48, 109 (1990)
1,2,3-Tris(chloromethoxy)propane	15, 301 (1977); *Suppl. 7*, 73 (1987)
Tris(2,3-dibromopropyl)phosphate	20, 575 (1979); *Suppl. 7*, 369 (1987)
Tris(2-methyl-1-aziridinyl)phosphine oxide	9, 107 (1975); *Suppl. 7*, 73 (1987)
Trp-P-1	31, 247 (1983); *Suppl. 7*, 73 (1987)
Trp-P-2	31, 255 (1983); *Suppl. 7*, 73 (1987)
Trypan blue	8, 267 (1975); *Suppl. 7*, 73 (1987)
Tussilago farfara L. (*see* Pyrrolizidine alkaloids)	

U

Ultraviolet radiation	40, 379 (1986)
Underground haematite mining with exposure to radon	1, 29 (1972); *Suppl. 7*, 216 (1987)
Uracil mustard	9, 235 (1975); *Suppl. 7*, 370 (1987)
Urethane	7, 111 (1974); *Suppl. 7*, 73 (1987)

V

Vat Yellow 4	48, 161 (1990)
Vinblastine sulphate	26, 349 (1981) (*corr.* 42, 261); *Suppl. 7*, 371 (1987)
Vincristine sulphate	26, 365 (1981); *Suppl. 7*, 372 (1987)
Vinyl acetate	19, 341 (1979); 39, 113 (1986); *Suppl. 7*, 73 (1987)
Vinyl bromide	19, 367 (1979); 39, 133 (1986); *Suppl. 7*, 73 (1987)
Vinyl chloride	7, 291 (1974); 19, 377 (1979) (*corr.* 42, 258); *Suppl. 7*, 373 (1987)
Vinyl chloride-vinyl acetate copolymers	7, 311 (1976); 19, 412 (1979) (*corr.* 42, 258); *Suppl. 7*, 73 (1987)
4-Vinylcyclohexene	11, 277 (1976); 39, 181 (1986); *Suppl. 7*, 73 (1987)
Vinyl fluoride	39, 147 (1986); *Suppl. 7*, 73 (1987)

Vinylidene chloride	*19*, 439 (1979); *39*, 195 (1986); *Suppl. 7*, 376 (1987)
Vinylidene chloride–vinyl chloride copolymers	*19*, 448 (1979) (corr. *42*, 258); *Suppl. 7*, 73 (1987)
Vinylidene fluoride	*39*, 227 (1986); *Suppl. 7*, 73 (1987)
N-Vinyl-2-pyrrolidone	*19*, 461 (1979); *Suppl. 7*, 73 (1987)

W

Welding	*49*, 447 (1990)
Wollastonite	*42*, 145 (1987); *Suppl. 7*, 377 (1987)
Wood industries	*25* (1981); *Suppl. 7*, 378 (1987)

X

Xylene	*47*, 125 (1989)
2,4-Xylidine	*16*, 367 (1978); *Suppl. 7*, 74 (1987)
2,5-Xylidine	*16*, 377 (1978); *Suppl. 7*, 74 (1987)

Y

Yellow AB	*8*, 279 (1975); *Suppl. 7*, 74 (1987)
Yellow OB	*8*, 287 (1975); *Suppl. 7*, 74 (1987)

Z

Zearalenone	*31*, 279 (1983); *Suppl. 7*, 74 (1987)
Zectran	*12*, 237 (1976); *Suppl. 7*, 74 (1987)
Zinc beryllium silicate (*see* Beryllium and beryllium compounds)	
Zinc chromate (*see* Chromium and chromium compounds)	
Zinc chromate hydroxide (*see* Chromium and chromium compounds)	
Zinc potassium chromate (*see* Chromium and chromium compounds)	
Zinc yellow (*see* Chromium and chromium compounds)	
Zineb	*12*, 245 (1976); *Suppl. 7*, 74 (1987)
Ziram	*12*, 259 (1976); *Suppl. 7*, 74 (1987)

PUBLICATIONS OF THE INTERNATIONAL AGENCY FOR RESEARCH ON CANCER
Scientific Publications Series

(Available from Oxford University Press through local bookshops)

No. 1 **Liver Cancer**
1971; 176 pages (*out of print*)

No. 2 **Oncogenesis and Herpesviruses**
Edited by P.M. Biggs, G. de-Thé and L.N. Payne
1972; 515 pages (*out of print*)

No. 3 ***N*-Nitroso Compounds: Analysis and Formation**
Edited by P. Bogovski, R. Preussman and E.A. Walker
1972; 140 pages (*out of print*)

No. 4 **Transplacental Carcinogenesis**
Edited by L. Tomatis and U. Mohr
1973; 181 pages (*out of print*)

No. 5/6 **Pathology of Tumours in Laboratory Animals, Volume 1, Tumours of the Rat**
Edited by V.S. Turusov
1973/1976; 533 pages; £50.00

No. 7 **Host Environment Interactions in the Etiology of Cancer in Man**
Edited by R. Doll and I. Vodopija
1973; 464 pages; £32.50

No. 8 **Biological Effects of Asbestos**
Edited by P. Bogovski, J.C. Gilson, V. Timbrell and J.C. Wagner
1973; 346 pages (*out of print*)

No. 9 ***N*-Nitroso Compounds in the Environment**
Edited by P. Bogovski and E.A. Walker
1974; 243 pages; £21.00

No. 10 **Chemical Carcinogenesis Essays**
Edited by R. Montesano and L. Tomatis
1974; 230 pages (*out of print*)

No. 11 **Oncogenesis and Herpesviruses II**
Edited by G. de-Thé, M.A. Epstein and H. zur Hausen
1975; Part I: 511 pages
Part II: 403 pages; £65.00

No. 12 **Screening Tests in Chemical Carcinogenesis**
Edited by R. Montesano, H. Bartsch and L. Tomatis
1976; 666 pages; £45.00

No. 13 **Environmental Pollution and Carcinogenic Risks**
Edited by C. Rosenfeld and W. Davis
1975; 441 pages (*out of print*)

No. 14 **Environmental *N*-Nitroso Compounds. Analysis and Formation**
Edited by E.A. Walker, P. Bogovski and L. Griciute
1976; 512 pages; £37.50

No. 15 **Cancer Incidence in Five Continents, Volume III**
Edited by J.A.H. Waterhouse, C. Muir, P. Correa and J. Powell
1976; 584 pages; (*out of print*)

No. 16 **Air Pollution and Cancer in Man**
Edited by U. Mohr, D. Schmähl and L. Tomatis
1977; 328 pages (*out of print*)

No. 17 **Directory of On-going Research in Cancer Epidemiology 1977**
Edited by C.S. Muir and G. Wagner
1977; 599 pages (*out of print*)

No. 18 **Environmental Carcinogens. Selected Methods of Analysis. Volume 1: Analysis of Volatile Nitrosamines in Food**
Editor-in-Chief: H. Egan
1978; 212 pages (*out of print*)

No. 19 **Environmental Aspects of *N*-Nitroso Compounds**
Edited by E.A. Walker, M. Castegnaro, L. Griciute and R.E. Lyle
1978; 561 pages (*out of print*)

No. 20 **Nasopharyngeal Carcinoma: Etiology and Control**
Edited by G. de-Thé and Y. Ito
1978; 606 pages (*out of print*)

No. 21 **Cancer Registration and its Techniques**
Edited by R. MacLennan, C. Muir, R. Steinitz and A. Winkler
1978; 235 pages; £35.00

No. 22 **Environmental Carcinogens. Selected Methods of Analysis. Volume 2: Methods for the Measurement of Vinyl Chloride in Poly(vinyl chloride), Air, Water and Foodstuffs**
Editor-in-Chief: H. Egan
1978; 142 pages (*out of print*)

No. 23 **Pathology of Tumours in Laboratory Animals. Volume II: Tumours of the Mouse**
Editor-in-Chief: V.S. Turusov
1979; 669 pages (*out of print*)

Prices, valid for January 1990, are subject to change without notice

List of IARC Publications

No. 24 Oncogenesis and Herpesviruses III
Edited by G. de-Thé, W. Henle and F. Rapp
1978; Part I: 580 pages, Part II: 512 pages (*out of print*)

No. 25 Carcinogenic Risk. Strategies for Intervention
Edited by W. Davis and C. Rosenfeld
1979; 280 pages (*out of print*)

No. 26 Directory of On-going Research in Cancer Epidemiology 1978
Edited by C.S. Muir and G. Wagner
1978; 550 pages (*out of print*)

No. 27 Molecular and Cellular Aspects of Carcinogen Screening Tests
Edited by R. Montesano, H. Bartsch and L. Tomatis
1980; 372 pages; £29.00

No. 28 Directory of On-going Research in Cancer Epidemiology 1979
Edited by C.S. Muir and G. Wagner
1979; 672 pages (*out of print*)

No. 29 Environmental Carcinogens. Selected Methods of Analysis. Volume 3: Analysis of Polycyclic Aromatic Hydrocarbons in Environmental Samples
Editor-in-Chief: H. Egan
1979; 240 pages (*out of print*)

No. 30 Biological Effects of Mineral Fibres
Editor-in-Chief: J.C. Wagner
1980; Volume 1: 494 pages; Volume 2: 513 pages; £65.00

No. 31 *N*-Nitroso Compounds: Analysis, Formation and Occurrence
Edited by E.A. Walker, L. Griciute, M. Castegnaro and M. Börzsönyi
1980; 835 pages (*out of print*)

No. 32 Statistical Methods in Cancer Research. Volume 1. The Analysis of Case-control Studies
By N.E. Breslow and N.E. Day
1980; 338 pages; £20.00

No. 33 Handling Chemical Carcinogens in the Laboratory
Edited by R. Montesano *et al.*
1979; 32 pages (*out of print*)

No. 34 Pathology of Tumours in Laboratory Animals. Volume III. Tumours of the Hamster
Editor-in-Chief: V.S. Turusov
1982; 461 pages; £39.00

No. 35 Directory of On-going Research in Cancer Epidemiology 1980
Edited by C.S. Muir and G. Wagner
1980; 660 pages (*out of print*)

No. 36 Cancer Mortality by Occupation and Social Class 1851-1971
Edited by W.P.D. Logan
1982; 253 pages; £22.50

No. 37 Laboratory Decontamination and Destruction of Aflatoxins B_1, B_2, G_1, G_2 in Laboratory Wastes
Edited by M. Castegnaro *et al.*
1980; 56 pages; £6.50

No. 38 Directory of On-going Research in Cancer Epidemiology 1981
Edited by C.S. Muir and G. Wagner
1981; 696 pages (*out of print*)

No. 39 Host Factors in Human Carcinogenesis
Edited by H. Bartsch and B. Armstrong
1982; 583 pages; £46.00

No. 40 Environmental Carcinogens. Selected Methods of Analysis. Volume 4: Some Aromatic Amines and Azo Dyes in the General and Industrial Environment
Edited by L. Fishbein, M. Castegnaro, I.K. O'Neill and H. Bartsch
1981; 347 pages; £29.00

No. 41 *N*-Nitroso Compounds: Occurrence and Biological Effects
Edited by H. Bartsch, I.K. O'Neill, M. Castegnaro and M. Okada
1982; 755 pages; £48.00

No. 42 Cancer Incidence in Five Continents, Volume IV
Edited by J. Waterhouse, C. Muir, K. Shanmugaratnam and J. Powell
1982; 811 pages (*out of print*)

No. 43 Laboratory Decontamination and Destruction of Carcinogens in Laboratory Wastes: Some *N*-Nitrosamines
Edited by M. Castegnaro *et al.*
1982; 73 pages; £7.50

No. 44 Environmental Carcinogens. Selected Methods of Analysis. Volume 5: Some Mycotoxins
Edited by L. Stoloff, M. Castegnaro, P. Scott, I.K. O'Neill and H. Bartsch
1983; 455 pages; £29.00

No. 45 Environmental Carcinogens. Selected Methods of Analysis. Volume 6: *N*-Nitroso Compounds
Edited by R. Preussmann, I.K. O'Neill, G. Eisenbrand, B. Spiegelhalder and H. Bartsch
1983; 508 pages; £29.00

No. 46 Directory of On-going Research in Cancer Epidemiology 1982
Edited by C.S. Muir and G. Wagner
1982; 722 pages (*out of print*)

List of IARC Publications

No. 47 Cancer Incidence in Singapore 1968-1977
Edited by K. Shanmugaratnam, H.P. Lee and N.E. Day
1983; 171 pages (*out of print*)

No. 48 Cancer Incidence in the USSR (2nd Revised Edition)
Edited by N.P. Napalkov, G.F. Tserkovny, V.M. Merabishvili, D.M. Parkin, M. Smans and C.S. Muir
1983; 75 pages; £12.00

No. 49 Laboratory Decontamination and Destruction of Carcinogens in Laboratory Wastes: Some Polycyclic Aromatic Hydrocarbons
Edited by M. Castegnaro, et al.
1983; 87 pages; £9.00

No. 50 Directory of On-going Research in Cancer Epidemiology 1983
Edited by C.S. Muir and G. Wagner
1983; 731 pages (*out of print*)

No. 51 Modulators of Experimental Carcinogenesis
Edited by V. Turusov and R. Montesano
1983; 307 pages; £22.50

No. 52 Second Cancers in Relation to Radiation Treatment for Cervical Cancer: Results of a Cancer Registry Collaboration
Edited by N.E. Day and J.C. Boice, Jr
1984; 207 pages; £20.00

No. 53 Nickel in the Human Environment
Editor-in-Chief: F.W. Sunderman, Jr
1984; 529 pages; £41.00

No. 54 Laboratory Decontamination and Destruction of Carcinogens in Laboratory Wastes: Some Hydrazines
Edited by M. Castegnaro, et al.
1983; 87 pages; £9.00

No. 55 Laboratory Decontamination and Destruction of Carcinogens in Laboratory Wastes: Some N-Nitrosamides
Edited by M. Castegnaro et al.
1984; 66 pages; £7.50

No. 56 Models, Mechanisms and Etiology of Tumour Promotion
Edited by M. Börzsönyi, N.E. Day, K. Lapis and H. Yamasaki
1984; 532 pages; £42.00

No. 57 N-Nitroso Compounds: Occurrence, Biological Effects and Relevance to Human Cancer
Edited by I.K. O'Neill, R.C. von Borstel, C.T. Miller, J. Long and H. Bartsch
1984; 1013 pages; £80.00

No. 58 Age-related Factors in Carcinogenesis
Edited by A. Likhachev, V. Anisimov and R. Montesano
1985; 288 pages; £20.00

No. 59 Monitoring Human Exposure to Carcinogenic and Mutagenic Agents
Edited by A. Berlin, M. Draper, K. Hemminki and H. Vainio
1984; 457 pages; £27.50

No. 60 Burkitt's Lymphoma: A Human Cancer Model
Edited by G. Lenoir, G. O'Conor and C.L.M. Olweny
1985; 484 pages; £29.00

No. 61 Laboratory Decontamination and Destruction of Carcinogens in Laboratory Wastes: Some Haloethers
Edited by M. Castegnaro et al.
1985; 55 pages; £7.50

No. 62 Directory of On-going Research in Cancer Epidemiology 1984
Edited by C.S. Muir and G. Wagner
1984; 717 pages (*out of print*)

No. 63 Virus-associated Cancers in Africa
Edited by A.O. Williams, G.T. O'Conor, G.B. de-Thé and C.A. Johnson
1984; 773 pages; £22.00

No. 64 Laboratory Decontamination and Destruction of Carcinogens in Laboratory Wastes: Some Aromatic Amines and 4-Nitrobiphenyl
Edited by M. Castegnaro et al.
1985; 84 pages; £6.95

No. 65 Interpretation of Negative Epidemiological Evidence for Carcinogenicity
Edited by N.J. Wald and R. Doll
1985; 232 pages; £20.00

No. 66 The Role of the Registry in Cancer Control
Edited by D.M. Parkin, G. Wagner and C.S. Muir
1985; 152 pages; £10.00

No. 67 Transformation Assay of Established Cell Lines: Mechanisms and Application
Edited by T. Kakunaga and H. Yamasaki
1985; 225 pages; £20.00

No. 68 Environmental Carcinogens. Selected Methods of Analysis. Volume 7. Some Volatile Halogenated Hydrocarbons
Edited by L. Fishbein and I.K. O'Neill
1985; 479 pages; £42.00

No. 69 Directory of On-going Research in Cancer Epidemiology 1985
Edited by C.S. Muir and G. Wagner
1985; 745 pages; £22.00

List of IARC Publications

No. 70 **The Role of Cyclic Nucleic Acid Adducts in Carcinogenesis and Mutagenesis**
Edited by B. Singer and H. Bartsch
1986; 467 pages; £40.00

No. 71 **Environmental Carcinogens. Selected Methods of Analysis. Volume 8: Some Metals: As, Be, Cd, Cr, Ni, Pb, Se Zn**
Edited by I.K. O'Neill, P. Schuller and L. Fishbein
1986; 485 pages; £42.00

No. 72 **Atlas of Cancer in Scotland, 1975-1980. Incidence and Epidemiological Perspective**
Edited by I. Kemp, P. Boyle, M. Smans and C.S. Muir
1985; 285 pages; £35.00

No. 73 **Laboratory Decontamination and Destruction of Carcinogens in Laboratory Wastes: Some Antineoplastic Agents**
Edited by M. Castegnaro et al.
1985; 163 pages; £10.00

No. 74 **Tobacco: A Major International Health Hazard**
Edited by D. Zaridze and R. Peto
1986; 324 pages; £20.00

No. 75 **Cancer Occurrence in Developing Countries**
Edited by D.M. Parkin
1986; 339 pages; £20.00

No. 76 **Screening for Cancer of the Uterine Cervix**
Edited by M. Hakama, A.B. Miller and N.E. Day
1986; 315 pages; £25.00

No. 77 **Hexachlorobenzene: Proceedings of an International Symposium**
Edited by C.R. Morris and J.R.P. Cabral
1986; 668 pages; £50.00

No. 78 **Carcinogenicity of Alkylating Cytostatic Drugs**
Edited by D. Schmähl and J.M. Kaldor
1986; 337 pages; £25.00

No. 79 **Statistical Methods in Cancer Research. Volume III: The Design and Analysis of Long-term Animal Experiments**
By J.J. Gart, D. Krewski, P.N. Lee, R.E. Tarone and J. Wahrendorf
1986; 213 pages; £20.00

No. 80 **Directory of On-going Research in Cancer Epidemiology 1986**
Edited by C.S. Muir and G. Wagner
1986; 805 pages; £22.00

No. 81 **Environmental Carcinogens: Methods of Analysis and Exposure Measurement. Volume 9: Passive Smoking**
Edited by I.K. O'Neill, K.D. Brunnemann, B. Dodet and D. Hoffmann
1987; 383 pages; £35.00

No. 82 **Statistical Methods in Cancer Research. Volume II: The Design and Analysis of Cohort Studies**
By N.E. Breslow and N.E. Day
1987; 404 pages; £30.00

No. 83 **Long-term and Short-term Assays for Carcinogens: A Critical Appraisal**
Edited by R. Montesano, H. Bartsch, H. Vainio, J. Wilbourn and H. Yamasaki
1986; 575 pages; £48.00

No. 84 **The Relevance of N-Nitroso Compounds to Human Cancer: Exposure and Mechanisms**
Edited by H. Bartsch, I.K. O'Neill and R. Schulte-Hermann
1987; 671 pages; £50.00

No. 85 **Environmental Carcinogens: Methods of Analysis and Exposure Measurement. Volume 10: Benzene and Alkylated Benzenes**
Edited by L. Fishbein and I.K. O'Neill
1988; 327 pages; £35.00

No. 86 **Directory of On-going Research in Cancer Epidemiology 1987**
Edited by D.M. Parkin and J. Wahrendorf
1987; 676 pages; £22.00

No. 87 **International Incidence of Childhood Cancer**
Edited by D.M. Parkin, C.A. Stiller, C.A. Bieber, G.J. Draper. B. Terracini and J.L. Young
1988; 401 pages; £35.00

No. 88 **Cancer Incidence in Five Continents Volume V**
Edited by C. Muir, J. Waterhouse, T. Mack, J. Powell and S. Whelan
1987; 1004 pages; £50.00

No. 89 **Method for Detecting DNA Damaging Agents in Humans: Applications in Cancer Epidemiology and Prevention**
Edited by H. Bartsch, K. Hemminki and I.K. O'Neill
1988; 518 pages; £45.00

No. 90 **Non-occupational Exposure to Mineral Fibres**
Edited by J. Bignon, J. Peto and R. Saracci
1989; 500 pages; £45.00

No. 91 **Trends in Cancer Incidence in Singapore 1968-1982**
Edited by H.P. Lee, N.E. Day and K. Shanmugaratnam
1988; 160 pages; £25.00

No. 92 **Cell Differentiation, Genes and Cancer**
Edited by T. Kakunaga, T. Sugimura, L. Tomatis and H. Yamasaki
1988; 204 pages; £25.00

List of IARC Publications

No. 93 **Directory of On-going Research in Cancer Epidemiology 1988**
Edited by M. Coleman and J. Wahrendorf
1988; 662 pages (*out of print*)

No. 94 **Human Papillomavirus and Cervical Cancer**
Edited by N. Muñoz, F.X. Bosch and O.M. Jensen
1989; 154 pages; £19.00

No. 95 **Cancer Registration: Principles and Methods**
Edited by O.M. Jensen, D.M. Parkin, R. MacLennan, C.S. Muir and R. Skeet
Publ. due 1990; approx. 300 pages

No. 96 **Perinatal and Multigeneration Carcinogenesis**
Edited by N.P. Napalkov, J.M. Rice, L. Tomatis and H. Yamasaki
1989; 436 pages; £48.00

No. 97 **Occupational Exposure to Silica and Cancer Risk**
Edited by L. Simonato, A.C. Fletcher, R. Saracci and T. Thomas
1990; 124 pages; £19.00

No. 98 **Cancer Incidence in Jewish Migrants to Israel, 1961–1981**
Edited by R. Steinitz, D.M. Parkin, J.L. Young, C.A. Bieber and L. Katz
1989; 320 pages; £30.00

No. 99 **Pathology of Tumours in Laboratory Animals, Second Edition, Volume 1, Tumours of the Rat**
Edited by V.S. Turusov and U. Mohr
Publ. due 1990; 740 pages; £85.00

No. 100 **Cancer: Causes, Occurrence and Control**
Editor-in-Chief L. Tomatis
1990; 352 pages; £24.00

No. 101 **Directory of On-going Research in Cancer Epidemiology 1989–90**
Edited by M. Coleman and J. Wahrendorf
1989; 818 pages; £36.00

No. 102 **Patterns of Cancer in Five Continents**
Edited by S.L. Whelan and D.M. Parkin
1990; 162 pages; £25.00

No. 103 **Evaluating Effectiveness of Primary Prevention of Cancer**
Edited by M. Hakama, V. Beral, J.W. Cullen and D.M. Parkin
1990; 250 pages; £32.00

No. 104 **Complex Mixtures and Cancer Risk**
Edited by H. Vainio, M. Sorsa and A.J. McMichael
1990; 442 pages; £38.00

No. 105 **Relevance to Human Cancer of N-Nitroso Compounds, Tobacco Smoke and Mycotoxins**
Edited by I.K. O'Neill, J. Chen, S.H. Lu and H. Bartsch
Publ. due 1990; approx. 600 pages

No. 108 **Environmental Carcinogens: Methods of Analysis and Exposure Measurement. Volume 11: Polychlorinated Dioxins and Dibenzofurans**
Edited by C. Rappe, H.R. Buser, B. Dodet and I.K. O'Neill
Publ. due 1991; approx. 400 pages; £45.00

No. 109 **Environmental Carcinogens: Methods of Analysis and Exposure Measurement. Volume 12: Indoor Air Contaminants**
Edited by B. Seifert, B. Dodet and I.K. O'Neill
Publ. due 1991; approx. 400 pages

No. 110 **Directory of On-going Research in Cancer Epidemiology 1991**
Edited by M. Coleman and J. Wahrendorf
1991; approx. 720 pages; £36.00

List of IARC Publications

IARC MONOGRAPHS ON THE EVALUATION OF CARCINOGENIC RISKS TO HUMANS

(Available from booksellers through the network of WHO Sales Agents*)

Volume 1 Some Inorganic Substances, Chlorinated Hydrocarbons, Aromatic Amines, N-Nitroso Compounds, and Natural Products
1972; 184 pages (*out of print*)

Volume 2 Some Inorganic and Organometallic Compounds
1973; 181 pages (out of print)

Volume 3 Certain Polycyclic Aromatic Hydrocarbons and Heterocyclic Compounds
1973; 271 pages (*out of print*)

Volume 4 Some Aromatic Amines, Hydrazine and Related Substances, N-Nitroso Compounds and Miscellaneous Alkylating Agents
1974; 286 pages;
Sw. fr. 18.-/US $14.40

Volume 5 Some Organochlorine Pesticides
1974; 241 pages (*out of print*)

Volume 6 Sex Hormones
1974; 243 pages (*out of print*)

Volume 7 Some Anti-Thyroid and Related Substances, Nitrofurans and Industrial Chemicals
1974; 326 pages (*out of print*)

Volume 8 Some Aromatic Azo Compounds
1975; 375 pages;
Sw. fr. 36.-/US $28.80

Volume 9 Some Aziridines, N-, S- and O-Mustards and Selenium
1975; 268 pages;
Sw.fr. 27.-/US $21.60

Volume 10 Some Naturally Occurring Substances
1976; 353 pages (*out of print*)

Volume 11 Cadmium, Nickel, Some Epoxides, Miscellaneous Industrial Chemicals and General Considerations on Volatile Anaesthetics
1976; 306 pages (*out of print*)

Volume 12 Some Carbamates, Thiocarbamates and Carbazides
1976; 282 pages;
Sw fr. 34.-/US $27.20

Volume 13 Some Miscellaneous Pharmaceutical Substances
1977; 255 pages;
Sw. fr. 30.-/US$ 24.00

Volume 14 Asbestos
1977; 106 pages (*out of print*)

Volume 15 Some Fumigants, The Herbicides 2,4-D and 2,4,5-T, Chlorinated Dibenzodioxins and Miscellaneous Industrial Chemicals
1977; 354 pages;
Sw. fr. 50.-/US $40.00

Volume 16 Some Aromatic Amines and Related Nitro Compounds - Hair Dyes, Colouring Agents and Miscellaneous Industrial Chemicals
1978; 400 pages;
Sw. fr. 50.-/US $40.00

Volume 17 Some N-Nitroso Compounds
1987; 365 pages;
Sw. fr. 50.-/US $40.00

Volume 18 Polychlorinated Biphenyls and Polybrominated Biphenyls
1978; 140 pages;
Sw. fr. 20.-/US $16.00

Volume 19 Some Monomers, Plastics and Synthetic Elastomers, and Acrolein
1979; 513 pages;
Sw. fr. 60.-/US $48.00

Volume 20 Some Halogenated Hydrocarbons
1979; 609 pages (*out of print*)

Volume 21 Sex Hormones (II)
1979; 583 pages;
Sw. fr. 60.-/US $48.00

Volume 22 Some Non-Nutritive Sweetening Agents
1980; 208 pages;
Sw. fr. 25.-/US $20.00

Volume 23 Some Metals and Metallic Compounds
1980; 438 pages (*out of print*)

Volume 24 Some Pharmaceutical Drugs
1980; 337 pages;
Sw. fr. 40.-/US $32.00

Volume 25 Wood, Leather and Some Associated Industries
1981; 412 pages;
Sw. fr. 60-/US $48.00

Volume 26 Some Antineoplastic and Immunosuppressive Agents
1981; 411 pages;
Sw. fr. 62.-/US $49.60

Volume 27 Some Aromatic Amines, Anthraquinones and Nitroso Compounds, and Inorganic Fluorides Used in Drinking Water and Dental Preparations
1982; 341 pages;
Sw. fr. 40.-/US $32.00

Volume 28 The Rubber Industry
1982; 486 pages;
Sw. fr. 70.-/US $56.00

Volume 29 Some Industrial Chemicals and Dyestuffs
1982; 416 pages;
Sw. fr. 60.-/US $48.00

List of IARC Publications

Volume 30 Miscellaneous Pesticides
1983; 424 pages;
Sw. fr. 60.-/US $48.00

Volume 31 Some Food Additives, Feed Additives and Naturally Occurring Substances
1983; 314 pages;
Sw. fr. 60.-/US $48.00

Volume 32 Polynuclear Aromatic Compounds, Part 1: Chemical, Environmental and Experimental Data
1984; 477 pages;
Sw. fr. 60.-/US $48.00

Volume 33 Polynuclear Aromatic Compounds, Part 2: Carbon Blacks, Mineral Oils and Some Nitroarenes
1984; 245 pages;
Sw. fr. 50.-/US $40.00

Volume 34 Polynuclear Aromatic Compounds, Part 3: Industrial Exposures in Aluminium Production, Coal Gasification, Coke Production, and Iron and Steel Founding
1984; 219 pages;
Sw. fr. 48.-/US $38.40

Volume 35 Polynuclear Aromatic Compounds: Part 4: Bitumens, Coal-tars and Derived Products, Shale-oils and Soots
1985; 271 pages;
Sw. fr. 70.-/US $56.00

Volume 37 Tobacco Habits Other than Smoking: Betel-quid and Areca-nut Chewing; and some Related Nitrosamines
1985; 291 pages;
Sw. fr. 70.-/US $56.00

Volume 38 Tobacco Smoking
1986; 421 pages;
Sw. fr. 75.-/US $60.00

Volume 39 Some Chemicals Used in Plastics and Elastomers
1986; 403 pages;
Sw. fr. 60.-/US $48.00

Volume 40 Some Naturally Occurring and Synthetic Food Components, Furocoumarins and Ultraviolet Radiation
1986; 444 pages;
Sw. fr. 65.-/US $52.00

Volume 41 Some Halogenated Hydrocarbons and Pesticide Exposures
1986; 434 pages;
Sw. fr. 65.-/US $52.00

Volume 42 Silica and Some Silicates
1987; 289 pages;
Sw. fr. 65.-/US $52.00

Volume 43 Man-Made Mineral Fibres and Radon
1988; 300 pages;
Sw. fr. 65.-/US $52.00

Volume 44 Alcohol Drinking
1988; 416 pages;
Sw. fr. 65.-/US $52.00

Volume 45 Occupational Exposures in Petroleum Refining; Crude Oil and Major Petroleum Fuels
1989; 322 pages;
Sw. fr. 65.-/US $52.00

Volume 46 Diesel and Gasoline Engine Exhausts and Some Nitroarenes
1989; 458 pages;
Sw. fr. 65.-/US $52.00

Volume 47 Some Organic Solvents, Resin Monomers and Related Compounds, Pigments and Occupational Exposures in Paint Manufacture and Painting
1990; 536 pages;
Sw. fr. 85.-/US $68.00

Volume 48 Some Flame Retardants and Textile Chemicals, and Exposures in the Textile Manufacturing Industry
1990; 345 pages;
Sw. fr. 65.-/US $52.00

Volume 49 Chromium, Nickel and Welding
1990; 677 pages;
Sw. fr. 95.-/US$76.00

Volume 50 Pharmaceutical Drugs
1990; 415 pages;
Sw. fr. 65.-/US$52.00

Supplement No. 1
Chemicals and Industrial Processes Associated with Cancer in Humans (IARC Monographs, Volumes 1 to 20)
1979; 71 pages; (*out of print*)

Supplement No. 2
Long-term and Short-term Screening Assays for Carcinogens: A Critical Appraisal
1980; 426 pages;
Sw. fr. 40.-/US $32.00

Supplement No. 3
Cross Index of Synonyms and Trade Names in Volumes 1 to 26
1982; 199 pages (*out of print*)

Supplement No. 4
Chemicals, Industrial Processes and Industries Associated with Cancer in Humans (IARC Monographs, Volumes 1 to 29)
1982; 292 pages (*out of print*)

Supplement No. 5
Cross Index of Synonyms and Trade Names in Volumes 1 to 36
1985; 259 pages;
Sw. fr. 46.-/US $36.80

Supplement No. 6
Genetic and Related Effects: An Updating of Selected IARC Monographs from Volumes 1 to 42
1987; 729 pages;
Sw. fr. 80.-/US $64.00

Supplement No. 7
Overall Evaluations of Carcinogenicity: An Updating of IARC Monographs Volumes 1-42
1987; 434 pages;
Sw. fr. 65.-/US $52.00

Supplement No. 8
Cross Index of Synonyms and Trade Names in Volumes 1 to 46 of the IARC Monographs
1990; 260 pages;
Sw. fr. 60.-/US $48.00

List of IARC Publications

IARC TECHNICAL REPORTS*

No. 1 **Cancer in Costa Rica**
Edited by R. Sierra,
R. Barrantes, G. Muñoz Leiva,
D.M. Parkin, C.A. Bieber and
N. Muñoz Calero
1988; 124 pages;
Sw. fr. 30.-/US $24.00

No. 2 **SEARCH: A Computer Package to Assist the Statistical Analysis of Case-control Studies**
Edited by G.J. Macfarlane,
P. Boyle and P. Maisonneuve (in press)

No. 3 **Cancer Registration in the European Economic Community**
Edited by M.P. Coleman and
E. Démaret
1988; 188 pages;
Sw. fr. 30.-/US $24.00

No. 4 **Diet, Hormones and Cancer: Methodological Issues for Prospective Studies**
Edited by E. Riboli and
R. Saracci
1988; 156 pages;
Sw. fr. 30.-/US $24.00

No. 5 **Cancer in the Philippines**
Edited by A.V. Laudico,
D. Esteban and D.M. Parkin
1989; 186 pages;
Sw. fr. 30.-/US $24.00

No. 6 **La genèse du Centre International de Recherche sur le Cancer**
Par R. Sohier et A.G.B. Sutherland
1990; 104 pages
Sw. fr. 30.-/US $24.00

No. 7 **Epidémiologie du cancer dans les pays de langue latine**
1990; 310 pages
Sw. fr. 30.-/US $24.00

No. 8 **Comparative Study of Anti-smoking Legislation in Countries of the European Economic Community**
Edited by A. Sasco
1990; c. 80 pages
Sw. fr. 30.-/US $24.00
(English and French editions available) (in press)

DIRECTORY OF AGENTS BEING TESTED FOR CARCINOGENICITY
(Until Vol. 13 Information Bulletin on the Survey of Chemicals Being Tested for Carcinogenicity)*

No. 8 Edited by M.-J. Ghess,
H. Bartsch and L. Tomatis
1979; 604 pages; Sw. fr. 40.-

No. 9 Edited by M.-J. Ghess,
J.D. Wilbourn, H. Bartsch and
L. Tomatis
1981; 294 pages; Sw. fr. 41.-

No. 10 Edited by M.-J. Ghess,
J.D. Wilbourn and H. Bartsch
1982; 362 pages; Sw. fr. 42.-

No. 11 Edited by M.-J. Ghess,
J.D. Wilbourn, H. Vainio and
H. Bartsch
1984; 362 pages; Sw. fr. 50.-

No. 12 Edited by M.-J. Ghess,
J.D. Wilbourn, A. Tossavainen
and H. Vainio
1986; 385 pages; Sw. fr. 50.-

No. 13 Edited by M.-J. Ghess,
J.D. Wilbourn and A. Aitio
1988; 404 pages; Sw. fr. 43.-

No. 14 Edited by M.-J. Ghess,
J.D. Wilbourn and H. Vainio
1990; c. 370 pages;
Sw. fr. 45.-

NON-SERIAL PUBLICATIONS †

Alcool et Cancer
By A. Tuyns (in French only)
1978; 42 pages; Fr. fr. 35.-

Cancer Morbidity and Causes of Death Among Danish Brewery Workers
By O.M. Jensen 1980;
143 pages; Fr. fr. 75.-

Directory of Computer Systems Used in Cancer Registries
By H.R. Menck and D.M. Parkin 1986; 236 pages;
Fr. fr. 50.-

---

* Available from booksellers through the network of WHO sales agents.

†Available directly from IARC

www.ingramcontent.com/pod-product-compliance
Ingram Content Group UK Ltd.
Pitfield, Milton Keynes, MK11 3LW, UK
UKHW051258180426
11947UKWH00020B/1777